STEM CELLS – LABORATORY AND CLINICAL RESEARCH

PERSPECTIVES IN STEM CELL RESEARCH

Stem Cells – Laboratory and Clinical Research

Additional books in this series can be found on Nova's website under the Series tab.

Additional E-books in this series can be found on Nova's website under the E-books tab.

STEM CELLS – LABORATORY AND CLINICAL RESEARCH

PERSPECTIVES IN STEM CELL RESEARCH

BRENDA M. DAVIS
AND
CHRISTOPHER B. HALTON
EDITORS

Nova Science Publishers, Inc.
New York

For permission to use material from this book please contact us:
Telephone 631-231-7269; Fax 631-231-8175
Web Site: http://www.novapublishers.com

LIBRARY OF CONGRESS CATALOGING-IN-PUBLICATION DATA

Perspectives in stem cell research / editors, Brenda M. Davis and
Christopher B. Halton.
p. cm.
Includes index.
ISBN 978-1-61122-985-1 (hardcover)
1. Stem cells. I. Davis, Brenda M. II. Halton, Christopher B.
QH588.S83P475 2010
616'.02774--dc22
2010047112

Published by Nova Science Publishers, Inc. † New York

CONTENTS

PREFACE

Stem cells are cells found in all multi cellular organisms. They are characterized by the ability to renew themselves through mitotic cell division and differentiate into a diverse range of specialized cell types. This book presents and discusses current research in the study of stem cell research, including cancer and prostate stem cells; neural stem cells and taurine; interactions between transplanted neural stem cells and host tissue; retrovirus vector silencing in stem cells and moral and scientific consideration in embryonic stem cell research.

Chapter 1 - Embryonic stem cells have the ability to develop into virtually any cell in the body, and may have the potential to treat medical conditions such as diabetes and Parkinson's disease. In August 2001, President Bush announced that for the first time federal funds would be used to support research on human embryonic stem cells, but funding would be limited to "existing stem cell lines." The National Institutes of Health (NIH) has established the Human Embryonic Stem Cell Registry which lists stem cell lines that are eligible for use in federally funded research. Although 78 cell lines are listed, 21 embryonic stem cell lines are currently available. Scientists are concerned about the quality, longevity, and availability of the eligible stem cell lines. For a variety of reasons, many believe research advancement requires new embryonic stem cell lines, and for certain applications, stem cells derived from cloned embryos may offer the best hope for progress in understanding and treating disease. A significant cohort of pro-life advocates support stem cell research; those opposed are concerned that the isolation of stem cells requires the destruction of embryos. Letters from Congress, one signed by 206 Members of the House and a second signed by 58 Senators, have been sent urging President Bush to expand the current federal policy concerning embryonic stem cell research.

Chapter 2 - Emerging evidence suggests that cancers contain a rare and biologically distinct subpopulation of cells with the ability to self-renew and to sustain tumor growth, termed "cancer stem cells". Cancer stem cells share many characteristics with normal stem cells including self-renewal, asymmetric division, indefinite proliferative capacity, and self-protection mechanisms. The cancer stem cell concept is best understood in hematologic malignancies. In solid tumors, breast cancer stem cells have been the most explored. Several techniques have been described, allowing the identification or isolation of cancer stem cells by either expression of specific cell surface markers, their differential ability to efflux dyes, or by a distinct enzymatic activity. More recent studies also established the crucial role of cancer stem cells in multistage cancer progression and metastasis which has important implications for the design of novel targeted therapies. Since most of the conventional chemotherapies only affect differentiated cancer cells, initial reduction in tumor mass is often followed by a rapid relapse. In order to achieve durable remissions, it will be imperative to eradicate cancer stem cells.

Chapter 3 - The aim of this article is to provide an up-to-date review of an area of biological research in its infancy, namely the identification of stem and tumor initiating cells from the prostate gland.

Chapter 4 - Mesenchymal stem cells (MSCs) constitute a heterogeneous population of undifferentiated and committed multipotential cells. They serve in vitro and in vivo as precursors for bone marrow stroma, bone, fat, cartilage, muscle (smooth, cardiac and skeletal) and neural cells. They are able to home upon engraftment to a number of microenvironments, capable of extensive proliferation and of producing large number of differentiated progenitors to repair functionally tissue after injury. MSCs are usually isolated from adult bone marrow but can also be isolated from several other tissues, such as fetal liver, adult circulating blood, umbilical cord blood, placenta or adipose tissue. Furthermore, MSCs present several immuno-regulatory characteristics with immuno-suppressive effects that induce a tolerance and could be therapeutic for reduction of graft-versus-host disease, rejection and modulation of inflammation.

Since MSCs follow a vascular smooth muscle differentiation pathway, their therapeutic potential has been widely investigated in the treatment of vascular diseases. Indeed, MSCs can participate in the development of new vessels from pre-existing vascular walls (angiogenesis), in the induction of new vascular networks (vasculogenesis), in the collateral artery growth (arteriogenesis) or in plastic and reconstructive surgery applications. These cells can promote vascular growth by incorporating into vessels' wall, but they also may function as supporting factors by producing paracrine vascular promoting factors. In this chapter, the mesenchymal stem cells isolation, culture and characterization, but also their potential use in vascular therapy, in both human and animal models, are reported and discussed, whereas perspectives in angiogenesis, vasculogenesis, arteriogenesis or vascular engineering are explored.

Chapter 5 - Taurine is a β-amino acid that serves important functions in mammalian brain development. However, no data are available about its distribution and possible roles in neural precursors from a non-retinal origin. Neural stem cells (NSC) with self-renewal and multilineage potential are an important tool to study the signals involved in the regulation of brain development. The aim of this study was to investigate the role played by taurine during the differentiation of NSC from fetal rat striatum. Taurine content was analyzed in the cultures by HPLC at different times post-plating. Between 2 and 24 hours taurine was detected at a basal value of 7 nmol/mg protein. As cells were maintained in culture, this value increased to reach 40 nmol/mg protein at 10 days post-plating. Taurine immunoreactivity was found in nestin, A2B5, β-tubulin III and O1 positive cells. The addition for 1 to 3 days of 2 mM taurine to recently seeded neurospheres increased its intracellular content by 28 fold, and high taurine levels were maintained even 7 days after taurine withdrawal. By contrast, cultures treated with 2 mM of the high-affinity taurine transporter inhibitor guanidine-oethanesulfonic acid (GES) showed a sharp decrease in taurine content. When taurine was applied in combination with GES, taurine levels were significantly higher than those observed after GES treatment. Taurine treatment did not affect the relative amount of neurons and oligodendrocytes in the cultures, but promoted the differentiation of O1-positive cells that showed an increase in the length and number of their processes. The authors conclude that NSC develop specific taurine uptake mechanisms at early stages differentiation. Since taurine was not present in the feeding medium, they suggest that NSC and their progeny have the machinery for taurine synthesis. Present results also indicate that taurine might influence the development of NSC oligodendroglial progeny.

Chapter 6 - The recent identification of endothelial progenitor cells (EPCs) in the peripheral blood of adult individuals has highlighted the possibility that vasculogenesis can take place in the postnatal life. It has been reported that circulating EPCs can be recruited and incorporated into sites of active neovascularization but they can also play a role in replacing lost endothelial cells on the vessel wall mediating a mechanism of maintenance of the normal vascular homeostasis. An accurate and unique phenotypical and functional characterization of circulating EPC subsets is still matter of debate; infact, neither a precise and unique panel of cell surface markers nor universally accepted protocols are available up to now for their in vitro growth.

Methods for the identification and characterization of circulating endothelial cells able to participate to postnatal vasculogenesis and endothelial repair will be part of our review, that will be focused mainly on physiological and pathological conditions characterized by a spontaneous increase of the number of circulating EPCs. The possible role of a number of soluble factors able to induce the mobilization of EPCs from the bone marrow into the peripheral blood will be also discussed.

Chapter 7 - Among main toxicities of standard myeloablative conditioning (MAC) regimens for allogeneic stem cell transplantation (allo-SCT), anemia is a well recognised complication, and virtually every patient would require red blood cells support. In the last few years, in an attempt to reduce treatment-related morbidity and mortality associated with standard MAC allo-SCT, different reduced intensity and less ablative conditioning regimens (RIC) have been developed with encouraging results in regards to feasibility and engraftment. In the RIC setting, the burden of disease eradication is shifted towards the graft-versus-tumor effect, while reduced myelosuppression creates a different pattern of post-transplant hemopoeitic reconstitution. Although RIC regimens are usually highly immunosuppressive, the toxicity profile may still vary from one regimen to another because of variability in the degree of myeloablation. The aim of this work is to analyse the available research evidence related to red blood cell transfusions (RBCT) in the era of RIC allo-SCT. An ever-growing body of data suggests that RIC allo-SCT is associated with decreased transfusion requirements and a different pattern of RBC recovery in comparison to MAC allo-SCT. Recently, we demonstrated that the intensity of the conditioning (RIC vs. MAC; $P=.0005$) and graft source (PBSC vs. BM; $P<.0001$) independently predicted RBCT requirements. Hb recovery was accelerated after RIC when compared to MAC allo-SCT ($P=0.02$). In RIC patients the number of RBCTs was inversely correlated with Hb level prior to conditioning ($P<.0001$) and the dose of anti-thymocyte globulin used as a part of the RIC preparative regimen ($P=.009$). Moreover, Hb level prior to allo-SCT significantly influenced Hb recovery kinetics after RIC but had no impact on RBCT requirements and Hb recovery after MAC. This data suggests that Hb recovery pattern is different after RIC and may represent a setting for the use of rHuEPO, even if its use after MAC allo-SCT has been associated with only marginal effects on Hb recovery and the number of RBCTs.

In this perspective, the authors initiated a pilot trial of rHuEPO administration early after matched sibling RIC allo-SCT. RHuEPO treatment was analyzed in terms of toxicity, impact on the frequency of RBCTs and kinetic of Hb recovery within the 60 days post-allo-SCT. Results were compared with a matched population who did not receive EPO. In the first 2 months after allo-SCT, all patients with rHuEPO (100%) achieved an Hb level>11 g/dL at a median of 30 (15-35) days post-allo-SCT, as compared to only 63% of the patients without rHuEPO (P=.007) at a median of 35 (20-55) days (P=.03). Seventy percent (95% CI, 50-90%) of rHuEPO patients maintained an Hb over 11 g/dL for the second month as compared to only 19% (95% CI, 4-34) in the other group (P=.0004). In patients receiving RBCTs, the use of rHuEPO was associated with a trend towards reduced RBCT requirements, highlighting the potential benefit of early administration of rHuEPO after RIC allo-SCT on early erythropoietic recovery.

Overall, the use of RIC regimens creates a different pattern of erythropoietic recovery as compared with standard regimens warranting further studies aimed at a further reduction of RBCT requirements and acceleration of Hb recovery.

Chapter 8 - Research on stem cell transplantation as potential therapy for neurodegenerative disorders has increased dramatically in the last 5 years. However, the mechanism whereby transplanted cells might integrate 'appropriately' throughout the mammalian nervous system is still poorly understood. Recent studies have demonstrated that transplanted neural stem cells are capable of engrafting in a cytoarchitecturally and developmentally appropriate manner within the normal and abnormal central nervous system (CNS) following transplantation. Furthermore, studies have shown that the transplanted neural stem cells are capable of migrating to areas of the CNS affected by disease or injury; that is, these transplanted cells have the ability to 'hone in' on pathology, even over great distances. Given these recent reports, discussion on this chapter will include the phenomenon of how the host CNS environment instructs and influence the fate of transplanted neural stem cells migrating to areas of pathology and assuming the phenotype(s) of host cells that are affected by disease or injury. Moreover, the emerging data on the capability of transplanted cells to instruct and alter the fate of host CNS tissue will also be covered in this chapter. The growing evidence to support the notion that donor neural stem cells and host tissue communicate in a reciprocal fashion will also be discussed. For example, while it has been demonstrated that a given host CNS environment is instructive of donor stem cells, influencing their migration and differentiation patterns, the donor neural stem cells are apparently equally capable of manipulating their milieu. However, the signals generated by neural stem cells to comm.-unicate with the host tissue have yet to be identified but it is speculated that molecules such as growth factors, cell adhesion molecules, cytokines and chemokines are involved. This continuously evolving understanding of how the donor neural stem cells are interacting with host tissue in a regenerative or restorative manner will be the main focus of this chapter.

Chapter 9 - Retrovirus vectors suffer severe gene silencing in stem cells that hampers their use in stem cell gene therapy. Transduced retrovirus vector can be completely silenced, or dynamically silenced in a subset of cells resulting in variegation. Expressing retrovirus also can be extinguished during stem cell differentiation. Multiple epigenetic modifications including histone modifications and DNA methylation are functionally involved in establishing and maintaining retrovirus silencing via the formation of silent chromatin. A model is proposed that the balance of epigenetic effects at the integration site and retroviral silencer elements on the vectors determines the decision to be silent, variegated or expressing in stem cells. Silencing resistant retrovirus vectors have been developed by removal of these silencer elements, and silencing in stem cells may ultimately be blocked using appropriate insulator elements.

Chapter 10 - Hematopoietic stem/ progenitor cells (HSPC) are a rare population of cells within the bone marrow, which are capable to self-renew and which constantly reproduce all hematopoietic lineages. Transplantation of HSPC collected from peripheral mobilized blood or bone marrow has become more and more significant, e.g., for treatment of hematological diseases. Thereby, the homing and migration capacities of HSPC are of fundamental importance for successful transplantation since HSPC are usually administered intravenously. The multi-step process of HSPC homing, involving adhesion, transendothelial migration and migration across the bone marrow stroma, depends on active migration along a gradient of the chemokine SDF-1α. The potential of HSPC to undergo self-renewing cell divisions has stimulated investigations of *ex vivo* stem cell expansion, which would be valuable to improve the quality of stem cell transplants by increasing the number of stem cells. HSPC can be expanded *in vitro* by supplementation with hematopoietic cytokines, for instance, Flt3-Ligand and stem cell factor (SCF). However, analyses of migratory activity using a collagen matrix migration assay recently revealed a dramatic impact of various hematopoietic cytokines on the SDF-1α-directed migration of these *ex vivo* expanded HSPC.

Most hematopoietic progenitors reside in the bone marrow, however, a small fraction of these motile cells constantly circulate via the blood vessel system during steady state homeostasis. During inflammatory conditions, e.g., after (organ) tissue injury, the number of circulating HSPC increases dramatically. Inflammatory chemokines such as IL-8 and GROβ causes a rapid mobilization of HSPC from bone marrow. Conjointly, SDF-1α, released by endothelial cells, attracts HSPC to sites of injury, which thereupon participate in tissue repair. Due to their plasticity and pluripotency as well as their capacity to fuse with other cells, HSPC can transdifferentiate in various cell types such as liver, heart and skeletal muscle, or neurons. However, the directed migration and homing of HSPC to their target tissues underlies the influence of both *start* and *stop* signals. Recent observations indicate a modulating effect of the chemokine IL-8 and even the neurotransmitter GABA on the SDF-1α mediated migratory activity of HSPC. Further elucidation of these mechanisms may facilitate the selective manipulation of HSPC homing to their target tissues.

Thus, it appears that understanding the mechanisms influencing and regulating the migratory processes of HSPC, comprising homing, retention, release and mobilization, may allow the improvement of their clinical applications.

Chapter 11 - The science of human embryonic stem (hES) cells holds tremendous promise for the discovery of revolutionary cellular therapeutic options for the restoration and regeneration of damaged or destroyed cells and tissues. Yet the fact that the derivation of hES cells from embryos normally results in the destruction of the embryo poses ethical challenges, which for some, amounts to a veritable impasse to the further development of stem cell science. In this article, we review the scientific and ethics literature on hES cells including the use of somatic cell nuclear transfer to generate cloned hES cells for biomedical research and potential clinical applications. The article reviews the various normative theories on the moral status of the human embryo that capture issues ranging from the continuity of embryonic development to cognitive prerequisites for personhood such as sentience, rationality and self-awareness. The authors also discuss arguments for the symbolic value of human embryos and the need to respect human embryos as potential persons. Beyond issues related to the destruction of human embryos, a number of other ethical issues germane to embryonic stem cell science are also considered, such as the instrumentalization and commercialization of human materials for stem cell research, and the potential social and health risks to women in obtaining and donating oocytes or embryos for hES cell research. Finally, ethical questions arising from the relatively recent development of scientific methods to create new types of embryos for harvesting hES cells are also discussed.

Chapter 12 - With certain restrictions, the President has announced that federal funds may be used to conduct research on human embryonic stem cells. Federal research is limited to 64 existing stem cell lines that were derived (1) with the informed consent of the donors; (2) from excess embryos created solely for reproductive purposes; and (3) without any financial inducements to the donors. No federal funds will be used for the derivation or use of stem cell lines derived from newly destroyed embryos; the creation of any human embryos for research purposes; or cloning of human embryos for any purposes. Several lawsuits have been filed relating to stem cell research, and questions have been raised concerning access to existing stem cell lines by federal researchers.

Human Embryonic Stem Cells. Human embryonic stem cells are "master cells" and are able to develop into almost any cell in the human body. Building on earlier stem cell research, in 1998, researchers at the University of Wisconsin isolated cells from the inner cell mass of the early human embryo, called the blastocyst, and developed the first human embryonic stem cell lines. Research has focused on the potential that these cells can offer to treat or mitigate diseases and conditions and to generate replacement tissues for disfunctioning cells or organs. Research efforts have focused on spinal cord injury, multiple sclerosis, Parkinson's disease, Alzheimer's disease, diabetes, and other diseases or conditions. Scientists hope to use specialized cells to replace dysfunctional cells in the brain, spinal cord, pancreas, and other organs. The sources for stem cells include: one week old embryos (blastocysts) created via in vitro fertilization (IVF) to treat infertility; five to nine week old embryos or fetuses obtained through elective abortion; embryos created through IVF for research purposes; embryos created through cloning or somatic cell nuclear transfer (SCNT); and adult tissues (umbilical cord blood, bone marrow). Controversy surrounds the derivation of stem cells from human embryos and fetuses. In order to derive or extract the stem cells found within the embryo, the embryo is destroyed in the removal process. The earliest embryonic stem cells are called totipotent cells, which means they can develop into an entire organism, producing both the embryo and tissues required to support it in the uterus. At a later stage of development, pluripotent embryonic stem cells exist and can develop into almost any type of cell in the body. These stem cells cannot form the supporting tissues, as seen with totipotent cells. Human embryonic stem cells found in the early stage embryo are believed to have a greater ability to become different types of body cells and have more uses than adult stem cells.

Versions of these chapters were also published in *Stem Cell Research Journal* Volume 1, Numbers 1-4, edited by Frank Columbus, published by Nova Science Publishers, Inc. They were submitted for appropriate modifications in an effort to encourage wider dissemination of research.

In: Perspectives in Stem Cell Research ISBN: 978-1-61122-985-1
Editors: Brenda M. Davis and Christopher B. Halton

Chapter I

STEM CELL RESEARCH*

Judith A. Johnson and Erin Williams

SUMMARY

Embryonic stem cells have the ability to develop into virtually any cell in the body, and may have the potential to treat medical conditions such as diabetes and Parkinson's disease. In August 2001, President Bush announced that for the first time federal funds would be used to support research on human embryonic stem cells, but funding would be limited to "existing stem cell lines." The National Institutes of Health (NIH) has established the Human Embryonic Stem Cell Registry which lists stem cell lines that are eligible for use in federally funded research. Although 78 cell lines are listed, 21 embryonic stem cell lines are currently available. Scientists are concerned about the quality, longevity, and availability of the eligible stem cell lines. For a variety of reasons, many believe research advancement requires new embryonic stem cell lines, and for certain applications, stem cells derived from cloned embryos may offer the best hope for progress in understanding and treating disease. A significant cohort of pro-life advocates support stem cell research; those opposed are concerned that the isolation of stem cells requires the destruction of embryos. Letters from Congress, one signed by 206 Members of the House and a second signed by 58 Senators, have been sent urging President Bush to expand the current federal policy concerning embryonic stem cell research.

Some have argued that stem cell research be limited to adult stem cells obtained from tissues such as bone marrow. They argue that adult stem cells should be pursued instead of embryonic stem cells because they believe the derivation of stem cells from either embryos or aborted fetuses is ethically unacceptable. Other scientists believe adult stem cells should not be the sole target of research because of important scientific and technical limitations. Groups make ethical distinctions in the debate on how to proceed with stem cell research based upon

* Excerpted from CRS Report RL31015 updated August 13, 2004.

embryo protection, relief of suffering, viability, the purpose and timing of embryo creation and destruction, donor consent, scientific alternatives, federal funding, and cloning.

On February 27, 2003, the House passed H.R. 534 (Dave Weldon), which would ban the process of human cloning and the importation of any product derived from an embryo created via cloning. Cloning could not be used for reproductive purposes or for research on therapeutic purposes, which has implications for stem cell research. The House defeated a substitute amendment, H.Amdt. 5, that would have banned *only* human reproductive cloning; the ban would have sunset after 10 years. H.R. 801 (Greenwood) is similar to H.Amdt 5. S. 245 (Brownback) would ban reproductive cloning and research on therapeutic cloning; S. 303 (Hatch) would ban only reproductive cloning. Supporters of H.R. 534 argue that a partial ban on human cloning, such as S. 303 and H.R. 801, would be impossible to enforce. Critics argue that H.R. 534 would curtail medical research and prevent Americans from receiving life-saving treatments created overseas. President Bush has stated his support for the Weldon bill, but 40 Nobel Laureates, who are in favor of nuclear transplantation technology for research and therapeutic purposes, are strongly opposed to the legislation. H.R. 3960 (Millender-McDonald) and H.R. 4682 (Castle) would fund research on embryonic stem cell lines derived after the August 9, 2001, policy established by the Bush Administration. This report will be updated as needed.

Overview of Basic Research and Potential Applications

Most cells within an animal or human being are committed to fulfilling a single function within the body. In contrast, stem cells are a unique and important set of cells that are not specialized. Stem cells retain the ability to become many or all of the different cell types in the body and thereby play a critical role in repairing organs and body tissues throughout life. Although the term stem cells is often used in reference to these repair cells within an adult organism, a more fundamental variety of stem cells is found in the early stage embryo. Embryonic stem cells may have a greater ability to become different types of body cells than adult stem cells.

Stem Cells from Embryos or Fetal Tissue

Embryonic stem cells were first isolated from mouse embryos in 1981. Animal embryos were the only source for research on embryonic stem cells until November 1998, when two groups of U.S. scientists announced the successful isolation of human embryonic stem cells. One group, at the University of Wisconsin, derived stem cells from one-week-old embryos produced via *in vitro* fertilization (IVF).[1] The work is controversial, in the opinion of some individuals, because the stem cells are located within the embryo and the process of removing them destroys the embryo. The second group, at Johns Hopkins University, derived cells with very similar properties from five- to nine-week-old embryos or fetuses obtained through elective abortion.[2] Both groups reported the human embryos or fetuses were donated for research following a process of informed consent. The cells were then manipulated in the laboratory to create embryonic stem cell lines that may continue to divide for many months to years.

Another potential source of embryonic stem cells is somatic cell nuclear transfer (SCNT), also referred to as cloning.[3] In SCNT the nucleus of an egg is removed and replaced by the nucleus from a mature body cell, such as a skin cell. The cell created via SCNT is allowed to develop for a week and then the stem cells are removed. In 1996, scientists in Scotland used the SCNT procedure to produce Dolly the sheep, the first mammalian clone.[4] In February 2004, Korean scientists announced that they had created human embryos via the SCNT process and had succeeded in isolating human stem cells from a cloned embryo. This development and the unsubstantiated announcement by Clonaid in December 2002 of the birth of a cloned child have contributed to the controversy over research on human embryos.[5]

Stem Cells from Adult Tissue or Umbilical Cord Blood

Stem cells obtained from adult organisms are also the focus of research. There have been a number of recent publications on adult stem cells from a variety of different sources, such as bone marrow and the umbilical cord following birth. In addition, a number of private companies (such as MorphoGen, NeuralStem, Osiris Therapeutics, StemSource, ViaCell) are working on therapeutic uses of adult stem cells.

Some advocate that adult instead of embryonic stem cell research should be pursued because they believe the derivation of stem cells from either IVF embryos or aborted fetuses is ethically unacceptable. Others believe that adult stem cells should not be the sole target of research because of important scientific and technical limitations. Adult stem cells may not be as long lived or capable of as many cell divisions as embryonic stem cells. Also, adult stem cells may not be as versatile in developing into various types of tissue as embryonic stem cells, and the location and rarity of the cells in the body might rule out safe and easy access. For these reasons, many scientists argue that both adult and embryonic stem cells should be the subject of research, allowing for a comparison of their various capabilities.

Possible Sources of Stem Cells

— embryos created via IVF (for infertility treatment or for research purposes)
— embryos or fetuses obtained through elective abortion
— embryos created via SCNT (somatic cell nuclear transfer, or cloning)
— adult tissues (bone marrow, umbilical cord blood)

Potential Applications of Stem Cell Research

Stem cells provide the opportunity to study the growth and differentiation of individual cells into tissues. Understanding these processes could provide insights into the causes of birth defects, genetic abnormalities, and other disease states. If normal development were better understood, it might be possible to prevent or correct some of these conditions. Stem cells could be used to produce large amounts of one cell type to test new drugs for effectiveness and chemicals for toxicity. Stem cells might be transplanted into the body to treat disease (diabetes, Parkinson's disease) or injury (e.g., spinal cord). The damaging side effects of medical treatments might be repaired with stem cell treatment. For example, cancer chemotherapy destroys immune cells in patients, decreasing their ability to fight off a broad range of diseases; correcting this adverse effect would be a major advance.

Before stem cells can be applied to human medical problems, substantial advances in basic cell biology and clinical technique are required. In addition, very challenging regulatory decisions will be required on the individually created tissue-based therapies resulting from stem cell research. Such decisions would likely be made by the Center for Biologics Evaluation and Research (CBER) of the Food and Drug Administration (FDA). The potential benefits mentioned above would be likely only after many more years of research. Technical hurdles include developing the ability to control the differentiation of stem cells into a desired cell type (like a heart or nerve cell) and to ensure that uncontrolled development, such as a cancerous tumor, does not occur. If stem cells are to be used for transplantation, the problem of immune rejection must also be overcome. Some scientists think that the creation of many more embryonic stem cell lines will eventually account for all the various immunological types needed for use in tissue transplantation therapy. Others envision the eventual development of a "universal donor" type of stem cell tissue, analogous to a universal blood donor.

However, if the SCNT technique (cloning) was employed using a cell nucleus from the patient, stem cells created via this method would be genetically identical to the patient, would presumably be recognized by the patient's immune system, and thus would avoid any tissue rejection problems that could occur in other stem cell therapeutic approaches. Because of this, many scientists believe that the SCNT technique may provide the best hope of eventually treating patients using stem cells for tissue transplantation.

Current Federal Regulatory Landscape

The Dickey Amendment and Clinton Administration Stem Cell Policy. Prior to an August 2001 Bush Administration decision (see below), no federal funds had been used to support research on stem cells derived from either human embryos or fetal tissue.[6] The work at the University of Wisconsin and Johns Hopkins University was supported by private funding from the Geron Corporation. Private funding for experiments involving embryos was required because Congress attached a rider to legislation that affected FY1996 National Institutes of Health (NIH) funding. The rider, an amendment originally introduced by Representative Jay Dickey, prohibited HHS from using appropriated funds for the creation of human embryos for research purposes or for research in which human embryos are destroyed. The Dickey amendment language has been added to each of the Labor, HHS and Education appropriations acts for FY1997 through FY2004.[7] For FY2004, the provision is found in Section 510 of Division E, which is the Labor, HHS and Education division of the FY2004 Consolidated Appropriations bill (P.L. 108-199). It prohibits HHS from using FY2004 appropriated funds for

> (1) the creation of a human embryo or embryos for research purposes; or (2) research in which a human embryo or embryos are destroyed, discarded, or knowingly subjected to risk of injury or death greater than that allowed for research on fetuses in utero under 45 CFR 46.208(a)(2) and Section 498(b) of the Public Health Service Act (42 U.S.C. 289g(b)). For purposes of this section, the term "human embryo or embryos" includes any organism, not protected as a human subject under 45 CFR 46 [the Human Subject Protection regulations]... that is derived by fertilization, parthenogenesis, cloning, or any other means from one or more human gametes [sperm or egg] or human diploid cells [cells that have two sets of chromosomes, such as somatic cells].

There is no similar federal prohibition on fetal tissue research; however, other restrictions do apply.

Following the November 1998 announcement on the derivation of human embryonic stem cells, NIH requested a legal opinion from HHS on whether federal funds could be used to support research on human stem cells derived from embryos. The January 15, 1999, response from HHS General Counsel Harriet Rabb found that the Dickey amendment would not apply to research using human stem cells "because such cells are not a human embryo within the statutory definition." The finding was based, in part, on the determination by HHS that the statutory ban on human embryo research defines an embryo as an *organism* that when implanted in the uterus is capable of becoming a human being. Human stem cells are not and cannot develop into an organism; they lack the capacity to become organisms even if they are transferred to a uterus. As a result, HHS maintained that NIH could support research that uses stem cells derived through private funds, but could not support research that itself, with federal funds, derives stem cells from embryos because of the federal ban in the Dickey amendment.

Shortly after the opinion by the HHS General Counsel was released, NIH disclosed that the agency planned to fund research on stem cells derived from human embryos once appropriate guidelines were developed and an oversight committee established. NIH Director Harold Varmus appointed a working group that began drafting guidelines in April 1999. Draft guidelines were published in the *Federal Register* on December 2, 1999. About 50,000 comments were received during the public comment period, which ended February 22, 2000. On August 25, 2000, NIH published in the *Federal Register* final guidelines on the support of human embryonic stem cell research. The guidelines stated that studies utilizing "stem cells derived from human embryos may be conducted using NIH funds only if the cells were derived (without federal funds) from human embryos that were created for the purposes of fertility treatment and were in excess of the clinical need of the individuals seeking such treatment." Under the guidelines, NIH would not fund research directly involving the derivation of human stem cells from embryos; this was prohibited by the Dickey amendment.

Other areas of research ineligible for NIH funding under the guidelines include (1) research in which human stem cells are utilized to create or contribute to a human embryo; (2) research in which human stem cells are combined with an animal embryo; (3) research in which human stem cells are used for reproductive cloning of a human; (4) research in which human stem cells are *derived* using somatic cell nuclear transfer, i.e., the transfer of a human somatic cell nucleus into a human or animal egg; (5) research *utilizing* human stem cells that were derived using somatic cell nuclear transfer; and (6) research utilizing stem cells that were derived from human embryos created for research purposes, rather than for infertility treatment.

NIH began accepting grant applications for research projects utilizing human stem cells immediately following publication of the guidelines; the deadline for submitting a grant application was March 15, 2001. All such applications were to be reviewed by the NIH Human Pluripotent Stem Cell Review Group (HPSCRG), which was established to ensure compliance with the guidelines. James Kushner, director of the University of Utah General Clinical Research Center, served briefly as chair of the HPSCRG. Applications would also have undergone the normal NIH peer-review process.p8] The first meeting of the HPSCRG was scheduled for April 25, 2001. The HPSCRG was to conduct an ethical review of human pluripotent stem cell lines to determine whether the research groups involved had followed the NIH guidelines in deriving the cell lines. However, in mid April 2001, HHS postponed the meeting until a review of the Clinton Administration's policy decisions on stem cell research was completed by the new Bush Administration.[9] According to media sources, the 12 HPSCRG members, whose names were not made public, represented a wide range of scientific, ethical and theological expertise and opinion, as well as at least one "mainstream Catholic."[10]

The Bush Administration conducted a legal review of the policy decisions made during the Clinton Administration regarding federal support of stem cell research, as well as a scientific review, prepared by NIH, of the status of the research and its applications. The scientific review was released on July 18, 2001, at a hearing on stem cell research held by the Senate Appropriations Subcommittee on Labor, Health and Human Services and Education.[11] The NIH report did not make any recommendations, but argued that both embryonic and adult stem cell research should be pursued.

Bush Administration Stem Cell Policy. On August 9, 2001, President Bush announced that for the first time federal funds would be used to support research on human embryonic stem cells, but funding would be limited to "existing stem cell lines where the life and death decision has already been made."[12] President Bush stated that the decision "allows us to explore the promise and potential of stem cell research without crossing a fundamental moral line, by providing taxpayer funding that would sanction or encourage further destruction of human embryos that have at least the potential for life." The President also stated that the federal government would continue to support research involving stem cells from other sources, such as umbilical cord blood, placentas, and adult and animal tissues, "which do not involve the same moral dilemma."

Under the Bush policy, federal funds may only be used for research on existing stem cell lines that were derived (1) with the informed consent of the donors; (2) from excess embryos created solely for reproductive purposes; and (3) without any financial inducements to the donors.[13] NIH was tasked with examining the derivation of all existing stem cell lines and creating a registry of those lines that satisfy the Bush Administration criteria. According to the White House, this will ensure that federal funds are used to support only stem cell research that is scientifically sound, legal, and ethical. Federal funds will not be used for (1) the derivation or use of stem cell lines derived from newly destroyed embryos; (2) the creation of any human embryos for research purposes; or (3) the cloning of human embryos for any purpose.

Agency Regulation. Many entities and individuals that conduct research on humans ("human subjects" research) are both federally and institutionally regulated. Ex vivo embryos (those not in a uterus) are not considered "human subjects" for these purposes, though federally funded research on them is regulated by the Dickey Amendment as described above.

Stem cells and stem cell lines are not considered "human subjects," nor are they governed by the Dickey Amendment.

Two HHS agencies, FDA and NIH, regulate some aspects of stem cell research, even if research on stem cell lines is not classified as "human subjects" research. FDA, the agency that ensures the safety and efficacy of food, drugs, medical devices and cosmetics, regulates stem cell research aimed at the development of any "product" subject to its approval. NIH, the medical and behavioral research agency within HHS, regulates stem cell research that it funds in compliance with President Bush's 2001 policy. In accordance, NIH has created a Human Embryonic Stem Cell Registry that lists the human embryonic stem cell lines that meet the eligibility criteria as outlined in the Bush Administration stem cell policy.

FDA Regulation. All of the human embryonic stem cell lines listed on the NIH Human Embryonic Stem Cell Registry (see **Table 2**) have been grown on beds of mouse "feeder" cells. The mouse cells secrete a substance that prevents the human embryonic stem cells from differentiating into more mature cell types (nerve or muscle cells). Infectious agents, such as viruses, within the mouse feeder cells could transfer into the human cells. If the human cells were transplanted into a patient, these infected human cells may cause disease in the patient which could be transmitted to close contacts of the patient and eventually to the general population. Public health officials and regulatory agencies such as the FDA are specifically concerned about retroviruses, which may remain hidden in the DNA only to cause disease many years later, as well as any unrecognized agents which may be present in the mouse cells.

The FDA defines xenotransplantation as "any procedure that involves the transplantation, implantation, or infusion into a human recipient of either (a) live cells, tissues, or organs from a nonhuman source, or (b) human body fluids, cells, tissues or organs that have had ex vivo contact with live nonhuman animal cells, tissues or organs."[14] So transplantation therapy involving Bush approved stem cell lines, which all have been exposed to mouse feeder cells, would constitute xenotransplantation. Xenotrans-plantation products are subject to regulation by the FDA under Section 351 of the Public Health Service Act (42 USC 262) and the Federal Food, Drug and Cosmetic Act (21 USC 321 et. seq.). FDA has developed guidance documents and the U.S. Public Health Service has developed guidelines on infectious disease issues associated with xenotransplantation.[15]

During a Senate hearing on stem cell research held by the Health, Education, Labor and Pensions Committee on September 5, 2001, HHS Secretary Thompson stated that the FDA is overseeing 17 investigational protocols involving xenotransplantation in other areas of clinical research that involve patients. Therefore, the xenotransplantation-related public health concerns over the human embryonic stem cell lines may not necessarily preclude the development of treatments for patients. While the problems presented by xenotransplantation for clinical research are neither unique to stem cell research nor insurmountable, many scientists believe it will be preferable to use sterile cell lines when attempting to treat patients via stem cell transplantation, and scientists have been successful in developing human embryonic stem cells that can be maintained without the use of mouse feeder cells.[16]

NIH Research Funding and Stem Cell Registry. The Bush Administration's August 9, 2001, policy statement on stem cell research and the NIH Stem Cell Registry effectively replaced the NIH stem cell guidelines that were developed under the Clinton Administration and never fully implemented. Grant proposals for embryonic stem cell research undergo only the normal peer-review process without the added review of the HPSCRG as had been specified under the Clinton NIH stem cell guidelines. In February 2002, NIH announced the approval of the first expenditures for research on human embryonic stem cells. Funding for stem cell research by NIH is shown in **Table 1**. The NIH website provides additional information about current stem cell activities and funding opportunities.[17]

The NIH Human Embryonic Stem Cell Registry lists stem cell lines that are eligible for use in federally funded research and currently available to be shipped to scientists.[18] As shown in **Table 2**, the NIH registry originally listed universities and companies that had derived a total of 78 human embryonic stem cell lines which were eligible for use in federally funded research under the August 2001 Bush Administration policy.

Table 1. National Institutes of Health Funding ($ in millions).

	FY2001	FY2002	FY2003
Stem cell research	$306	$387	$521
Human embryonic stem cell	(0)	(10.7)	(25)

Source: NIH Budget Office, May 7, 2004.

Table 2. NIH List of Human Embryonic Stem Cell Lines Eligible for Use in Federal Research.

Names	Number of stem cell lines	
	Eligible	**Available**
BresaGen, Inc., Athens, GA	4	3
Cell & Gene Therapy Institute (Pochon CHA University), Seoul, Korea	2	
Cellaritis AB, Goteborg, Sweden	3	2
CyThera, Inc., San Diego, CA	9	0
ES Cell International, Melbourne, Australia	6	6
Geron Corporation, Menlo Park, CA	7	
Goteborg University, Goteborg,, Sweden	16	
Karolinska Institute, Stockholm, Sweden	6	0
Maria Biotech Co. Ltd. — Maria Infertility Hospital Medical Institute, Seoul, Korea	3	
MizMedi Hospital — Seoul National University, Seoul, Korea	1	1
National Center for Biological Sciences/Tata Institute of Fundamental Research, Bangalore, India	3	
Reliance Life Sciences, Mumbai, India	7	
Technion University, Haifa, Israel	4	2
University of California, San Francisco, CA	2	2
Wisconsin Alumni Research Foundation, Madison, WI	5	5
Total	**78**	**21**

a. Entities in gray do not have stem cell lines available for shipment to U.S. researchers because of a variety of scientific, regulatory and legal reasons. The zeros entered in the "Available" column indicate that "the cells failed to expand into undifferentiated cell cultures."

However, many of these stem cell lines were found to be either unavailable or unsuitable for research. As of August 11, 2004, the NIH registry listed a total of 21 stem cell lines available from seven sources as shown above.

Access to Stem Cell Lines. Many scientists, disease advocates and others remain concerned that federally supported research on human embryonic stem cells is limited to the number of cell lines that meet the criteria of the August 9, 2001 Bush policy. As stated above, currently 21 cell lines are available for research with federal dollars, and an unpublished NIH report indicates that under a best case scenario, a total of 23 human embryonic stem cell lines will ever be ready for use in research.[19] Because the pre-August 9 cell lines were developed in the early days of human stem cell research using older 1990s techniques, the cell lines not only have the problems of xenotransplantion described above, but they are harder to work with, not well characterized, and somewhat unstable.

In reaction to the limitations imposed by the Bush policy, some U.S. research groups have decided to develop additional human embryonic stem cell lines using private funding. In June 2004, a team of scientists at the Reproductive Genetics Institute, a private fertility clinic in Chicago, announced that they had isolated 50 new human embryonic stem cell lines from frozen embryos that were donated by patients following fertility treatment.[20] By using genetic diagnosis techniques, the Chicago team was able to create stem cell lines that carry the gene for muscular dystrophy as well as stem cell lines with the gene for six other diseases.[21] The new stem cell lines are to be used to understand the origins of disease-related symptoms and to develop and test new treatments.

In March 2004, a Harvard University laboratory headed by Douglas Melton announced that using private research dollars they had isolated 17 new human embryonic stem cell lines.[22] In order to perform this work it was necessary to build a new laboratory so that the group's federally funded research would be conducted separately from research on the new stem cell lines. Likewise, although the 17 stem cell lines are available for use by other laboratories, any research using the new stem cell lines must be performed at a facility that does not receive federal support. The Harvard group intends to raise $100 million in private funding to establish a stem cell center in order to continue the work begun by Melton and his group of scientists.

In December 2002, Stanford University announced that a gift of $12 million from an anonymous donor would be used to establish an institute that will use expertise in stem cell biology and cancer biology to develop novel treatments for cancer and other diseases.[23] The new institute is headed by Dr. Irving Weissman, a Professor in Cancer Biology at Stanford. Scientists at the Institute for Cancer/Stem Cell Biology and Medicine are developing new stem cell lines, some through the process of SCNT, to study the disease process of a wide range of disorders including cancer, diabetes, cardiovascular disease, autoimmune disease, allergies, and neurological disorders such as Parkinson's and Lou Gehrig's disease. Initial studies are performed in mice; however, the work may be extended to human cells and eggs. The new stem cell lines may allow investigators to better understand the biological and genetic basis of a disorder and thereby develop new treatments.

In August 2002, the University of California at San Francisco established the UCSF Developmental and Stem Cell Biology Program with a $5 million matching grant from Andy Grove, the chairman of Intel Corporation. The program funds basic studies (using both animal and human cells) in stem cell biology and their translation into clinical practice with a goal of developing treatments for such diseases as diabetes, cardiovascular disease, Parkinson's disease, Alzheimer's disease and spinal cord injury. UCSF and the University of Wisconsin are the only two universities in the United States that have derived human embryonic stem cell lines that qualified for inclusion on the NIH Stem Cell Registry. This past winter, the new UCSF stem cell program announced it had met the Grove "Stem Cell Challenge" and had raised the total funding for the program to more than $11 million in gifts and matching funds. The program recently awarded $50,000 grants to four scientists who are studying various aspects of stem cell biology.[24]

A worldwide survey of laboratories conducted by the Boston Globe found that as of May 23, 2004, 128 human embryonic stem cell lines had been created since August 9, 2001; all would be ineligible for use in federally funded research under the Bush policy on stem cell research.[25] More lines are being created in laboratories overseas than in the United States, according to the survey. The survey found that 94 were created in labs outside the United States and 34 were created in this country. Of the 128 lines, 51 of the new stem cell lines are currently available for use, the remaining cell lines are not available for a variety of technical or legal reasons. For example, some cell lines have not yet been fully characterized to determine their stability or suitability for research. However, eventually their status is to be determined by using laboratory techniques. In Japan, stem cell lines are not allowed to be shipped to laboratories in other countries. In the United Kingdom, stem cell lines cannot be shipped abroad until they have been processed by the new UK Stem Cell Bank.[26]

In response to concerns over access to human embryonic stem cell lines, in April 2004, a group of over 200 Members of the House of Representatives sent a letter to President Bush requesting that the Administration revise the current stem cell policy and utilize the embryos that are created in excess of need during the treatment of infertile couples.[27] The letter points out that an estimated 400,000 frozen IVF embryos[28] "will likely be destroyed if not donated, with informed consent of the couple, for research." According to the letter, "scientists are reporting that it is increasingly difficult to attract new scientists to this area of research because of concerns that funding restrictions will keep this research from being successful.... We have already seen researchers move to countries like the United Kingdom, which have more supportive policies. In addition, leadership in this area of research has shifted to the United Kingdom, which sees this scientific area as the cornerstone of its biotech industry."

Under the direction of the White House, NIH Director Elias A. Zerhouni sent a letter in response to the House Members which restates the Bush Administration position against using federal funds for research involving the destruction of human embryos.[29] The letter from NIH Director Zerhouni did contain the following sentence which some observers believe indicates a potential future policy shift: "And although it is fair to say that from a purely scientific perspective more cell lines may well speed some areas of human embryonic stem cell research, the president's position is still predicated on his belief that taxpayer funds should not 'sanction or encourage further destruction of human embryos that have at least the potential for life."[30] Although White House spokesperson Claire Buchan stated that the sentence does not indicate the president's position has changed, supporters of stem cell research point out that it concedes that science could benefit from additional stem cell lines and that the president's position now rests solely on ethical arguments.

A letter signed by 58 Senators urging President Bush to expand the current federal policy concerning embryonic stem cell research was sent on June 4, 2004.[31] The letter states that "despite the fact that U.S. scientists were the first to derive human embryonic stem cells, leadership in this area of research is shifting to other countries such as the United Kingdom, Singapore, South Korea and Australia."

On July 14, 2004, HHS Secretary Thompson announced in a letter to Speaker of the House Dennis Hastert that NIH would establish Centers of Excellence in Translational Stem Cell Research.[32] The new centers will be funded by $18 millions in grants over a four year period and will investigate how stem cells can be used to treat a variety of diseases. NIH will also create a National Embryonic Stem Cell Bank that will collect in one location many of the stem cell lines that are eligible for federal research funding. In the letter to Speaker Hastert, Secretary Thompson stated that "before anyone can successfully argue the stem cell policy should be broadened, we must first exhaust the potential of the stem cell lines made available with the policy."[33] In reaction to the announcement, the President of the Coalition for the Advancement of Medical Research stated that "creating a bank to house stem cell lines created before August 2001 does nothing to increase the wholly inadequate supply of stem cell lines for research."[34] The co-sponsors of the Stem Cell Research Enhancement Act (H.R. 4682), Representative Michael Castle and Representative Diana DeGette are quoted as saying that the plan is "a positive step forward but stops short of providing researchers the full support they need."[35]

State Legislation on Embryonic Stem Cell Research

The Dickey Amendment restricts federal funding for embryo research; however, states are the principal sources of direct regulation of non-federally funded embryo research. State laws vary widely in their application and content. Nebraska, New Jersey, California and New Hampshire have enacted legislation directly regarding stem cell research. Nebraska prohibits the use of state funds for embryonic stem cell research (Nebraska Health Care Funding Act §71-7606(3)). New Hampshire's Safety and Welfare statutes (Title VXII §168-B: 16 (I, II)) circumscribe the boundaries of permissible embryo research.[36] New Jersey and California encourage embryonic stem cell research, and permit state funding for it. Kansas restricts its bioscience funding to exclude research that would be "contrary to federal laws that are in effect on the date of enactment of [the] act."[37] New Hampshire, Massachusetts, Pennsylvania, Louisiana and Minnesota are currently considering pro-stem cell legislation.[38]

California's law, enacted in September 2002, was the nation's first to expressly permit and encourage research involving the derivation of human embryonic stem cells and cloned embryos (California Health and Safety Code § 123440, 24185, 12115-7, 125300-320). The law does not authorize practices that were previously proscribed, but instead provides assurances to researchers and sponsors hesitant to invest in embryonic stem cell research since the 2001 Bush policy took effect. The law has reportedly enticed several prominent researchers to move there from other states. A pro-stem cell coalition in California has placed an initiative on the November 2004 ballot that would generate $3 billion in state-bond funding for embryonic stem cell research over the next 10 years and the establishment of a California Institute for Regenerative Medicine.[39]

New Jersey's law, enacted in January 2004, specifically permits embryonic stem cell research, but bans human cloning for reproductive purposes (NJ Permanent Statutes, Title 26:2Z-2). Like the California law, New Jersey's stem cell statute provides assurances to researchers and sponsors and does not contradict the 2001 Bush policy. In May 2004, Governor James McGreevey signed a bill to create the first state-funded embryonic stem cell research center, a $25 million endeavor.[40] The legislature funded the measure on June 25, 2004, passing a state budget that allocates $9.5 million to the newly chartered Stem Cell Institute of New Jersey.41 The state money is supposed to attract private investment, which Dr. Ira Black, the Institute's founding Director, says has already happened.[42]

In an effort to discourage abortion, 15 states restrict research on fetuses and embryos that have been aborted, which may preclude some forms of stem cell research. Among the states with such restrictions are California, which encourages stem cell research in other law, Pennsylvania, which is considering pro-stem cell research legislation, and Nebraska, which prohibits the use of state funds for stem cell research. The restrictions on aborted fetal and embryonic tissue research vary in scope among the states. Arizona, Indiana, North Dakota, Ohio, Oklahoma, and South Dakota prohibit research on living and nonliving fetuses or embryos. Arkansas, California, Florida, Montana, and Nebraska prohibit research on aborted live fetuses. Massachusetts and Pennsylvania prohibit research on embryos and live fetuses. Illinois prohibits research on aborted living and nonliving fetuses. Missouri prohibits research on live fetuses before abortion. The remaining 35 states do not prohibit research using aborted fetal tissue.

Thirteen states have restrictions on research using fetal or embryonic tissue derived from processes other than abortion (such as in vitro fertilization (IVF) or cloning), which may also preclude some forms of stem cell research. Among them are Louisiana, which is considering pro-stem cell legislation, and North Dakota, South Dakota and Illinois, which also prohibit research on fetuses and embryos. Illinois prohibits research on fetuses and embryos. Louisiana prohibits research on fetuses and embryos in utero and in vitro. Maine, New Mexico, Rhode Island and Utah prohibit research on fetuses or embryos born or extracted alive. This restriction does not apply to pre-implantation in vitro fertilized embryos. South Dakota prohibits research on embryos outside of a woman's body or on cells or tissues derived from an embryo outside a woman's body. Minnesota prohibits research on fetuses and on some live embryos. Michigan and North Dakota prohibit research on live embryos and fetuses, or cloned embryos. The law in Virginia may prohibit research on cloned embryos or fetuses.[43] Arkansas and Iowa prohibit research on cloned embryos. Thirty-seven states have no such restrictions.

Congressional Actions

A number of hearings have been held by both House and Senate committees on the topic of stem cell research. With regard to legislation, Congress addressed the issue of stem cell research in the Consolidated Appropriations Act of 2004 (P.L. 108-199) by including the Dickey Amendment which bans almost all publically funded human embryo research. The act also bars the Patent and Trademark Office from spending money "to issue patents on claims directed to or encompassing a human organism." This restriction could potentially deter human stem cell research because researchers might not be able to claim ownership of their work.

P.L. 108-199 provides support for research using stem cells found in umbilical cord blood by making $10,000,000 available to establish a National Cord Blood Stem Cell Bank.

Two other bills, H.R. 2852 (Christopher Smith) and S. 1717 (Hatch), both titled the Cord Blood Stem Cell Act of 2003, would amend the Public Health Service Act to establish a National Cord Blood Stem Cell Bank Network to prepare, store, and distribute human umbilical cord blood stem cells for the treatment of patients and to support peer-reviewed research using this type of stem cell. H.R. 2852 was referred to the Committee on Energy and Commerce. S. 1717 was referred to the Committee on Health, Education, Labor and Pensions.

H.R. 3960 (Millender-McDonald), the Stem Cell Replenishment Act of 2004, was introduced on March 11, 2004. H.R. 3960 authorizes the use of federal funds for research on human embryonic stem cells irrespective of the date on which the derivation process for the stem cells was initiated or completed. The bill directs the Director of NIH to review the guidelines and notices published by NIH with respect to human embryonic stem cell research and revise the guidelines and notices to ensure the availability of not less than 60 stem cell lines that are able to be used for scientific research. H.R. 3960 was referred to the House Committee on Energy and Commerce on March 30, 2004.

H.R. 4682 (Castle), the Stem Cell Research Enhancement Act, was introduced on June 24, 2004. H.R. 4682 amends the Public Health Service Act and directs the Secretary of HHS, in consultation with the Director of NIH, to fund research on embryonic stem cell lines derived after the August 9, 2001 policy established by the Bush Administration. In accordance with the Dickey Amendment, no federal funds shall be used to derive stem cells or destroy embryos. Stem cell lines derived after enactment must meet ethical guidelines established by the NIH. Only embryos that were originally created for fertility treatment purposes and in excess of clinical need are eligible for stem cell derivation. Only embryos that the individuals seeking fertility treatments have determined will not be implanted in a woman and will be discarded are eligible for stem cell derivation. Written consent is required for embryo donation. The Secretary in consultation with the Director of NIH shall promulgate guidelines 60 days after enactment. These guidelines shall ensure that federally funded researchers adhere to ethical considerations. No federal funds shall be used to conduct research on unapproved stem cell lines. The Secretary shall annually report to Congress about stem cell research. H.R. 4682 has been referred to the House Committee on Energy and Commerce.

On February 27, 2003, the House passed H.R. 534 (Dave Weldon), the Human Cloning Prohibition Act of 2003 by a vote of 241-155. H.R. 534 amends Title 18 of the United States Code and would ban the process of human cloning as well as the importation of any product derived from an embryo created via cloning. Under this measure, cloning could not be used for reproductive purposes or for research on therapeutic purposes, which would have implications for stem cell research. H.R. 534 includes a criminal penalty of imprisonment of not more than 10 years and a civil penalty of not less than $1 million. H.R. 534 is essentially identical to the measure which passed the House in the 107th Congress (H.R. 2505).

During floor debate on H.R. 534, an amendment, H.Amdt. 4 (Robert Scott), was agreed to by voice vote. H.Amdt. 4 requires that the General Accounting Office (GAO), in consultation with the National Academy of Sciences, conduct a study on the impact of the cloning ban on medical technology and assess the need (if any) for modification of the cloning ban contained in the bill. A report to Congress with findings and recommendations would be required within two years of enactment. An amendment in the nature of a substitute, H.Amdt. 5 (Greenwood), failed by a vote of 174 to 231. The amendment would have prohibited human SCNT technology when used to initiate a pregnancy but allowed SCNT to be used in medical research. H.Amdt 5 is similar to H.R. 801 (Greenwood) (see below).

H.R. 534 was introduced on February 5, 2003, and reported (19-12 vote) by the House Judiciary Committee on February 12, 2003 (H.Rept. 108-18). During markup, four amendments were defeated by 12-19 or by voice vote. The amendments attempted to either limit the ban to three years, exempt the importation of medical treatments, exempt the use of cloning in research, or in the creation of additional stem cell lines. A fifth amendment that would add the GAO study was withdrawn when Chairman Sensenbrenner assured his support if it was added to the bill during floor debate.

A companion bill, S. 245 (Brownback), was introduced on January 29, 2003. It is similar to H.R. 534, except that (1) it does not contain the ban on importation of products derived from therapeutic cloning; and (2) it amends Title 4 of the Public Health Service Act (42 U.S.C. 289 et seq.) instead of Title 18 of the United States Code.[44] S. 245 includes a criminal penalty of imprisonment of not more than 10 years and a civil penalty of not less than $1 million. It requires the General Accounting Office to conduct a study to assess the need (if any) for any changes of the prohibition on cloning in light of new developments in medical technology, the need for SCNT to produce medical advances, current public attitudes and prevailing ethical views on the use of SCNT and potential legal implications of research in SCNT. The study is to be completed within four years of enactment. S. 245 has been referred to the Senate Health, Education, Labor, and Pensions Committee.

H.R. 801 (Greenwood), the Cloning Prohibition Act of 2003, was introduced on February 13, 2003. H.R. 801 would prohibit human reproductive cloning while allowing cloning for medical research purposes, including stem cell research. The bill includes a civil penalty of up to $10 million and a criminal penalty of up to 10 years in prison for those convicted of using SCNT for human reproductive purposes, or for importing the products of human cloning if the products would be used to initiate a pregnancy. The bill amends the Food, Drug and Cosmetic Act (21 U.S.C. 301 et seq.) and requires that all researchers performing SCNT on human cells must register their research activity with the HHS Secretary; such registration would most likely be submitted to the FDA.

H.R. 801 stipulates that all research involving human SCNT be conducted in accordance with Part 50 (Protection of Human Subjects) and Part 56 (Institutional Review Boards) of Title 21 of the Code of Federal Regulations (CFR). Under the bill, individuals whose cells are used for such research (presumably the donor of the unfertilized egg and the donor of the somatic cell) would be considered human subjects for the purposes of Parts 50 and 56 of 21CFR. In addition to the requirements under Parts 50 and 56 of 21CFR, the human cell donors must sign an informed consent statement declaring that (1) the cells are donated for research purposes; (2) the donor understands that federal law regulates SCNT and use of SCNT to initiate a pregnancy is a criminal act; and, (3) the individual does not intend for the donated cells to be used to initiate a pregnancy. A sunset provision states that the prohibition would expire 10 years after enactment.

H.R. 801 requires the Secretary of HHS to request a study reviewing the current state of knowledge on (1) the biological properties of stem cells obtained from embryos, fetal tissue, and adult tissue; (2) any biological differences of such stem cells and the consequences for research and medicine; and (3) the ability of stem cells to generate different types of tissue and their potential clinical uses. The study must be conducted by the Institute of Medicine or another appropriate public or nonprofit private entity.

S. 303 (Hatch), the Human Cloning Ban and Stem Cell Research Protection Act of 2003, was introduced on February 5, 2003. Although S. 303 and H.R. 801 amend different titles of the United States Code (S. 303 amends Title 18 and H.R. 801 amends Title 21), both bills would have the same effect: human reproductive cloning would be banned, but cloning for medical research purposes would be allowed, including stem cell research.[45] S. 303 includes a criminal penalty of imprisonment of not more than 10 years and a civil penalty of not less than $1 million.

S. 303 requires the Comptroller General to prepare a report within one year of enactment that describes the actions taken by the Attorney General to enforce the prohibition on human reproductive cloning, the personnel and resources used to enforce the prohibition, and a list of any violations of the prohibition. The Comptroller General must also prepare a report within one year of enactment on similar state laws that prohibit human cloning and actions taken by the states' attorney general to enforce the provisions of any similar state law along with a list of violations. A report on the coordination of enforcement actions among the federal, state and local governments must also be prepared by the Comptroller General within one year of enactment, as well as a report on laws adopted by foreign countries related to human cloning.

S. 303 also would amend the Public Health Service Act by requiring that human SCNT be conducted in accordance with the ethical requirements (such as informed consent, examination by an Institutional Review Board, and protections for safety and privacy) contained in subpart A of [45CFR4646], or Parts 50 and 56 of 21CFR.[47] In contrast, H.R. 801 requires that all such research shall be conducted in accordance with Part 50 and 56 of 21CFR and does not refer to subpart A of 45CFR46.[48]

S. 303 contains a prohibition on conducting SCNT on fertilized human eggs (oocytes), and states that "unfertilized blastocysts" shall not be maintained after more than 14 days from its first cell division, aside from storage at temperatures less that zero degrees centigrade. S. 303 stipulates that a human egg may not be used in SCNT research unless the egg is donated voluntarily with the informed consent of the woman donating the egg; H.R. 801 contains a similar egg donation and informed consent provision. S. 303 also specifies that human eggs or unfertilized blastocysts may not be acquired, received or otherwise transferred for valuable consideration if the transfer affects interstate commerce. Under S. 303, SCNT may not be conducted in a laboratory in which human eggs are subject to assisted reproductive technology treatments or procedures, such as in vitro fertilization for the treatment of infertility.

Violation of these provisions in S. 303 regarding ethical requirements would result in a civil penalty of not more than $250,000. S. 303 has been referred to the Senate Judiciary Committee.

Supporters of a total ban on human cloning, such as that contained in H.R. 534, argue that a partial ban on human cloning, like the one in H.R. 801 or S. 303, would be impossible to enforce. Critics of the total ban on human cloning argue that SCNT creates a "clump of cells" rather than an embryo, and that the ban would curtail medical research and prevent Americans from receiving life-saving treatments created overseas.

The U.S. Supreme Court has recognized in past cases certain personal rights as being fundamental and protected from government interference.[49] Some legal scholars believe a ban on human cloning may be struck down by the Supreme Court because it would infringe upon the right to make reproductive decisions which is "protected under the constitutional right to privacy and the constitutional right to liberty."[50] Other scholars do not believe that noncoital, asexual reproduction, such as cloning, would be considered a fundamental right by the Supreme Court. A ban on human cloning research may raise other constitutional issues: scientists' right to personal liberty and free speech. In the opinion of some legal scholars, any government limits on the use of cloning in scientific inquiry or human reproduction would have to be "narrowly tailored to further a compelling state interest."[51] However, no case involving these issues is scheduled to come before the Supreme Court this term.

International Actions on Embryonic Stem Cell Research

The international community has taken a variety of action regarding stem cell research. Action by the United Nations, which was considering a restrictive human cloning treaty, is currently on hold until 2005. The European Union (EU) clarified its stem cell rules in November 2003, smoothing the path for EU funding and support for human embryonic stem cell research.[52] Under the terms of its sixth research framework program(FP6), the EU may fund embryonic stem cell research regardless of the date that the stem cells were procured from embryos. A cut-off date, which would have created a restriction similar to the one in the 2001 Bush policy, was under consideration, but was dropped.[53] FP6 allows funding for research on tissue derived from "spontaneous or therapeutic abortion," but not for the creation of human embryos for the purpose of stem cell procurement.[54] FP6 implies but does not state that it will allow funding for research on embryos that remain after IVF, in that it "no longer requir[es] parental consent where embryos have to be destroyed in order to produce embryonic stem cell lines."[55] According to Members of the European Parliament, FP6 funding decisions should depend "both upon the contents of the scientific proposal and the legal framework of the Member States involved."[56]

EU member states are considering a range of legislation on the subject. In Italy, a proposal would prohibit any experiments on human embryos, the production of embryos for research purposes, and any destruction of human embryos. By contrast, a proposal before the Spanish Parliament would allow research using surplus frozen embryos that can no longer be used for reproductive purposes, provided that the consent of the donor is given. Sweden's parliamentary committee on genetic integrity reviewed the country's regulation of stem cell research and proposed that no prohibition relating to the production of fertilized eggs for research be introduced.

Other countries' activities designed to regulate and promote stem cell research have come to the attention of Congress.[57] For example, in March 2004, the Canadian government enacted legislation allowing stem cell and other research to be conducted on donated embryos created but no longer needed for reproductive purposes.[58] Australia permits the use of spare IVF embryos for stem cell research,[59] and its government has reportedly allotted $57.9 million to its National Stem Cell Centre.[60] Singapore, which allows scientists to clone human embryos and keep them alive for up to 14 days to extract the stem cells, is reported to have "research-friendly policies and generous government funding have already helped jump-start the tiny city-state's nascent stem cell sector.... Singapore and the New York-based Juvenile Diabetes Research Foundation International launched a $3 million funding program to support stem cell research [in Singapore],... [and in May 2004, Singapore unveiled] its resort-like Biopolis, created to give biotech researchers and their families a place to live and work."[61] The United Kingdom's Human Fertilisation and Embryology Authority can issue licences permitting research on embryos less than 14 days old as well as cloning for research purposes.[62] The UK "founded a new £16.5 million (USD $30 million) stem cell center in Cambridge this week with a commitment to fundamental research on both human embryonic and adult stem cells as a precursor to studying therapeutic applications."[63] South Korea, the home of the doctor who announced in February 2004 that he had cloned human embryos and extracted stem cells from them, subsequently enacted legislation to regulate and license reproductive cloning.[64]

Ethical Issues

Stem cell research is controversial not because of its goals, but rather because of the means of obtaining some of the cells. Research involving most types of stem cells, such as those derived from adult tissues and umbilical cord blood, is uncontroversial, except when its effectiveness as an alternative to embryonic stem cells is debated. The crux of the debate centers around embryonic stem cells, which enable research that may facilitate the development of medical treatments and cures, but which require the destruction of an embryo to derive. In addition, because cloning is one method of producing embryos for research, the ethical issues surrounding cloning are also relevant.

As previously mentioned, the Bush Administration, a group of Representatives, a group of Senators, and a group of Nobel Laureates have each presented their respective positions on embryonic stem cell research. In addition, various other organizations, individuals, and councils have issued opinions and reports on the topic. Some groups, such as the Christian Legal Society,[65] Focus on the Family,[66] and the Christian Coalition,[67] support the 2001 Bush policy. Others, such as the National Academies,[68] the Coalition for the Advancement of Medical Research (CAMR),[69] former First Lady Nancy Reagan,[70] and former Presidents Gerald Ford, Jimmy Carter, Bill Clinton[71] favor more embryonic stem cell research than the Bush policy allows. Still others, such as the National Right to Life Committee[72] and the United States Conference of Catholic Bishops,[73] oppose all embryonic stem cell research.

Two presidential bioethics advisory panels have considered the issues involved in embryonic stem cell research. The President's Council on Bioethics (President's Council)[74] published one report directly on the topic, *Monitoring Stem Cell Research*,[75] in which it sought to characterize the issues. While the Council made no recommendations there, in two other reports it has recommended that "Congress should... [p]rohibit the use of human embryos in research beyond a designated stage in their development (between 10 and 14 days after fertilization),"[76] and unanimously recommended "a ban on cloning-to-produce-children," with a 10-member majority also favoring "a four-year moratorium on cloning-for-biomedical-research," and a seven-member minority favoring "regulation of the use of cloned embryos for biomedical research."[77] A predecessor to the President's Council, the National Bioethics Advisory Committee (NBAC),[78] recommended federal funding for stem cell research using "embryos remaining after infertility treatments," but not for the "derivation or use of embryos... made for research purposes."[79]

Detailed review of the assorted reports and statements reveals that, while positions on embryonic stem cell research may be broadly categorized as *for* or *against*, there is an array of finer distinctions present. These finer distinctions in turn reveal the variation in ethical and moral as well as factual beliefs. The following discussion breaks down the arguments about embryonic stem cell research according to these finer distinctions, demonstrating both the complexity of the issues and the points of resonance among the groups.

Embryo Destruction and Relief of Human Suffering. Most positions on embryonic stem cell research rest at least in part on the relative moral weight accorded to embryos and that accorded to the prospect of saving, prolonging, or improving others' lives. For some, the inquiry begins and ends with this question. For instance, one opponent of the research, the American Life League, posits that "human life begins at conception / fertilization and that there is never an acceptable reason for intentionally taking an innocent human life."[80] Similarly, the United States Conference of Catholic Bishops states that the research is immoral because it "relies on the destruction of some defenseless human beings for the possible benefit to others."[81]

Some groups explore the moral standing of human embryos, and also consider the "duty to relieve the pain and suffering of others."[82] Others take the position that embryos do not have the same moral status as persons. They acknowledge that embryos are genetically human, but hold that they do not have the same moral relevance because they lack specific capacities, including consciousness, reasoning and sentience.[83] They conclude that performing research to benefit persons justifies the destruction of embryos. Acceptance of the notion that the destruction of embryos can be justified in some circumstances forms the basis of pro-stem cell research opinions, and is usually modified with some combination of the distinctions and limitations that follow.

Viability of Embryos. Some proponents of embryonic stem cell research draw distinctions based upon whether an embryo is viable. The idea behind this distinction is that it is morally preferable for embryos that will not grow or develop beyond a certain stage and/or those that would otherwise be discarded to be used for the purpose of alleviating human suffering. This distinction has led some, though not all, pro-life advocates to support embryonic stem cell research that does not destroy embryos that are viable, meaning pre-implantation embryos, those created via cloning that are incapable of full development, or those without a woman willing to carry them to term.

Most supporters of some type of embryonic stem cell research touch on the question of viability. The 2001 Bush policy requires, among other things, use of only excess (non-viable) embryos for federally-funded research. One report of the President's Council explores the moral significance of viability that is based upon "human choices" rather than an embryo's "own intrinsic nature," but draws no conclusions.[84] A second report broaches the subject of viability, recommending that Congress ban both the transfer of a human embryo to a woman's uterus for any purpose other than to produce a live-born child, and also research conducted on embryos more than 10 to 14 days after fertilization.[85] The NBAC report touches on the moral status of embryos in utero and those in vitro,[86] though NBAC does not specify whether viability was a key rationale for its recommendations. A group of Representatives, a group of Senators,[87] and CAMR imply but do not state a distinction based on viability by expressly calling for the use of "excess" embryos developed for IVF, and making no mention of those in utero.[88] By contrast, the National Academies and the group of Nobel Laureates more broadly support research on embryos, making no mention of viability.

Purpose of Embryo Creation. A separate distinction that often leads to the same conclusions as viability is the purpose for which embryos are created. This distinction draws an ethical line based upon the intent of the people creating embryos. In the view of some, it is permissible to create an embryo for reproductive purposes (such as IVF), but impermissible to create one with the intention of destroying it for research.

Most groups at least note the potential ethical significance of reproductive versus research motives for creating embryos. The 2001 Bush policy draws a motive distinction by including a requirement that federally funded research be conducted only on embryonic stem cell lines derived from embryos created solely for reproductive purposes. NBAC draws the same distinction by recommending that federal funding be used for embryos remaining after infertility treatment but not for research involving the derivation or use of stem cells from embryos made for research purposes or from embryos made using cloning (SCNT).[89] The President's Council recommends that Congress ban attempts at conception by any means other than the union of egg and sperm (essentially banning cloning via SCNT), but does not specify whether embryos might be created in vitro specifically for research purposes.[90] A group of Representatives, a group of Senators, and CAMR imply but do not state that embryos should not be created for research purposes. They overtly call for the use of "excess" embryos developed for IVF, and make no mention of embryos created expressly for research.[91] By contrast, the National Academies supports the creation of embryos for research purposes, including via cloning (SCNT), to "ensure that stem cell-based therapies can be broadly applied for many conditions and people [by] overcoming the problem of tissue rejection."[92] Mrs. Nancy Reagan, her supporters, and the group of Nobel Laureates also take this position.

New and Existing Cell Lines. A further distinction has been drawn based upon the timing of the creation of embryonic stem cell lines. Here, the premise is that it is unacceptable to induce the destruction of embryos for the creation of new lines. However, in cases in which embryos have already been destroyed and the lines already exist, it is morally preferable to use those lines for research to improve the human condition.

This was one central distinction drawn in the 2001 Bush policy, which limited the use of federal funding to research on lines derived on or before the date of the policy. Supporters of the Bush policy on both sides of the issue favor this distinction as a compromise. It allows research on some embryonic stem cell lines. It deters the future destruction of embryos for research. The President's Council writes that the Bush policy mixes "prudence" with "principle, in the hope that the two might reinforce (rather than undermine) each other."[93] The Council notes that the policy is supported by what it titles a *moralist's* notion of when one may benefit from prior bad acts (referring to embryo destruction): it prevents the government from complying in the commission of or encouraging the act in the future, and it reaffirms the principle that the act was wrong.[94] The same report also contains analyses of the Bush policy that characterize distinction between new and existing cell lines as "arbitrary," "unsustainable," and "inconsistent."[95] The Council itself takes no position in the report on this or any other issue.

Opponents of the Bush policy on both sides of the issue view the distinction between new and existing stem cell lines with reproach. One side, which includes The National Right to Life Committee and the United States Conference of Catholic Bishops, objects because the distinction validates destruction of embryos, and in fact rewards those who did so first with a monopoly. The other side, which includes the National Academies, a group of Representatives, a group of Senators, Nancy Reagan and her supporters, Gerald Ford, CAMR, and the group of Nobel Laureates, objects because the distinction limits the number of embryonic stem cell lines available for research, particularly since the number of authorized lines are dwindling and are "contaminated with mouse feeder cells."[96] Likewise, though NBAC recognized the distinction between destroying embryos and using ones previously destroyed (e.g., "derivation of [embryonic stem] cells involves destroying the embryos, whereas abortion precedes the donation of fetal tissue and death precedes the donation of whole organs for trans-plantation"[97]), it still recommended future development of embryonic stem cell lines.

Consent of Donors. There is consensus throughout a wide array of viewpoints about embryonic stem cell research that embryos should only be obtained for research with the consent of their biological donors. This consent requirement necessitates that embryos be taken only with donors' knowledge, understanding, and uncoerced agreement. The donor consent requirement is consistent with the rules governing human beings' participation in research, and with individuals' general legal authority to make decisions regarding embryos they procreate. A drawback of the requirement is that it may restrict the number of embryos available for research purposes.

The 2001 Bush policy contains a donor consent requirement. It limits approved stem cell lines to those derived with the informed consent of the donors, and obtained without any financial inducements to the donors. The NBAC and the President's Council also favor donor consent requirements. The National Academies notes the importance of informed consent in its discussion of stem cell research oversight requirements.[98] A group of Representatives and a group of Senators mention and imply their support for donor consent requirements.[99]

Effectiveness of Alternatives. One factual distinction that has been used to support competing ethical viewpoints is the efficacy of alternatives to embryonic stem cell research. The promise of stem cell therapies derived from adult tissue and umbilical cord blood have buttressed opposition to embryonic stem cell research. These opponents argue that therapies and cures can be developed without the morally undesirable destruction of embryos. However, not all scientists agree that adult stem cells hold as much potential as embryonic stem cells. Most supporters of embryonic stem cell research believe that it is the quickest and, perhaps in some cases, the only path that will yield results. Supporters also stress that embryonic and other stem cell research should be conducted collaboratively, so that they can inform one another.

Findings regarding the effectiveness of alternatives to embryonic stem cell research are mixed. The President's Council notes that there is a "debate about the relative merits of embryonic stem cells and adult stem cells."[100] Focus on the Family cites promising non-embryonic stem cell research: "adult stem cells may be as "flexible" as embryonic ones and equally capable of converting into various cell types for healing the body."[101] By contrast, the National Academies finds that the "best available scientific and medical evidence indicates that research on both embryonic and adult human stem cells will be needed."[102] NBAC finds in its deliberations that "the claim that there are alternatives to using stem cells derived from embryos is not, at the present time, supported scientifically."[103] CAMR supports both embryonic and adult stem cell research, and adds that "many scientists believe and studies show that embryonic stem cells will likely be more effective in curing diseases because they can grow and differentiate into any of the body's cells and tissues and thus into different organs."[104] Mrs. Nancy Reagan and her supporters favor expedient approaches including embryonic stem cell research.[105]

Use of Federal Funding. Some division over the support for and opposition to embryonic stem cell research focuses on the question of whether the use of federal funding is appropriate. Those who oppose federal funding argue that the government should not be associated with embryo destruction.[106] They point out that embryo destruction violates the “deeply held moral beliefs of some citizens,” and suggest that “funding alternative research is morally preferable.”[107] Proponents of federal funding argue that it is immoral to discourage life-saving research by withholding federal funding. They point out that consensus support is not required for many federal spending policies, as it “does not violate democratic principles or infringe on the rights of dissent of those in the minority.”[108] They argue that the efforts of both federally supported and privately supported researchers are necessary to keep the United States at the forefront of what they believe is a very important, cutting edge area of science. Furthermore, supporters believe that the oversight that comes with federal dollars will result in better and more ethically controlled research in the field.

Groups’ positions on federal funding tend to mirror their positions on stem cell research generally. The Bush policy authorizes federal funding for some embryonic stem cell research. The President’s Council does not take a position on the issue, but notes the pros and cons, and stresses that there is a “difference between *prohibiting* embryo research and *refraining from funding* it.”[109] Focus on the Family generally supports the President Bush and his policy, but is “disappointed by his decision to allow federal funding of research on the existing stem cell lines.”[110] NBAC finds the arguments in favor of federal funding more persuasive than those against it.[111] The National Academies, a group of Representatives, a group of Senators, Mrs. Nancy Reagan and her supporters, CAMR, and the Nobel Laureates favor federal funding for embryonic stem cell research.[112]

References

[1] The IVF embryos were originally created for the treatment of infertility. Excess embryos are often frozen in liquid nitrogen for future use. A couple may elect to discard their excess embryos, donate the embryos for research, or allow another couple to adopt an embryo.

[2] Scientists and physicians use the term embryo for the first eight weeks after fertilization, and fetus for the ninth week through birth. In contrast, the Department of Health and Human Services (HHS) regulations define fetus as “the product of conception from the time of implantation.” (45 CFR 46.203)

[3] A somatic cell is a body cell. In contrast, a germ cell is an egg or sperm cell.

[4] Dolly was euthanized in Feb. 2003 after developing a lung infection. Some claim her death at six years was related to being a clone, but her ailment may also have occurred because she was raised indoors (for security reasons) rather than as a pastured sheep, which often live to 12 years of age. G. Kolata, “First Mammal Clone Dies,” *New York Times*, Feb. 15, 2003, p. A4.

[5] For further information, see CRS Report RL31358, *Human Cloning*, by Judith A. Johnson.

[6] However, federal funds have been provided for research on both human and animal adult stem cells and animal embryonic stem cells.

[7] The rider language has not changed significantly from year to year. The original rider can be found in Section 128 of P.L. 104-99; it affected NIH funding for FY1996 contained in P.L. 104-91. For subsequent fiscal years, the rider is found in Title V, General Provisions, of the Labor, HHS and Education appropriations acts in the following public laws: FY1997, P.L. 104-208; FY1998, P.L. 105-78; FY1999, P.L. 105-277; FY2000, P.L. 106-113; FY2001, P.L. 106-554; FY2002, P.L. 107-116, and FY2003, P.L. 108-7.

[8] According to media sources, as of Apr. 2001 only three grant applications had been submitted to NIH, and one was subsequently withdrawn. (*Washington FAX*, Apr. 19, 2001.) Presumably, scientists were reluctant to invest the time and effort into preparing the necessary paperwork for the NIH grant application process when the prospects of receiving federal funding were uncertain under the new Bush Administration. (P. Recer, "Stem Cell Studies said Hurt by Doubt." *AP Online*, May 2, 2001.) In a related development, one of the leading U.S. researchers on stem cells, Roger Pederson of the University of California, San Francisco, decided to move his laboratory to the United Kingdom for "the possibility of carrying out my research with human embryonic stem cells with public support." (Aaron Zitner, "Uncertainty Is Thwarting Stem Cell Researchers." *Los Angeles Times*, July 16, 2001, pp. A1, A8.) Human embryonic stem cell research was approved overwhelmingly by the House of Commons in Dec. 2000 and the House of Lords in Jan. 2001.

[9] Rick Weiss, "Bush Administration Order Halts Stem Cell Meeting; NIH Planned Session To Review Fund Requests." *The Washington Post*, Apr. 21, 2001, p. A2.

[10] ibid.

[11] National Institutes of Health, Department of Health and Human Services. *Stem Cells: Scientific Progress and Future Research Directions*, June 2001. The NIH scientific report can be found at [*http://stemcells.nih.gov/info/scireport/*]

[12] The Aug. 9, 2001, *Remarks by the President on Stem Cell Research* can be found at [*http://www.whitehouse.gov/news/releases/2001/08/20010809-2.html*].

[13] The White House, *Fact Sheet on Embryonic Stem Cell Research,* Aug. 9, 2001, found at [*http://www.whitehouse.gov/news/releases/2001/08/20010809-1.html*].

[14] Xenotransplantation Action Plan: FDA approach to the regulation of xenotr-ansplantation. Available at [*http://www.fda.gov/cber/xap/xap.htm*].

[15] These documents are available at [*http://www.fda.gov/cber/xap/xap.htm*].

[16] National Institutes of Health, Department of Health and Human Services, *Stem Cells: Scientific Progress and Future Research Directions*, June 2001, pp. 95-96.

[17] See [*http://stemcells.nih.gov/research/funding/*].

[18] Information about the NIH Human Embryonic Stem Cell Registry is available at [*http://stemcells.nih.gov/research/registry/index.asp*].

[19] Farhad Manjoo, "Thou Shalt Not Make Scientific Progress," *Salon.com*, Mar. 25, 2004, [*http://www.salon.com/tech/feature/ 2004/03/25/stem_cells/index_np.html*].

[20] Gareth Cook, "Clinic in U.S. Isolates 50 Lines of Stem Cells," *Boston Globe*, June 9, 2004, p. A1.

[21] The six diseases are beta thalassemia, neurofibromatosis type 1, Marfan's syndrome, myotonic dystrophy, fragile X syndrome, and Fanconi's anemia.

[22] Rick Weiss and Justin Gillis, "New Embryonic Stem Cells Made Available," *The Washington Post*, Mar. 4, 2004, p. A2.

[23] For further information, see the Stanford University Medical Center website at [*http://mednews.stanford.edu/stemcellQA.html*].

[24] UCSF News Office, *UCSF Names First Director of its Stem Cell Biology Program*, Apr. 26, 2004. See [*http://pub.ucsf.edu/newsservices/releases/200404261/*].

[25] Gareth Cook, "94 New Cell Lines Created Abroad Since Bush Decision," *Boston Globe*, May 23, 2004, p. A14.

[26] For further information on the UK Stem Cell Bank, see [*http://www.nibsc.ac.uk/divisions/ cbi/stemcell.html*].

[27] See [*http://www.house.gov/degette/news/releases/040428.pdf*].

[28] A survey conducted in 2002 and published in 2003 by the Society for Assisted Reproductive Technology and RAND determined that nearly 400,000 frozen embryos are stored in the United States, but most are currently target for patient use. See David I. Hoffman et al., "Cryopreserved Embryos in the United States and Their Availability for Research," *Fertility and Sterility*, v. 79, May 2003, p. 1063-1069.

[29] Rick Weiss, "Bush's Stem Cell Policy Reiterated, but Some See Shift," *The Washington Post*, May 16, 2004, p. A18.

[30] Letter from Elias A. Zerhouni, Director, National Institutes of Health, to The Honorable Diana DeGette and The Honorable Michael Castle, May 14, 2004.

[31] See [*http://feinstein.senate.gov/04Releases/r-stemcell-ltr.pdf*].

[32] Andrew J. Hawkins, "NIH Stem Cell Bank, Centers of Excellence Will Fast-Track Translational Research, Says Thompson," *Washington FAX*, July 15, 2004.

[33] ibid.

[34] ibid.

[35] ibid.

[36] New Hampshire Safety and Welfare statutes (Title VXII §168-B: 16 (I, II) prohibit "noncryo-preserved" embryos from being maintained for more than 14 days post-fertilization, and prohibit embryos "donated for use in research" from being "transferred to a uterine cavity."

[37] HB 2647 (2004); 12-1770a (Supp) (2004). It is unclear whether the 2001 Bush stem cell policy would be interpreted to be a "law" for purposes of Kansas' HB 2647. If so, Kansas' funding of stem cell research would be limited to those lines approved for federal funding under the Bush policy.

[38] John T. Softcheck, "Massachusetts Measure Would Permit Use of State Funds for Stem Cell Research," *The Washington Fax*, Dec. 11, 2002; "U.S. States Making Stem Cell Policies," *Bionews*, no. 258, May 5, 2004.

[39] *Stem Cell Research, Funding, Bonds, Initiative Constitutional Amendment and Statute, 1021*,(SA03RF0055, Amdt. #1-NS), at [*http://www.ss.ca.gov/elections/elections_j.htm #2004General*].

[40] "U.S. States Making Stem Cell Policies," *Bionews*, no. 258, May 5, 2004.

[41] Barbara Mantel, "Analysis: New Jersey Is First State to Fund Research on Stem Cell,"*NPR: All Things Considered*, June 25, 2004.

[42] ibid.

[43] "Virginia law does not expressly prohibit research on cloned embryos, but it is forbidden to possess the product of human cloning. Under the state human cloning

statute human cloning is defined as the creation of or attempt to create a human being by transferring the nucleus from a human cell from whatever source into an oocyte from which the nucleus has been removed. Human being is not defined as to whether it includes neonates, embryos or fetuses only." Alissa Johnson, "State Embryonic and Fetal Research Laws," *National Council of State Legislatures*, Jan.27, 2004, at [*http://www.ncsl.org/programs/health/ genetics/embfet.htm#b*], visited May 17, 2004.

[44] By seeking to amend Title 18 of the U.S. Code rather than the Public Health Service Act, S. 245 would likely be subject to different committee jurisdiction.

[45] ibid.

[46] This provision specifies protections due to human beings who participate in research conducted or supported by HHS and many other departments.

[47] This provision specifies protections due to human beings who participate in research involved in testing a drug or medical device for FDA approval.

[48] Often referred to as the Common Rule, 45CFR46, Subpart A, "applies to all research involving human subjects conducted, supported or otherwise subject to regulation by any federal department or agency which takes appropriate administrative action to make this policy applicable to such research." The Common Rule covers 18 federal agencies by force of law or Executive Order. FDA has regulatory authority over research on the products the agency regulates (food, drugs, medical devices) and applies its own set of regulations on the protection of human subjects, 21CFR 50 and 56, that are generally but not entirely the same as subpart A of 45CFR46. For further information, see National Bioethics Advisory Commission, *Ethical and Policy Issues in Research Involving Human Participants*, Appendix C: The Current Oversight System: History and Description, Aug. 2001.

[49] For further discussion of these issues and their relationship to human cloning, see CRS Report RL31422, *Substantive Due Process and a Right to Clone*, by Jon O. Shimabukuro.

[50] L.B. Andrews, "Is There a Right to Clone? Constitutional Challenges to Bans on Human Cloning," *Harvard Journal of Law and Technology*, summer 1998, pp. 643-680.

[51] ibid., p. 667.

[52] Committee on Industry, External Trade, Research and Energy, "Integrating and Strengthening the European Research Area" (2002-2006) (COM(2003) 390 —C5-0349/2003 — 2003/0151(CNS)) European Parliament, (A5-0369/2003) (Nov. 4, 2003).

[53] John T. Softcheck, "European Union Moves Close to Funding Stem Cell Research with Two Parliament Votes," *Washington Fax*, Nov. 10, 2003.

[54] ibid.

[55] "Sixth Framework Programme," *Bulletin EU 11-2003, Research and technology (8/10)*, Nov. 26, 2003, at [*http://europa.eu.int/abc/doc/off/bull/en/200311/p103069.htm*].

[56] John T. Softcheck, "European Union Moves Close to Funding Stem Cell Research with Two Parliament Votes," *Washington Fax*, Nov. 10, 2003.

[57] *See, e.g.,* Letter from 58 Senators to President George W. Bush, June 4, 2004; Letter from 206 Members of the House of Representatives to President George W. Bush, Apr. 28, 2004.

[58] Assisted Human Reproduction Act (Canadian Bill No. C-6, 2004), LS-466E.

[59] Research Involving Human Embryos Act, No. 145, 2002.

[60] "The National Stem Cell Centre," *Commonwealth of Australia's Department of Education, Science and Training*, Jun. 2, 2004, at [*http://backingaus.innovation.gov.au/2004/commercial/stem_cell.htm*], visited July 15, 2004.

[61] "Singapore Hosts Stem Cell Meeting" *MSNBC*, May 19, 2004, at the MSNBC website [*http://msnbc.msn.com/id/3341644/*], visited July 15, 2004.

[62] Human Fertilisation and Embryology (Research Purposes) Regulations 2001, S1 2001 No.188.

[63] Philip Hunter, "UK to Open Stem Cell Center," *The Scientist*, June 22, 2004 at [*http://www.biomedcentral.com/news/20040622/04*], visited July 15, 2004.

[64] "Stem Cells Extracted from Human Clone," *MSNBC*, Feb. 12, 2004, at [*http://www.msnbc.msn.com/id/4244988/*], visited July 12, 2004; Dr. Hwuang, the South Korean scientist referenced herein, stated on July 13, 2004 that he is still awaiting his license from the South Korean Government to continue his cloning and stem cell research. Dr. Wu-Suk Hwuang, *Press conference on stem cell research*, Gijon, Spain, July 13, 2004, 10:30 AM.

[65] The Christian Legal Society is a "national grassroots network of lawyers and law students, committed to... advocating biblical conflict reconciliation, public justice, religious freedom and the sanctity of human life." [*http://www.clsnet.org/ clsPages/vision.php*].

[66] *Focus on the Family* was founded in 1977 by Dr. James Dobson to promote teachings of Jesus Christ. [*http://www.family.org*].

[67] The Christian Coalition is "the largest and most active conservative grassroots political organization in America," [*http://www.cc.org*].

[68] The National Academies brings together "committees of experts in all areas of scientific and technological endeavor" as "advisors to the Nation." For statements on embryonic stem cell research and cloning, see National Research Council, Institute of Medicine, National Academies, *Stem Cells and the Future of Regenerative Medicine* (Washington: National Academies, 2001); Committee on Science, Engineering and Public Policy and Global Affairs Division et al., *Scientific and Medical Aspects of Human Reproductive Cloning,*(Washington National Academy Press, 2002) at [*http://www.nationalacademies.org/ about/#org*].

[69] CAMR is a nonprofit organization comprised of patient organizations, universities, scientific societies, foundations, and individuals with life-threatening illnesses and disorders, [*http://www.camradvocacy.org/ fastaction/*]. For a statement on embryonic stem cell research, see Coalition for the Advancement of Medical Research, "Embryonic Stem Cell Research," talking points [*http://www.camradvocacy.org/fastaction/news.asp?id=167*], visited May 14, 2004.

[70] "Nancy Reagan Urges Stem Cell Research," *MSNBC*, May 9, 2004, at [*http://www.msnbc. msn.com/id/4937850/*], visited May 14, 2004.

[71] ibid.

[72] The National Right to Life Committee was founded in 1973 to "restore legal protection to innocent human life," at [*http://www.nrlc.org/Missionstatement.htm*].

[73] The United States Conference of Catholic Bishops is "is an assembly of the hierarchy of the United States and the U.S. Virgin Islands who jointly exercise certain pastoral functions on behalf of the Christian faithful of the United States," at [*http://www.nccbuscc.org/ whoweare.htm*].

[74] The *President's Council* was created by President Bush in Nov. 2001 to "advise the President on bioethical issues that may emerge as a consequence of advances in biomedical science and technology." George W. Bush, "Creation of The President's Council on Bioethics," *Executive Order 13237*, Nov. 28, 2001, at [*http://www.bioethics.gov/reports/ executive.html*].

[75] The President's Council on Bioethics, *Monitoring Stem Cell Research*, Jan. 2004.

[76] The President's Council on Bioethics, Reproduction and Responsibility, Mar. 2004, p.xlviii.

[77] President's Council on Bioethics, Human Cloning and Human Dignity, July 2002, pp. xxxv- xxxviii). Note: At the June 20, 2002, meeting, nine of 17 Council members voted to support cloning for medical research purposes, without a moratorium, provided a regulatory mechanism was established. Because one member of the Council had not attended the meetings and was not voting, the vote seemed to be nine to eight in favor of research cloning. However, draft versions of the Council report sent to Council members on June 28, 2002, indicated that two of the group of nine members had changed their votes in favor of a moratorium. Both made it clear that they have no ethical problem with cloning for biomedical research, but felt that a moratorium would provide time for additional discussion. The changed vote took many Council members by surprise, and some on the Council believe that the moratorium option, as opposed to a ban, was thrown in at the last minute and did not receive adequate discussion. In addition, some on the Council believe that the widely reported final vote of 10 to 7 in favor of a moratorium does not accurately reflect the fact "that the majority of the council has no problem with the ethics of biomedical cloning." (Transcripts of the Council meetings and papers developed by staff for discussion during Council meetings can be found at [*http://www.bioethics.gov*]; S.S. Hall, "President's Bioethics Council Delivers," Science, v. 297, July 19, 2002, pp. 322-324.) "Wise Words from Across the Pond?," BioNews, no. 252, Mar. 29, 2004.

[78] In 1995, President Clinton created the National Bioethics Advisory Commission by Executive Order, to advise him on bioethical issues. The Order expired in 2001. "Former Bioethics Commissions," *President's Commission on Bioethics* website, at [*http://www. bioethics.gov/reports/past_commissions/index.html*], visited Jun. 30, 2004.

[79] National Bioethics Advisory Commission, *Ethical Issues in Human Stem Cell Research*, vol. 1, Sept. 1999, pp. 70-71.

[80] American Life League, *Analysis of George W. Bush's Stem Cell Decision*, 2001, at [*http://www.all.org/issues/scanalyz.htm*] visited May 11, 2004.

[81] Office of Communications, United States Conference of Catholic Bishops, *Catholic Bishops Criticize Bush Policy on Embryo Research*,(Aug. 9, 2001) at [*http://www.usccb. org/comm/archives/ 2001/01-142.htm*] accessed May 11, 2004.

[82] The President's Council on Bioethics, *Monitoring Stem Cell Research*, Jan. 2004, pp.58,62.

[83] Presentation by B. Steinbock, Dept. Of Philosophy, SUNY, Albany, NY, NIH Human Embryo Research Panel Meeting, Feb. 3, 1994.

[84] The President's Council on Bioethics, *Monitoring Stem Cell Research*, Jan. 2004, p. 87.

[85] The President's Council on Bioethics, *Reproduction and Responsibility*, Mar. 2004.

[86] National Bioethics Advisory Commission, *Ethical Issues in Human Stem Cell Research, vol. 1,* Sept. 1999, p. 50.

[87] Letter from 58 Senators to President George W. Bush, June 4, 2004. (Hereafter cited as Letter from 58 Senators.)
[88] Letter from 206 Members of the House of Representatives to President George W. Bush, Apr. 28, 2004. (Hereafter cited as Letter from 206 Members of the House of Representatives.)
[89] National Bioethics Advisory Commission, *Ethical Issues in Human Stem Cell Research*, vol. 1, Sept. 1999, pp. 70-72.
[90] The President's Council on Bioethics, *Reproduction and Responsibility,* Mar. 2004, p. xlviii.
[91] Letter from 206 Members of the House of Representatives; Letter from 58 Senators.
[92] National Research Council, Institute of Medicine, National Academies, *Stem Cells and the Future of Regenerative Medicine* (Washington: National Academies, 2001), p. 58.
[93] The President's Council on Bioethics, *Monitoring Stem Cell Research*, Jan. 2004, pp. 33-34.
[94] ibid.
[95] The President's Council on Bioethics, *Monitoring Stem Cell Research*, Jan. 2004, pp. 63-67.
[96] Letter from 206 Members of the House of Representatives; Letter from 58 Senators.
[97] National Bioethics Advisory Commission, *Ethical Issues in Human Stem Cell Research*, vol. 1, Sept. 1999, p. 49.
[98] National Research Council, Institute of Medicine, National Academies, *Stem Cells and the Future of Regenerative Medicine* (Washington: National Academies, 2001), p. 53.
[99] Letter from 206 Members of the House of Representatives; Letter from 58 Senators.
[100] The President's Council on Bioethics, *Monitoring Stem Cell Research*, Jan. 2004, p. 10.
[101] Carrie Gordon Earll, "Talking Points on Stem Cell Research," *Focus on the Family*, Sept. 17, 2003 at [*http://www.family.org/cforum/fosi/bioethics/faqs/a0027980.cfm*], visited May 14, 2003.
[102] National Research Council, Institute of Medicine, National Academies, *Stem Cells and the Future of Regenerative Medicine* (Washington: National Academies, 2001), p. 56.
[103] National Bioethics Advisory Commission, *Ethical Issues in Human Stem Cell Research*, vol. 1, Sept. 1999, p. 53.
[104] Coalition for the Advancement of Medical Research, "Embryonic Stem Cell Research," talking points [*http://www.camradvocacy.org/ fastaction/news.asp?id=167*], visited May 14, 2004.
[105] "Nancy Reagan Urges Stem Cell Research," *MSNBC*, May 9, 2004, at [*http://www.msnbc.msn.com/id/4937850/*], accessed May 14, 2004.
[106] National Bioethics Advisory Commission, *Ethical Issues in Human Stem Cell Research*, vol. 1, Sept. 1999, p. 57.
[107] ibid.
[108] ibid.
[109] The President's Council on Bioethics, *Monitoring Stem Cell Research*, Jan. 2004, p. 37.
[110] Carrie Gordon Earll, "Talking Points on Stem Cell Research," *Focus on the Family*, Sept. 17, 2003 at [*http://www.family.org/cforum/fosi/ bioethics/faqs/a0027980.cfm*], visited May 14, 2003.

[111] National Bioethics Advisory Commission, *Ethical Issues in Human Stem Cell Research*, vol. 1, Sept. 1999, p. 70.

[112] See e.g., National Research Council, Institute of Medicine, National Academies, *Stem Cells and the Future of Regenerative Medicine* (Washington: National Academies, 2001), p. 49.

In: Perspectives in Stem Cell Research ISBN: 978-1-61122-985-1
Editors: Brenda M. Davis and Christopher B. Halton

Chapter II

CANCER STEM CELLS

Saranya Chumsri[1] and Angelika M. Burger[1, 2]
[1] Marlene and Stewart Greenebaum Cancer Center
[2]Department of Pharmacology and Experimental Therapeutics,
University of Maryland, School of Medicine, Baltimore, Maryland, USA

ABSTRACT

Emerging evidence suggests that cancers contain a rare and biologically distinct subpopulation of cells with the ability to self-renew and to sustain tumor growth, termed "cancer stem cells". Cancer stem cells share many characteristics with normal stem cells including self-renewal, asymmetric division, indefinite proliferative capacity, and self-protection mechanisms. The cancer stem cell concept is best understood in hematologic malignancies. In solid tumors, breast cancer stem cells have been the most explored. Several techniques have been described, allowing the identification or isolation of cancer stem cells by either expression of specific cell surface markers, their differential ability to efflux dyes, or by a distinct enzymatic activity. More recent studies also established the crucial role of cancer stem cells in multistage cancer progression and metastasis which has important implications for the design of novel targeted therapies. Since most of the conventional chemotherapies only affect differentiated cancer cells, initial reduction in tumor mass is often followed by a rapid relapse. In order to achieve durable remissions, it will be imperative to eradicate cancer stem cells.

INTRODUCTION

Cancer is the third leading cause of death worldwide and only preceded by cardiovascular disease and infection [1]. Despite improvements of existing and the development of novel treatment modalities, the majority of cancer patients still have a poor prognosis. Although chemotherapy and/or radiation can induce initial tumor shrinkage, a high proportion of cancer patients will inevitably relapse and ultimately die of their disease. It was not until recently that advances in molecular biology and embryonic stem cell research have shed more light on the biology of cancer recurrence. There is emerging evidence that a rare and biologically distinct population of cancer cells exists that has exclusive self-renewal ability and limitless proliferative capacity. These characteristics are analogous to those of normal stem cells and hence this population was termed "cancer stem cells". Most conventional chemotherapies affect differentiated cancer cells that make up the bulk of a tumor, but are often ineffective against cancer stem cells [2,3]. Thus, a critical challenge in anti-cancer drug development is to target and eradicate cancer stem cells together with the bulk tumor mass. In this chapter, we will review the discovery of cancer stem cells, the available evidence of their origin, and novel strategies to target cancer stem cells [4].

STEM CELLS

While the concept of a stem cell has been proposed since the early 1900s, stem cells were actually identified in the early 1960's by two Canadian scientists, Ernest A. McCulloch and James E. Till. They pioneered the field by injecting bone marrow cells into sub-lethally irradiated mice and noticed that visible nodules formed in the spleens. These nodules were described as "spleen colonies". Initially, they postulated that each nodule arose from a single marrow cell and perhaps a stem cell. Subsequently, they were able to demonstrate that each nodule did indeed arise from a single cell [5,6]. This work illustrated the fundamental characteristics of stem cells, namely their ability to self-renew and to differentiate into multiple lineages [7].

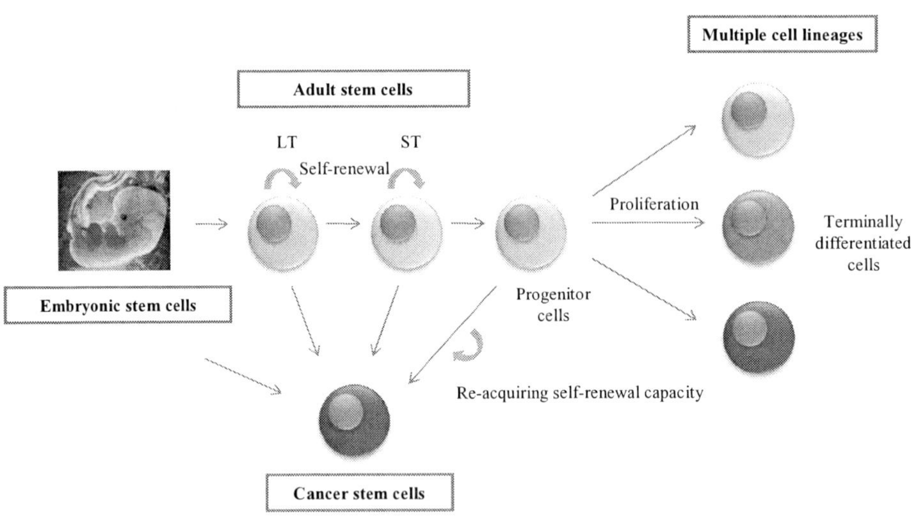

Figure 1. The origin of cancer stem cells. Embryonic stem cells (ES) are pleuripotent and capable of recapitulating multiple lineages of adult stem cells. Long-term repopulating stem cells (LT) are slowly cycling and long-lasting through the life span. Short-term repopulating stem cells (ST) mobilize out of the niches and become more rapidly cycling. ST can give rise to progenitor cells that actively proliferate. Unlike LT and ST, progenitor cells have lost self-renewal capacity and are only able to produce terminally differentiated cells. Recent evidence suggests that cancer stem cells may derive from either ES, LT, ST or progenitor cells that re-acquire self-renewal capacity.

Self-renewal is a unique characteristic of stem cells and is distinct from proliferation (Figure 1). Unlike progenitor cells which have extensive proliferative capacity, stem cells are mostly quiescent (long term stem cells). Owing to their self-renewal gene signature, stem cells can produce the identical daughter cells that preserve stem cell properties [8]. Moreover, stem cells are capable of dividing asymmetrically and possess an axis of polarity.

Polarity is the unequal spatial distribution of cellular constituents. For example, there are two types of polarity in simple epithelia: planar cell polarity and apicobasal polarity. After asymmetric division, one daughter cell will retain stem cell characteristics and the other daughter cell will become a committed progenitor which will give rise to differentiated cells. There is evidence that disruption of the process of asymmetric cell division and loss of polarity induces a cancer-like state in neuronal stem cells [9,10].

Cancer Stem Cells

The stochastic model of cell division assumes that cancer cells are homogenous and that each cancer cell can give rise to the entire tumor. However, recent studies have provided strong evidence that cancer cells are in fact heterogeneous and exhibit a hierarchical arrangement similar to their normal counterparts, and that only a rare and biologically distinct subset of cancer cells is capable of recapitulation of the entire tumor [7,9]. Prior to the molecular definition of cancer stem cells, experiments in the 1960s [11] have shown that only a small fraction (0.77%) of murine lymphoma cells was able to form colonies in the spleens of mice and that 1 in 10,000 mouse myeloma cells was capable of forming colonies in clonal *in vitro* colony-forming assays [10,12]. It was further proposed that for successful control of tumor growth, these tumor stem cells must be eradicated. In absence of means to isolate and classify cancer stem cells, it still remained possible that all cells have clonogenic capacity, but that they are unable to proliferate under the assay conditions used. In order to demonstrate that cancer cells are in fact heterogeneous and that only a distinct subset of cells has clonogenic capacity, it was essential to separate the different populations and define one subset of cancer cells that has extensive proliferating capacity. This was accomplished in 1997, when it was demonstrated that only cells with a $CD34^+/CD38^-$ phenotype were able to initiate human acute myelogenous leukemia in non-obese diabetic/severe combined immunodeficient (NOD/SCID) mice [13]. These cells were capable of self-renewal and recapitulation of the leukemia similar to the parental tumor phenotype *in vivo.* It was further demonstrated that leukemic stem cells are not functionally homogeneous but consist of a distinct hierarchically arranged class similar to normal hematopoietic stem cells [14]. Likewise, solid tumors have been demonstrated to possess a phenotypically distinct and rare population of cancer cells with self-renewal capacity [15].

Al-Hajj and colleagues [16] were the first to isolate and describe a distinct cell population in solid cancers and demonstrated self-renewal properties, namely for $CD44^+/CD24^{-/low}/lineage^-$ cells in breast cancer. As few as 100 cells of this particular phenotype were capable of generating a phenotypically diverse breast tumor similar to the original patient tumor in NOD/SCID mice, whereas as many as 20,000 cells with the $CD44^+/CD24^+$ phenotype were unable to generate a tumor [16,17]. NOD/SCID mouse repopulation capabilities were also demonstrated for $CD133^+/Nestin^+/Lineage^-$ cells from human brain tumors [18,19], a $CD138^-$ population in multiple myeloma [20], and cells with a $CD44^+/\alpha_2\beta_1^{hi}/CD133^+$ phenotype in prostate cancers [21]. Most recently, cancer stem cells exhibiting a $CD44^+CD24^+ESA^+$ phenotype were also described in pancreatic cancer.

Since the discovery of cancer stem cells some decades ago, their existence and significance have been continously debated. Work that has been accepted as proof of cancer stem cell properties was based on the ability of a distinct subpopulation of cancer cells that can form a tumor in sublethally irradiated NOD/SCID mice. The latter is complicated however by the interactions between cancer cells and their microenvironment. It is possible that only a rare subpopulation of cancer cells can acclimatize and grow in a foreign or mouse microenvironment. Kelly *et al* [22] have recently demonstrated that as few as 10 of primary pre-B/B lymphoma cells from Eμ-*myc* transgenic mice of every phenotype can form a tumor in non-irradiated congenic mice. This observation challenges the concept that only a rare cancer stem cell subpopulation can sustain the tumor growth. Moreover, Kern and Shibata suggested that the mathematical model for the concept of cancer stem cells in solid tumor is weak and even may be invalid [23].

In February 2006, the American Association for Cancer Research (AACR) had a workshop on cancer stem cells to discuss the definition, importance, and implications of this rapid emerging field. Currently, cancer stem cells have been defined as "a small subset of cancer cells within a cancer that constitute a reservoir of self-sustaining cells with the exclusive ability to self-renew and to cause the heterogeneous lineages of cancer cells that comprise the tumor" [24,25]. While a normal stem cell is considered to be multipotent or capable of differentiating into different cell phenotypes across all lineages, the current definition of a cancer stem cell does not include multipotency. In fact, the extent to which cancer stem cells share the characteristics of normal stem cells, including self-renewal properties, remains unclear. Therefore, although the term "cancer stem cell" may be attractive, it may be illusory and suitable only in a limited sense. Some groups have proposed that it may be more appropriate to use a functional definition such as "tumor-initiating cell" or "cancer-initiating cell" [26-28].

ORIGIN OF CANCER STEM CELLS

Cancer stem cells and "normal" (embryonic and adult) stem cells share several common features. At the molecular level, distinct sets of genes have emerged that can be associated with "stemness". In particular the Wnt- (Wnt-3, β-catenin), Notch- (Notch-1) and Hedgehog- (Gli1 and 2, PTCH1, SMO) signaling pathways, the polycomb family transcriptional repressor Bmi-1, octamer-binding transcription factor Oct-4, the drug efflux pump breast cancer resistance protein (BCRP), and human telomerase reverse transcriptase (hTERT) have been associated with stem cells [17,29-32]. Biological similarities that are governed by these genes include the ability to self-renew, the ability to differentiate, limitless proliferative capacity, the ability to activate anti-apoptotic pathways, resistance to cytotoxic agents, and the ability to migrate [33]. This has led to the thought that cancer stem cells may derive from mutated and/or dysregulated stem cells.

Most of the published data regarding the origin of cancer stem cells has been described in leukemia. Leukemic stem cells (LSCs) express CD34 and lack markers of lineage commitment such as CD38. In addition, LSCs can develop at each step in the hierarchy of the hematopoietic stem cell system; it has therefore been hypothesized that most human leukemias arise from transformation of HSCs [13,34]. For example it has been demonstrated that transduction of the MLL-ENL or MOZ-TIF2 fusion genes into HSCs, common myeloid progenitors (CMPs), and granulocyte-macrophage progenitors (GMPs) resulted in identical leukemia [35]. These results indicate that committed progenitors with little long-term replicative potential may acquire self-renewal capability and transform into LSCs. Nevertheless, it is currently uncertain what proportion of human myeloid leukemia arise from committed progenitors or a single oncogenic event such as MLL-ENL and MOZ-TIF2 tanslocations.

Further support of the hypothesis that tumors may derive from the transformation of a progenitor and/or stem cell are studies which showed that soft-tissue sarcoma cells and bone marrow derived mesenchymal progenitor cells share a common phenotype [36,37]. By transfecting with the oncogenic fusion protein ETS–FLI-1, mesenchymal progenitor cells could be converted into Ewing's sarcoma [38] There is also evidence suggesting an epithelial tumor type, namely gastric cancer, may arise from progenitor cells of non-epithelial origin [39]. Together, these results raise the possibility that a small subset of cancer stem cells may originate from normal stem cells, progenitor cells, or even different cell lineages as illustrated in figure 1.

Identification and Isolation of Cancer Stem Cells

Self-renewal and lineage capacity are the hallmarks of any stem cell, including cancer stem cells. Assays for identifying cancer stem cells are thus based on both self-renewal capability and tumor recapitulation. The current assay that is considered as the "gold standard", and that tests these cancer stem cell criteria best, is serial transplantation in animal models, most commonly NOD/SCID mice. Limiting dilutions of selected cancer cells are injected into sublethally irradiated immunodeficient mice to evaluate which phenotype of cancer cells can best recapitulate the tumor *in vivo*.

Cell Surface Markers: The majority of the described methods for the identification and isolation of viable cancer stem cells are based on the ability in the cell surface markers between stem and bulk cancer cells. The basis for detecting the different subtype of cancer cells by cell surface markers was pioneered by John E. Dick and colleagues in leukemia [13]. As described earlier, only the $CD34^+/CD38^-$ phenotype was able to initiate human AML in NOD/SCID mice. Subsequently, several other groups also used differences in cell surface markers between stem and differentiated cells to identify cancer stem cells in solid tumor types. These markers include CD44, α_6 integrin, β_6 integrin, and CD133.

Side Population: The side population (SP) is a particular cell population enriched in primitive stem/progenitor cells and undifferentiated cells [40-42]. The work was originally pioneered by Goodell *et al.* in 1996 [40]. The assay is based on the capability of stem cells to efflux the vital dye, Hoechst 33342. This particular dye simultaneously emits at two wavelengths (red 675 nm and blue 450 nm). A distinct, small, non-stained cell population, which comprises approximately 0.1% of all cells in bone marrow from mice, and which resides in the left lower quadrant of a Flow Activated Cell Sorter (FACS) profile, was first described as the side population. This population expressed murine bone marrow stem cells markers ($Sca1^{+}lin^{neg/low}$) and was enriched at least 1,000-fold for *in vivo* reconstitution activity. The differential ability of stem cells to efflux the vital dye H33342 is based on the high expression level of several members of the ABC transporter family, such as MDR1 (multidrug resistance 1, or P-glycoprotein) and BCRP (breast cancer resistance protein), which are also responsible for drug resistance. Although the SP is not "pure", but only enriched for putative stem cells, it is considered as an alternative assay, particularly in situations where stem cells molecular markers are unknown [43]. However, some authors remain skeptical about the existence of stem cells in the SP. Triel et al.[44] demonstrated that the SP of dermal epithelial cells did not express stem cells markers and identified high expression of BCRP in the secretory duct epithelium of the sweat glands instead of the basal layer of the epidermis.

Aldehyde Dehydrogenase (ALDH): Aldehyde dehydrogenases (ALDH) are a family of enzymes involved in the oxidization of intracellular aldehydes. ALDH are thought to have an important role in oxidation of alcohol and vitamin A as well as in resistance to cyclophosphamide [45,46]. Cytosolic ALDH1A1 is highly expressed in human and murine hematopoietic stem and progenitor cells [47,48]. More recently, a technique has been developed for the assessment of ALDH activity in viable cells by flow cytometric analysis and has been made commercially available as Aldeflour kit (StemCell Technologies). This non cytotoxic method uses a cell-permeable fluorescent substrate to identify cells with high ALDH activity [49]. The substrate converted by ALDH is a charged molecule and is unable to leave the cell as freely as the parent substrate. Therefore, the cells with high ALDH activity will accumulate fluorescent ALDH substrate which can be quantified by FACS and used for FACS sorting of viable cells for functional studies. This method has been used mainly to study hematopoietic and leukemic stem cells. $CD34^{+}ALDH^{bright}$ (ALDHbr) cells from human umbilical cord blood (UCB) have been shown to contain all the NOD/SCID engrafting cells in the $CD34^{+}$ fraction [49]. In leukemia, the $ALDH^{br}$ cell population was found to coexpress $CD34^{+}$ and engraft significantly better in NOD/SCID mice [50].

Tumor Spheres: In 1996, Reynolds and Weiss described a method to culture undifferentiated multipotent neural cells in suspension or on non-adherent surfaces with growth factors, termed the "neurosphere assay"[51]. Neurospheres were shown to consist of 4%–20% stem cells, the rest of the population representing progenitor cells in various stages of differentiation. A similar concept was also applied to normal human mammary epithelial cells and is known as the mammosphere assay. Mammospheres have been shown to be enriched in early progenitor/stem cells and are able to differentiate along all three mammary epithelial lineages and to clonally generate complex functional structures in reconstituted 3D culture systems. Furthermore, gene expression analysis of cells isolated from these mammospheres seems to be similar to genetic programs in other stem and progenitor cells [17]. This technique is frequently used as a model to enrich a cancer stem cell population *in vitro* for functional and molecular studies.

Although there are several described methods to identify and isolate cancer stem cells, most of the current methods are flow cytometry-based assays that often require fresh and substantial amounts of tumor tissue, which clearly limits their clinical application for example as a diagnostic tool. Hence, novel methods to identify cancer stem cells by other techniques such as blood based stem cell markers and ultra-sensitive assays that can measure low-abundance proteins are urgently needed. The identification of circulating cancer stem cell markers would allow the monitoring of thc cfficacy of therapy and disease relapse.

More recently, a gene expression analysis by Clarke and colleagues [52] identified a 186-gene signature differentially expressed in $CD44^{+}CD24^{-/low}$ breast cancer cells that can serve as a better prognostic marker for both overall survival and metastasis-free survival in patients with breast cancer independent of conventional clinical and pathological factors. Furthermore, several groups demonstrated that self-renewal pathways as well as multiple "stemness" genes are highly expressed in $CD44^{+}CD24^{-/low}$ breast cancer cells. These include hedgehog signaling components such as *PTCH1*, *Gli1*, *Gli2*, the polycomb gene *Bmi-1*, Notch homolog 3, Msh homeobox homolog 1, cyclin-dependent kinase inhibitor 1A, Chordin, H19, and Insulin-like growth factor binding protein 7 (IGFBP-7/IGFBP-rP1) [29,53].

Cancer Stem Cell-Targeted Therapies

The vast majority of the over 100 registered and clinically utilized anticancer drugs are "classical" cytotoxic agents. Their common mechanism of action is the preferential killing of rapid dividing bulk tumor cells by either interruption of their cytoskeletal integrity or targeting of DNA-synthesis. To date, only about 4% of advanced cancers that require systemic treatment are curable [33]. The failure of cytotoxic chemotherapy could best be explained by the inability to eradicate cancer stem cells. Similar to their normal counterparts, cancer stem cells are quiescent and primarily persist in the G_0 phase; therefore, cancer stem cells are resistant to cell cycle specific drugs such as those targeting DNA-synthesis [54]. In addition, the over expression of drug efflux pumps in cancer stem cells limits a drug's availability to achieve cell kill.

In an approach similar to the culture and sensitivity assays used in infectious disease, Salmon and Hamburger pioneered the concept of targeting cancer stem cells and concomitantly individualizing cancer therapy in the late 1970s [55]. Single cell suspensions from patients' tumor tissues or malignant effusions were cultured in multilayered soft agar and treated with anticancer drugs. This technique was termed "clonogenic assay" or "human tumor stem cell assay" (HTCA) and was based on the observation that only 0.001-0.1% of tumor cells grow in soft agar comparable to the extent of colony formation by pluripotent cells in bone marrow. Additionally, the homogenous appearance of tumor colonies as well as the staining of these colonies with cell type specific dyes was consistent with a hypothesis that they were stem cells [55,56]. The HTCA was used in a first approach to personalize cancer medicine by assessing a patient's prognosis and response to chemotherapy. However, in prospective clinical studies and a meta analysis of all available data, the HTCA was found to be a better predictor for clinical resistance than sensitivity [55,57]. This outcome could be explained by the fact that the HTCA was largely used to test drugs (standard chemotherapy) that are substrates of drug efflux pumps expressed on the cell surface by cancer stem cells.

Owing to the limitations of standard chemotherapy, pathways that regulate the self-renewal of normal stem cells [17,58] including Wnt, Notch, and Hedgehog, and that have also been found to play an important role in human carcinogenesis offer interesting new targets for anticancer therapies [17]. Deregulation of developmental pathways has been reported in colon, pancreatic, gastric, prostate [59], cervical, leukemia, skin [60] and breast [61] cancers

[17,62]. Several groups are now focusing their efforts on targeting these self-renewal pathways in cancer stem cells. Whilst these essential pathways are shared by normal stem cells and cancer stem cells alike, multiple studies in animal models have shown that interdicting a particular self-renewal pathways may selectively target cancer stem cells [17]. Inhibitors of the Hedgehog pathway, such as cyclopamine, were identified and have a therapeutic window with remarkable activity against a wide range of human cancer cell lines and tumor xenografts including ovarian cancer [45], medulloblastoma [63], gastrointestinal neuroendocrine carcinomas [64], and prostate cancer [59]. Similarly, gamma secretase inhibitors such as LY-411,575, which block Notch activation, were found to have activity in Kaposi's sarcoma [65], breast cancers [66], and melanoma [67].

Another possibility to target the self-renewal capacity of cancer stem cells is to force them to differentiate [68]. Retinoic acid can induce differentiation in embryonic stem cells [69]. All-trans retinoic acid (ATRA) has been used with great success in combination chemotherapy in acute promyelocytic leukemia (APL), a disease with a cure rate of more than 70 %. This suggests that cancer stem cells are being successfully eliminated in this particular disease [70-72]. Arsenic trioxide, an agent that may function through telomere targeting, has recently been demonstrated to further improve the rate of cure in patients with APL. Histone deacetylases (HDACs) regulate transcriptional gene activity. HDAC inhibitors can be used for epigenetic reprogramming of silenced genes and thus, induce cell differentiation. The HDAC inhibitor, vorinostat (SAHA), has been found to have activity in multiple malignancies including leukemia [24], lymphoma [73], thyroid cancer [74], myeloma [75], and hepatocellular carcinoma [76].

Vascular endothelial growth factor (VEGF) has been validated as a target for anti-cancer therapeutics and demonstrated clinical efficacy in colon, lung and breast cancers when the monoclonal anti-VEGF antibody bevacizumab was combined with cytotoxic chemotherapy [77-79]. Initially, the driving hypothesis for this approach was that tumors could not grow beyond a certain size without generating a new blood supply and therefore inhibition of the blood supply would destroy the malignancy. Another hypothesis is that anti-VEGF therapy results in "normalization " of blood supply to the tumor by decreasing interstitial pressures and ultimately by increasing the flow of chemotherapy to the tumor [80]. More recently, a third, stem cell-related hypothesis has emerged . It has become apparent that cancer stem cells live in vascularized lacunae and that anti-VEGF therapy may destroy these sites and consequently improve outcome [81].

Finally, cancer stem cells within a tumor may change their phenotype as the tumor progresses, and also may exhibit a hierarchy, in which different populations of stem cells have a different response to treatment. Treatments targeted against a certain phenotype of cancer stem cells may not be effective against another type of cancer stem cells in a tumor. Thus, multifaceted approaches may be required similar to polychemotherapy of bulk tumor masses in order to eradicate "all" cancer stem cells [25].

Conclusion

Recent evidence strengthens the hypothesis that cancer stem cells exist. Further investigations into the origin and characteristics of cancer stem cells will increase our understanding of tumor initiation and progression and provide selective drug targets. Future development of new drugs that target cancer stem cells will require the implementation of new paradigms in investigating these agents in a clinical setting since we may not be able to determine their effectiveness by using currently employed tumor regression endpoints. Because chronic treatment of cancer patients is likely to be necessary for the eradication of cancer stem cells, long-term toxicity studies will also be necessary that determine whether side effects are associated with the depletion of a particular stem cell pool in normal tissues.

References

[1] Mathers CD, Shibuya K, Boschi-Pinto C, et al: Global and regional estimates of cancer mortality and incidence by site: I. Application of regional cancer survival model to estimate cancer mortality distribution by site. *BMC Cancer* 2:36, 2002.

[2] Al-Hajj M, Becker MW, Wicha M, et al: Therapeutic implications of cancer stem cells. *Curr. Opin. Genet Dev.* 14:43-7, 2004.

[3] Jordan CT: Targeting the most critical cells: approaching leukemia therapy as a problem in stem cell biology. *Nat. Clin. Pract. Oncol.* 2:224-5, 2005.

[4] Abbott A: Cancer: the root of the problem. *Nature* 442:742-3, 2006.

[5] Wikipedia tfe: Ernest McCulloch, 2006.

[6] Becker AJ, Mc CE, Till JE: Cytological demonstration of the clonal nature of spleen colonies derived from transplanted mouse marrow cells. *Nature* 197:452-4, 1963.

[7] Reya T, Morrison SJ, Clarke MF, et al: Stem cells, cancer, and cancer stem cells. *Nature* 414:105-11, 2001.

[8] Ramalho-Santos M, Yoon S, Matsuzaki Y, et al: "Stemness": transcriptional profiling of embryonic and adult stem cells. *Science* 298:597-600, 2002.

[9] Clevers H: Stem cells, asymmetric division and cancer. *Nat. Genet.* 37:1027-8, 2005.

[10] Caussinus E, Gonzalez C: Induction of tumor growth by altered stem-cell asymmetric division in Drosophila melanogaster. *Nat. Genet.* 37:1125-9, 2005.

[11] Bruce WR, Van Der Gaag H: A Quantitative Assay for the Number of Murine Lymphoma Cells Capable of Proliferation in Vivo. *Nature* 199:79-80, 1963.

[12] Park CH, Bergsagel DE, McCulloch EA: Mouse myeloma tumor stem cells: a primary cell culture assay. *J. Natl. Cancer Inst.* 46:411-22, 1971.

[13] Bonnet D, Dick JE: Human acute myeloid leukemia is organized as a hierarchy that originates from a primitive hematopoietic cell. *Nat. Med.* 3:730-7, 1997.

[14] Hope KJ, Jin L, Dick JE: Acute myeloid leukemia originates from a hierarchy of leukemic stem cell classes that differ in self-renewal capacity. *Nat. Immunol.* 5:738-43, 2004.

[15] Fidler IJ, Hart IR: Biological diversity in metastatic neoplasms: origins and implications. *Science* 217:998-1003, 1982.

[16] Al-Hajj M, Wicha MS, Benito-Hernandez A, et al: Prospective identification of tumorigenic breast cancer cells. *Proc. Natl. Acad. Sci. USA* 100:3983-8, 2003.

[17] Dontu G, Abdallah WM, Foley JM, et al: In vitro propagation and transcriptional profiling of human mammary stem/progenitor cells. *Genes Dev.* 17:1253-70, 2003.

[18] Singh SK, Hawkins C, Clarke ID, et al: Identification of human brain tumour initiating cells. *Nature* 432:396-401, 2004.

[19] Singh SK, Clarke ID, Hide T, et al: Cancer stem cells in nervous system tumors. *Oncogene* 23:7267-73, 2004.

[20] Matsui W, Huff CA, Wang Q, et al: Characterization of clonogenic multiple myeloma cells. *Blood* 103:2332-6, 2004.

[21] Collins AT, Berry PA, Hyde C, et al: Prospective identification of tumorigenic prostate cancer stem cells. *Cancer Res*. 65:10946-51, 2005.

[22] Kelly PN, Dakic A, Adams JM, et al: Tumor growth need not be driven by rare cancer stem cells. *Science* 317:337, 2007.

[23] Kern SE, Shibata D: The fuzzy math of solid tumor stem cells: a perspective. *Cancer Res*. 67:8985-8, 2007.

[24] Clarke MF, Dick JE, Dirks PB, et al: Cancer Stem Cells--Perspectives on Current Status and Future Directions: AACR Workshop on Cancer Stem Cells. *Cancer Res* 66:9339-44, 2006.

[25] Hill RP, Perris R: "Destemming" cancer stem cells. *J. Natl. Cancer Inst*. 99:1435-40, 2007.

[26] Neuzil J, Stantic M, Zobalova R, et al: Tumour-initiating cells vs. cancer 'stem' cells and CD133: what's in the name? *Biochem. Biophys. Res. Commun*. 355:855-9, 2007.

[27] Phillips TM, McBride WH, Pajonk F: The response of CD24(-/low)/CD44+ breast cancer-initiating cells to radiation. *J. Natl. Cancer Inst*. 98:1777-85, 2006.

[28] Ricci-Vitiani L, Lombardi DG, Pilozzi E, et al: Identification and expansion of human colon-cancer-initiating cells. *Nature* 445:111-5, 2007.

[29] Liu S, Dontu G, Mantle ID, et al: Hedgehog signaling and Bmi-1 regulate self-renewal of normal and malignant human mammary stem cells. *Cancer Res*. 66:6063-71, 2006.

[30] Doyle LA, Yang W, Abruzzo LV, et al: A multidrug resistance transporter from human MCF-7 breast cancer cells. *Proc. Natl. Acad. Sci. USA* 95:15665-70, 1998.

[31] Patrawala L, Calhoun T, Schneider-Broussard R, et al: Highly purified CD44+ prostate cancer cells from xenograft human tumors are enriched in tumorigenic and metastatic progenitor cells. *Oncogene* 25:1696-708, 2006.

[32] Ponti D, Costa A, Zaffaroni N, et al: Isolation and in vitro propagation of tumorigenic breast cancer cells with stem/progenitor cell properties. *Cancer Res*. 65:5506-11, 2005.

[33] Chumsri S, Phatak P, Edelman MJ, et al: Cancer stem cells and individualized therapy. *Cancer Genomics Proteomics* 4:165-74, 2007.

[34] Ravandi F, Estrov Z: Eradication of leukemia stem cells as a new goal of therapy in leukemia. *Clin. Cancer Res*. 12:340-4, 2006.

[35] Cozzio A, Passegue E, Ayton PM, et al: Similar MLL-associated leukemias arising from self-renewing stem cells and short-lived myeloid progenitors. *Genes Dev*. 17:3029-35, 2003.

[36] Gazziola C, Cordani N, Wasserman B, et al: Malignant fibrous histiocytoma: a proposed cellular origin and identification of its characterizing gene transcripts. *Int. J. Oncol*. 23:343-51, 2003.

[37] Tirode F, Laud-Duval K, Prieur A, et al: Mesenchymal stem cell features of Ewing tumors. *Cancer Cell* 11:421-9, 2007.

[38] Riggi N, Cironi L, Provero P, et al: Development of Ewing's sarcoma from primary bone marrow-derived mesenchymal progenitor cells. *Cancer Res*. 65:11459-68, 2005.

[39] Houghton J, Stoicov C, Nomura S, et al: Gastric cancer originating from bone marrow-derived cells. *Science* 306:1568-71, 2004.

[40] Goodell MA, Brose K, Paradis G, et al: Isolation and functional properties of murine hematopoietic stem cells that are replicating in vivo. *J. Exp. Med.* 183:1797-806, 1996.

[41] Hadnagy A, Gaboury L, Beaulieu R, et al: SP analysis may be used to identify cancer stem cell populations. *Exp. Cell Res.* 312:3701-10, 2006.

[42] Camargo FD, Chambers SM, Drew E, et al: Hematopoietic stem cells do not engraft with absolute efficiencies. *Blood* 107:501-7, 2006.

[43] Challen GA, Little MH: A side order of stem cells: the SP phenotype. *Stem Cells* 24:3-12, 2006.

[44] Triel C, Vestergaard ME, Bolund L, et al: Side population cells in human and mouse epidermis lack stem cell characteristics. *Exp. Cell Res.* 295:79-90, 2004.

[45] Wang JS, Fang Q, Sun DJ, et al: Genetic modification of hematopoietic progenitor cells for combined resistance to 4-hydroperoxycyclophosphamide, vincristine, and daunorubicin. *Acta Pharmacol. Sin.* 22:949-55, 2001.

[46] Duester G: Families of retinoid dehydrogenases regulating vitamin A function: production of visual pigment and retinoic acid. *Eur. J. Biochem.* 267:4315-24, 2000.

[47] Kastan MB, Schlaffer E, Russo JE, et al: Direct demonstration of elevated aldehyde dehydrogenase in human hematopoietic progenitor cells. *Blood* 75:1947-50, 1990.

[48] Storms RW, Trujillo AP, Springer JB, et al: Isolation of primitive human hematopoietic progenitors on the basis of aldehyde dehydrogenase activity. *Proc. Natl. Acad. Sci. USA* 96:9118-23, 1999

[49] Storms RW, Green PD, Safford KM, et al: Distinct hematopoietic progenitor compartments are delineated by the expression of aldehyde dehydrogenase and CD34. *Blood* 106:95-102, 2005.

[50] Cheung AM, Wan TS, Leung JC, et al: Aldehyde dehydrogenase activity in leukemic blasts defines a subgroup of acute myeloid leukemia with adverse prognosis and superior NOD/SCID engrafting potential. *Leukemia* 21:1423-30, 2007.

[51] Weiss S, Reynolds BA, Vescovi AL, et al: Is there a neural stem cell in the mammalian forebrain? *Trends Neurosci.* 19:387-93, 1996.

[52] Liu R, Wang X, Chen GY, et al: The prognostic role of a gene signature from tumorigenic breast-cancer cells. *N. Engl. J. Med.* 356:217-26, 2007.

[53] Shipitsin M, Campbell LL, Argani P, et al: Molecular definition of breast tumor heterogeneity. *Cancer Cell* 11:259-73, 2007.

[54] Venezia TA, Merchant AA, Ramos CA, et al: Molecular signatures of proliferation and quiescence in hematopoietic stem cells. *PLoS Biol.* 2:e301, 2004.

[55] Salmon SE, Hamburger AW, Soehnlen B, et al: Quantitation of differential sensitivity of human-tumor stem cells to anticancer drugs. *N. Engl. J. Med.* 298:1321-7, 1978.

[56] Schrag D, Garewal HS, Burstein HJ, et al: American Society of Clinical Oncology Technology Assessment: chemotherapy sensitivity and resistance assays. *J. Clin. Oncol.* 22:3631-8, 2004.

[57] Fiebig HH, Maier A, Burger AM: Clonogenic assay with established human tumour xenografts: correlation of in vitro to in vivo activity as a basis for anticancer drug discovery. *Eur. J. Cancer* 40:802-20, 2004.

[58] Liu S, Dontu G, Wicha MS: Mammary stem cells, self-renewal pathways, and carcinogenesis. *Breast Cancer Res.* 7:86-95, 2005.

[59] Karhadkar SS, Bova GS, Abdallah N, et al: Hedgehog signalling in prostate regeneration, neoplasia and metastasis. *Nature* 431:707-12, 2004.

[60] Gailani MR, Stahle-Backdahl M, Leffell DJ, et al: The role of the human homologue of Drosophila patched in sporadic basal cell carcinomas. *Nat. Genet* 14:78-81, 1996.

[61] Dievart A, Beaulieu N, Jolicoeur P: Involvement of Notch1 in the development of mouse mammary tumors. *Oncogene* 18:5973-81, 1999.

[62] Olsen CL, Hsu PP, Glienke J, et al: Hedgehog-interacting protein is highly expressed in endothelial cells but down-regulated during angiogenesis and in several human tumors. *BMC Cancer* 4:43, 2004.

[63] Romer JT, Kimura H, Magdaleno S, et al: Suppression of the Shh pathway using a small molecule inhibitor eliminates medulloblastoma in Ptc1(+/-)p53(-/-) mice. *Cancer Cell* 6:229-40, 2004.

[64] Shida T, Furuya M, Nikaido T, et al: Sonic Hedgehog-Gli1 Signaling Pathway Might Become an Effective Therapeutic Target in Gastrointestinal Neuroendocrine Carcinomas. *Cancer Biol. Ther.* 5, 2006.

[65] Lan K, Choudhuri T, Murakami M, et al: Intracellular activated Notch1 is critical for proliferation of Kaposi's sarcoma-associated herpesvirus-associated B-lymphoma cell lines in vitro. *J. Virol.* 80:6411-9, 2006.

[66] Pece S, Serresi M, Santolini E, et al: Loss of negative regulation by Numb over Notch is relevant to human breast carcinogenesis. *J. Cell Biol.* 167:215-21, 2004.

[67] Nickoloff BJ, Hendrix MJ, Pollock PM, et al: Notch and NOXA-related pathways in melanoma cells. *J. Investig Dermatol. Symp. Proc.* 10:95-104, 2005.

[68] Massard C, Deutsch E, Soria JC: Tumour stem cell-targeted treatment: elimination or differentiation. *Ann. Oncol.* 17:1620-4, 2006.

[69] Motohashi T, Aoki H, Chiba K, et al: Multipotent cell fate of neural crest-like cells derived from embryonic stem cells. *Stem Cells,* 2006.

[70] Sanz MA, Lo Coco F, Martin G, et al: Definition of relapse risk and role of nonanthracycline drugs for consolidation in patients with acute promyelocytic leukemia: a joint study of the PETHEMA and GIMEMA cooperative groups. *Blood* 96:1247-53, 2000.

[71] Sanz MA, Martin G, Gonzalez M, et al: Risk-adapted treatment of acute promyelocytic leukemia with all-trans-retinoic acid and anthracycline monochemotherapy: a multicenter study by the PETHEMA group. *Blood* 103:1237-43, 2004.

[72] Sanz MA, Martin G, Rayon C, et al: A modified AIDA protocol with anthracycline-based consolidation results in high antileukemic efficacy and reduced toxicity in newly diagnosed PML/RARalpha-positive acute promyelocytic leukemia. PETHEMA group. *Blood* 94:3015-21, 1999.

[73] O'Connor OA: Developing new drugs for the treatment of lymphoma. *Eur. J. Haematol.* Suppl:150-8, 2005.

[74] Luong QT, O'Kelly J, Braunstein GD, et al: Antitumor activity of suberoylanilide hydroxamic acid against thyroid cancer cell lines in vitro and in vivo. *Clin. Cancer Res.* 12:5570-7, 2006.

[75] Yaccoby S, Wezeman MJ, Zangari M, et al: Inhibitory effects of osteoblasts and increased bone formation on myeloma in novel culture systems and a myelomatous mouse model. *Haematologica* 91:192-9, 2006.

[76] Ocker M, Alajati A, Ganslmayer M, et al: The histone-deacetylase inhibitor SAHA potentiates proapoptotic effects of 5-fluorouracil and irinotecan in hepatoma cells. *J. Cancer Res. Clin. Oncol.* 131:385-94, 2005.

[77] Hurwitz H, Fehrenbacher L, Novotny W, et al: Bevacizumab plus irinotecan, fluorouracil, and leucovorin for metastatic colorectal cancer. N. *Engl. J. Med.* 350:2335-42, 2004.

[78] Sandler A, Gray R, Perry MC, et al: Paclitaxel-carboplatin alone or with bevacizumab for non-small-cell lung cancer. *N. Engl. J. Med.* 355:2542-50, 2006.

[79] Wedam SB, Low JA, Yang SX, et al: Antiangiogenic and antitumor effects of bevacizumab in patients with inflammatory and locally advanced breast cancer. *J. Clin. Oncol.* 24:769-77, 2006.

[80] Jain RK: Normalization of tumor vasculature: an emerging concept in antiangiogenic therapy. *Science* 307:58-62, 2005.

[81] Calabrese C, Poppleton H, Kocak M, et al: A perivascular niche for brain tumor stem cells. *Cancer Cell* 11:69-82, 2007.

In: Perspectives in Stem Cell Research ISBN: 978-1-61122-985-1
Editors: Brenda M. Davis and Christopher B. Halton

Chapter III

PROSTATE STEM CELLS

Aamir Ahmed, Isabelle Bisson, Charlotte L. Foley and John R. W. Masters*
Prostate Cancer Research Centre, Institute of Urology and Nephrology,
University College London, London, UK

ABSTRACT

The aim of this article is to provide an up-to-date review of an area of biological research in its infancy, namely the identification of stem and tumor initiating cells from the prostate gland.

THE PROSTATE GLAND

The prostate in a young adult human male weighs about 20g. The main boost for growth of the prostate arrives with the onset of puberty associated with the increased availability of testosterone. The tissue thereafter is dependent upon the availability of androgens for its growth and development [1]. Indeed, the dependency for growth and maintenance of the prostate on androgens is a feature that is utilized as therapy for prostate cancer [1,2].

The anatomy of the prostate is illustrated in Figure 1. It can be described as an inverted pyramid surrounding the urethra as it exits the bladder; the apex of the pyramid pointing towards the penis and the base adjacent to the bladder. The urethra runs through the anterior prostate exiting proximal to the apex. The ejaculatory ducts, the conduits of sperm from the testes to the urethra, also pass through the prostate gland, meeting the urethra at the verumontanum.

A thin pseudo-capsule of smooth muscle, collagen and elastin surrounds the external surface of the prostate. This capsule blends internally with prostatic stroma and externally

* Corresponding author: j.masters@ucl.ac.uk

with Denonvilliers fascia and the endopelvic fascia. However at the junction of the prostate and the bladder the prostate merges into the striated muscle of the urethral sphincter. The prostatic urethra is divided into proximal and distal parts by the verumontanum, where many of the prostatic ducts drain into urethra. A sinus like structure, the prostatic utricle (considered to be a remnant of the Mullerian duct) is situated at the peak of the verumontanum. The ejaculatory ducts arising from the seminal vesicles and vas deferens enter the prostate posteriorly and drain into the urethra on either side of the prostatic utricle.

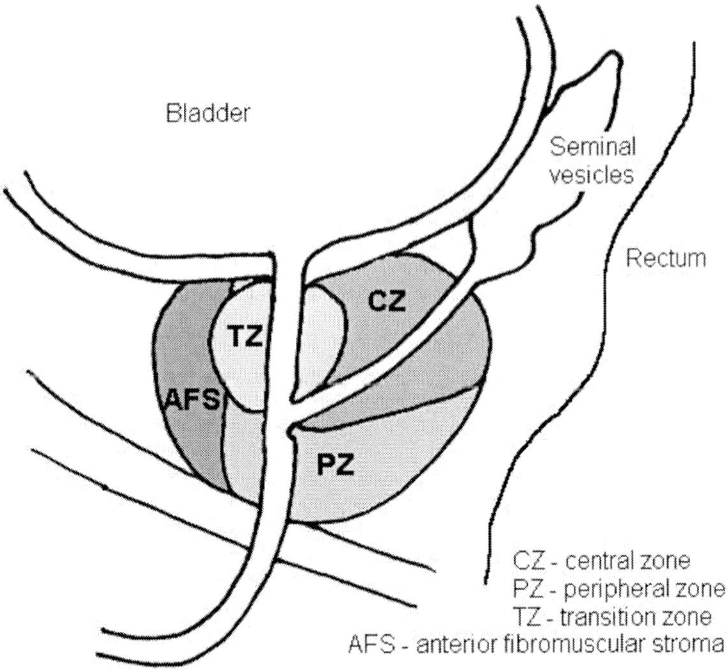

Figure 1. Diagrammatic representation of the anatomy of the human prostate, based on the nomenclature described by McNeal [6]. This sagittal plane drawing shows the three glandular zones of the prostate in a representation of a man standing vertically and facing towards the left.

The prostate gland is made up of epithelial ducts and acini surrounded by stroma (Figure 2). The prostate epithelium is a two layered structure comprising an apical layer of columnar, secretory cells which are separated by a flattened layer of basal cells from the basement membrane. The two layers can be distinguished by immunochemical staining using specific site markers such as integrins and cytokeratins [3]. Serotonin and chromogranin A staining has also been shown in the epithelium of the prostate [4] due to the neuroendocrine cells scattered through the epithelial layer. The apical cells are columnar, with cytoplasm containing secretory granules containing prostate specific antigen (PSA, a serine protease belonging to the kallikrein family) and prostatic acid phosphatase (PAP) [5]. The stroma contains smooth muscle cells, fibroblasts, myofibroblasts, nerves, capillaries and lymphatics.

Anatomy - The Zonal Model of the Prostate

McNeal [6] described the currently accepted anatomical model of the prostate (Figure 1). According to this model, the prostate, in addition to the anterior fibromuscular stroma, is divided into the anterior fibromuscular stroma and three glandular zones: the peripheral, transition and central zones [6]. Evidence supporting this model of the prostate has been gathered from histochemical analysis [7,8,9], limited studies of protein expression [10,11,12,13,14,15] and observations using various imaging techniques [16,17,18,19].

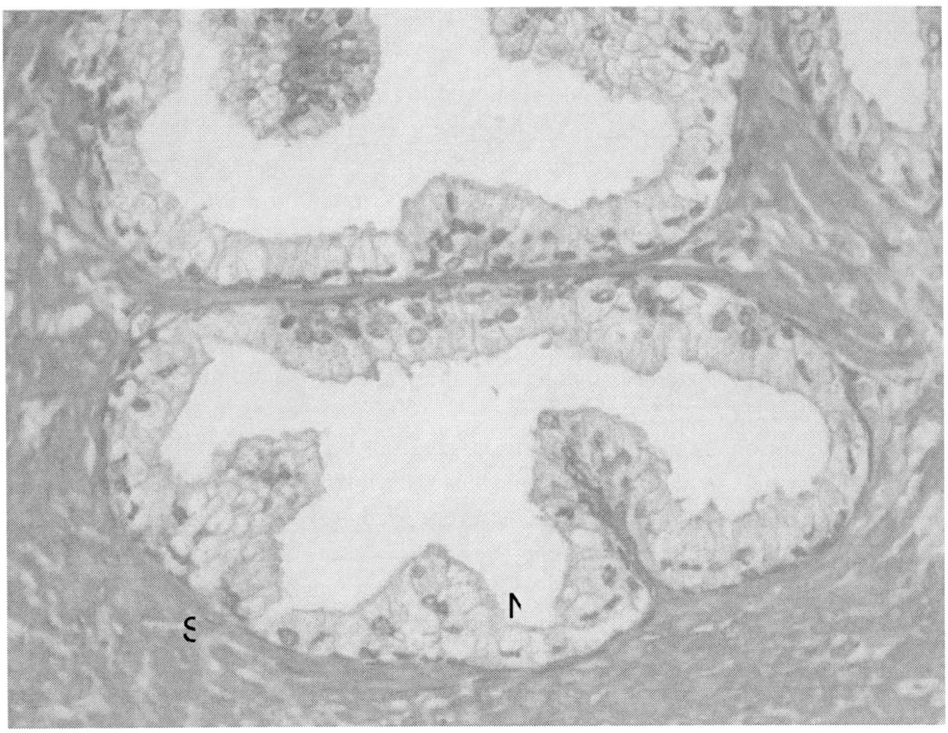

Figure 2. A hematoxylin and eosin (H&E) stained transverse section of the human prostate viewed at 40x. A complete acinus, embedded within the stroma (S), is visible comprising two layers of epithelial cells. Above a flattened layer of basal layers is a layer of PSA-producing columnar cells (N) lining the lumen.

Peripheral Zone

The peripheral zone almost surrounds the prostate, forming a horseshoe shape with the thickest region at the back (Fig1). The largest by volume of the three zones, the peripheral zone constitutes around 70% of the glandular prostate. Histologically, it is seen as a disc of tissue whose ducts radiate laterally from the urethra, lateral and distal to the verumontanum [6].

Central Zone

The central zone comprises approximately 25% of the glandular tissue [6] surrounding the ejaculatory ducts at the back of the prostate (Figure 1). Its ducts arise near to the openings of the ejaculatory ducts, following these ducts proximally and branching laterally near the base of the prostate [6].

Transition Zone

The transition zone makes up about 5% of the glandular prostate (Figure 1). This zone surrounds the urethra proximal to the ejaculatory ducts and verumontanum. Duct development is limited in this zone.

Physiology of the Prostate

The main role of the prostate gland is believed to be its contribution to semen production. The prostate contributes 0.5 to 1ml (~20% of semen volume) of fluid to the human ejaculate, the remainder provided by the seminal vesicles, Cowper's glands, vas deferens, epididymi and testes. A curious observation regarding the function of the prostate is its ability to produce high quantities of citrate (21μmol/g wet wt; see [20] for a review) and also its high accumulation of zinc (relative to other human tissues) with an estimated concentration of zinc of ~150μg/g wet wt of prostate tissue [21]. Why such high quantities of citrate and zinc are found in prostate is not known. However, as the concentration of both citrate and zinc is reduced in malignant prostate, it is thought that there may be some link between malignancy and these compounds [22].

The prostate surrounds the urethra as it passes from the bladder to the penis (Figure 1). The fibromuscular part of the prostate may thus contribute towards regulating the flow of urine. Another function of the prostate is its role in the expulsion of the semen into the ejaculate. During ejaculation, the seminal vesicles, prostate and the neck of the bladder contract; this contraction forces the semen into the prostatic urethra. Subsequent relaxation of the distal prostatic sphincter and rhythmic bulbocavernosal muscle contractions then expel the sperm.

Prostatic Hyperplasia and Cancer

It is estimated that in 2004 in the US, prostate cancer accounts for nearly 33% of all new cancers diagnosed in men [23]. This figure represents about 230,000 men resulting in over 30,000 deaths due to prostate cancer [23]. The incidence and death rates due to prostate cancer are two fold higher in African-Americans compared to Caucasian-Americans [23]. Although prostate cancer has a higher probability of occurrence in men over 60 years of age (1 in 7 men over 60 will develop prostate cancer in their lifetime), the probability of developing invasive prostate cancer increases by 230 fold in men 40 to 60 years of age compared to men aged under 40 [23]. Prostate cancer is a significant problem in an aging population, as is the trend in most developed nations.

Benign Prostatic Hyperplasia (BPH)

BPH is a non-malignant growth of the prostate. A frequent consequence of this overgrowth is decreased flow of urine as the urethra passes through the prostate. Clinically, BPH is a condition defined by the presence of lower urinary tract symptoms (LUTS), prostate enlargement and bladder outflow obstruction [24]. The incidence of BPH increases with age and over 40% of men in their 50s, and 90% of men in their 80s have histopathological evidence of BPH [25].

BPH is largely associated with the transition zone [25]. The initial phase of BPH is asymptomatic and is characterized by a progression from microscopic to macroscopic disease. Microscopic BPH develops in all men (if they live long enough), however, only half progress to macroscopic BPH.

Prostatic Intraepithelial Neoplasia

Lesions within the prostate epithelium called prostatic intraepithelial neoplasia (PIN) are thought to be the precursor of prostate cancer [26]. PIN is predominantly seen in the peripheral zone and is rarely seen in the transition zone [27]. PIN is categorized into low and high-grade PIN, although low grade PIN largely remains unreported. The presence of high-grade PIN is often associated with prostate cancer. PIN is characterized by dramatic cytological changes in the prostate. An interesting observation, which could be highly relevant to the isolation of adult prostate stem cells, is that in normal prostate and BPH, 70 to 80% of the proliferative cells are seen in the basal layer [28]. In low-grade PIN nearly 70% of the proliferative cells are in the luminal layer [28].

Prostate Cancer

Prostate cancer is an adenocarcinoma derived from the glandular epithelium and in its most well differentiated form can only be distinguished from normal epithelium by the absence of a basal layer. The most frequent site of prostate cancer is the peripheral zone [8,29]. The cellular characteristics of this adenocarcinoma include nuclear enlargement, hyperchromasia (with single prominent nucleolus) dark cytoplasm and mitotic figures [8]. The presence of perineural invasion serves as a diagnostic feature. Prostatic adenocarcinoma demonstrates distinct lack of a basal cell layer, frequently used to verify the diagnosis of cancer [30,31]. Grading of the cancer is based upon the gland morphology [32]. PSA serum levels are also a useful marker for the diagnosis and monitoring of prostate cancer [33].

Another type of carcinoma identified in the prostate is the small cell carcinoma (SCC) which makes up less than2% of all prostatic malignancies. SCCs of the prostate are thought to arise from malignant transformation of neuroendocrine cells [34,35]. These cancers are PSA negative and show evidence of neuroendocrine differentiation [34].

Adult Stem Cells – A Short History and Properties

An original observation in the 1950s [36] led to the development of the stem cell as a biological concept in the 1960s and 1970s [37,38,39] and later to the establishment of primary cultures of stem cells. Adult stem cells are the small fraction of cells within a specialized tissue that are thought to be responsible for regeneration, maintenance and replenishing the cells within that tissue [37,40]. Although the characteristics of stem cells is a matter of considerable debate, two minimum criteria are used to define stem cells, namely self-renewal capacity and pluripotency (the ability to differentiate into specialized cells and/or tissues) [41,40]. These two properties will serve as guiding principles in this chapter regarding adult prostate stem cells.

Self-renewal of Stem Cells

If the adult stem cells regenerate, maintain and repair a specific tissue over its life-time, how could the stem cells achieve this feat without being depleted? The answer probably lies in a trait considered to be specific to stem cells, and to the exclusion of other specialized or differentiated cells, namely self-renewal. As a consequence of self-renewal, one or both daughter cells retain the genetic and functional properties of the parent cell rather than becoming further specialized [42]. It follows that by opting for self-renewal and limiting cell division (an inherently error prone process with accumulation of mutations during DNA replication) [42] the stem cells may avoid high rates of malignancy [42].

Most of the evidence substantiating the concept of adult stem cells comes from the hematopoietic system (see [42] for review). In the hematopoietic system a probabilistic model has been proposed. In this model hematopoietic stem cells (HSCs) sit at the apex of a hierarchy of lineage-committed, specialized cells, with four probable fates for HSCs i.e. depletion, maintenance, expansion and death [42]. In the depletion mode both the daughter cells become committed to specialization resulting in an initial reduction and subsequent extinction of the stem cell pool. So HSCs are thought to generate at least one daughter cell that retains the property of the parent stem cell via the maintenance or expansion mode, thus preserving the stem cell pool within the hematopoietic system [42].

Pluripotency of Adult Stem Cells

The second property that distinguishes stem cells experimentally is their ability to give rise to all the differentiated cells within that tissue lineage *in vitro* and/or *in vivo* [43]. Pluripotency (the ability to differentiate into different cells or tissue types) is best characterized in the hematopoietic/bone marrow system, where HSCs have been demonstrated to have the ability to reconstitute all the cells of the blood (see [43] for a review). Stem cells from bone marrow seem to have the capacity to differentiate into all cells in the body like embryonic stem cells [44] The second best characterized system for the demonstration of pluripotency of stem cells is the central nervous system (CNS). Stem cells from the CNS have been shown to be able to differentiate into neurons, astrocytes and oligodendrocytes both *in vitro* and *in vivo* [45,46,47,48,49].

These two properties of self-renewal and pluripotency distinguish stem cells from other cell types in the hematopoietic/bone marrow and central nervous systems. These are now accepted to be the criteria by which putative stem cells from other adult tissues must be assessed. These characteristics are the criteria by which investigation of prostate stem cells are judged in this chapter.

Two further issues, important for this discussion, are how should self-renewal and pluripotency be assessed? There are now established protocols to measure these features in individual cells (e.g. see [45,50,48]). These methods are briefly discussed in the next section followed by comparisons of the published reports of putative adult prostate stem cells against these two criteria.

Techniques of Isolation of Adult Stem Cell from Tissues other than Prostate

Adult stem cells have been isolated, in addition to the HSCs, from solid tissues such as the brain, skin, breast and eye [51,52,53,54,55]. A common approach for the isolation of stem cells from these tissues is enzymatic (either collagenase or trypsin) digestion of the tissue followed by mechanical dissociation and *in vitro* culture of dissociated cells at variable density to permit sphere formation in media specifically developed for this purpose [45]. These spheres do not attach to the plastic and float in the culture medium. This approach has become a standard for the isolation and purification of stem cells from various solid tissues [45,50,56,54,57,53]. Self-renewal is assessed by dissociation of primary spheres into single cells that are plated out individually into 96 well plates. The generation of new spheres from the individual cell from the primary sphere providing the evidence for self-renewal [45]. This procedure is repeated at least up to the fourth generation to validate self-renewal capability of individual cells.

Various methods have been utilized to study pluripotency, including studies of differentiation following cell attachment to ionically charged glass [45], growth in semi-solid matrices such as matrigel [58] and inoculation of putative stem cells or enriched cell fractions into animals [51,50,59,60]. To be considered pluripotent, the cells must show the ability to differentiate into specialized cells [51]. For example, the self-renewing spheres from the adult brain tissue have the potential to differentiate into neurons, astrocytes, and oligodendrocytes demonstrating their pluripotency [51]. This procedure is performed, for example in the case of neural and utrical stem cells, by plating these cells on poly-L-orinithine coated coverslips and allowed to grow for 1 to 8 days [45,50].

Different terms are used in the stem cell literature to describe various cells that demonstrate differentiation short of pluripotency. Thus the term "progenitor" refers to a cell with a more restricted potential than a stem cell. "Precursor" is a less stringent term that refers to any cell that is earlier in a developmental pathway than another [51].

Recently, certain proteins (e.g. nestin, Bmi-1and Bcrp-1) have been identified as markers of stem cells in certain tissues [45,56,61]. It has been suggested that proteins such as Bmi-1 (an oncogene that causes neoplastic proliferation when over-expressed in lymphocytes [62]) are required for self-renewal of stem cells but not for survival or differentiation (thus distinguishing stem cells from progenitors during the isolation of stem cells from the CNS

[63]). Although these markers (gene or protein) may not be identical in stem cells from different tissues, these reports provide evidence of differential expression of such markers between stem and non-stem cells that may facilitate the isolation of the former.

Isolation of Adult Stem Cells from the Prostate

This area of research is at an early stage of development. A search (March 2004) of the ISI Web Science (Thomson, ISI) with the terms ‘prostate/prostatic epithelial/ stem cells’ yields a handful of citations [64,65,66,67,68,69,70,71,72], compared to the thousands of hits using the terms ‘hematopoietic stem cells’ or ‘neural stem cells’. Various factors have contributed to inertia in the field of prostate stem cells. One of the first reports extending the concept of stem cells to the prostate was that of Isaacs and Coffey [73]. In this study [73] castration in male rats resulted in the involution of the prostate gland with persistence of the basal layer. The authors observed that upon replacement of androgens, the prostate regains its original size [73]. It was concluded that a population of cells in the basal layer is capable of reconstituting the prostate in presence of androgens.

Bonkhoff and Remberger [74] also proposed a stem cell model for the prostate, suggesting that a small population in the basal cell layer gives rise to all epithelial cell lineages encountered in the normal, hyperplastic and neoplastic prostate. This population of cells was characterized mainly on the basis of staining with PSA, high molecular weight and basal specific cytokeratins, and proliferation associated antigens (such as Ki-67, PCNA and MiB-1). The authors suggested that the putative prostate stem cells reside in the basal layer. Although these reports [73,74] provided useful concepts regarding prostate stem cells, no direct evidence of either self-renewal or pluripotency was provided.

Some studies have tried to identify the subpopulation containing the stem cells. Liu et al [75] separated the epithelial cells from the basal and luminal layers and studied these in isolation and with stromal cells. When the $CD44^+$ basal cells, isolated using flow cytometry, were co-cultured with stromal cells [75], they produced PSA, suggesting differentiation into luminal cells. As the Bonkhoff and Remberger [74] model of prostate stem cells suggests that stem cells are likely to be present in the basal compartment, the authors reasoned that the $CD44^+$ basal cells possess characteristics of stem cells and are the candidate progenitors of luminal cells. However, no direct evidence for either formation of epithelial like structures or more importantly demonstration of self-renewal was provided.

In two further studies, the ability of single cells to proliferate and form colonies was equated with stem and transit amplifying (progenitor or precursor) cells [76,77]. Peehl et al [78] first described the colony forming ability of primary cultures of human prostate epithelial cells. Hudson et al [68] extended this work by identifying two distinct colony types on the basis of morphology, i.e. small irregular (90% of the total number of colonies formed on a plate) and large regular (10% of the total number of colonies formed on a plate). Evidence of a very high proliferative capacity of the large colonies, coupled with indications of pluripotency based on matrigel assays of isolated colonies was provided [68]. However, no attempt was made to test whether the cells from the large colonies possess the ability to self-renew.

Also using colony forming ability in vitro, Collins et al [65] suggested that putative prostate stem cells pre-selected on the basis of CD44 expression, express higher levels of α_2-

integrin subunit than other cells within the basal layer. About 1% of basal cells were integrin 'bright', and these cells could be selected directly from the tissue on the basis of rapid adhesion to type I collagen.

The study by Collins et al [64] provided the strongest evidence of pluripotency of a cell population isolated from adult prostate. When a basal cell population ($1x10^5$ to $1x10^6$ cells) from the prostate was xenografted in immunosuppressed mice, glandular structures developed that stained for PSA and PAP [65]. Although it is possible that self-renewing, pluripotent adult prostate stem cells may be present in the cell fraction used in the xenografts, various other committed progenitor and differentiation cells present in this fraction may also be argued to have given rise to the glandular structures. Furthermore, like other previous attempts to isolate prostate stem cells, no direct evidence of self-renewal (as that demonstrated for stem cells from other solid tissues, see section 3.1) of individual cells within this heterogeneous cell fraction was provided.

Bhatt et al [64] used a fluorescent dye (Hoechst 33342) exclusion approach to identify side populations of prostate cells. The principle behind this approach is that Hoechst 33342 binds to DNA in live cells and is therefore an indicator of cell cycle as it relates to DNA content. Hoechst 33342 is extruded by stem cells via the multi-drug resistance protein (MDR-1) [79] by an active process. Based upon this reasoning, Bhatt et al [64] suggested that a sub-population that accounts for less than 2% of the total cell population, could contain the prostate stem cells. Again, experiments to demonstrate either self-renewal or pluripotency were not performed.

Paradis et al [80] performed a study that identified a subpopulation of prostate cells assumed to contain putative prostate stem cells. The reasoning behind their approach was that within a heterogeneous cell population, stem cells are likely to have greater longevity. The expression of telomerase was used as an indicator for longevity of cells. Telomeres are repetitive, non-coding, DNA sequences at the end of human chromosomes. Erosion of telomeres with successive cell divisions is considered to be one of the mechanisms regulating cell senescence [81]. Telomerase, a ribonucleoprotein, prevents telomere shortening by adding TTAGGG repeats to the 3' end of chromosomes [82]. In most somatic cells, telomerase activity is undetectable, leading to the progressive erosion of telomeres with each cell division. In most somatic cells, telomerase activity is undetectable [80,81]. Conversely, longer living or immortalized cells have been shown to have higher levels of telomerase [83]. Paradis et al [80] demonstrated that telomerase activity was localized to the prostate epithelial basal cells and not to luminal cells. The authors did not isolate this population for further analysis of self-renewal or pluripotency, but by using the telomerase assay this study validates the likelihood of stem cell population being localized to the basal layer.

The reports claiming isolation of putative stem cells add to the body of knowledge regarding the prostate gland, but none of the cell populations were simultaneously shown to have the two essential properties of self renewal and pluripotency. Thus the definitive identification and characterization of adult human prostate stem cells has yet to be achieved.

Tumor Initiating Cells (TICs) from Normal Human Prostate

There is relatively little information regarding 'normal' prostate stem cells in the literature, and almost no information on the tumor initiating cells in the prostate. Our knowledge of the concepts of TICs is therefore derived almost entirely from other tissues.

It has been suggested by Dontu et al [52] that common genes are up-regulated in stem cells from different tissues. These include genes involved in TGF-ß signalling, growth hormone and thrombin receptor signalling as well as up-regulation of membrane transporters belonging to the ABC family [52]. Other authors have suggested that stem cells may be the targets for transformational events that lead to tumorigenesis [41,84]. A model has been developed that suggests that mutations in adult stem cells may be the initiating steps in cancer [52,85,41].

Like most of the literature in the field of stem cells, the models for tumor initiating cells or cancer stem cells have been tested mainly in the hematopoietic malignancies [62]. An important factor in the advancement of tumor initiating cell research in the hematopoietic field is the depth of understanding of normal hematopoietic development and the availability of *in vitro* and *in vivo* assays and markers for HSCs and the more differentiated cells they give rise to [86]. This understanding has allowed detailed characterization of normal development of the hematopoietic system and how it is disrupted in leukaemia [85].

More recently, evidence for stem cells in pediatric brain tumors [87] and breast cancer has been published [41,52,88]. Al-Hajj and colleagues [88] provided the first identification of the breast tumor initiating cells. A key to their approach, where others for solid tumors had failed, was the development of a reliable xenograft assay that enabled the injection of small numbers of single cells into NOD/SCID (non-obese diabetic/severe combined immune-odeficiency) mice.

There are two areas of controversy regarding cancer stem cells. The first is whether they exist and the second is from which cell are they derived? Evidence is mounting from the hematopoietic, brain and breast cancers for a stem cell fraction in cancer, analogous to that in normal tissue (see [41,52] for a review).

The greatest controversy exists over the origin of the cancer stem cell. Theoretically, it is possible that the cancer stem cell arises at any point in the differentiation pathway. However, if it is correct that it is only stem cells that have a long life span, then it is unlikely that the more differentiated cells live long enough to accumulate the mutations necessary to give rise to cancer. Nevertheless, the cancer stem cell will pass on all the genetic changes it has acquired to its more differentiated offspring, and therefore it is likely that later steps in the progression of the cancer may be due to additional genetic changes in a more differentiated fraction of the cancer.

The most important consequence of the stem cell theory for the individual with prostate or some other cancer is that by targeting the cancer stem cells, it may be possible to cure the cancer [67]. For this to be applied to prostate cancer requires that both normal and prostate cancer stem cells be isolated, cultured and characterised, but also specific markers need to be identified, ideally on the cell surface, that will enable the stem cells to be targeted.

Future Perspectives

The identification and characterization of adult prostate stem cells is at an early stage. Nevertheless, there have been significant advances in the identification and characterization of stem cells from tissues such as brain, skin, eye and breast [51,52,53,54,55]. The improvement in adult tissue stem cell isolation techniques and identification of common stem cell markers from these tissues should also help to accelerate progress in the isolation of adult prostate stem cells. However, due to the distinct anatomical and cellular make up of the prostate (see sections 1 and 2) there may be complexities associated with the isolation of stem cells. For example, are the cells from the various anatomical zones (section 1) maintained by independent stem cells or is there an adult master prostate epithelial stem cell that maintains all these zones? If so, where do these stem cells reside? Are the differences observed in different malignancies associated with these zones reflective of independent TICs? These and many more fundamental questions await what we hope to be a vigorous period of research in the field of adult prostate stem cells. There remains much work to be done, but it should be possible to make rapid progress based on the advances in other tissue and tumor types.

References

[1] Lieberman, Ronald. Androgen deprivation therapy for prostate cancer chemoprevention: current status and future directions for agent development. *Urology* 58: 83-90, 2001.

[2] Huggins, C., Stevens, R. E., and Hodges, C. V. Studies on prostatic cancer II - The effects of castration on advanced carcinoma of the prostate gland. *Arch.Surg.* 43: 209-223, 1941.

[3] Wojno, K. J. and Epstein, J. I. The utility of basal cell-specific anti-cytokeratin antibody (34 beta E12) in the diagnosis of prostate cancer. A review of 228 cases. *Am.J.Surg.Pathol.* 19: 251-260, 1995.

[4] Rojas-Corona, R. R., Chen, L. Z., and Mahadevia, P. S. Prostatic carcinoma with endocrine features. A report of a neoplasm containing multiple immunoreactive hormonal substances. *Am.J.Clin.Pathol.* 88: 759-762, 1987.

[5] Kuriyama, M., Loor, R., Wang, M. C., Lee, C., Killian, C. S., Papsidero, L. D., Inaji, H., Nishiura, T., Slack, N. H., Murphy, G. P., and Chu, T. M. Prostatic acid phosphatase and prostate-specific antigen in prostate cancer. *Int.Adv.Surg.Oncol.* 5: 29-49, 1982.

[6] McNeal, J. E. The zonal anatomy of the prostate. *Prostate* 2: 35-49, 1981.

[7] Leung, C. S. and Srigley, J. R. Distribution of lipochrome pigment in the prostate gland: biological and diagnostic implications. *Hum.Pathol.* 26: 1302-1307, 1995.

[8] McNeal, J. E., Redwine, E. A., Freiha, F. S., and Stamey, T. A. Zonal distribution of prostatic adenocarcinoma. Correlation with histologic pattern and direction of spread. *Am.J.Surg.Pathol.* 12: 897-906, 1988.

[9] Arenas, M. I., Romo, E., de, Gaspar, I, de Bethencourt, F. R., Sanchez-Chapado, M., Fraile, B., and Paniagua, R. A lectin histochemistry comparative study in human normal

prostate, benign prostatic hyperplasia, and prostatic carcinoma. *Glycoconj.J.* 16: 375-382, 1999.

[10] Reese, J. H., McNeal, J. E., Redwine, E. A., Samloff, I. M., and Stamey, T. A. Differential distribution of pepsinogen II between the zones of the human prostate and the seminal vesicle. *J.Urol.* 136: 1148-1152, 1986.

[11] Reese, J. H., McNeal, J. E., Redwine, E. A., Stamey, T. A., and Freiha, F. S. Tissue type plasminogen activator as a marker for functional zones, within the human prostate gland. *Prostate* 12: 47-53, 1988.

[12] Reese, J. H., McNeal, J. E., Goldenberg, S. L., Redwine, E. A., and Sellers, R. G. Distribution of lactoferrin in the normal and inflamed human prostate: an immunohistochemical study. *Prostate* 20: 73-85, 1992.

[13] Kobayashi, S., Demura, T., Nonomura, K., and Koyanagi, T. Autoradiographic localization of alpha 1-adrenoceptors in human prostate: special reference to zonal difference. *J.Urol.* 146: 887-890, 1991.

[14] Kobayashi, S., Tang, R., Wang, B., Opgenorth, T., Stein, E., Shapiro, E., and Lepor, H. Localization of endothelin receptors in the human prostate. *J.Urol.* 151: 763-766, 1994.

[15] Krill, D., DeFlavia, P., Dhir, R., Luo, J., Becich, M. J., Lehman, E., and Getzenberg, R. H. Expression patterns of vitamin D receptor in human prostate. *J.Cell Biochem.* 82: 566-572, 2001.

[16] Mirowitz, S. A. and Hammerman, A. M. CT depiction of prostatic zonal anatomy. *J.Comput.Assist.Tomogr.* 16: 439-441, 1992.

[17] Hricak, H., Jeffrey, R. B., Dooms, G. C., and Tanagho, E. A. Evaluation of prostate size: a comparison of ultrasound and magnetic resonance imaging. *Urol.Radiol.* 9: 1-8, 1987.

[18] Koslin, D. B., Kenney, P. J., Koehler, R. E., and Van Dyke, J. A. Magnetic resonance imaging of the internal anatomy of the prostate gland. *Invest. Radiol.* 22: 947-953, 1987.

[19] Villers, A., Terris, M. K., McNeal, J. E., and Stamey, T. A. Ultrasound anatomy of the prostate: the normal gland and anatomical variations. *J.Urol.* 143: 732-738, 1990.

[20] Costello, L. C. and Franklin, R. B. Citrate metabolism of normal and malignant prostate epithelial cells. *Urology* 50: 3-12, 1997.

[21] Costello, L. C. and Franklin, R. B. Novel role of zinc in the regulation of prostate citrate metabolism and its implications in prostate cancer. *Prostate* 35: 285-296, 1998.

[22] Costello, L. C. and Franklin, R. B. The intermediary metabolism of the prostate: A key to understanding the pathogenesis and progression of prostate malignancy. *Oncology* 59: 269-282, 2000.

[23] Jemal, A., Tiwari, R. C., Murray, T., Ghafoor, A., Samuels, A., Ward, E., Feuer, E. J., and Thun, M. J. Cancer statistics, 2004. *CA Cancer J.Clin.* 54: 8-29, 2004.

[24] Hald, T. Urodynamics in benign prostatic hyperplasia: a survey. *Prostate Suppl* 2: 69-77, 1989.

[25] Berry, S. J., Coffey, D. S., Walsh, P. C., and Ewing, L. L. The development of human benign prostatic hyperplasia with age. *J.Urol.* 132: 474-479, 1984.

[26] Bostwick, D. G. and Brawer, M. K. Prostatic intra-epithelial neoplasia and early invasion in prostate cancer. *Cancer* 59: 788-794, 1987.

[27] Bostwick, D. G. Prospective origins of prostate carcinoma. Prostatic intraepithelial neoplasia and atypical adenomatous hyperplasia. *Cancer* 78: 330-336, 1996.

[28] Bonkhoff, H., Stein, U., and Remberger, K. Multidirectional differentiation in the normal, hyperplastic, and neoplastic human prostate: simultaneous demonstration of cell-specific epithelial markers. *Hum.Pathol.* 25: 42-46, 1994.

[29] McNeal, J. E., Price, H. M., Redwine, E. A., Freiha, F. S., and Stamey, T. A. Stage A versus stage B adenocarcinoma of the prostate: morphological comparison and biological significance. *J.Urol.* 139: 61-65, 1988.

[30] Shah, I. A., Schlageter, M. O., Stinnett, P., and Lechago, J. Cytokeratin immunohistochemistry as a diagnostic tool for distinguishing malignant from benign epithelial lesions of the prostate. *Mod.Pathol.* 4: 220-224, 1991.

[31] Ronnett, B. M. and Epstein, J. I. A case showing sclerosing adenosis and an unusual form of basal cell hyperplasia of the prostate. *Am.J.Surg.Pathol.* 13: 866-872, 1989.

[32] Gleason, D. F. and Mellinger, G. T. Prediction of prognosis for prostatic adenocarcinoma by combined histological grading and clinical staging. *J.Urol.* 111: 58-64, 1974.

[33] Stein, B. S., Vangore, S., Petersen, R. O., and Kendall, A. R. Immunoperoxidase localization of prostate-specific antigen. *Am.J.Surg.Pathol.* 6: 553-557, 1982.

[34] di Sant'Agnese, P. A. Neuroendocrine differentiation in carcinoma of the prostate. Diagnostic, prognostic, and therapeutic implications. *Cancer* 70: 254-268, 1992.

[35] di Sant'Agnese, P. A. Neuroendocrine differentiation in human prostatic carcinoma. *Hum.Pathol.* 23: 287-296, 1992.

[36] Stevens, L. C. Studies on transplantable testicular teratomas of strain 129 mice. *J.Natl.Cancer Inst.* 20: 1257-1275, 1958.

[37] Till, J. E. and McCulloch, E. A. A direct measurement of the radiation sensitivity of normal mouse bone marrow cells. *Radiat.Res.* 14: 213-222, 1961.

[38] Metcalf, D., Moore, A. S., and Shortman, K. Adherence column and buoyant density separation of bone marrow stem cells and more differentiated cells. *J.Cell Physiol.* 78: 441-450, 1971.

[39] Stevens, L. C. The development of transplantable teratocarcinomas from intratesticular grafts of pre- and postimplantation mouse embryos. *Dev.Biol.* 21: 364-382, 1970.

[40] Blau, H. M., Brazelton, T. R., and Weimann, J. M. The evolving concept of a stem cell: entity or function? *Cell* 105: 829-841, 2001.

[41] Reya, T., Morrison, S. J., Clarke, M. F., and Weissman, I. L. Stem cells, cancer, and cancer stem cells. *Nature* 414: 105-111, 2001.

[42] Dick, J. E. Stem cells: Self-renewal writ in blood. *Nature* 423: 231-233, 2003.

[43] Weissman, I. L. Stem cells: units of development, units of regeneration, and units in evolution. *Cell* 100: 157-168, 2000.

[44] Jiang, Y., Jahagirdar, B. N., Reinhardt, R. L., Schwartz, R. E., Keene, C. D., Ortiz-Gonzalez, X. R., Reyes, M., Lenvik, T., Lund, T., Blackstad, M., Du, J., Aldrich, S., Lisberg, A., Low, W. C., Largaespada, D. A., and Verfaillie, C. M. Pluripotency of mesenchymal stem cells derived from adult marrow. *Nature* 418: 41-49, 2002.

[45] Rietze, R. L., Valcanis, H., Brooker, G. F., Thomas, T., Voss, A. K., and Bartlett, P. F. Purification of a pluripotent neural stem cell from the adult mouse brain. *Nature* 412: 736-739, 2001.

[46] Gage, F. H. Mammalian neural stem cells. *Science* 287: 1433-1438, 2000.

[47] Reynolds, B. A. and Weiss, S. Generation of neurons and astrocytes from isolated cells of the adult mammalian central nervous system. *Science* 255: 1707-1710, 1992.

[48] Qian, X., Shen, Q., Goderie, S. K., He, W., Capela, A., Davis, A. A., and Temple, S. Timing of CNS cell generation: a programmed sequence of neuron and glial cell production from isolated murine cortical stem cells. *Neuron* 28: 69-80, 2000.

[49] Morshead, C. M. and van der Kooy, D. Disguising adult neural stem cells. *Curr. Opin. Neurobiology* 14: 125-131, 2004.

[50] Li, H., Liu, H., and Heller, S. Pluripotent stem cells from the adult mouse inner ear. *Nat.Med.* 9: 1293-1299, 2003.

[51] McKay, R. Stem cells in the central nervous system. *Science* 276: 66-71, 1997.

[52] Dontu, G., Al Hajj, M., Abdallah, W. M., Clarke, M. F., and Wicha, M. S. Stem cells in normal breast development and breast cancer. *Cell Prolif.* 36 Suppl 1: 59-72, 2003.

[53] Dontu, G., Abdallah, W. M., Foley, J. M., Jackson, K. W., Clarke, M. F., Kawamura, M. J., and Wicha, M. S. In vitro propagation and transcriptional profiling of human mammary stem/progenitor cells. *Genes Dev.* 17: 1253-1270, 2003.

[54] Tropepe, V., Coles, B. L., Chiasson, B. J., Horsford, D. J., Elia, A. J., McInnes, R. R., and van der, Kooy D. Retinal stem cells in the adult mammalian eye. *Science* 287: 2032-2036, 2000.

[55] Toma, J. G., Akhavan, M., Fernandes, K. J., Barnabe-Heider, F., Sadikot, A., Kaplan, D. R., and Miller, F. D. Isolation of multipotent adult stem cells from the dermis of mammalian skin. *Nat.Cell Biol.* 3: 778-784, 2001.

[56] Molofsky, A. V., Pardal, R., Iwashita, T., Park, I. K., Clarke, M. F., and Morrison, S. J. Bmi-1 dependence distinguishes neural stem cell self-renewal from progenitor proliferation. *Nature* 425: 962-967, 2003.

[57] Carpenter, M. K., Cui, X., Hu, Z. Y., Jackson, J., Sherman, S., Seiger, A., and Wahlberg, L. U. In vitro expansion of a multipotent population of human neural progenitor cells. *Exp.Neurol.* 158: 265-278, 1999.

[58] Aarum, J., Sandberg, K., Haeberlein, S. L., and Persson, M. A. Migration and differentiation of neural precursor cells can be directed by microglia. *Proc.Natl.Acad.Sci.U.S.A* 100: 15983-15988, 2003.

[59] Bjornson, C. R. R., Rietze, R. L., Reynolds, B. A., Magli, M. C., and Vescovi, A. L. Turning brain into blood: A hematopoietic fate adopted by adult neural stem cells in vivo. *Science* 283: 534-537, 1999.

[60] Mezey, E., Chandross, K. J., Harta, G., Maki, R. A., and McKercher, S. R. Turning blood into brain: Cells bearing neuronal antigens generated in vivo from bone marrow. *Science* 290: 1779-1782, 2000.

[61] Zhou, S., Schuetz, J. D., Bunting, K. D., Colapietro, A. M., Sampath, J., Morris, J. J., Lagutina, I., Grosveld, G. C., Osawa, M., Nakauchi, H., and Sorrentino, B. P. The ABC transporter Bcrp1/ABCG2 is expressed in a wide variety of stem cells and is a molecular determinant of the side-population phenotype. *Nat.Med.* 7: 1028-1034, 2001.

[62] Haupt, Y., Bath, M. L., Harris, A. W., and Adams, J. M. bmi-1 transgene induces lymphomas and collaborates with myc in tumorigenesis. *Oncogene* 8: 3161-3164, 1993.

[63] Krishnamurthy, P., Ross, D. D., Nakanishi, T., Bailey-Dell, K., Zhou, S., Mercer, K. E., Sarkadi, B., Sorrentino, B. P., and Schuetz, J. D. The stem cell marker Bcrp/ABCG2 enhances hypoxic cell survival through interactions with heme. *J.Biol.Chem.* 279: 24218-24225, 2004.

[64] Bhatt, R. I., Brown, M. D., Hart, C. A., Gilmore, P., Ramani, V. A. C., George, N. J., and Clarke, N. W. Novel method for the isolation and characterisation of the putative prostatic stem cell. *Cytometry Part A* 54A: 89-99, 2003.

[65] Collins, A. T., Habib, F. K., Maitland, N. J., and Neal, D. E. Identification and isolation of human prostate epithelial stem cells based on alpha(2)beta(1)-integrin expression. *J.Cell Sci.* 114: 3865-3872, 2001.

[66] Signoretti, S., Waltregny, D., Dilks, J., Isaac, B., Lin, D., Garraway, L., Yang, A., Montironi, R., McKeon, F., and Loda, M. p63 is a prostate basal cell marker and is required for prostate development. *Am. J.Pathol.* 157: 1769-1775, 2000.

[67] Anderson, K. M., Bonomi, P., and Harris, J. E. Does an inability to eradicate normal stem cells preclude the cure of some cancers? *Medical Hypotheses* 47: 31-34, 1996.

[68] Hudson, D. L., O'Hare, M., Watt, F. M., and Masters, J. R. Proliferative heterogeneity in the human prostate: evidence for epithelial stem cells. *Lab. Invest.* 80: 1243-1250, 2000.

[69] Foster, C. S., Dodson, A., Karavana, V., Smith, P. H., and Ke, Y. Prostatic stem cells. *J.Pathol.* 197: 551-565, 2002.

[70] De Marzo, A. M., Nelson, W. G., Meeker, A. K., and Coffey, D. S. Stem cell features of benign and malignant prostate epithelial cells. *J.Urol.* 160: 2381-2392, 1998.

[71] De Marzo, A. M., Meeker, A. K., Epstein, J. I., and Coffey, D. S. Prostate stem cell compartments - Expression of the cell cycle inhibitor p27(Kip1) in, normal, hyperplastic, and neoplastic cells. *Am. J.Pathol.* 153: 911-919, 1998.

[72] Bonkhoff, H. and Remberger, K. Morphogenesis of benign prostatic hyperplasia and prostate carcinoma. *Pathologe* 19: 12-20, 1998.

[73] Isaacs, J. T. and Coffey, D. S. Etiology and disease process of benign prostatic hyperplasia. *Prostate Suppl* 2: 33-50, 1989.

[74] Bonkhoff, H. and Remberger, K. Differentiation pathways and histogenetic aspects of normal and abnormal prostatic growth: a stem cell model. *Prostate* 28: 98-106, 1996.

[75] Liu, A. Y., True, L. D., LaTray, L., Nelson, P. S., Ellis, W. J., Vessella, R. L., Lange, P. H., Hood, L., and van den, Engh G. Cell-cell interaction in prostate gene regulation and cytodifferentiation. *Proc.Natl.Acad.Sci.U.S.A* 94: 10705-10710, 1997.

[76] Buick, R. N. and Pollak, M. N. Perspectives on clonogenic tumor cells, stem cells, and oncogenes. *Cancer Res.* 44: 4909-4918, 1984.

[77] Popova, N. V., Teti, K. A., Wu, K. Q., and Morris, R. J. Identification of two keratinocyte stem cell regulatory loci implicated in skin carcinogenesis. *Carcinogenesis* 24: 417-425, 2003.

[78] Peehl, D. M., Wong, S. T., and Stamey, T. A. Clonal growth characteristics of adult human prostatic epithelial cells. *In Vitro Cell Dev.Biol.* 24: 530-536, 1988.

[79] Goodell, M. A., Brose, K., Paradis, G., Conner, A. S., and Mulligan, R. C. Isolation and functional properties of murine hematopoietic stem cells that are replicating in vivo. *J.Exp.Med.* 183: 1797-1806, 1996.

[80] Paradis, V., Dargere, D., Laurendeau, I., Benoit, G., Vidaud, M., Jardin, A., and Bedossa, P. Expression of the RNA component of human telomerase (hTR) in prostate cancer, prostatic intraepithelial neoplasia, and normal prostate tissue. *J.Pathol.* 189: 213-218, 1999.

[81] Levy, M. Z., Allsopp, R. C., Futcher, A. B., Greider, C. W., and Harley, C. B. Telomere end-replication problem and cell aging. *J.Mol.Biol.* 225: 951-960, 1992.

[82] Morin, G. B. The human telomere terminal transferase enzyme is a ribonucleoprotein that synthesizes TTAGGG repeats. *Cell* 59: 521-529, 1989.

[83] Kim, N. W., Piatyszek, M. A., Prowse, K. R., Harley, C. B., West, M. D., Ho, P. L., Coviello, G. M., Wright, W. E., Weinrich, S. L., and Shay, J. W. Specific association of human telomerase activity with immortal cells and cancer. *Science* 266: 2011-2015, 1994.

[84] Tu, S. M., Reyes, A., Maa, A., Bhowmick, D., Pisters, L. L., Pettaway, C. A., Lin, S. H., Troncoso, P., and Logothetis, C. J. Prostate carcinoma with testicular or penile metastases. Clinical, pathologic, and immunohistochemical features. *Cancer* 94: 2610-2617, 2002.

[85] Dick, J. E. Breast cancer stem cells revealed. *Proc.Natl.Acad.Sci.U.S.A* 100: 3547-3549, 2003.

[86] Weissman, I. L. Translating stem and progenitor cell biology to the clinic: barriers and opportunities. *Science* 287: 1442-1446, 2000.

[87] Hemmati, H. D., Nakano, I., Lazareff, J. A., Masterman-Smith, M., Geschwind, D. H., Bronner-Fraser, M., and Kornblum, H. I. Cancerous stem cells can arise from pediatric brain tumors. *Proc.Natl.Acad.Sci.U.S.A* 100: 15178-15183, 2003.

[88] Al Hajj, M., Wicha, M. S., Benito-Hernandez, A., Morrison, S. J., and Clarke, M. F. Prospective identification of tumorigenic breast cancer cells. *Proc.Natl.Acad.Sci.U.S.A* 100: 3983-3988, 2003.

In: Perspectives in Stem Cell Research ISBN: 978-1-61122-985-1
Editors: Brenda M. Davis and Christopher B. Halton

Chapter IV

MESENCHYMAL STEM CELLS IN VASCULAR THERAPY

Gael Y. Rochefort*
LAB.P.ART., EA3852, IFR 135
UFR Medecine, Universite François Rabelais
10 Bd Tonnelle, BP 3223, 37032 TOURS Cedex
France

ABSTRACT

Mesenchymal stem cells (MSCs) constitute a heterogeneous population of undifferentiated and committed multipotential cells. They serve in vitro and in vivo as precursors for bone marrow stroma, bone, fat, cartilage, muscle (smooth, cardiac and skeletal) and neural cells. They are able to home upon engraftment to a number of microenvironments, capable of extensive proliferation and of producing large number of differentiated progenitors to repair functionally tissue after injury. MSCs are usually isolated from adult bone marrow but can also be isolated from several other tissues, such as fetal liver, adult circulating blood, umbilical cord blood, placenta or adipose tissue. Furthermore, MSCs present several immuno-regulatory characteristics with immuno-suppressive effects that induce a tolerance and could be therapeutic for reduction of graft-versus-host disease, rejection and modulation of inflammation.

Since MSCs follow a vascular smooth muscle differentiation pathway, their therapeutic potential has been widely investigated in the treatment of vascular diseases. Indeed, MSCs can participate in the development of new vessels from pre-existing vascular walls (angiogenesis), in the induction of new vascular networks (vasculogenesis), in the collateral artery growth (arteriogenesis) or in plastic and reconstructive surgery applications. These cells can promote vascular growth by incorporating into vessels' wall, but they also may function as supporting factors by producing paracrine vascular promoting factors. In this chapter, the mesenchymal stem cells isolation, culture and characterization, but also their potential use in vascular therapy, in both human and animal models, are reported and discussed, whereas

* Tel. (+33) 247 366 091; gael.rochefort@gmail.com

perspectives in angiogenesis, vasculogenesis, arteriogenesis or vascular engineering are explored.

I. Introduction

The biology of stem cells and progenitors is currently one of the most promising fields of investigation, with a very broad potential of application in the field of regenerative medicine. Most of the stem cell and progenitor studies were initially focused on the contribution of a mixed cell population, composed of poorly characterized stem cells among a larger population of support cells, on the tissue regeneration after injection. Next, the specific role of characterized and defined stem cell populations like mesenchymal stem cells (MSCs) was assessed *in-situ* or after local injections, with in particular the role of MSCs during cardiopulmonary remodeling. At last, many recent studies were focused on the stem cell angiogenic potential and on their paracrine action during the initial development of pathologies. This is particularly true in the vascular biology field, where many studies were interested in the participation of various stem cell types, such as MSCs, in angiogenesis and the revascularization of specific organs, like lungs, heart or peripheral vessels.

Arterial remodeling, characterized either by an expansive remodeling (by widening) or by a constrictive remodeling (by a diameter reduction), is an important factor that can be observed under various pathological conditions involving a lot of different cells, such as smooth muscle cells. The origin of the smooth muscle cells in several vascular remodeling is not clearly established. These cells can indeed come from a local proliferation of the smooth muscle cells that are present in the vessel media at the lesion level, but these cells can also come from the differentiation of stem cells or progenitors that are also present in the vessel media or from circulating progenitors. The therapeutic use of stem cells to repair an organ or tissue degenerative lesion becomes thus a very attractive possibility.

Adult stem cells are constitutively present in most tissues and organs, including the skin, lungs, the liver, the heart and the bone marrow, thus authorizing local tissue regeneration during physiological or pathological processes. The bone marrow is composed of hematopoietic stem cells (HSCs) closely associated to a bone marrow stroma responsible for their survival, their proliferation, their self-renewal and their differentiation into mature blood cells. This stromal tissue is mainly made up of stromal cells, which follow a vascular smooth muscle differentiation, osteoblasts, adipocytes and endothelial cells, all deriving from the differentiation of MSCs. These multipotent stem cells have also the capacity to give rise to chondrocytes and to differentiate into other cell types, such as hepatocytes or nervous-related cells. These stem cells represent a heterogeneous population of cells having very variable characteristics according to studies, culture conditions and species. Moreover, MSCs have a strong proliferation potential as well as immuno-modulating capacity allowing these cells to become powerful tools in the treatment of pathologies by cell therapy.

II. What Is a Stem Cell?

A. Definitions and Ontogenesis

Definition: The classic definition of a stem cell is an entity that meets the basic characteristics of self-renewal, clonality, multi-potentiality, generation of differentiated cells, and *in vivo* functional reconstitution of a given tissue [1]. Admittedly, this definition may be satisfactory for embryonic stem cells (ES) or the primordial stem cells, the zygote, but this definition is not applicable in all occurrences and is best used as a guide to help describe cellular attributes.

Indeed, stem cells have varying degrees of potential, ranging from the totipotency (ability to form the whole embryo and its annexes, i.e. the trophoblast of the placenta or the amnios) of the fertilized oocyte (the zygote), to the pluripotency (ability to form all tissues from the three germ layers) of ES cells, to the multipotency (capacity to differentiate into a limited range of cell lineages appropriate to their location) of most tissues derived stem cells, and at last to the unipotency (only able to generate one cell type) of progenitor cells such as intestinal epithelial precursors, gastric epithelial precursors or spermatogonial cells of the testis [2]. Thus, a more complete description of a stem cell includes a consideration of replication capacity, clonality, and potency.

Self-renewal: Stem cells are often described with expressions such as "immortal", "unlimited", "continuous", and "capable of extensive proliferation". All these terms, used to describe the stem cell's replicative or proliferative capacity, must be probably best used sparingly if at all.

Clonality: This important characteristic is the idea that stem cells are clonogenic entities, where a single stem cell has the capacity to create more stem cells with the same capacities. Indeed, the best cellular preparation would be a high purified clonal population of stem cells, but it must be recognized that most cellular stem cell preparations, that do not derive from a single cell, may be a mixed population containing stem cells and a separate population of "supportive" cells required for the propagation of the purported stem cells.

Potency: This basic and widely accepted characteristic is supported by the idea of a lineage hierarchy of each cell type. Thus, the primordial totipotent stem cell generates among other things multipotent stem cells, which then generate multiple types of differentiated cells with distinct morphologies and gene expression patterns.

Plasticity: This idea is based on the fact that restrictions in cell fates are not permanent but are flexible and reversible. In that way, a terminally differentiated somatic cell can be reverse to another committed cell fate by dedifferentiation. A related concept is that of trans-differentiation, where a functional cells from a tissue, organ, or lineage can be generated from another cell type that is distinct from that of the founding stem cell. Important issues are to known whether the cells supposed to dedifferentiate and trans-differentiate are clonal or not, and whether the mechanism by which they form the functional cell requires fusion.

Tissue reconstitution: The best assessment of this characteristic is to purify a population of cells, transplant a single cell into an acceptable host without any intervening *in vitro* culture, and observe self-renewal and tissue, organ, or lineage reconstitution. Admittedly, this type of *in vivo* reconstitution assay is not well defined for many types of adult stem cells, but this developmental potential remains to be accurately defined for *in vitro* assays. Nevertheless, this clonal assay should be the standard by which fetal and adult stem cells should be evaluated because it removes doubts about contamination with other cell types.

Ontogenesis: The concept of stem cells came from the hematopoietic system where the short blood cells lifetime and the high need of renewal require a quick, high and continuous generation of blood cells to avoid aplasia. This blood cells production is provided by the bone marrow hematopoietic stem cells (HSC) that are able to self-renew and to engender the whole blood lineage.

B. Totipotent Stem Cells

The first cell of life, the zygote (the fertilized egg) is also the first totipotent stem cell and has the exclusive ability to generate an entire organism from the three germ layers to the embryonic annexes. This totipotency is retained by early progeny of the zygote up to the eight-cell stage of the morula. Subsequently, cell differentiation results in the formation of a blastocyst composed of two cell types. The first one, the outer trophoblast cells, is composed of multipotent cells and generates the embryonic annexes. Indeed, trophectoderm stem cells have been isolated, and these only generate cells of the trophectoderm lineage. The second cell type, the undifferentiated inner cells commonly referred to as the "inner cell mass", generates ES cells and embryonic germinal stem cells (EG) that are no longer totipotent but pluripotent and retain the ability to develop into all cell types of the embryo proper [3]. ES and EG cells generate all somatic lineages as well as germ cells but rarely if ever contribute to the trophectoderm, extra-embryonic endoderm, or extra-embryonic mesoderm. Importantly, no totipotent stem cell has been isolated from early embryo.

C. Pluripotent Stem Cells

Researches on pluripotent stem cells, which are able to form all tissues from the three germ layers, dates back to the early 1970s with mouse ES cells, and is now widely extended to other species. Pluripotent stem cell lines have been generated from human livestock (review in [4]) but also from model organisms, such as chicken [5, 6], hamster [7], rabbit [8, 9] and rat [10-13]; however, only mouse and chicken ES cells have proven capable of colonizing the germ line. The establishment of ES cell lines from nonhuman primates, including rhesus monkey [14, 15], common marmoset (*Callithrix jacchus* [16]), and cynomolgus monkey (*Macaca fascicularis* [3, 17]) is also of major importance for human stem cell research.

To date, three pluripotent stem cell types have been fully establish, including embryonic carcinoma cells (EC), embryonic stem (ES) cells and primordial germ (PG) cells.

EC: Embryonic carcinoma cells were firstly generated from a mouse germ-line tumor, called teratocarcinomas [18], and were then established as cell lines [19-21] in the early 1970s. This "funny little tumor" produced benign teratomas or malignant teratocarcinomas [22, 23] after transplantation to extra-uterine sites of appropriate mouse strains. When clonally isolated, EC cells retained the differentiation capacity and could produce derivatives of all three primary germ layers, including ectoderm, mesoderm, and endoderm. Furthermore, when introduced into the inner cell mass of early embryos, EC cells were able to participate in embryonic development and to generate chimeric mice [24].

However, EC cells demonstrated chromosomal aberrations [25], lost their ability to differentiate [26], or differentiated *in vitro* only under specific conditions [27] and with chemical inducers such as dimethyl sulphoxide or retinoic acid [28]. The undifferentiated state maintenance was also relied only on cultivation with feeder cells [29]. Furthermore, EC cells only sporadically colonized the germ line after transfer into early blastocysts [30]. All these data suggested that the EC cells had undergone cellular changes during the transient tumorigenic state *in vivo*, and thus partially retain the pluripotent capacities of early embryonic cells (see [31] for review).

ES: Embryonic stem cell lines are originated from the inner cell mass and can be maintained *in vitro* without any apparent or significant loss of differentiation potential, even after several hundred divisions. The demonstration of their pluripotency was made *in vivo* by their introduction into a mouse blastocyst in the early 1980s. The resulting mouse chimera demonstrated that the introduced ES cells could contribute to all cell lineages including the germ line [32]. *In vitro*, mouse ES cells also showed the capacity to generate various somatic cell types from the three germ layers [33-35]. ES cells were finally found to generate germ cell lines *in vitro* only in the early 2000s [36-38]. ES cells are characterized by the high proliferation ability, by *in vitro* differentiation capacities [39], by the presence of stem cell markers typical of other stem cell lines, and by the capacity to erase gene imprints.

PG: The third embryonic cell type with pluripotent capabilities is the primordial germ cells, which form normally within the developing genital ridges. Isolation and cultivation of mouse PG cells on feeder cells led to the establishment of mouse embryonic germ cell lines [40-42]. Once transferred into blastocysts, these cells can contribute to somatic and germ cell lineages in chimeric animals [40-43]. Finally, PG cells retain the capacity to erase gene imprints.

D. Multipotent Stem Cells

Multipotent stem cells have the fundamental capacity to differentiate into a limited range of cell lineages appropriate to their location. Most tissues derived stem cells self-renew and generate single stem cell-derived daughter cells that are able to differentiate *in vitro* and *in vivo* into more than one cell type. Several examples are now known, include hematopoietic stem cells (HSC), neural stem cells (NSC), endothelial progenitor cells (EPC), or mesenchymal stem cells (MSC). Multipotent stem cells also contribute to the generation of differentiated progeny *in vivo* even in the absence of tissue damage [44].

HSC: Hematopoietic stem cells, the first tissue-specific stem cells to be prospectively isolated [45], are one of the most stem cells used in routine clinical, with extensive use of grafts and transplantations in the treatment of a variety of blood cell diseases such as leukemias or autoimmune disorders [46]. In fact, HSCs were extensively reported to repopulate the tissue of origin when transplanted in a damaged recipient. In the hematopoietic system, HSCs reside at the top of the hematopoietic hierarchy and give rise to several functional cells. All these distinct types are produced from HSCs in successive differentiation processes, producing intermediary increasingly committed progenitor cells. Because of the very short life span of most cells, mature blood cell production is an ongoing process and the estimated production reaches 1.5 x 10^6 blood cells every second in an adult human. In that case, this high turnover rate necessitates profound homeostatic control mechanisms where the primary level is the HSC itself.

EPC: As epithelial tissue comprises 60% of the differentiated tissue types in mammals, epithelial stem cells and EPCs need to reach a high proliferative potential when a broad array of diseases, injuries and wounds are surrounded [47]. EPCs were first identified in the late 1990s as a population of postnatal mononuclear blood cells that adopted an adherent, endothelial morphology when cultured for 7 days in endothelial growth medium [48]. Like endothelial cells, these isolated cells incorporated acetylated DiI-LDL, expressed several markers in common with endothelial cells such as CD34, CD31, vascular endothelial growth factor receptor 2 and Tie2. To date, the circulating EPC contributions to angiogenesis in tumors, ischaemic injury or other diseases, and their usefulness in the repair of wounded hearts and limbs remain under intense investigation.

NSC: Neural stem cells can generate neural tissue or are derived from the nervous system, have the ability to self-renew, and can generate other cells than themselves through asymmetric cell division [49]. Neural stem cells are more frequent in the developing mammalian nervous system but are retained in the adult nervous system of all mammalian organisms, including humans. A variety of neural dysfunctions are now candidates for NSC-based cell therapy, including many neurodegenerative diseases such as Parkinson's disease, Alzheimer's diseases, and genetic disorders such as Batten's, Gaucher's, and Tay Sach's diseases. The potential for tissue repair is not restricted to the replacement of neurons, and a promising approach is the generation of oligodendrocytes from stem cells to promote repair in diseases such as multiple sclerosis [50].

MSC: mesenchymal stem cells are multipotent stem cells that can be differentiated into several cells types, including fibroblasts, osteoblasts, chondroblasts, and adipocytes. More information regarding this multipotent cell type is given below.

E. Unipotent Stem Cells

Unipotent stem cells are probably best described as progenitors. Indeed, progenitors are typically the descendants of stem cells; they are more constrain in their differentiation potential or capacity for self-renewal and can only produce one type of differentiated descendant that is no more a stem cell. Intestinal epithelial precursors, gastric epithelial precursors or satellites cells, which conduct to the formation of muscle fibers, are some example of progenitors.

F. Between Differentiation and Self-Renewing: The Stem Cell Niche

The first stem cell niche, the bone marrow HSC niche, was first formally laid by Schofield in 1978 after an analysis of findings on the spleen colony-forming cell (CFU-S) [51]. Schofield proposed that stem cells are fixed tissue cells that are prevented from differentiation and continue to proliferate as stem cells within a functionally and spatially characterized "niche", where the micro-anatomic environment, composed of neighboring stromal cells, supports and instructs stem cells. However, the stem cell niche concept was largely neglected until its recent resurgence with Drosophila studies [52].

A stem cell niche is an interactive structural unit, composed of tissue cells, extracellular substrates and micro-environmental cells that nurture stem cells and enable them to maintain their undifferentiated state capacities and tissue homeostasis [53]. An appropriate spatio-temporal dialog occurs between stem cells and niche cells in order to fulfill lifelong demands for differentiated cells and to facilitate cell-fate decisions in a proper spatiotemporal manner. Niche cells provide a sheltering environment that sequesters stem cells from differentiation, apoptotic, or other stimuli that would challenge stem cell reserves. The niche also safeguards against excessive stem cell production that could lead to cancer. Stem cells must be periodically activated to produce progenitors or transit amplifying cells that are committed to produce mature cell lineages. Thus, the hallmark of a functional niche is to maintain a balance between stem cell quiescence and activity, with key signaling and molecular cross-talk events that occurred in the right place at the right time [54, 55]. Interactions with other cell types and the components of the extracellular matrix are believed to control the stem cell survival and self-renewal, the progeny production and the generation of the committed cells.

G. Stemness

The core stem cell properties of self-renewal and common molecular processes underlying the generation of differentiated progeny are referred in the literature by "stemness". Although stems cells in different cellular microenvironments or niches will by necessity have different physiological demands and therefore distinct molecular programs, there are likely certain genetic characteristics specific to and shared by all stem cells.

Stem cells appear to have the capacity to sense a broad range of growth factors and signaling molecules and to express many of the downstream signaling components involved in the transduction of these signals, including TGFβ, Notch, Wnt, and Jak/Stat family members. Stem cells also express many molecules according to the establishment of their specialized cell cycles. Thus, most quiescent adult stem cells express compounds related to maintaining cell cycle arrest, whereas stem cells rapid cycling, as is the case for example for ES cells, depends on molecules connected to progression through cell cycle checkpoints. There is considerable evidence that stem cells express high levels of telomerase enzyme and with higher activity, and present significantly remodeled chromatin involving DNA methylases or transcriptional repressors of histone deacetylase. Finally, most stem cells have the molecular and functional characteristic to be resistant to stress mediated by the expression of multi-drug resistance transporters, protein-folding machinery, ubiquitin, and detoxifier systems [3].

Identification of cell surface and molecular markers has proven critical to define the molecular basis of stem cell balance between self-renewal and determination/commitment toward lineages. In the future, it may be possible to define stem cells as a whole and individually entity by their molecular identities, and thus to precisely describe the stemness concept [3].

III. Mesenchymal Stem Cells

A. Origin

1. Historical Identification

Mesenchymal stem cells (MSC) were first identified by Alexander Friedenstein who described undifferentiated progenitors cells in adult bone marrow [56-58]. When seeding at low density in liquid medium containing serum, bone marrow cells from rabbits or rodents, formed after few days discrete colonies containing plastic-adherent, non phagocytic, elongated cells that resemble to fibroblasts. Such colony being generated from a single cell was called colony-forming unit-fibroblasts (CFU-F). When seeded individually under the renal capsule of semi-syngeneic animals, each colony generated after a few weeks fibrous tissue, bone and bone-containing bone marrow. Friedenstein also observed by using chimerical animals that fibrous tissue and bone cells were of donor origin, while marrow hematopoietic cells within the bony spaces were provided by the host. He hypothesized that the bone marrow contains a population of progenitors capable to generate *in vivo* fibrous tissue and bone, and that the CFU-F-generated bone-containing tissue express cellular and/or molecular components proving the adequate microenvironment for HSC homing and growth. Friedenstein was thus the first to conjecture the existence of stem cell niches within the bone marrow.

Then in the early 1990s, Arnold Caplan defined MSCs as cells that would give rise not only to bone and marrow stroma, but also to cartilage, tendon, and muscle [59]. During the course of the years, these cells received several designations and abbreviations. Maureen Owen used in 1988 the term of “Stromal Stem Cells” to underline the fact that MSCs are generated from the stromal layer of long-term bone marrow cultures [60, 61]. In 1997, Darwin Prockop proposed that the abbreviation of MSC could stands for either “Mesenchymal Stem Cell” or “Marrow Stromal Cell”, because of their capacity to serve also as niche for other types of stem cells such as HSCs [62]. James Dennis used in 1999 the term of “Mesenchymal Progenitor Cell” to indicate that this cell type may not represent an authentic category of stem cells but be closer to progenitor/transit amplifying cells situated downstream of the stem cell compartment [63]. Pamela Gehron Robey and Paolo Bianco used in the early 2000s the term of “Skeletal Stem Cell” to emphasize the specificity for MSCs to give rise to the different cellular components of skeletal tissues [64-67]. Finally, Catherine Verfaillie’s team described a cell population that may represent a more primitive cell type with differentiation potential larger than that of MSCs, and they designated it as “Mesodermal Progenitor Cells” [68] and “Multipotent Adult Progenitor Cells” (MAPCs) [69].

2. Source

a) Various Species

MSC, or progenitor cells with similar features, can be isolated from many different species.

The best characterized are those of human [67, 70-75], murine [76-78] and rat [79-81] origin but MSCs from guinea pigs, cats [82], baboons [83], sheep [84], dogs [85], pigs [86,

87], cows [88] and horses [89, 90] provide a better opportunity to test their therapeutic potential in large mammal systems.

b) Tissue Localization

MSCs are widely distributed with a variable proportion in several fetal and adult tissues. However, MSCs are often a rare population in these tissues.

Adult bone marrow: The most well studied and accessible source of MSCs is the adult bone marrow [70, 76, 78, 91]. MSCs are a rare population of the bone marrow microenvironment, present in a low frequency that may represent 0.01-0.0001% of the adult human bone marrow nucleated cells [74, 75].

Other adult tissues: To date, cells with mesenchymal stem cell characteristics were isolated from several tissues such as spleen [92], liver [92, 93], kidney [92], pancreas [92, 94], lung [92], smooth muscle [92], skeletal muscle [91, 95, 96], aorta [92], vena cava [92], brain [92], thymus [92], dental pulp [97], deciduous teeth [96], scalp tissue and hair follicle [98, 99], periosteum [95, 96], trabecular bone [96], adipose tissue [95, 96, 100] and synovium [95, 96].

Fetal tissues: MSCs have also been isolated from several fetal tissues including fetal liver [101-103], fetal bone marrow [102, 103], fetal thymus [104], fetal lung [102], fetal spleen [102] and fetal pancreas [105]. MSCs can also be isolated with a variable proportion from several parts of the placenta including chorionic villi of the placenta [73-75, 106], amniotic fluid [107], umbilical cord blood collections [108] and umbilical cord vein [72, 109].

Blood sample: Blood samples are of particular importance because of the facility to be obtained. Thus, MSCs were described in the peripheral blood of normal adults [71, 110] and healthy women during or following pregnancy [111], where they may be of fetal origin and may persist for more than 60 years [56, 112]. MSCs can also been isolated from fetal blood [71, 103] and from fresh umbilical cord blood [108, 113, 114] and cryopreserved cord blood [115].

c) Mobilization

The term of mobilization indicates the recruitment into the bloodstream after treatment (chemotherapy, cytokine injection) or physiopathological events, and the enhancement of the physiological release of stem cells and progenitors from reservoirs, such as the bone marrow, in response to stress signals during injury and inflammation. Currently, mobilized cells are the preferable and major source of stem and progenitor cells because of the higher yield of these cells and decreased procedural risks compared with harvested BM cells [116]. Less known than the HSC mobilization, the MSC specific mobilization process might be initiated by repeated stimulation with cytokines such as granulocyte colony-stimulating factor (G-CSF) or granulocyte-macrophage colony-stimulating factor (GM-CSF) [110, 117, 118], or recently by several physiopathological circumstances, such as chronic hypoxia [79], myocardial infarction or encephalopathy [119].

Thus, after injection of G-CSF during the development of hypoxic encephalopathy in mice, MSCs were found mobilized in the blood system, homed into damaged zones and committed into specialized elements [119]. After myocardial infarction and G-CSF treatment in lethally irradiated mice, MSCs were found mobilized and expressed cardiomyogenic markers [120]. Finally, chronic hypoxia has been shown to increase the circulating concentration of MSCs without increasing the circulating hematopoietic progenitor cells concentration [79].

B. Culture

1. Isolation

There are as many different isolation procedures as there are tissue sources, species and publications, but we have summarized the MSC procedure outlines.

The bone marrow-derived MSCs are obtained from bone shafts. Typically, cells are aspirated into a syringe containing anticoagulant, wash with medium or with phosphate-buffered saline and cultured at a density of 10^4 to 10^5 cells/cm^2. The first change of medium is performed between 2 and 3 days after initial plating and adherent cells are cultured during 2 to 3 weeks until they reach 80%–90% confluence. Tissue-derived MSCs are usually obtained after enzymatic digestion. The tissue is washed several times, mechanically minced and then enzymatically digested (with trypsin and/or collagenase). Digested tissue is filtered through cell strainer to eliminate undigested fragments, washed and then cultured at a density of 10^5 to 10^6 cells/cm^2. At last, blood-derived MSCs (from umbilical cord blood or from peripheral blood) are obtained after a low-density fraction separation (e.g. Ficoll). The mononuclear cell fraction is washed and then cultured at a density of 10^6 to 10^7 cells/cm^2.

Some authors also optimize their isolation procedures with a subpopulation fraction enrichment (depletion or enrichment), with red cells disruption, with dish coating (e.g. fibronectin, gelatin or collagen), or with growth factor and cytokine supplementation.

2. CFU-F

Contributions to our understanding of stromal precursor cells were provided by Friedenstein, Owen, and colleagues. Indeed, they demonstrated the growth of colonies of cells morphologically resembling to fibroblasts when single cell suspensions of bone marrow were explanted at low densities (10^4 to 10^5 cells/cm^2). In liquid cultures generated from single-cell suspensions, colonies were formed, each derived from a single precursor cell termed the colony-forming-unit fibroblast (CFU-F) and described as rapidly adherent, non-phagocytic clonogenic cells capable of extended proliferation in vitro [58, 121]. When these cells were plated at higher densities, the colonies merged early and grew as monolayer.

To visualize and enumerate CFU-F, cells are usually stained with Giemsa solution, washed and then air-dried. CFU-F colonies are typically between 1 and 8mm in diameter and are scored macroscopically.

3. A Heterogeneous Population

When grown *in vitro* in fetal calf serum, culture-expanded MSCs form characteristic adherent, fibroblast-like colonies that may be expanded further in the presence of various growth factors [122, 123] and thus appear to be homogeneous according to a number of criteria. The morphology is usually that of elongated cells with, in particular in murine cultures, thin filopodial extensions. However, the homogeneity of the cultured cell population depends on culture conditions.

Initial cell growing populating is consisted of cells with two different morphologies: one population with a fibroblastic, spindle-shaped morphology and another with an epithelioid, polygonal morphology. After passaging, the epithelioid population disappears rapidly from culture and it is no longer found thereafter. The fibroblastic population of cells continues to proliferate, even after numerous passages [75]. These single-cell derived colonies are morphologically heterogeneous and contain a mixture of small and larger cells [68, 124]. The proliferative activity of MSC appears to be directly proportional to their differentiation potential but both cell types are similarly efficient in supporting cultures of hematopoietic stem cells [56]. Small cells, about 7μm in diameter and spindle-shaped with large nuclear-to-cytoplasmic ratio, are in the G0-G1 phase of the cell cycle and, after a lag phase, these cells rapidly renew; whereas large cells, about 15μm in diameter and widespread, slowly renew [124, 125]. The selection of adherent cells by day 2-4 [70] and the passages, required to get rid of contaminating hematopoietic cells (usually 1-2 passages for human, but 4-6 for murine cultures), may lead to a more homogeneous population.

The population heterogeneity is better assessed on freshly isolated cells or, at least, on cells cultured for short spans of time. The proliferative capacity and differentiation potential heterogeneity were greatly revealed by clonal studies of human bone marrow cells. Thus, Pittenger and co-workers [70] but also Muraglia and collaborators [126] both proved that only one third of the human MSC clones studied were tripotential and were able to differentiate into osteoblasts, chondrocytes and adipocytes, whereas the clones generated by the team of Phinney differed widely in their expression of alkaline phosphatase, an osteoblast marker [76]. In 2002 and using immortalized human MSCs, Okamoto *et al.* found that only a minority of the generated clones were multipotential [127]. At last, the generation of bone-like tissue *in vitro* did not appear to reflect the capacity of forming bones *in vivo* [128] and only 50% of these clones had the ability to form bone *in vivo* [123]. However, this apparent heterogeneity is not translated into a distinctive and specific phenotype (see below) and only few phenotypical studies report heterogeneity. Thus, Gronthos and collaborators used the membrane expression of alkaline phosphatase within a human Stro-1$^+$ MSC subset to discriminate a population of cells with a restricted differentiation potential into osteoblastic cells [129]. Finally, the human STRO-1$^+$ MSC subpopulation was also reported to have a higher engraftment potential in spleen, bone marrow and kidneys, a lower engraftment potential in lungs, and a lesser hematopoiesis-supportive capacity than the Stro-1$^-$ MSC subset [130].

Taken together, all these data indicate that MSCs constitute a heterogeneous cell population that may reflects a hierarchy of stem and transit amplifying cells as described for HSCs. In 2000, Muraglia *et al.* proposed a hierarchy model based on clonogenic studies, where early tripotent mesenchymal progenitors display a sequential loss of lineage potentials and generate osteo-chondrogenic progenitors, which, in turn, give rise to osteogenic precursors [126].

4. Phenotype

To date, no specific immuno-phenotypic markers have been identified to allow the phenotypic isolation of MSCs, but in contrast, MSCs express a wide variety of antigens presented by many other cell types. Therefore, the MSC identification is based on an extensive panel of markers, including differentiation and lineage specific markers, adhesion molecules, extracellular matrix, and growth factor receptors [122, 131, 132]. MSCs are most homogeneously accepted positive for CD13, CD29, CD44, CD49a, CD49e, CD73 (SH3 and SH4), CD90, CD105 (SH2), CD106, CD166 and HLA ABC but are negative for the hematopoietic and/or endothelial markers CD31, CD34, CD45 and HLA DR [70, 74, 133,

134]. Nevertheless, few antigens appear to be present on cell subsets only [135, 136], and to add confusion to the issue of MSC specific markers, there are evidences that some molecules are variably expressed depending on time in culture and the extent of MSC multipotency [56, 137].

C. Properties

1. Growth and Self-Renewing

The proliferation potential: *In vitro*, human CFU-Fs show extensive proliferation capacity, giving rise to colonies that can reach several millimeters in diameter, but the MSC proliferation is restricted by the Hayflick's limit of 50 cell doublings [70, 138], with shortened telomeres and lacking telomerases [139]. Although, when transfected with the catalytic unit of the telomerase, MSCs then obtained are displaying improved proliferation, hematopoiesis-supportive capacity and differentiation potential *in vitro* [131, 140]. *In vivo*, extensive proliferation can be observed only in models with intense mesenchymal turnover such as osteogenesis imperfecta [141].

Tritiated thymidine continuous labeling of fresh bone marrow harvested cell reveals that CFU-Fs are not cycling *in vivo* [57], and their subsequent development into colonies and their entry into the cell cycle depend on serum growth factors *in vitro* [142]. In fact, higher cell doublings might be achieved when adding specific growth factors (e.g., fibroblast growth factor-2) to the basal culture medium [143]. Cell seeding density also plays a critical role in the MSC expansion capacity, because a higher expansion profile (2,000-fold expansion) is obtained when MSCs are plated at very low density (1.5-3 cells/cm^2) whereas a lower expansion profile (60-fold expansion) is observed when cells are plated at higher density (12 cells/cm^2) [124].

The self-renewal capacity: This ability to generate identical copies of themselves through mitotic division over extended periods is one of the defining characteristics of a stem cell and the MSC absolute self-renewal potential remains unclear, due in large part to the different methods employed to derive MSC populations. *In vitro*, some CFU-Fs can be expanded many times, and *in vivo*, ossicle formation capacity is transferable for up to five passages [144]. However, the demonstration of the self-renewal capacity of multipotential cells can be made only in models with sufficient and systemic cell renewal such as osteogenesis imperfecta. To date, there are no experiments in such models where cells from reconstituted tissues (e.g. cartilage, bone, or other tissues) from a primary recipient were injected into a secondary recipient to show that the multipotential reconstituting activity had been maintained in the primary recipient and transferable to the second.

2. The Bone Marrow Microenvironment and Hematopoiesis Support

The bone marrow hematopoiesis niche can be subdivided into a hematopoietic cell compartment and a stroma compartment, which is mainly composed of fibroblasts, adipocytes, nerves, and the bone marrow's vascular system [54, 56]. However, mesenchymal cells are always found in fetal liver and in fetal bone marrow as early as 9 weeks of gestation before the onset of definitive hematopoiesis [145-148]. MSCs are also reported to circulate in fetal blood in high numbers from at least 7 weeks gestation. The circulating fetal MSC rate is at its highest level early in the first trimester and declines to around 0.0001% during the second trimester [103]. Thus, MSCs might contribute to the establishment of hematopoiesis [56].

The supporting role of marrow stromal cells in hematopoiesis was firstly evidenced by Friedenstein, who reported the formation of bone-like structures ("ossicles") when marrow stromal cells were transplanted under the capsule kidney, and where the donor stroma was colonized by hematopoietic cells deriving from the host [149]. Furthermore, donor HSCs engrafted in the host stromal microenvironment during clinical bone marrow transplantation *in vivo*, whereas MSCs supported hematopoiesis *in vitro* for periods longer than 6 months in Dexter cultures [150] and thus allowed the generation of all lineage, including myeloid, lymphoid, and megakaryocytic cells [56].

The hematopoietic bone marrow microenvironment is composed of osteoblasts and their extra-cellular products, adipocytic cells and several ad-luminal mural stromal cells with smooth muscle characteristics, including endothelial cells, capillary pericytes, parasinusal myoid cells, adventitial reticular cells, barrier cells [54, 151-155]. All these cells might derive from MSCs since they are able to differentiate into osteoblasts, adipocytes, vascular smooth muscle-like stroma, and more controversially into endothelial cells [156, 157].

3. Lineage Differentiation

During the embryonic development, the neuron-ectodermal lineage gives rise to the peripheral and central nervous systems, but also to the epithelial lineage which will become epidermal tissue, and partially to muscles (muscles of the iris, the arrector pili muscles attached to hairs, and the myoepithelial cells of the lacrimal, salivary, sweat and mammary glands) [158, 159]. Mesoderm gives rise to muscles (skeletal, cardiac, visceral and vascular smooth muscles), bone, cartilage, blood and connective tissue [160]. Pancreas and liver cells derive from the endoderm layer [3, 161, 162].

a) Mechanism

Adult stem cells are able to differentiate into cells of the tissue in which they reside; however, this committed fate dogma has been extended during the last few years with several evidences for the multi-lineage differentiation potential of many stem cell types including MSCs [163]. In fact, MSCs are not only able to differentiate into limb-bud mesodermal tissues, including osteoblasts, chondroblasts, adipocytes, fibroblasts and skeletal myoblasts [62, 70, 133, 164, 165], but they are also able to acquire characteristics of cell lineages outside the limb-bud, such as endothelial cells [69, 166], neural cells [167-169], and cells of the endoderm [1, 69, 170, 171], *in vitro* and *in vivo* [172-174].

In the early 2000s, Markus Loeffler and his team proposed a single cell-based stochastic model to describe the stem cell organization and to explain the cell kinetic and functional stem cell heterogeneity, flexibility and reversibility of cellular properties, self-organized regeneration after damage, fluctuating activity and competition of stem cell clones, and microenvironment dependency of stem cell quality [175-177]. To illustrate the flexibility and reversibility concept, they postulated that stem cells might change their proliferative status, change their lineage specification, lose and subsequently re-acquire their self-renewal potential. In fact, the MSC differentiation potential does not appear to be an irreversible process because cells apparently terminally differentiated may shift their differentiation pathway when placed in specific *in vitro* conditions [178]. Thus, for examples adipocytes may turn into osteoblasts, osteoblasts into chondrocytes, chondrocytes into adipocytes, and so on [179].

This lineage reversibility does not result from the selection of a subset because it has been reported at the single cell (clonal) level; and furthermore several lineage characteristics are reported to be expressed at the same time indicating an intermediate state between several lineages. Indeed, MSCs express simultaneously, at the mRNA or protein level, adipocytic and chondrocytic and/or osteoblastic or vascular smooth muscle markers [178], but also present structures specific for vascular smooth muscle cells and adipocytes [180]. This property of plasticity, implying de-differentiation and reprogramming, might be explained by the stimulation of several distinct lineage-specific transcription factors already activated in primitive stem cells and thus by making cells receptive to extrinsic factors (hormones, cytokines, cell contacts…).

Recently, the bone marrow stem cells trans-differentiation was discussed after the observation of spontaneous fusion of stem cells to adopt the phenotype of the recipient cells. Moreover, cell fusion is reported to be a frequent rather than rare event and up to 1% of human MSCs were recovered as bi-nucleated cells [181, 182]. However, other studies demonstrated that stem-cell plasticity is a true characteristic of stem cells and can be achieved without cell fusion [173, 183].

Whatever the degree of differentiation of the cell undergoing the differentiation shift, plasticity has major functional consequences: it removes the theoretical requirement of hierarchy and self-renewal since it makes possible for a daughter cell to recover the full differentiation potential of the mother MSC at the origin of the clone.

b). Ectodermal Tissues

The ectoderm is the start of a tissue that covers the body surface. It emerges first and forms the outermost of the germ layers. The ectoderm forms several tissues, including the central nervous system, retina and lens, cranial bones, ganglia and nerves, pigment cells, head connective tissue, epidermis, hair, mammary glands.

Skin-related tissue: The skin, perhaps the largest organ in the body, is composed by three layers, the dermis, the epidermis and the hypodermis, and has several physiological functions. Indeed, skin keeps organs in place, stops pathogens entering, helps in the prevention of getting burnt, prevents unregulated water loss, is almost waterproof, is sensitive to touch and pain, regulates body temperature through homeostasis, makes vitamin D and melanin, and finally has an excretory role in removing urea.

When co-cultured directly or indirectly with heat-shocked human sweat gland cells, human MSCs differentiate into gland cells. Indeed, carcinoembryonic antigen, a specific marker of the sweat gland which is not expressed elsewhere in the normal skin [184, 185], and cytokeratin 19, a structural protein of intermediate filaments which is expressed in both ductal and secretory cells of normal human sweat glands [184], are both expressed by MSCs after both the direct and indirect co-culture differentiation conditions [186]. When implanted subcutaneously into nude mice, human MSCs produce E-cadherin and contribute to the development of hair follicles by forming epithelial-like cells *in vitro* and *in vivo*, by following a mesenchymal to epithelial transition [187, 188]. Furthermore, the hair follicle may represent a suitable, accessible source for MSCs [99, 187].

Like other stem cells, MSCs are also widely and successfully used in the treatment of extensive wounds and deep burn injury [189, 190]. Indeed, the transplantation of bone marrow MSCs allows the regeneration of the dermis in wound healing and the reduction of scar formation [191-193]. In addition, MSCs are able to migrate *in vivo*, proliferate and differentiate into either matrix epithelial cells (which form the hair shaft) or cornified keratinocytes (which form skin) in response to epidermal damage [187]. At last, here are several protocols that allow stem cells to differentiate into the keratinocyte lineage *in vitro* [194].

Central nervous system-related tissue: During the brain development, neurons migrate from the neural tubes and differentiate into various neural cells and satellite cells. It has long been established that mature neurons lack their proliferation potential, but in 1992, Reynolds and Weiss [195] isolated for the first time the multipotential stem cells from the striatum of adult human brain and induced them into neural cells *in vitro*. Although further researchers showed that only a very few sites, such as the sub-ventricular zone, may contain neural stem cells (NSC), this discovery necessitated revision of classical assumptions of neuronal theory and problems associated with regeneration. Indeed, NSCs are present in the brain during the entire life span of mammals and humans; they can be isolated and differentiated into all three types of neural cells. NSCs might offer some wonderful perspectives for cell therapy of neurodegenerative diseases and injuries of the central nervous system, but on the other hand, the problems of immunological compatibility of allogeneic NSCs remain unsolved, as are the ethical problems. Recently, MSCs were reported to possess the potential of *in vitro* differentiation into NeuN-expressing neurons and astrocytes expressing glial fibrillary acidic protein (GFAP) when cultured under appropriate conditions [168], but also *in vivo*, after implantation into the brain tissue [167, 169].

As a matter of fact, MSCs were reported to express neural markers at baseline [196-198], and their neural differentiation into glial and neuron-like cells can be easily obtained after co-culturing with NSCs or with stimulating culture media and factors [196-203], whereas some groups failed to show glial and neural markers [204, 205]. Several methods of induction were developed to differentiate human or rodent MSCs into neuron-like cells [168, 196, 204, 206], including combinations of different growth factors and retinoic acid [207]. MSCs thus acquired new morphological characteristics, neural markers, and electrophysiological properties compatible with a neuronal differentiation [208].

After infusion into a rat brain, MSCs can engraft, migrate and survive without any evidence of an inflammatory response or rejection [202]. Injected MSCs react to brain microenvironment signals, differentiate into glia and neurons [202, 203], and promote restoration and regeneration of the nervous tissue after brain or spinal cord injuries [203, 209-211].

Eye-related tissue: The retinal pigment epithelium (RPE) is the pigmented cell layer just outside the retina that contains retinal visual cells, and is firmly attached to the underlying choroid and overlying retinal visual cells. The RPE is composed of a single layer of hexagonal cells that are densely packed with pigment granules. When viewed from the outer surface, these cells are smooth and hexagonal in shape. When seen in section, each cell consists of an outer non-pigmented part containing a large oval nucleus and an inner-pigmented portion, which extends as a series of straight thread-like processes between the rods, this being especially the case when the eye is exposed to light.

When co-cultured *in vitro* with retina or sub-retinal cells, or when cultured with epidermal growth factor and activin A, MSCs were able to generate cells expressing markers for photoreceptors like opsin [212], rhodopsin and recoverin [213]. Recently, MSCs were also reported to have the ability to adopt a RPE-like morphology *in* vivo after sub-retinal grafting into normal adult rats and into RPE degenerative rat model. MSCs thus adopted the hexagonal morphology of RPE cells, and expressed the epithelial marker cytokeratin after transplantation [214]. Finally, MSCs made contacts with adjacent recipient cells, expressed the tight junction protein ZO-1 [215], and retinal cell-specific markers including calbindin and rhodopsin [216].

c) Mesodermal Tissues

The mesoderm germ layer is forming in triploblastic animals during gastrulation, where some of the cells migrating inward to contribute an additional layer between the endoderm and the ectoderm. The formation of a mesoderm led to the formation of a coelom where organs formed inside can freely move, grow, and develop independently of the body wall while fluid cushions protects them from shocks. The mesoderm forms several tissues, including skeletal muscles, skeleton, dermis of skin, connective tissue, urogenital system, heart, blood (lymph cells), and spleen.

Adipocytic lineage: The primary role of adipocytes is to store energy and to break down this stored lipid into free fatty acids when energy is required. Adipocytes also play a major role in the control of metabolism through secretion of paracrine and endocrine hormones that have effects on feeding behavior, metabolism, insulin sensitivity and secretion, and reproductive and immune functions [217]. Finally, adipose tissue has a major impact on energy flux, plasma lipid levels, and rates of glucose uptake.

During the embryonary development, the adipose lineage arises from a multipotent stem cell population of mesodermal origin residing in the vascular stroma of adipose tissue, and undergoes a multi-step differentiation process, comprising an initial commitment step and then a subsequent activation program resulting in the adipocyte phenotype. Factors that initiate this process are now identified and secreted by the vascular stromal population and/or adipocytes. These factors are now used *ex vivo* to induce the commitment of MSCs to the adipose lineage [218, 219].

MSCs express small amounts of the crucial transcription factors that promote adipogenesis, such as CCAAT-enhancer-binding protein α (C/EBPα) and peroxisome proliferator-activated receptor γ (PPARγ) [220-224], but also osteogenic factors such as RUNX2, MSX2, DLX5, and osterix [225-227]. As factors of one lineage repress factors of the other lineages, thereby maintaining the undifferentiated state, the balance may be tipped under appropriate conditions leading to a cascade that promotes one cell fate while repressing other possible fates. Indeed, RUNX2 represses adipogenesis, and furthermore cells with suppressed Runx2 show enhanced adipocyte development [228], whereas mice lacking PPARγ have increased bone mass while PPARγ agonists decrease bone density in normal mice [229-231].

C/EBPα and PPARγ proteins, already present in uncommitted MSCs [232, 233], may be induced after the treatment with a differentiation cocktail and promote the adipocytic differentiation [234]. Insulin is classically viewed as a promoter of adipogenesis when using low concentrations, whereas high concentrations of insulin activate the IGF-I receptor, have a mitogenic effect and slightly inhibit adipogenesis [235]. Serums, insulin, dexamethasone, indomethacin and 3-isobutyl-1-methylxanthine (IBMX) are thus classically used to induce the differentiation of MSCs into the adipose lineage. Then, the adipogenic differentiation is usually shown by cellular accumulation of large lipid vacuoles, visualized after Oil Red O staining that has an excitation wavelength of 485 and an emission wavelength of 595 nm. The gene and protein expression of all factors that are involved in regulation of the differentiation process during adipogenic conversion may also be assessed by reverse-transcription and Western blotting [79, 236-238].

Osteogenic lineage: Bones are rigid organs that form part of the skeleton of vertebrates. One of the first functions of the skeleton is to hold up the body and supports muscles and soft organs. Bones enclose and protect the brain, spinal cord, lungs, heart, pelvic viscera and bone marrow. Bones provide the rigid attachment and leverage that allow skeletal muscle movements. Red bone marrow is the major producer of blood cells, including most cells of the immune system. The skeleton is also the body's main mineral reservoir; it stores calcium and phosphate and releases them according to the body's physiological needs. Finally, bones buffer the blood against excessive pH changes by absorbing or releasing alkaline mineral salts.

During early development, neural crest cells give rise to the cranio-facial skeleton whereas the axial skeleton (spine, sternum, rib cage) is derived from sclerotome cells that came from somites, and finally, the lateral-plate mesoderm give rise to the appendicular skeletal components (limbs) [239]. In the postnatal state, cells with osteogenic potential like MSCs persist in the bone marrow and play an integral part in bone growth and remodeling, as well as bone repair. After migration of cells with osteogenic potential (mesenchymal cells) to the site of future skeletogenesis, the process of bone development is followed by mesenchymal-epithelial interactions that lead to condensation or aggregation of MSCs and subsequent differentiation into either the chondrogenic or osteogenic lineage.

Thus, several strategies were extensively used to direct the *in vitro* differentiation of MSCs into the osteogenic and chondrocytic lineages for tissue repair [134, 240, 241]. The first of them was to develop a defined culture medium for directing osteogenic differentiation of MSCs *in vitro*. Thus, several exogenous cytokines and growth factors were used, including various isoforms of bone morphogenic protein (BMP) which are all members of the transforming growth factor-β (TGF-β) superfamily [242-245], interleukin-6 (IL-6) [246], growth hormone [247], leptin [248], sortilin [249], and transglutaminase [250]. In addition to cytokines and growth factors, several non-proteinaceous chemical compounds have also been used to promote stem cell differentiation into the osteogenic lineage *in vitro*, including prostaglandin E_2 (a natural eicosanoid) [251, 252], 1,25-dihydroxyvitamin D3 (the active form of vitamin D3 also known as calcitriol) [253], L-ascorbic acid (vitamin C) [254], dexamethasone (a synthetic steroid) [254-257], β-glycerol phosphate [257], the synthetic potent inducer TAK-778 [258, 259], and statins [260-262]. Another strategy to direct osteogenic differentiation of MSCs *in vitro* was to co-culture the stem cells with a different stem cell population. Indeed, co-culture with chondrocytes is reported to have a positive effect on the osteogenic differentiation of MSCs [250, 263, 264], but also co-culture with myeloma cells [265], vascular endothelial cells [266, 267], calvarial dura mater cells [268, 269], non-adherent bone marrow cells [270] and differentiated osteoblasts [254, 262], bone sialoprotein [271], osteopontin [272], osteocalcin [273], osteonectin [254] and osteocrin [274].

To promote osteogenic differentiation *in vivo*, MSCs were firstly seeded *in vitro* on extracellular matrices such as hydroxyapatite and then subcutaneously implanted *in vivo* into NOD/SCID mice, subsequently observing bone formation [275]. Next, MSCs were used to repair segmental bone defects of critical size in various animal models, including rabbit, sheep, rat, mice, goat, pig and dog [276-285]. Then, MSCs infused *in situ* into irradiated mice with osteogenesis imperfecta were able to promote the formation of functional bone and cartilage [141]. Similarly, with children suffering of osteogenesis imperfecta, infused MSCs were not only able to engrafted without any side effect, but they also increased the osteoblast number three months after, the formation of new lamellar bone and the total body mineral content [286]. After that and especially for orthopedic applications, natural or synthetic biomaterials were used as carriers for MSC delivery [287], with the use of nonporous, biologically inert materials (ceramics or titanium), and porous, resorbable and osteoconductive biomaterials (hydroxyapatite and tricalcium phosphate) [288, 289]. The next step was to use cell-matrix compounds, composed of MSCs seeded on hydroxyapatite/ tricalcium phosphate ceramics [290] or poly-L-lactide-co-glycolide [291], which were successfully used *in vivo* to repair critical segmental bone defects in animals but also in humans with large bone defects [292], to reconstruct a phalanx [293], or to repair a mandible [294].

Chondrogenic lineage: Cartilage is a type of dense connective tissue composed of collagenous fibers and/or elastic fibers, and chondrocytes, all embedded in a matrix of gel-like ground substance. Cartilage is avascular and serves several functions, including providing a framework for bone deposition, and supplying smooth surfaces for the movement of articulating bones. Cartilage is found in many places in the body including joints, rib cage, ear, nose, bronchial tubes and between inter-vertebral discs. During embryonic development, cartilage is enclosed in a dense connective tissue called the perichondrium, which also contains the cartilage cell precursors (chondroblasts), and is afterward replaced by bone (ossification) or remains unossified during the whole of life (joint cartilage).

To promote the chondrogenic differentiation of MSCs *in vitro*, two different strategies were adapted from the original method of the "pellet" culture system [295, 296]. This system is based on the aggregation of MSCs into a conical tube and the culture of pelleted cells with a defined serum-free medium. Indeed, "alginate bead" culture system, that maintained the differentiated phenotype of encapsulated cells over times, allows freshly isolated articular chondrocytes but also MSCs to synthesize *in vitro* a matrix similar to that of native articular cartilage and to maintain their chondrogenic phenotype for as long as eight months [297-299]. The second strategy to induce chondrogenesis *in vitro* is to allow MSCs to form a compact cell pellet in conical tubes (by gently centrifugation) and to incubate them with a chemically defined serum-free medium, consisting of high-glucose Dulbecco modified Eagle medium supplemented with insulin, transferrin, selenious acid, linoleic acid, ascorbate 2-phosphate, dexamethasone and TGF-β [295, 296]. The chondrogenic differentiation is finally checked by the Safranin O or toluidine blue specific staining of cartilage glycosaminoglycans on formalin-fixed paraffin or resin embedded aggregates, whereas up-regulation of both type II and X collagens is also usually confirmed.

In vivo, undifferentiated MSCs have been used to repair full-thickness, joint cartilage defects in animal models using various carrier matrices [300-304] since local injections of chondrocyte suspension inducing clinical benefits were described [305], allowing the development of MSC-based strategies to induce *in situ* differentiation of mesenchymal progenitors into cartilage [306, 307]. Thus, evidence of regeneration of the injured knee meniscus after medial denisciectomy and resection of the anterior crucial ligament was observed when allogeneic MSCs were injected into goats in combination with hyaluronan carrier [308]. Furthermore, goats treated in that way showed a significant decrease of bone resorption with subchondral bone remodeling, osteophyte formation and cartilage destruction, and a better preservation of the joint lining, without any signs of inflammation or immune rejection [308]. This kind of cartilage regeneration is also reported in rabbit with the full reparation of joint cartilage defect after injection of autologous MSCs dispersed in a type I collagen gel [302], or with the reparation of osteochondral defects after injection of MSC-loaded phosphate and hyaluronan deriving from sponges [309]. Like with the osteogenic lineage differentiation, the chondrogenic differentiation is promoted when using poly-L-lactic acid and poly-L-lactide-co-glycolide synthetic polymers [310, 311]. In a rat model, MSCs have been successfully used to repair intervertebral discs after local injection with a reported 100% cell viability [312]. Autologous MSC injection was also successfully realized to treat patients with osteoarthritis [303], showing the feasibility of MSC therapy for cartilage repair in human.

Finally, the mostly effective strategy to treat joint cartilage defects might be to use the combination of bioactive tridimensional matrices and scaffolds, osteoinductive growth factors and cytokines (such as the bone morphogenetic protein-2), and injection of MSCs [313-317].

Tendon: A tendon is a tough band of fibrous connective tissue that connects muscle to bone, or muscle to muscle and that is designed to withstand tension. Tendons are similar to ligaments except that ligaments join one bone to another. Tendons and muscles work together and can only exert a pulling force. Tendons are composed mainly of water, type-I collagen and tenocytes or tendinocytes, which are inactive fibrocytes. Minor fibrillar collagens, fibril-associated collagens and proteoglycans are present in small quantities and are critical for tendon structure. Most of the strength of tendon is due to the vertical, hierarchical arrangement of densely packed collagen fibrils. Tenocytes are specialized fibroblasts responsible for the maintenance of collagen structure; they produce collagen molecules that aggregate end-to-end and side-to-side to produce collagen fibrils. Blood vessels may be visualized within the endotendon running parallel to collagen fibers, with occasional branching transverse anastomoses. After tendon injury, rehabilitation and repair are long processes that could easily last eight to twelve weeks. During this time, immobilization and protected motion are required because the inability to return to full function early puts the healing tendon at risk of complications.

Recently, several animal and human studies have evaluated the efficiency of MSC local injections in tendon repair [318, 319]. Indeed, local injection of autologous MSCs in a type I collagen gel significantly improved tendon repair [320]. Unexpectedly almost 30% of the MSC grafted tendons demonstrated evidences of ectopic tendon formation in the regenerating repair site [320], but unfortunately, the maximum force and maximum stress for the MSCs grafted repairs were only around 30% of normal control [320]. When implanted into long gap defects in the rabbit Achilles tendon, biochemical and histological analysis revealed that MSCs collagen composites improved biomechanical properties, tissue architecture and functionality of the tendon after injury [321]. Furthermore, 12 weeks after surgery, the repaired tissue presented a modulus and maximum stress around one third of normal values [321].

Tendon and ligament tissue regeneration may be enhanced by using exogenous growth or differentiation factors (GDF), members of the TGF-beta factor super-family implicated in tendon formation, including GDF-5, GDF-6 and GDF-7 [322]. Scaffold alone, but also scaffolds seeded with poly-lactide-co-glycolide have also the potential to regenerate and repair gap defect of Achilles tendon and to restore structure and function [323, 324]. MSC viability in culture, but also biomechanics and histological appearance 12 weeks after surgery, may as well be improved by have an adequate cell-to-collagen ratio (around 40.10^3 cells/mg collagen) [325]. Finally, 12 weeks after surgery, biomechanics and cellular organization of patellar tendon repairs may be significantly improved by the introduction of MSCs into a gel-sponge composite, and by the mechanical stimulation with a matched strain signal [325].

Skeletal muscle lineage: Skeletal muscle is the contractile and voluntary tissue of the body deriving from the mesodermal layer. Its function is to produce force and cause motion, either locomotion or movement within internal organs. The skeletal muscle cell or fiber, which is the main compound of the muscle, contains myofibrils and sarcomeres, composed of actin and myosin. Muscle fibers, surrounded by endomysium, are bound together by perimysium into bundles called fascicles, whereas bundles are enclosed in a sheath of epimysium and grouped together to form muscle. The body musculature, composed of approximately 650 muscles in the human body, is thus arranged in discrete muscles and attached to skeletal tissue by tendons.

Skeletal mature muscles also contain mononuclear progenitor cells, referred as satellite cells, which are localized between the basal lamina and sarcolemma. Satellite cells are able to re-enter the cell cycle, to differentiate and fuse to augment existing muscle fibers and to form new fibers. These cells are involved in the normal growth of muscle, as well as regeneration following injury or disease [326, 327]. In addition to satellite cells, others progenitor cells, known to be involved in muscle regeneration, are present in skeletal muscle [328, 329]. Indeed, side population progenitors, MSCs and HSCs may play a role during the muscle regeneration process [330-332]. Furthermore, several studies have reported that MSCs have the potential to differentiate into muscle fibers but also to contribute to the replenishment of the satellite cell compartment [333-337].

In vitro, differentiation of MSCs into skeletal muscle cells may be obtained after incubation with various chemical compounds, including 5-azacytidine, basic fibroblast growth factor, forskolin, platelet-derived growth factor or neuregulin [81, 211, 338-340], but also vascular endothelial growth factor, insulin-like growth factor [338] or amphotericin B [76, 341]. During the skeletal differentiation process, adjacent MSCs fused, formed multinucleated myotubes [64, 76, 341-343] and express several markers, including Pax3, Pax7, Myo-D, myogenin, Myf5 and the myogenic regulatory factor 4 [64, 338, 339, 344, 345]. Finally, after differentiation *in vitro*, MSCs were able to differentiate into contractile myotubes [333, 346]. Although the conversion of MSCs into skeletal muscle cells *in vitro* is a rare event [338], this allows the establishment of the differentiation mechanism and thus allows a better understanding of the regeneration muscle process performed by satellite cells, particularly in the awareness of the local signals released by damaged muscles [81].

Differentiation of MSCs into skeletal muscle was also widely reported after infusion *in vivo*. Ferrari et al. thus have demonstrated for the first time in 1998 that, after infusion, BM-derived stem cells (i.e. a majority of HSC) migrate into muscle degeneration areas, differentiate into myogenic cells contribute to the skeletal muscle regeneration [334]. After that, Gussoni *et al.* reported that infused adult BM stem cells in the mdx mouse, an animal model of Duchenne's muscular dystrophy, were able to migrate into skeletal muscles, incorporate and partial restore the dystrophin expression in the affected muscle [328]. This benefit from HSC transplantation to restore muscle structure and function has opened several perspectives in the treatment of congenital skeletal muscle defects, such as muscular dystrophy and other myopathies, and numerous authors have intended to explore the specific muscle restoration potential of MSCs *in vivo* [172, 347]. Adult MSCs contributed to myofibers, restored sarcolemmal expression of dystrophin, acted as long-term persisting functional satellite cells when administrated into mdx mouse muscle and thus providing evidences for their potential clinical use in human Duchenne muscular dystrophy [337, 348], but also during muscle regeneration after injury [347]. Although, like *in vitro*, the *in vivo* conversation of MSCs into satellite cells or skeletal muscle only occurs in a limited amount of fibers, varying between less than 1 and to a maximum of 10% [349-352], all data clearly indicated a significant muscle regeneration providing hopes for the treatment of muscle degenerative disorders using MSCs transplantation therapy.

Cardiac muscle lineage: Cardiac muscle is a type of involuntary mononucleated and striated muscle found exclusively within the heart. Its function is to pump blood through the circulatory system by contracting. Whereas skeletal muscle contracts in response to nerve stimulation, cardiac muscle is myogenic and is able of self-excitable stimulating contraction without a requisite electrical impulse coming from the central nervous system. Indeed, an isolated cardiac muscle cell will contract rhythmically at a steady rate, and if two or more cardiac muscle cells are in contact, whichever one contracts first will stimulate the other to contract, and so on. This transmission of impulses is allowed by specialized intercellular connections, called intercalated discs, which conduct electrochemical potentials directly between the cytoplasms of adjacent cells via gap junctions. Since cardiac muscle is myogenic, specialized pacemaker cells in the sinoatrial node normally determine the overall rate of contractions, with an average resting pulse of 72 beats per minute, and serve only to modulate and coordinate contractions. This inherent contractile activity is heavily regulated by the autonomic nervous system. Thus, the central nervous system does not directly create the impulses that contract the heart, but only sends modulatory signals to speed up (sympathetic nervous system) or slow down (parasympathetic nervous system) the heart rate. If synchronization of cardiac muscle contraction is disrupted for some reason (e.g. during a heart attack), uncoordinated contraction can result, leading to fibrillation.

The cardiovascular system begins to develop during the third week in human embryonic development, in the extra-embryonic mesoderm of the yolk sac. Thus, blood islands in the splanchnopleuric mesoderm of the yolk sac wall begin to anastamose and form the initial vascular network. After that, embryonic vasculature, forming a primitive vascular network, extends towards and anastamoses to establish a primitive circulatory system. The heart is thus materialized initially in the embryonic disc as a simple paired tube inside the forming pericardial cavity. When the embryonic disc folds, the embryonic heart is carried into the correct anatomical position in the chest cavity, whereas small regions differentiate into "blood islands" throughout the mesoderm, which supply both blood vessels (walls) and fetal red blood cells. A key aspect of heart development is the septation of the heart into separate chambers. Indeed, the initial primitive heart tube develops a series of constrictions and expansions, and then loops and folds into a characteristic “S” shape, whereas it is internally divided by septae into four separate chambers.

After birth, the adult mammalian heart is not able to regenerate extensively the large number of cardiomyocytes lost after diseases (e.g. infarction). After adaptative mechanisms, such as hypertrophy that is initially beneficial but becomes detrimental at the end, the only curative option is the heart transplantation that is limited by donor availability and transplant rejection. Thus, stem cell-based strategies, including differentiation of stem cells or reactivation of resident myocardial cells, are currently investigated for their potential to reconstitute the myocardium and regenerate the heart.

Several studies have shown that MSCs, once exposed to a variety of physiologic or non-physiologic stimuli, differentiate into cells displaying several features of cardiomyocytes-like cells [333, 342, 353-359]. Thus, after culturing with chemicals, including 5-azacytidine, amphotericin B or oxytocin, or after co-culturing with cardiomyocytes, *in vitro* differentiated MSCs exhibit a myotubes-like structure spontaneously beating. The cardiomyocytes-like phenotype was demonstrated by the exhibition of a characteristic ultrastructure with typical sarcomeres, atrial granules and a centrally positioned nucleus, and by the production of peptides and the expression of multiple structural and contractile proteins, including myosin heavy chain, beta-actin, desmin, phospholamban, adrenergic and muscarinic receptors, connexin 43, titin, and troponins C, I and T [342, 354-361]. Thus, co-culture experiments demonstrated that a cell-to-cell contact with cardiomyocytes *in vitro* might relay a "cardiac environmental signals" that promote extensively the MSC differentiation into a cardiomyogenic lineage [358, 359, 362, 363]. At last, differentiated MSCs into cardio-myogenic lineage cells display gap junction with a cell-to-cell coupling, but also sinus node–like and ventricular cell–like action potentials [333, 364, 365].

In vivo, injected MSCs can be tracked with the help an iron fluorophore-particle labeling and the use of magnetic resonance fluoroscopy, or using after transfection with a tag gene (e.g. luciferase or GFP). Indeed, after cardiac damage, injected MSCs into the myocardium of experimental models (e.g. myocardial cryoinjury, infarction) were able to engraft, to differentiate into cardiomyocytes and induce angiogenesis [342, 366-370]. Furthermore, some groups have reported improved cardiac function and myocardial perfusion after injection of autologous MSCs in a myocardial infarction pig model [355, 366, 367]. Following animal studies, the first randomized clinical trial assessing the effect of intra-coronary infusion of autologous BM-derived progenitor cells was carried out in 2004. Sixty patients with myocardial infarction were thus enrolled and 30 of them received autologous BM cells. After 6 month, the left ventricular systolic function was enhanced, with increased left ventricular ejection fraction and reduced end-systolic volume, only in the BM cell group, without adverse clinical events (e.g. pro-arrhythmic effects or in-stent restenosis) [371]. Also in 2004, another randomized clinical trial was carried out in 69 patients with acute myocardial infarction. Thirty-four of them received an intra-coronary injection of autologous BM-derived MSCs during the percutaneous coronary intervention procedure. Three months after, the left ventricular function was improved in the BM-derived MSC injection group, with an improved left ventricle perfusion and decreased perfusion defects, suggesting that MSCs may improve the ventricle remodeling by supplying viable cardiomyocytes or paracrine factors [372]. Finally, Miyahara and colleagues have reported in 2006 that purified and fully characterized MSCs were able to form a thick striatum containing newly formed vessels, undifferentiated cells and few cardiomyocytes, after transplantation onto the coronary ligated scarred myocardium, and improved cardiac function [373].

Hematopoietic supporting stroma and vascular-smooth muscle-like lineage: In the bone marrow, the structural and physiological support for hematopoietic cells is provided by the bone marrow stroma, which consists of a heterogeneous population of cells following a vascular smooth muscle cell differentiation pathway [374]. Within the bone marrow stromal niche, MSCs provide cell contacts and release growth factors, chemokines and extracellular matrix molecules that regulate the survival, self-renewal, migration and differentiation of HSCs into all hematopoietic lineages [56].

In fact, MSC-derived long-term cultures but also immortalized stromal lines express cytoskeletal and extracellular matrix proteins specific for vascular smooth muscle cells [375-380]. The earliest reported and constitutively expressed markers in culture are the α-smooth muscle actin (ASMA) and the fibronectin isoforms, both strongly express in smooth muscle cells [381-383]. Then, other cytoskeletal vascular smooth muscle cell-specific markers appear later, including vinculin, metavinculin, h-caldesmon, l-caldesmon, h1-calponin, SM22α and smooth muscle actinin [380-382, 384]. Finally, when fully differentiated into a vascular smooth muscle cell phenotype, MSCs express contractile protein, including desmin and smooth muscle myosin heavy chain 1 and 2 [384]. MSCs also express extracellular matrix proteins observed on vascular smooth muscle cells, including thrombospondin and laminin [380, 384]. Indeed, MSC differentiation in culture appears to recapitulate the developmental program of vascular smooth muscle cells differentiation.

Kidney and urogenital-related tissues: Part of the urinary system, the kidneys are bean-shaped excretory organs in and filter wastes (such as urea and uric acid) from the blood and excrete them, along with water, as urine. The kidneys also regulate the pH, by eliminating H ions concentration, the water composition of the blood, and the plasma volume. They regulate the blood pressure by a homeostatic process involving the rennin-angiotensin system and aldosterone. At last, the kidneys secrete a variety of hormones, including erythropoietin, urodilatin and vitamin D.

In humans, the two kidneys are located in the posterior part of the abdomen on each side of the spine, with the right just below the liver and the left below the diaphragm and adjacent to the spleen. An adrenal gland (also called the suprarenal gland) is found above each kidney. Kidney development, also called nephrogenesis, proceeds from the intermediate mesoderm through a series of three successive phases, each marked by the development of a more advanced pair of kidneys. The first of them, the pronephros, appears approximately on day 22 of human gestation and is considered nonfunctional in mammals because it cannot excrete waste from the embryo. The second, the mesonephros, is similar to the kidneys of aquatic amphibians and fishes. At last, the third, the metanephros, develops during the fifth week of gestation to form the ureteric bud, the metanephric duct and the ureter, and undergoes a series of branching to form the collecting duct system of the kidney [385].

The kidneys may be affected by several congenital diseases and disorders, including congenital hydronephrosis, congenital obstruction of urinary tract, duplicated ureter, horseshoe kidney, polycystic kidney disease, renal dysplasia or unilateral small kidney, and acquired diseases and disorders, including diabetic nephropathy, glomerulonephritis, hydronephrosis, interstitial nephritis, kidney stones, kidney tumors, lupus nephritis, nephrotic syndrome, pyelonephritis or renal failure. In the early 2000s, some experiments have reported that BM-derived cells were able to give rise to renal cells *in vitro* and *in vivo* [386]. Indeed, after transplantation of GFP-labeled BM-derived cells (i.e. a majority of HSCs), Imasawa *et al.* but also Ito *et al.* were able to trace and localized the GFP-positive cells in glomeruli, in the periglomerular space, and in the kidney interstitium, and to demonstrate that BM-derived cells differentiate into mesangial cells [387, 388]. After detection of Y chromosome in female kidney after sex-mismatched transplantation, Poulsom *et al.* and Krause *et al.* reported that BM cells exhibited a tubular epithelial phenotype, expressed the epithelial markers CAM5.2 and may thus partially contribute to the renal cell turnover [389, 390]. Then, the MSC contribution in kidney remodeling was first suggested by Iwano *et al.* and El Kossi *et al.* [391, 392]. Then, the presence of cytokeratin expressing and Y chromosome containing tubular epithelial cells in female kidneys of male recipients was confirmed *in vivo* supporting the hypothesis that extra-renal stem cells participate in the injured kidney regeneration [393]. After intravenous infusion, MSCs were monitored *in vivo* [394, 395], engrafted into the damaged kidney and differentiated into tubular epithelial cells, thereby restoring renal structure and function after acute renal failure [174, 396, 397].

d) Endodermal Tissues

Endoderm is one of the germ layers forming the inner layer of the gastrula during animal embryogenesis. Endoderm forms several tissues, including whole digestive tube epithelial lining (excepting part of the mouth, pharynx and the terminal part of the rectum, which are lined by involutions of the ectoderm), all digestive tube glands lining cells (liver and pancreas), auditory tube epithelium, tympanic cavity, trachea, bronchi, and lungs air cells, urinary bladder, thyroid gland follicles and thymus.

Gastrointestinal tract related tissues: The gastrointestinal tract is the system of organs that takes in food, digests it to extract energy and nutrients, and expels the remaining waste. The major functions of the gastrointestinal tract are digestion and excretion. The gastrointestinal tract is connected with other endoderm-derived digestion related organs, including the liver, which secretes bile into the small intestine via the biliary system and employs the gall-bladder as a reservoir, and the pancreas, which secretes bicarbonate and several enzymes, including trypsin, chymotrypsin, lipase, and pancreatic amylase, as well as nucleolytic enzymes (deoxyribonuclease and ribonuclease), into the small intestine.

In a normal human adult male, the gastrointestinal tract is approximately 6.5 meters long (20 feet) and consists of the upper and lower gastrointestinal tracts, but it may also be divided into foregut, midgut, and hindgut, reflecting the endoderm-derived embryological origin of each segment of the tract. The upper gastrointestinal tract, consisting of the mouth, pharynx, esophagus, and stomach, roughly corresponds to the derivatives of the foregut, with the exception of the first part of the duodenum. The lower gastrointestinal tract, comprising the intestines and anus, derives from the midgut for the lower duodenum and the first half of the transverse colon, and from the hindgut for the second half of the transverse colon and the upper part of the anal canal.

Since the epithelial cell lineage turnover within the gastrointestinal tract is a constant process, occurring every 2–7 days, it must be highly regulated by multipotent stem cells, which give rise to all gastrointestinal epithelial cell lineages and can regenerate the entire intestinal crypts and gastric glands under normal homeostasis but also after damage [398]. Next to the gastrointestinal side population cells [395, 398-400], recent reports illustrated that BM-derived cells were also able to incorporate into the small intestine pericryptal fibroblast region and to contribute to the intestinal regeneration after sex-mismatched BM transplants in human [399-401] and in animals [395, 402, 403] by forming myofibroblasts, fibroblasts, epithelial cells, smooth muscle cells and endothelial cell lineages. At last, BM-derived stem cells were also reported to express cytokeratin vimentin in the damage area and to be involved in the stomach regeneration in rats after ethanol-induced mucosal injury [404].

Liver lineage: The liver plays a major role in metabolism and has a number of functions in the body, including glycogen storage, plasma protein synthesis, and drug detoxification. Coming from an endoderm-derived part of the foregut called hepatic diverticulum, the liver produces bile and performs several functions, including the carbohydrate metabolism regulation (gluconeogenesis, glycogenolysis and glycogenesis), lipid and cholesterol metabolism, the detoxification and the production of insulin and coagulation factors. The liver, composed of hepatocytes that act as unipotential stem cells, and of bipotential stem cells, called oval cells that can differentiate into either hepatocytes or cholangiocytes, is among the few internal human organs capable of natural regeneration of lost tissue, and only 25% of remaining liver is enough to regenerate a whole liver.

Aside the different types of fetal and adult liver (stem) cells already identified, several types of BM-derived stem cells were reported to have the capacity to differentiate towards hepatocytic cells under appropriate *in vitro* conditions. A liver specific gene expression (cytokeratins 8 and 18, alpha-feto-protein, albumin, tryptophan-2,3-dioxygenase, tyrosine amino-transferase and the c-Met receptor for hepatocyte growth factor) was thus observed after induction by the hepatocyte growth factor HGF or the epidermal growth factor EGF, in culture with MSCs [405-412], for HSCs [413, 414], and for MAPCs from rat, mouse or human [170]. After co-cultures with hepatocytes, BM-derived stem cells were shown to express hepatic specific markers as well, and to adopt a metabolic activity [114, 408, 410, 415, 416].

In vivo, BM and liver transplantation were used to trace the origin of the liver repopulating cells during liver regeneration, and thus to observe that BM-derived HSCs may under certain conditions act as the progenitors of several types of liver cells, including oval cells, hepatocytes and cholangiocytes [93, 417]. At last, the *in vivo* differentiation of MSCs was also confirmed recently [406, 416].

Pancreas lineage: Deriving from two separate ventral and dorsal buds of the duodenum, the pancreas is an organ in the digestive and endocrine system which is both exocrine (secreting pancreatic juice containing digestive enzymes) and endocrine (islets of Langerhans that product several important hormones, including insulin, glucagon, and somatostatin). Due to the importance of its enzyme contents, injuring the pancreas is a very dangerous situation and several diseases or disorders may affect the pancreas, including tumors and cancer, insulinoma, cystic fibrosis, diabetes, exocrine pancreatic insufficiency, hemosuccus pancreaticus, pancreatitis and pancreatic pseudocyst. Among them, diabetes is one of the leading causes of morbidity and mortality in many countries caused by absolute insulin deficiency due to an autoimmune destruction of insulin secreting pancreatic β cells (type 1) or by a relative insulin deficiency due to decreased insulin sensitivity (type 2). Replacement of pancreatic β-cells, with the transplantation of islets of Langerhans, is already representing an ideal treatment [418, 419] but is restricted to a limited number of patients due the lack human islet donor tissues. Generation of insulin-producing cells from stem cells may thus represent an attractive alternative.

Within pancreatic islets and in non-endocrine compartments of the pancreas, some multipotent stem cells have been described [105, 420-422] and have the capacity to differentiate into pancreatic islet-like structures [423, 424]. Furthermore, cells that do not reside within the pancreas have been differentiated into pancreatic endocrine hormone-producing cells *in vitro* and *in vivo*, including embryonic stem cells [161, 423, 425], hepatic oval cells [426, 427], spleen-derived cells [428] or the central nervous system [429]. BM-derived stem cells could also play a supportive role in pancreas regeneration *in vivo* rather than participate in the differentiation of endocrine cells themselves [430]. However, human or rodent MSCs were reported to have the potential to differentiate *in vitro* into insulin, glucagon and somatostatin-secreting cells but also *in vivo* to reverse hyperglycemia in animal models of diabetes [431, 432], and to express the islet pancreatic transcription factors Nkx-2.2, Nkx-6.1, Pax-4, Pax-6, Isl-1 and Ipf-1 [412, 421, 432].

Lung-related tissue: In mammalians, the lung has the largest surface area, which reaches a final gas diffusion area of 70 m^2 in human lung, compared to the next largest epithelial organ, the skin, which has a surface area of about 40 times less. This essential respiration organ in air-breathing vertebrates is able to transport oxygen from the atmosphere into the bloodstream, to excrete carbon dioxide from the bloodstream into the atmosphere, and thus to support a systemic oxygen consumption ranging between 250 mL/min at rest to 5,500 mL/min during exercise. This gaze exchange is accomplished in the mosaic of specialized cells that form millions of tiny, exceptionally thin-walled air sacs called alveoli. A matching capillary network is also developed in close apposition to the alveolar surface, which can accommodate a blood flow rising from 4 to 40 L/min during the transition from rest to maximal exercise.

Coming from a ventral appendage of the endodermal epithelium lining the floor of the primitive embryonic anterior pharynx, the lung divides laterally into two buds and begins dichotomous branching into the surrounding splanchnic mesenchyme. The lung development is divided into four chronological stages, with the pseudoglandular stage (bronchial and respiratory tree development, undifferentiated primordial system formation), the canalicular stage (terminal sacs and vascularization development), the terminal sac stage (terminal sac number and vascularization increase, type I and II cells differentiation), and the alveolar stage (terminal sacs development into mature alveolar ducts and alveoli) [433, 434]. The mature lung comprises at least 40 morphologically differentiated cell lineages [435]. Thus, the larynx is lined with squamous epithelium and the upper airways are lined with ciliated columnar cells and mucus-secreting cells. Clara cells line the lower airways and alveolar type 1 and 2 epithelial cells line the alveoli and surround some pulmonary neuroendocrine cells situated in small foci. The pulmonary interstitium contains several specialized lineages of mesenchymal origin, including fibroblasts, myofibroblasts, and smooth muscle cells. At last, the lung also contains vascular, lymphatic and neuronal components [436]. Therefore, the development of the conducting airway and alveolar regions are suggested to be derived from different populations of stem cells, an airway stem cell population and a lung parenchyma stem cell population [92, 437-440].

Resident stem/progenitor cells have been described in specific regions in the proximal airway of the lung, including proximal airway epithelial progenitor cells [441, 442], bronchiolar epithelial progenitor cells [439] and alveolar epithelial stem cells [438, 443]. However, several groups have recently described the capacity of non-resident stem cells to differentiate into alveolar epithelial cells *in vitro*. For example, Rippon *et al.*, reported the differentiation of murine ES cells into distal airway epithelium after a three-step differentiation protocol incorporating an activin A treatment, a serum-free medium incubation and a commercially available lung-specific medium [444]. The MSC ability to differentiation into airway epithelium *in vitro* was described by Wang *et al.* when co-cultured with airway epithelial cells [445]. Moreover, when transduced with a virus construct expressing the cystic fibrosis trans-membrane regulator (CFTR), the gene corrected autologous MSCs were demonstrated to contribute to apical chloride secretion in response to cAMP agonist stimulation, suggesting the possibility of developing cell-based therapy for human cystic fibrosis [445]. At last, after intravenous injection into bleomycin-induced pulmonary fibrosis sex-mismatched animals, BM-derived bleomycin-resistant MSCs were reported to engraft the lung, to exhibit an epithelium-like morphology, to express type 1 alveolar epithelial cell specific markers (*Lycopersicon esculentum* lectin, aquaporin-5 and T1α) and to reduce inflammation and collagen deposition in lung tissue [446, 447].

4. Immunosuppressive Properties

In recent years, several observations reported that MSCs could exert immuno-regulatory activity, such as immuno-suppression by inhibiting T-cell responses to both polyclonal stimuli and their cognate peptide [448-450]. On study state, MSCs constitutively express low surface densities of MHC class I molecules and are negative for MHC class II and for co-stimulatory molecules (e.g. CD40, CD80 and CD86), both up-regulated by inflammatory stimuli [451, 452]. Indeed, because MSCs are generally considered as poorly immunogenic cells, they are of great importance in the view of potential utilization for therapeutic purposes (e.g. hematopoietic stem/progenitor cell engraftment or graft-versus-host disease).

<u>MSCs and T-lymphocytes:</u> In 1984, the group of Ildstad was the first to postulate that the transplantation of incompatible BM-derived stem cells into a mismatched recipient could induce tolerance to allogeneic or xenogeneic grafts [453]. However, the clear demonstration of T cells proliferation inhibition induced by MSCs was only reported in 2002 [448, 454]. After that, other reports showed that the MSC anti-proliferative activity does not appear to be antigen specific and targets both primary and secondary T-cell responses, but may still exert some selectivity because it appears to discriminate between cellular responses to allo-antigens and recall antigens [449, 454, 455]. Both suppression of T cell proliferation and their accumulation in the G0 phase of the cell cycle did not require MHC restriction, but could also be mediated by allogeneic MSCs [450]. Suppression of T cells proliferation induced by MSCs depends on a cross talk between the two cell populations, on the production of inflammatory cytokines, such as IFN-γ and IL-1β [448, 455, 456], and on the decreased production of Th1 cytokines [457]. Several MSC-derived molecules have been proposed to exert immuno-modulatory activity on T cell responses, including TGF-β1, HGF, IL-10, indoleamine 2,3-dioxygenase and prostaglandin E2 [448, 456, 458-461].

<u>MSCs and B-lymphocytes:</u> Only few studies addressed the effects of MSCs on B cell function. However, in 2005, Glennie *et al.* but also Augello *et al.* both reported that MSCs inhibit B cell proliferation, instigated in part by a physical contact between the 2 cell types and in part by a soluble factors released by MSCs in the culture supernatant [450, 457]. Deng *et al.* also reported that allogeneic MSC inhibited B cell activation, proliferation and IgG secretion, with enhanced CD40 and CD40 ligand expression, on BXSB-derived B cells, which is an experimental model for human systemic lupus erythematosus [462]. Finally, Corcione *et al.* described a study in which proliferation of B cells, stimulated and activated with anti-Ig antibodies, soluble CD40 ligand and cytokines (IL-2 and IL-4), was inhibited by MSCs in a manner depending on MSC-derived soluble factors released upon their cross talk with B cells [463].

<u>MSCs and NK cells:</u> As for T and B cells, interactions between MSCs and NK cells, which are major effectors in the elimination of virus-infected and malignant cells, induced an inhibition of the IL-2- or IL-15-driven NK proliferation, but also a reduced production of IL-15-induced cytokines (IFN-c, IL-10 and TNF-α) [456, 464, 465]. Similarly, soluble factors, including TGF-β1 and prostaglandin E2 have been suggested to play a role in the MSC-mediated suppression of NK cell proliferation [466].

MSCs and dendritic cells: The main function of dendritic cells is to process antigen material and present it on their surface to other cells of the immune system. The antigen presenting capacity might thus be altered by MSCs to promote their immuno-modulatory effects. Indeed, MSCs have been reported to inhibit the maturation of monocyte-derived myeloid dendritic cells, by down-regulating the surface expression of CD11c, CD83, MHC class II and co-stimulatory molecules, and by reducing the production of IL-12 [461, 465, 467, 468]. Ones again, the MSC-induced inhibition of dendritic cells differentiation and function is mediated by soluble factors (prostaglandin E2) and cell-to-cell contacts [459, 468, 469]. Thus, the MSC-induced inhibition of T lymphocyte proliferation may not only be the result of a direct suppressive effect on T cells, but may also be caused by an inhibitory effect on dendritic cell maturation, activation and antigen presentation.

MSC immunological effects in vivo: Several *in vivo* studies have reported the immuno-modulatory effects of MSCs. Indeed, infusion of MSCs delayed the rejection of skins allografts in a non-human model of organ transplantation [454], attenuates experimental autoimmune encephalomyelitis (a model of human multiple sclerosis) [470], and has beneficial effects in different human diseases including graft-versus-host disease, breast cancer, osteogenesis imperfecta, metachromatic leukodystrophy, Hurler syndrome, hematological malignancies and stroke [471-475]. However, some doubts rose from recent *in vivo* experiments about the reported MSC immuno-privilege, indicating that in some cases, administration of allogeneic MSCs into an MHC-mismatched host may result in their rejection or failed to prevent graft-versus-host disease [452, 475-477].

D. Capacities

1. Homing and Domiciliation

After systemic administration, MSCs are detected in bone, bone marrow, spleen, and cartilage, which localization is in agreement with the *in vitro* differentiation potential, but also in liver, lungs, kidneys [80, 478-480]. When intravenously injected, the donor MSC contribution in recipient bone and BM was estimated in mice and represent 5% of the total cell content after 5 months [141]. Labeled MSCs were also collected and recovered from BM and spleen 6 weeks after transplantation of galactosidase labeled human MSCs into pre-immune fetal sheep [172]. After transplantation into sub-lethally irradiated mice, more than half injected GFP-labeled MSCs were recovered from BM after 24 hours [480], and around 10-20% in BM within 3-10 weeks after infusion [481]. After infusion, MSCs were still detected after 12 weeks in NOD/SCID mice in lungs, kidneys, liver, intestine and brain, in addition to bone, bone marrow and spleen [130] but also after 1 year in baboons [83]. At last, differentiated human MSCs were detected after birth in a number of tissues, with tissue-specific differentiation into myocytes, cardiomyocytes and thymic stroma, in addition to bone marrow stroma, chondrocytes and adipocytes, after intraperitoneal injected in pre-immune sheep fetus [172].

All these studies allowed several issues to be raised. Firstly, after intravenous injection, MSCs are immediately trapped in the lungs [80, 478], suggesting that the number of cells arriving to the target organ, in particular bone marrow and bone, might be extremely limited, while the intra-BM route was not reported to be more effective [482]. Secondly, the steady state MSC turnover in the mesenchymal system is small (years are for example needed to the complete bone renewal), but it may dramatically increase in normal period of growth or after injury [59, 138]. Therefore, the recipient condition is a critical parameter in the MSC homing capacity, such as irradiation, which allows a significant MSC homing increase [341, 357, 480]. Thirdly, the MSC detection in a given tissue after infusion does not necessarily mean engraftment, but at least indicate cell survival in tissue [66, 483]. Finally, some of the detected cells after transplantation might be the result of cell fusion with *in situ* cells, such as striated myocytes, cardiomyocytes, Purkinje cells and hepatocytes [182, 343, 347, 348, 484], whereas specific differentiation of MSC without fusion are reported for hepatocytes [173].

2. Tissue Regeneration

Tissue regeneration is a cardinal stem cell property that has been partially confirmed for MSCs, especially for bone repair. Transgenic mice, with mutated collagen 1 gene leading to a phenotype of fragile bones resembling osteogenesis imperfecta, were reported to have a significant increase in bone collagen and mineral content 1 month after transplantation with BM-derived MSC from normal mice [485]. Similarly in human, local administration of autologous MSCs allows the healing of large bone defects [292] and increase the growth velocity of body length of young patients with osteogenesis imperfecta 4-6 weeks after transplantation [286, 486]. MSCs may also be used in several other diseases because of their assumed large differentiation potential as described above, including for example vascular diseases or skeletal and cardiac muscle disorders.

3. Oxygen Sensing

Oxygen concentration, and particularly hypoxia, is associated with critical role in the placenta development [487], during the early human embryogenesis [488], at birth (ductus arteriosus and foramen ovale closures) [489], in adult to optimize the matching of regional blood flow and ventilation in the lung with a physiological mechanism called hypoxic pulmonary vasoconstriction, and during virtually all known diseases. Within the BM, adult stem cells are also exposed to low oxygen and the mean oxygen concentration of the BM has been reported to be around 7% at steady state [490]. Mathematical models have indicated the existence of a gradient across the marrow from the rather well oxygenated sinuses to the relatively hypoxic areas near the bone endosteum [491], and HSCs are reported to be in an undifferentiated state in BM hypoxic niches and to expanse and differentiate along an oxygen gradient [492]. Furthermore, hypoxia has been shown to improve HSC survival, enhance self-renewal [493] and stimulate the formation of granulocytic-monocytic progenitors [494]. The BM is also the residence place of MSCs and oxygen has been shown to modulate some MSC characteristics as well. In particular, culturing MSCs at reduced oxygen tension (5-8%) increased *in vitro* their bone-forming potential [495], their adipogenesis potential [496, 497], their chondrogenesis potential [498, 499], and promote their mobilization into peripheral blood [79]. On the other hand, a hypoxic condition (2% of oxygen or less) compared to the physiological condition (7% of oxygen), is reported to inhibit strongly MSC chondrogenesis and osteogenesis *in vitro* [500] and to induce apoptosis [501].

Finally, since oxygen might have a regulatory role in growth kinetic and some differentiation pathways, several precautions should be taken when reading nearly all MSC-related reports, especially when *in vitro* experiments are set up at an oxygen concentration corresponding to that of the ambient air, because such oxygen level conditions probably several-fold surpass those found under physiological conditions [502, 503].

IV. Vascular Therapies

There are a number of clinical situations where the recipient site may not be amenable to a direct MSC transplantation, such as vascular diseases. Moreover, several factors limit the vascular tissue engineering, such as the availability of a suitable and abundant source of tissue. Since MSCs are multipotent and their number can be expanded in culture, there has been much interest in their clinical potential for tissue repair, especially as a potential source for generating mesenchyme cells in the vascular wall such as smooth muscle cells (SMC) or for the construction of vascular grafts. When transplanted into the heart, MSCs can differentiate into SMCs and contribute to vascular remodeling *in vivo* [504, 505], suggesting that some micro-environmental signals may be important in promoting differentiation to a SMC phenotype. However, the effects of vascular micro-environmental factors on MSCs or the *in vitro* factors needed to undergo SMC differentiation are not yet fully understood.

Several physiological or pathological processes may contribute to modify the normal vessel. Arteriogenesis refers to an increase in the diameter of existing arterial vessels. Angiogenesis is a physiological and normal process, involving the growth of new blood vessels from pre-existing vessels, which can be observed in a normal process such as in growth and development, as well as in wound healing, but also during the tumors transition from a dormant state to a malignant state. At last, vasculogenesis is the process of blood vessel formation occurring by a *de novo* production of endothelial cells, when endothelial precursor cells (angioblasts) migrate and differentiate in response to local signals to form new blood vessels. Vasculogenesis is thus observed during the embryologic development but also in adult during the neo-vascularization of a tumor or during the revascularization process of an avascularized area following trauma (e.g. cardiac ischemia).

A. The Normal Vessel

The normal arterial wall, consisting of concentric layers that surround the arterial lumen, is divided into three well-defined layers having each distinctive composition of cells and extracellular matrix, including the layer immediately adjacent to the lumen called the intima, the middle layer known as the media, and the outermost layer referred as the arterial adventitia. Two concentric layers of elastin demarcate these three layers, known as the internal elastic lamina that separates the intima from the media, and the external elastic lamina that separates the media from the adventitia. Lining the luminal surface of arteries, a single contiguous layer of endothelial cells sits on a basement membrane of extracellular matrix and proteoglycans that is bordered by the internal elastic lamina. Although some SMCs are occasionally found in the intima, the principal cellular component, forming a functional barrier between flowing blood and the arterial wall stroma, is constituted by endothelial cells of this anatomic layer. The media layer is composed principally by SMCs arranged in layers, where the number of layers is depending on the arterial size. SMCs are held together by an extracellular matrix, composed of elastic fibers, collagen and proteoglycans, which may be supplied by an increasing content of elastin typically observed within larger arteries. At last, the outermost layer of the artery, the adventitia, is typically composed of a loose matrix of elastin, SMCs, fibroblasts, and collagen, where most of the neural input into blood vessels also traverses through the adventitia. Previously considered inactive with respect to vascular homeostasis, the adventitia is now playing an important role in controlling vascular remodeling and nitric oxide bioactivity, through the production of reactive oxygen species.

Like all the other organs, cells of the vessels must receive nutrients and oxygen and reject wastes. Most of the time, vascular cells directly carry out their exchanges with circulating blood, but for vessels of larger diameter, the nutrition of cells constituting the vascular wall can be assured at the same time by blood circulating in the vessel but also starting from a capillary system: the vasa vasorum. This capillary network, bringing nutrients to cells furthest away from the vessel lumen, is present in all arteries comprising more than 29 lamellate units. The vasa vasorum can moreover bring a certain number of mediators and hormones in more or less direct contact with SMCs of largest arteries.

B. Mesenchymal Stem Cells Implication in Vascular Remodeling

Within the framework of a vascular therapy, MSCs could be integrated into the muscular layer of the vascular wall and they may be differentiated into in smooth muscular cells. They may also transdifferentiate into endothelial cells and thus contribute to the vessel intima. At last, these cells could incorporate the arterial adventitia like pericytes and secrete cytokines and growth factors to act in an indirect way on a more extended portion of the vessel by paracrine stimulation.

1. MSCs and the Smooth Muscle Differentiation

a) Bone Marrow Stroma and Vascular Smooth Muscle Phenotype

Within the bone marrow, the structural and physiological support of hematopoietic cells is provided by the bone marrow stroma, which is composed of a heterogeneous population of cells that follow a vascular smooth muscle differentiation pathway [374]. In the bone marrow stroma niche *in vivo*, MSCs provide cellular contacts and produce growth factors, chemokines and extracellular matrix molecules that control survival, self-renewal, transfer and differentiation of HSCs into all hematopoietic cells [56]. *In vitro*, after long-term culture, MSCs but also MSCs derived cell-lines express cytoskeleton-associated and extracellular matrix specific proteins that are found on smooth muscle cells [375-380]. In MSC culture, the first and most constitutively expressed markers are the alpha-smooth muscle actin and fibronectin isoforms, which are both strongly expressed in smooth muscle cells [382, 383]. Then, other cellular markers found in smooth muscle cells appear belatedly in MSCs under culture, including the vinculin, the metavinculin, the h-caldesmon, the l-caldesmon, the h1-calponin, SM22α and the smooth muscle actinin [380, 381, 384]. At last and more lately, MSCs express smooth muscle specific contractile proteins, such as desmin or smooth muscle heavy chains 1 and 2 [384]. Moreover, MSCs produce a smooth muscle-like extracellular matrix, made up of thrombospondin 1 and laminin [384]. Thus, after long-term culture, MSCs seem to acquire a smooth muscle phenotype with the sequential expression of developmental markers.

This differentiation pathway might seem to be astonishing for the hematopoietic stroma and not related to a known function of the smooth muscle cells. However, some analyzes revealed a functional significance. Indeed, hematopoietic supporting stroma cells synthesize a great number of cytokines and adhesion molecules that are essential to hematopoiesis, but these cells also play a critical role in the hematopoietic cell migration by modifying the endothelial cell junction organization [266, 506] and by producing a SDF-1 gradient [507]. This dual role, the mediator synthesis and the progenitor traffic control, is a reminiscence of the two functions described for smooth muscle cells, passing from a synthetic to a contractile phenotype [384]. Thus, the synthetic phenotype would be characteristic of an immature cell (MSCs under the differentiation course), while the contractile phenotype would be characteristic of a mature and completely differentiated cell, such as smooth muscle cells from the vascular media layer.

b) The Smooth Muscle Differentiation

In vivo, mediators expressed and/or secreted by endothelial cells seem to play a role in the smooth muscle cell recruitment and differentiation [384, 508-510]. The cell recruitment might be induced by several released factors, such as PDGF, tissue factor and endoglin [511], and by the expression of transcription factors, such as MEF-2C (myocyte-specific enhancer-binding Factor-2C) [512]. The future smooth muscle differentiation cell would be controlled by a balance between activators (TGF-β, IGF, endothelin I, angiotensin II, heparan sulfate, laminin, type IV collagen, retinoic acid) and inhibitors (PDGF, interferon γ, fibronectin) [374]. Moreover, the cellular aspect seems to be important in the differentiation process since the alpha-smooth muscle actin and other cytoskeletal proteins are expressed in response to an extracellular matrix and to stretching [513].

Smooth muscle markers (alpha-smooth muscle actin, vimentin, desmin, myosins, calponin, metavinculin) are classically induced *in vitro* when culturing MSCs in a Dexter-type medium (basic medium supplemented with in particular fetal calf serum, horse serum and cortisol) [377]. However, other studies reported a smooth muscle phenotype induction after incubating stromal cells in another differentiation medium (basic medium supplemented with fetal calf serum and β-mercaptoethanol) [514], with the induction of various markers (alpha-smooth muscle actin, SM22α, h-caldesmon, h1-calponin). Moreover, these authors also showed that the ascorbic acid was a potential smooth muscle differentiation inductor [514]. On the other hand, the dimethyl sulfoxide was reported to inhibit the MSC to smooth muscle differentiation [515].

Studies about the MSC *in vitro* culture conditions had allow to point out the importance of many cytokines (TGF-β, EGF, IL-1, IL-6, TNF-α, bFGF, PDGF) in these stromal cells long-term maintenance and differentiation [122, 123, 516]. Moreover, these cytokines induce a variety of effects according to culture conditions (presence or not of serum, presence or not of adhesion molecules covering the dish, liquid or semi-solid culture medium, sorted-cells or not). Although few specific studies were specifically interested in the MSC to smooth muscle differentiation, it is probable that autocrine secreted TGF-β [517] and PDGF both play a modulating role in coordination with extracellular matrix molecules [346]. Thus, TGF-β and a TGF-β activator, the thrombospondin 1, would stimulate of the production of alpha-smooth muscle actin in fibroblasts and myofibroblasts [375, 380, 518], while PDGF-β would reduce the alpha-smooth muscle actin expression [346].

c) Markers of the Smooth Muscle Differentiation

The MSC *in vitro* acquisition of a smooth muscle phenotype, with the acquisition of specific markers, is currently well established. However, the presence of various markers is only one stage towards the acquisition of a complete smooth muscle phenotype and it is necessary to determine if MSC differentiated in smooth muscle cells have the fundamental capacity of the smooth muscle: the contraction.

One of the methods allowing the evaluation the contraction capacity is to place cells into a collagen or glycosaminoglycan matrix and to measure its shortening. Thus, Young and colleagues reported the rabbit MSC contraction capacity in a collagen matrix [321]; however, the contraction degree was not evaluated. Then, a quantitative analysis of the MSC contraction within a collagen and glycosaminoglycan composite matrix was reported where authors showed without ambiguity the contraction capacity of rabbit and dog bone marrow-derived MSC after culture into a Dexter-type medium (smooth muscle differentiation medium) [519]. At last, Kinner and collaborators showed in 2002 that human MSCs (characterized by their differentiation capacity along the three reference lineages) had a contraction capacity correlated to their alpha-smooth muscle actin content [346]. These authors also reported that the MSC contraction within a collagen matrix after culture into a Dexter-type medium was completely inhibited by cytochalasin-D (a cytoskeletal actin depolymerizing agent), partially inhibited by PDGF-β and potentiated by TGF-β [346].

Many studies remain to be carried out to determine whether all MSCs have this contraction capacity or if a particular cell fraction is selected during *in vitro* cultures. Moreover, since contractile proteins associated to the smooth muscle phenotype, such as the alpha-smooth muscle actin or myosins, are not sufficient to obtain contractile smooth muscle cells from MSCs, it would be important to study the presence of other markers associated with the smooth muscle cell functionality, such as the calcium homeostasis or the electrophysiological profile.

Some teams were thus interested in the calcium-signaling pathway in MSCs [140, 520-522]. In undifferentiated MSCs, the cytosolic calcium is thus reported to be released mainly from endoplasmic reticulum stocks. Moreover, this calcium is preferentially released through inositol-1,4,5-triphosphate sensitive endoplasmic receptors and not or little through ryanodine sensitive endoplasmic receptors. At last, a little part of the intracellular calcium might come inside cells mainly through plasma membrane calcium channels (store-operated calcium channels) [521]. Undifferentiated MSCs were also reported to show calcium oscillations mainly from sodium-calcium exchangers (NCX1, 2 and 3) and plasma membrane calcium pumps [140, 521], but not from plasma membrane voltage-operated calcium channels [522]. However, no specific study regarding the calcium-signaling pathway was made concerning the particular context of the MSC to smooth muscle differentiation.

The study of the MSC electrophysiological profile characterizing the membrane potential at rest and their capacity to be depolarized authorizing the contraction, could allow to determine which smooth muscle cell type might be obtained after differentiation. Thus, ionic channels usually reported on smooth muscle cells, such as the large-conductance calcium-activated potassium channel (BKca), and Kv2.1 or Kv1.5 sub-units, ionic exchanges (e.g. NCX-1, 2 or 3), are also found within the MSC membrane [521, 523, 524]. However, since these ionic channels are largely expressed in the majority of smooth muscle cell types (vascular, mesenteric, bronco-tracheal or uterine), they do not allow any discrimination.

2. MSCs and Endothelial Trans-Differentiation

Beside their integration in the vessel media layer and their smooth muscle differentiation, MSCs could also participate to the vessel intima layer and (trans)-differentiate into endothelial cells. Likewise, studies showed that endothelial cells and progenitors could differentiate into smooth muscle cells under TGF-β induction [525-527]; it was brought back a MSC "trans-differentiation" into endothelial cells *in vitro* coming from human bone marrow [528] or from human umbilical cord blood [529]. Even if the conversion of a cellular type towards another seems to be a rare event, with a conversion frequency estimated between 0,01 and 0,03% [530], it was also reported cells presenting at the same time an endothelial phenotype (von Willebrand factor expression), and a smooth muscle phenotype (alpha-smooth muscle actin expression) [526, 530].

This *in vitro* trans-differentiation was associated with a epithelial to mesenchymal transition, characterized by a cell-to-cell contact disruption [530], an endothelial markers differential expression (VE-cadherin, von Willebrand factor, Tie-1 and 2, VCAM-1) and by the capacity to form a tubular network structure [528, 529]. At last, various growth factors were also associated to this endothelial trans-differentiation, such as VEGF, TGF-β, EGF, PDGF or hydrocortisone [528, 529, 531]. Thus, this capacity adds a clinical advantage to the MSC use with an aim of vascular therapy.

3. Growth Factor Release and Paracrine Effects of MSCs

Practically all information regarding the cytokine production by stromal cells and MSCs come from *in vitro* studies on cultured cells. Indeed, it is currently difficult to correlate these *in vitro* results with a potential *in vivo* role of each cytokine. Moreover, it is currently not clearly established if MSCs, coming from various tissue sources, are presenting a specific cytokine production profile, and if there is a cytokine regionalization within the same tissue [56].

One of the first observations was to show the MSC capacity to produce cytokines maintaining HSCs in quiescence or inducing their self-renewal rather than their differentiation. Indeed, MSCs are reported to excrete the following molecules: SCF, LIF, SDF-1, BMP-4, Flt-3 ligand, TGF-β [74, 532-534]. MSCs produce a broad variety of interleukins (IL-1, IL-6, IL-7, IL-8, IL-11, IL-12, IL-14, and IL-15) and, when they are cultivated in the presence of IL-1a, MSCs also produce cytokines acting on more mature hematopoietic progenitors, such as the GM-CSF and G-CSF [534]. Studies also brought back the existence of a "dialog" between HSCs and MSCs, osteoblasts and stromal cells, allowing the regulation the hematopoietic cells production [535-537].

MSC paracrine secretions thus play a fundamental role in the bone marrow microenvironment; however, these cytokine secretions can also play an important role during angiogenesis and arteriogenesis. In 2004, Kinnaird and colleagues showed that MSCs could secrete angiogenic factors *in vitro*, such as VEGF, bFGF, PGF and MCP-1 [538, 539]. These authors also reported a beneficial effect of the MSC local injection on the vascular perfusion in a model of lower limb ischemia by MSC paracrine secretions *in situ* of VEGF and bFGF. Furthermore, this ischemia protection mechanism, characterized by an apoptosis reduction and an angiogenesis increase after injection of MSC, was also reported with a bFGF and TGF-α secretion in a model of acute renal ischemia [174] or in a model of myocardial infarction [373, 540, 541]. Thus, even if a low number of MSCs integrates the new vessels architecture [174, 373, 538-541], MSCs are capable of long-term survival after injection, to exhibit immunosuppressive activities, to reduce fibrosis (scar formation), to inhibit apoptosis, to induce angiogenesis and to stimulate mitosis and differentiation of cells leading to tissue repair by their of bioactive molecule secretion [542].

C. Stem Cell Implication during Angiogenesis, Vasculogenesis and Arteriogenesis

Vascular remodeling and in particular arterial remodeling can be observed under various pathological conditions whatever the touched organ, causing the widening (expansive remodeling) or the reduction (constrictive remodeling) of the vessel diameter. All vascular remodeling are important physiological and pathological mechanisms in the tissue perfusion adaptation that lead to structural and functional modifications of the vascular wall. These processes are characterized by a smooth muscle cell hypertrophy or hyperplasia within the media layer of preexistent vessels, but also by a complete remodeling of the vasculature with disappearance of some vessels by apoptose and with appearance of new vessels by angiogenesis or vasculogenesis.

Smooth muscle cells that play a critical role during these vascular remodeling may have a variable origin. Indeed, these cells can come from the local proliferation of smooth muscle cells that are already present in the vessel media layer at the lesion level, but these cells may also come from the differentiation of endogenous stem cells and progenitors that are present in the vessel media layer or from circulating progenitors.

1. Stem Cell Implication during Pulmonary Remodeling

a) Mechanisms of the Pulmonary Vascular Development

The pulmonary vascularization is formed according to two distinct mechanisms: angiogenesis and vasculogenesis. During vasculogenesis, local endogenous progenitors proliferate to form a loose complex of cells being used as starting point to the development of new vessels. After the cellular network formation, proliferative cells are assembled to form tubular structures, while the later development by angiogenesis leads to the formation of the final vascular tree. Angiogenesis is the process by which new vessels emergent starting from preexistent vessels. It is a complex process directed by growth factors that stimulate the endothelial cell proliferation, which control the vascular lumen formation, and which direct the recruitment of perivascular components (pericytes and smooth muscle cells) towards the vascular wall [543, 544]. Angiogenesis thus allows the extension of preexistent vessels but also the establishment of links between close structures.

Although there is a debate regarding the exact chronology of the pulmonary vascular network formation mechanisms, both angiogenesis and vasculogenesis play essential roles. Many studies actually showed that proximal vessels were initially formed by budding starting from a preexistent vessel (angiogenesis), while the distal vessels were formed *de novo* starting from splanchnopleuric-derived mesenchymal progenitors (vasculogenesis) [545, 546].

The stem cell and progenitor participation during the vascular vessel formation starts to be supported since Summer and his team has successfully isolated a stem cell population from embryonic lungs [440]. After characterization, this heterogeneous population was composed of hematopoietic cells and non-hematopoietic cells, and allowed endothelial and smooth muscle cells to be obtained. HSC- and MSC-like stem cells were also brought back as being present within the pulmonary tissue where they could participate to the constitutive replacement of the pulmonary parenchyma, the epithelium and pulmonary vessels, but also during several pathologies like pulmonary hypertension, pulmonary fibrosis or emphysema.

b) Stem Cells and Pulmonary Vascular Pathologies

The purpose of several studies was to show the stem cell contribution to the pathogenesis of many adult pulmonary diseases by contributing to a hyper-proliferative response with phenotypical and functional differentiations into alveolar, endothelial or smooth muscle cells. On the other hand, the stem cell contribution to the pulmonary tissue remodeling can also be defective, thus contributing to decrease the tissue repair.

Pulmonary arterial hypertension: Pulmonary hypertension is characterized by an abnormal function of endothelial cells, causing a sustained vasoconstriction and a pulmonary vessel remodeling [547], but it is also characterized by a high pulmonary blood pressure with a pulmonary vascular resistance increase, leading to a right cardiac insufficiency. In addition to an abnormal endothelial cell functionality, the pulmonary vascular remodeling is characterized by an intima thickening, a media hypertrophy, a smooth muscle cell hyperplasia and by plexiform lesions blocking pulmonary capillaries [548]. The pulmonary vessel sustained vasoconstriction was a long time considered as the principal cause of the pulmonary pressure rise; however, during the 10 last years, many data gave evidences that an exuberant angiogenesis also contributed to the development of the pathology. Thus, Tuder and collaborators were among the first to bring back the expression of angiogenic molecules within plexiform lesions from patients suffering of severe pulmonary arterial hypertension, with a VEGF over-expression leading to an excessive proliferation of local or circulating endothelial cells [549-551].

Then, as the pulmonary mesenchyme is a vascular precursor source [552] and as various types of progenitors capable of vascular differentiation are circulating constitutively in the bloodstream, the contribution of these stem cells during the plexiform lesion development was suspected but not yet clearly established [553]. Thus, Hashimoto and collaborators showed in 2004 that some pulmonary fibroblasts came from bone marrow derived progenitors [554], while Davie reported the presence of c-kit$^+$ progenitors (probably HSCs) around remodeled pulmonary arteries in a bovine model of hypoxia-induced pulmonary hypertension [555]. At last, even if Sca-1$^+$ c-kit$^+$ vascular progenitors not coming from bone marrow were detected in the mouse vessel adventitia [556], Hayashida concluded that bone marrow stem cells (i.e. HSCs) were mobilized into the peripheral blood and could contribute to pulmonary vascular remodeling in a model of hypoxia-induced pulmonary hypertension in the bone marrow transplanted transgenic GFP mouse [557].

The intravenous injection of MSCs or endothelial progenitors genetically modified to express the endothelial nitric oxide synthase attenuated the monocrotaline-induced pulmonary hypertension, with improvement of the animal survival and restoration of the pulmonary microvasculature structure and function [558, 559].

Asthma: Contrary to the pulmonary hypertension, the pulmonary angiogenesis contribution was brought back since more than one ten years in the airway remodeling of the patients suffering from bronchial asthma [560]. Indeed, bronchial biopsies coming from children and adult patients suffering from moderate to severe asthma showed a vessel number increase that was correlated to the expression of several angiogenic factors and their receptors

[561, 562]. In the same way, asthmatic patients presented an airways chronic inflammation whose severity is correlated to the disease severity [563]. Thus, great concentrations of angiogenesis and inflammation related growth factors, such as VEGF or angiopoietin 1 [564], were found in pulmonary tissue and were reported to cause a vascular patency variation but also modifications of the vessels fenestration [565].

MSCs, but also HSCs, that both have the capacity to differentiate into endothelial cells [166, 528], could intervene in the asthmatic angiogenesis. Moreover, bone marrow hematopoiesis sites can be stimulated by circulating factors produced during the airways inflammation [566], leading to the mobilization of inflammatory cells and various progenitors. Such cells could play an important role in the airway chronic inflammatory response by attenuating immunological responses [476], or by initiating the epithelium [567], collagen [554], blood vessels [568] and muscular cells smooth [569] remodeling.

Idiopathic pulmonary fibrosis and emphysema: The idiopathic pulmonary fibrosis and the emphysema are two pulmonary pathology examples where the stem cells contribution is defective in the local cellular regeneration with in particular an abnormal localization and differentiation of these stem cells within the pulmonary tissue.

The idiopathic pulmonary fibrosis could be the result of an initial lesion, inducing an inflammatory response or an activation of alveolar epithelial cells leading to a rise in the cytokine rate, an inappropriate signalization of the epithelial and mesenchymal cells and a disorganization of tissue repair [570, 571]. Although this disease is usually characterized by a small artery muscularization, Cosgrove and collaborators reported a strong reduction in the vessel density associated with an aberrant angiogenesis after pulmonary tissue histological observation [572]. In the same way, Ebina and collaborators reported an absence of vessels in pulmonary fibrosis zone with fibroblastic proliferation [573]. These myofibroblasts could also derive from preexistent intra-pulmonary mesenchymal precursors, but also from circulating progenitors such as MSCs or HSCs [574].

Emphysema and chronic obstructive pulmonary disease are also characterized they by a pulmonary blood vessel rarefaction, with a parenchyma destruction, an apoptose increase and an airway widening and fibrosis [575-577]. The origin of the cells contributing to the final fibrosis is discussed, with a pulmonary origin [578] or a bone marrow origin [554, 579]. The treatment would consist in the stimulation of an intact epithelium formation and in the fibroblastic proliferation suppression with in particular a correction of the local or bone marrow derived stem cell deficiency.

2. Stem Cell Implication during Cardiac Remodeling

The cardiomyocyte loss after a myocardial infarction causes a contractile function loss, since the necrotic area is replaced by fibroblasts forming an uncontractile scar tissue. Furthermore, the surrounding myocardium remodeling is itself critical and raise the cardiac insufficiency [580]. The fetal cardiomyocyte or skeletal myoblasts transplantation was proposed as a future method to treat myocardial infarctions [581-584].

a) Cellular Therapy of Myocardial Infarction

Several authors showed that the direct injection, within the coronary arteries, of a bone marrow derived heterogeneous stem cell population or MSCs could represent a simple but effective approach in the heart attack treatment. Thus, Strauer reported in 2002 a clinical study with 20 patients in the treatment of myocardial infarction [585]. After right and left catheterization, coronary angiography and left ventriculography, patients underwent a balloon angioplasty. Five to 9 days after the acute infarction, bone marrow cells were aspired and the mononuclear fraction, able to generate MSCs *in vitro*, was transplanted within the infarcted zone using a small balloon angioplasty. Tree months after, the comparison of both groups, treated by standard therapy or by cell transplantation, showed a significant positive effect of the cellular treatment on the cardiac function and on the infarcted zone regression. At last, the perfusion defect within the myocardium, detected by thallium scintigraphy, was considerably decreased in the cell treated group [585].

Another study on the use of the cellular therapy for the treatment of the myocardium acute infarction was carried out by the team of Chen in 2004 [372]. Sixty-nine patients, presenting a beginning of infarction since less than 12 hours and undergoing emergency angiography and angioplasty, were recruited in a randomized clinical study to receive or not autologous MSCs after bone marrow aspiration realized during the urgency examination. Ten days after the cardiac event, the adherent mononuclear fraction, cultivated *in vitro* to obtain MSCs, was injected through the coronary artery near the infarcted zone, while the other group of patients received a physiological solution. After a regular echocardiogram, echo-cardiography and positron emission tomography, the percentage of hypokinetic, akinetic, and dyskinetic segments significantly decreased in the cell-treated group after 3 months in comparison with the control group and with the beginning of the study. At last, the left ventricular ejection fraction was higher in the cell treated group compared to patients who received a physiological solution [372].

A randomized clinical study reported by the group of Wollert allowed to evaluate by echocardiography the effectiveness of the local injection of autologous adherent bone marrow cells (mainly MSCs) for the acute myocardial infarction treatment [371]. After angioplasty, patients were randomly separated in two groups to receive the traditional post-infarction treatment or an *in situ* injection of autologous cells cultivated *in vitro* during 4 to 8 days. Although authors could not highlight significant differences between the two groups regarding the left ventricular volumes in systole and diastole, they reported after 6 months a significant beneficial effect of the cellular therapy on the right ventricular ejection fraction and on the mobility of the ventricular wall surrounding the infarcted zone. Authors thus suggested that autologous adherent bone marrow cells could be injected *in situ* to improve the restoration of the ventricular function among patients presenting a myocardial infarction [371].

However, while experimental and clinical studies tend to support an improvement of cardiac repair by the cellular therapy, many points remain to be clear up; including 1/the optimal cellular type corresponding to the patient clinical profile, 2/the mechanism inducing the cardiac function improvement, 3/the cell survival optimization, 4/the development of less traumatic administration techniques, and 5/the potential benefits of cell transplantation in non-ischemic heart failure. Moreover, recent studies showed that adult stem cells (cardiomyocytes or bone marrow stem cells) fail to integrate electromechanically within the recipient heart, while cardiac stem cells and cardiac-precommitted ES cells could allow a true regeneration of the necrotic myocardium [586].

b) Mechanisms of Cardiac Repair

All these results, as well as others presenting similar studies [587, 588], show that the bone marrow stem cell therapy is feasible and sure, and could contribute to the tissue regeneration after myocardial infarction. Nevertheless, several aspects remain controversial: what kind of stem cells is appropriate to the patients? When these cells should be transplanted to patients? How the transplanted cell viability may be supervised? What is the action mechanism of the transplanted stem cells: secretion of growth factors or cell-to-cell interactions?

Some studies were thus interested in the cell type allowing the post-infarction cardiac function improvement after transplantation. Based on the cell therapeutic effectiveness and on the fact that an unpurified mononuclear cell population avoided cell expansion problems but was inevitably composed of a small percentage of pluripotent cells diluted among an enormous quantity of committed cells, some authors supposed that the preliminary culture of a bone marrow cell population composed of MSCs and endothelial progenitors could support at the same time the cardiomyogenesis (by MSCs) and the angiogenesis (by endothelial progenitors) on the level of the infarcted zone [589]. These authors thus enrolled patients presenting a recent or old myocardial infarction treated by angioplasty. Autologous MSCs and endothelial progenitors, selected *in vitro* during 7 days, were injected into the left coronary artery during catheterization and allowed a heart contractility improvement in one or more myocardial segments previously nonviable, while this improvement was not found in the group controls. Results indicated that the two cell type used (MSCs and endothelial progenitors) had a positive effect on the myocardial contractility mainly with patients presenting a recent myocardial infarction [589].

Perin *et al.* have evaluated the potential effect of a bone marrow-derived mononuclear cell transplantation on neo-vascularization and on the cardiac functionality loss prevention leading to the myocardial infarction in patients with cardiac ischemia [590]. They thus treated chronic coronary patients, who had a left ventricular ejection fraction lower than 40% and who were ineligible for a percutaneous or surgical revascularization, by cell therapy. Patients received local injections of bone marrow-derived mononuclear autologous cells during the cardiac catheterization intervention with electromechanical cartography of the ventricle right allowing the viable ventricular zone identification. Two and 4 months after, patients treated by cell therapy presented a cardiac function improvement [590] and an increased myocardial perfusion and exercise capacity [591].

At last, to determine if the myocardial regeneration observed after a stem cell injection was due to a cardiomyocyte differentiation or to the formation of new vessels, two animal studies reported the MSC effects on cardiac cytoprotection. The first study, based on a myocardial infarction experimental model after ligation of the left anterior descending coronary artery in rats, showed that the injection of MSCs in the infarcted myocardial zone increased the release of angiogenic factors, such as SDF-1, bFGF or VEGF [540]. Moreover, these authors reported a capillary density rise in animals treated with MSCs. Thus, this team supposed that the cardiac cytoprotection effects caused by the MSC injection were mainly due to a paracrine-induced angiogenesis [540]. The second study was interested in the angiogenic roles of MSCs in the myocardium regeneration after experimental infarction in rats [373]. A MSC monolayer, cultured *in vitro* on a detachable support and transplanted onto the scarred myocardium, allowed the formation of a thick stratum that included newly formed vessels, undifferentiated cells and few cardiomyocytes. Moreover, the stem cell layer secreted paracrine factors inducing angiogenesis. Thus, authors evidenced that MSCs could regenerate the myocardium by acting on angiogenesis and cardiac cytoprotection induced by paracrine factors. Furthermore, MSCs were also reported to be integrated into tissue and to be differentiated in cardiomyocytes and vascular cells [373].

3. Stem Cell Implication during Systemic Vascular Remodeling

Beside cardiopulmonary pathologies with an abnormal vascularization, ischemic effects can touch other organs or tissues inducing a reduction of the blood circulation by obstruction (atherosclerosis and obliterating arteriopathy of the lower limbs, renal ischemia). The treatment consists in tracking techniques, in angioplasty, in arterial bypass surgery or at last in the member amputation. Since many years, studies patients touched by vascular ischemia showed the spontaneous development of a collateral vascularization replacing the normal circulation [592-596]. Several approaches emerged to stimulate these spontaneous reparation mechanisms, in particular by activating the growth of compensatory blood vessels attenuating a too weak blood flow. Thus, most studies had concentrated on the stem and progenitor cell participation in two distinct types to reduce ischemia, such as the formation of new collateral vessels starting from preexistent vascular structures (angiogenesis) [597] or the growth and the enlargement of thin capillaries already present and functional (arteriogenesis) [598].

a) Atherosclerosis

Atherosclerosis is a phenomenon physiological of blood vessel ageing with loss of elasticity that begins with the embryonic life and that is considerably accelerated by cardiovascular risk factors (smoking, cholesterol, arterial hypertension, diabetes, sedentary, alcohol, heredity, age and gender). Thin arterial lesions can be observed as early as 20 years of age, while several various development stages were identified involving an intimal remodeling of the large and medium blood vessels (aorta and its branches, coronary, cerebral or lower limbs arteries) and an accumulation of lipids, complex carbohydrates, blood and blood products, fat tissues and mineral deposits.

The traditional hypothesis [599], which assumes that the smooth muscle cells forming atherosclerotic lesions would come from the vessel media layer after migration towards a neointimal space, is currently questioned since there are many evidence showing that these smooth muscle cells could also come from circulating progenitors [600]. The HSC participation in the atherosclerosis development was reported in 2002 by Sata [601] who gave the bases for the development of new strategies in the vascular pathology treatment by directing the mobilization, the domiciliation, the differentiation and the proliferation of bone marrow derived progenitors. Then other authors explored the immunophenotypical profile of cells found in atherosclerotic lesions of Apo-E mice [556]. They thus reported that a great number of these cells exhibited stem cell markers (Sca-1, C-kit, CD34, Flk1), indicating that many stem cell types, including endothelial progenitors, MSCs and HSCs, may participate in the formation of atherosclerotic vascular remodeling. Moreover, when Sca-1^{+} cells were injected onto the adventitia surrounding remodeled zones, these cells were found within atherosclerotic intimal lesions, thus showing their migration and their participation in the development of atherosclerotic lesions [556].

Recent studies reported the migration of stem cells coming from the vascular wall towards atherosclerotic lesion sites [602, 603], such as MSCs [604]. Since MSCs have the capacities to modulate the proliferation and the migration of smooth muscle cells and to differentiate into endothelial cells [605], MSCs could thus contribute to the atherosclerotic smooth muscle layer and could contribute to form a fibromuscular cap stabilizing the vulnerable atherosclerotic plaque. After bone marrow transplantation [606] or in an atherosclerosis mouse model [607], donor cells were found in vascular zones with atherosclerotic plaques but not in normal zones, indicating that this cell domiciliation could require inflammatory signals. Thus, since stem cells participate in the renewal and the generation of vascular tissues, a deregulation of these stem cells could play a part in the atherosclerosis development.

b) Vascular Stenosis

Arterial (re)stenosis is a physiopathological phenomenon that may occur after an angioplasty, an arteriotomy, or a bypass in human and in experimental animal models of vascular lesions, that induces a partial or complete occlusion of the arterial lumen and thus often requires a new revascularization procedure. The vascular damage, with intimal and medial cell loss, the internal elastic lamina fragmentation and the architectural tissue lesions, leads to an excessive repair and to the proliferation and the migration of smooth muscle cells, inducing a neointimal hyperplasia [608, 609]. Recent studies evidenced that the vascular function depended not only on the cells within the vessels, but also that stenosis and restenosis were also significantly modulated by bone marrow-derived stem cells [610]. Thus, some authors supposed that restenosis could be prevented by an early vessel repair under the influence of stem cells, such as endothelial progenitors or MSCs.

An interesting study was carried out by using endogenous endothelial progenitors where authors surgically implanted anti-CD34 coated stents and reported that circulating endothelial progenitors were captured on the stent surface leading to a prevention of a thrombus formation and restenosis [611]. A similar study in clinical situation was initiated in 2006 to determine the effects of the endothelial progenitor capture on stents, coupled with a statine-induced mobilization [612].

Many studies were also interested in the potential role of MSCs in the restenosis vascular process. Indeed, MSCs injected into the blood circulation 15 minutes before the induction of a vascular lesion were reported to have the capacity to domiciliate at the site lesion and in particular in vasa vasorum containing adventitial zones, in a rat coronary arteriotomy model [608]. Moreover, Han reported in 2001 the contribution of MSCs to a neointimal formation in a mouse model of iliac artery scratch lesion [613]. These authors also showed that 56% of the alpha-smooth muscle actin positive cells from the neointima were bone marrow stem cells. At last, these results, regarding the MSC acquisition of a smooth muscle profile during vascular lesions, were also confirmed by Tanaka *et al.* [610].

4. Stem Cell Implication during Tumor Vasculature Development

At the opposite of beneficial effects of such mechanisms reducing ischemia, the formation of the tumor vasculature is harmful since it allows the tumor to grow and leads to metastasis.

In 1971, Folkman was the first to postulate that the tumor growth and the development of metastases were angiogenesis dependant processes [614]. After what, various stages of the tumor development were reported [615] and showed that several genetic and epigenetic changes occurred in tumor cells, and revealed the microenvironment role in the malignity development. Indeed, tumors are made up of neoplastic cells and a stroma composed of fibroblasts, myofibroblasts, endothelial cells, pericytes and infiltrated hematopoietic cells. These tumor associated cells are supposed to control critical processes in the tumor progression, such as the tumor cell evolution, the anti-tumor immunity, the extracellular matrix remodeling, the angiogenesis and the metastasis invasion [616-619]. Thus, hematopoietic cells exhibit several functions in the tumor development, by decreasing the tumor immunogenicity and by stimulating the neoplastic progression [620].

In addition to stimulate the tumor cell growth and migration, the hematopoietic cells were reported to secrete factors inducing the tumor angiogenesis, allowing the generation of blood vessels with the tumor and providing nutrients and oxygen needed to the tumor growth. Angiogenesis was for a long time considered as a critical stage in the tumor growth, thus representing a key target in anti-tumor strategies [621, 622]. Many studies brought back the bone marrow-derived stem cell participation in the tumor angiogenesis, including MSCs, HSCs and endothelial progenitors. However, the specific stem cell type accused and the exact function of these cells in the tumor vessel formation remain irresolute and discussed.

The endothelial progenitor contribution to the tumor angiogenesis was reported in 2001 by Lyden, when he used a tumor xenograft murine model [623]. Other authors also proposed that this endothelial progenitor mobilization, from the bone marrow towards tumor sites, required the activation of the matrix metalloproteinase-9 [624]. However, De Palma reported that only a few number of endothelial progenitors integrated within new vessels was really detected and that a majority of bone marrow-derived cells found in tumor vessels was found localized in perivascular zones, attesting of a preferentially paracrine role rather than structural [625]. At last, another study reported that 4.9% of the total endothelial cells in tumor vessels came from the bone marrow [626].

Recently, some studies also studied the MSC potential role in the tumor angiogenesis. One pioneer study thus evidenced that MSCs could be integrated in tumor vessels [627]. MSCs were also reported to support the tumor growth *in vivo* [628]. Then, MSCs were suggested to have a positive role on the development of preexistent tumors, but also to have a tumor-initiating role. According to this concept, MSCs would fuse with muted cells leading to a tumor formation. In this case, bone marrow stem cells would be at the same time tools and targets for an anti-tumor therapy.

5. MSCs and Vascular Engineering

The increasing request for vascular grafts, in particular for vessels with a diameter lower than 5 mm, generated a growing interest for the artificial vascular prosthesis engineering. During 30 years, several synthetic materials, such as expanded polytetrafluoroethylene (ePTFE) and polyurethane, have been used to engineer small diameter vessels, but unfortunately, they did not lead to satisfactory patency, mainly because of a strong thrombosis [629]. This approach was then improved by seeding the prosthesis internal face with endothelial cells, thus reducing thrombosis [630-632]. Furthermore, vascular prosthesis seeded with smooth muscle and endothelial cells revealed a higher patency than unseeded covered prosthesis [633, 634], but thrombosis and restenosis of these prosthesis however remained notable [635]. The reasons could be a loss of the smooth muscle or endothelial cell functions during their *ex vivo* expansion, or a loss of cells *in vivo* by prosthesis partial washing caused by vascular flow.

Endothelial progenitors were first used to seed prosthesis, with an excellent patency after 130 days in a ovine carotid graft model [636]. However, these endothelial progenitors were not able to generate smooth muscle cells, indicating that this lonely cell type was not sufficient to regenerate a complete vascular structure. An alternative approach was then initiated by using MSCs to replace smooth muscle or endothelial cells. In 2005, Cho reported the use of bone marrow-derived adherent stem cells, differentiated in culture into smooth muscle or endothelial cells, to seed a vascular prosthesis [637, 638], while Kanki-Horimoto used β-galactosidase transduced MSCs to seed the internal face of a small diameter vascular prosthesis [639]. Taken together, these results evidenced that both MSC derived smooth muscle and endothelial cells contributed to the regeneration of the three vascular layers (intima, media and adventitia) and improved the small diameter vessel patency. However, we do not know yet if undifferentiated MSCs seeding on vascular prosthesis can differentiate *in vivo* into smooth muscle and endothelial cells.

a) Various Materials

Most of materials used currently to develop small diameter vascular grafts consist of synthetic or natural polymers with variable thickness, porosity, elasticity and density degrees. One of the first studies interested in the impact of these several parameters on the vascular patency showed that a low pore diameter promoted the cell growth and the vascular graft patency [629]. Thus, several studies were conducted with microporous vascular substitutes, such as the expanded polytetrafluoroethylene, allowing small diameter vessels (a few millimeters) to be successfully seeded with bone marrow derived stem cells [637]. A polypropylene carbonate matrix seeded with MSCs was also used to form small diameter vessels (2 mm) [640] because of its excellent compatibility its biological resorption [641].

Other materials, such as poly-glycolic acid polymers, were also reported to have a good MSC adhesion capacity and a gradual degradation allowing its physiological replacement by tissue [642]. Various resorbable materials were thus successfully seeded by MSCs, such as poly-L-lactic acid polymers [643], poly-lactic-Co-glycolic acid polymers [644, 645] or sodium arginate matrix [645]. Other new bioabsorbable matrices were used as cell culture support before being implanted *in vivo*. These synthetic polymer vascular substitutes, composed of 4-hydroxy-butyric acid, supported cell culture *in vitro* and after may be colonized by vascular cells after *in vivo* implantation [646]. Moreover, this substitute allowed the concentric cell growth of several overlaid layers. At last, authors reported a complete resorption of the synthetic material after 169 days, allowing the establishment of vascular structures without the long-term foreign material presence [646].

Other authors also reported the use of biological matrices where endogenous cells were eliminated by detergents (Triton) [638]. The resulting biological matrix, composed of collagen fibers, elastin and extracellular matrix molecules, was seeded with bone marrow-derived stem cells *in vitro* differentiated into smooth muscle and endothelial cells. After *in vivo* implantation, this vascular substitute conducted to a complete and functional vascular wall [638]. The major advantage of this substitute is its biological source (sometimes autologous), but above all this decellularized material limits the inflammation risk [647].

b) The Mechanical Stress Impact

Many studies showed that a mechanical environment controlled the smooth muscle cell characteristics. *In vivo*, smooth muscle cells within vascular walls reside typically in a dynamic environment with a vascular flow where they are guided in a particular direction and where they exhibit a contractile phenotype, which is crucial for the vascular tissue properties [648]. However, vascular smooth muscular tissues, produced *in vitro* with conventional culture techniques, could not be functional since cells are not lined up [649, 650] and exhibit a synthetic phenotype instead of a contractile phenotype [651, 652].

Several mechanical constraints can be found into vascular walls according to their localization. For example, the blood vessel rectilinear part is mainly subjected to a cyclic mechanical force following a circumferential direction, while junction or diameter change zones (e.g. aneurism) are subjected to isotropic constraints. To determine the relative contribution of each mechanical force on smooth muscle cell effects and regulation mechanisms, several equipments were developed. Thus, cells were cultured on two dimension deformable substrates (e.g. silicone membranes) where mechanical forces can be applied to stretch the substrate according to only one or several axes in the same plan. Three dimension systems were then used to mimic the pulsatile nature of the blood flow into a vascular substitute tube whose internal face was seeded with cells. These studies evidenced the importance of mechanical signals in the smooth muscle cell phenotype regulation in two dimensions systems [653-655] and in the smooth muscle cell proliferation and migration in three dimensions systems [648, 656, 657]. Thus, the design of vascular substitutes under mechanical constraints led to the improvement of the vascular patency, with an enhancement of the collagen production and with an increased protection against mechanical strains [633, 658].

At last, the induction the expression of smooth muscle-related properties were reported for MSC when cultured under mechanical stresses produced in these culture systems [659, 660]. Thus, the contractile protein expression (actin and myosin) was preferentially induced by the pressure constraints whereas shear-stress forces induced by the pulsatile component of flow did not induce this protein expression [659].

c) Towards the Realization of a Functional and Complete Vessel

Researches for a perfect complete and functional biocompatible vessel model started in 1986 when Weinberg and Bell designed for the first time an artery with multiple concentric layers around a Dacron mesh and where the vascular lumen was limited by endothelial cells [661]. Then in 1999, Niklason was among the first to report the *in vitro* constitution of a complete vessel starting from a poly-glycolic acid biodegradable matrix seeded with smooth muscle cells cultivated under pulsatile conditions [633]. After incubation during 8 weeks in a bioreactor under a radial pulsatile stress, this synthetic vessel presented concentric smooth muscle layers that could be recovered by an endothelial cell monolayer. At last, these authors also reported the absence of stenosis or dilation and an excellent patency up to 24 days after the substitution of a miniature swine femoral artery portion [633]. This *in vitro* engineered new concept of artificially vessels was also used by Hoerstrup who sequentially seeded fibroblasts and endothelial cells. Then, the resulting graft was placed under natural mechanical conditions of pulsatile flow, pressure and forces of shearing [662].

Taken together and considering our current knowledge regarding the MSC differentiation capacities into smooth muscle cells but also the technical possibilities to engineer arteries with several concentric layers, why a complete and functional vessel is not yet engineered and used in human? One of the problems could be the need to maintain a controlled growth of the new vessel allowing its growth and its remodeling capacities, but also preserving a biocompatibility [643, 663]. This difficulty could be overcome by using autologous stem cells, ensuring the biocompatibility and maintaining a proliferative potential. Another obstacle may be the requirement to cultivate these cells *in vitro* under an adequate flow in a growing medium containing animal-derived proteins and growth factors while these vascular substitutes will have to be implanted into men. However, this could be over-passed by the future arrival of serum-free culture medium.

Thus, the use of MSCs to engineer synthetic vessels is right at its beginning. Models currently used showed the utility to recreate conditions mimicking the morphological and the biological environment.

Conclusion

A better knowledge of the factors intervening in the MSC mobilization, domiciliation and differentiation is of obvious potential interest to use these cells in therapy. In the same way, the intrinsic roles of these cells in the vascular remodeling processes in response to chemotactic signals released by injured tissues remain to be determined. Lastly, MSCs improve significantly the biocompatibility of vascular prosthesis, and furthermore allow a complete and functional arterial wall to be recreated. Thus, the use of MSCs as a product for cell therapies remains a future prospect, since these cells exhibit a great plasticity and biocompatibility authorizing them to colonize many tissues, to survive and release many cytoprotective and angiogenic factors.

MSCs also exhibit a great capacity to domiciliate into several tissues. At last, their differentiation potential into vascular smooth muscle cells and their ability to response to mechanical stress authorize them to be used extensively for regenerative vascular therapies, like cardiac vascular endoprosthesis or valvular and vessel biocompatible prosthesis.

References

[1] Verfaillie, C.M., Adult stem cells: assessing the case for pluripotency. *Trends Cell Biol*, 2002. 12(11): p. 502-8.

[2] Preston, S.L., et al., The new stem cell biology: something for everyone. *Mol. Pathol.*, 2003. 56(2): p. 86-96.

[3] Wobus, A.M. and K.R. Boheler, Embryonic stem cells: prospects for developmental biology and cell therapy. *Physiol. Rev.*, 2005. 85(2): p. 635-78.

[4] Prelle, K., et al., Establishment of pluripotent cell lines from vertebrate species--present status and future prospects. *Cells Tissues Organs*, 1999. 165(3-4): p. 220-36.

[5] Pain, B., et al., Long-term in vitro culture and characterisation of avian embryonic stem cells with multiple morphogenetic potentialities. *Development,* 1996. 122(8): p. 2339-48.

[6] Chang, I.K., et al., Production of germline chimeric chickens by transfer of cultured primordial germ cells. *Cell Biol. Int.,* 1997. 21(8): p. 495-9.

[7] Doetschman, T., P. Williams, and N. Maeda, Establishment of hamster blastocyst-derived embryonic stem (ES) cells. *Dev. Biol.*, 1988. 127(1): p. 224-7.

[8] Graves, K.H. and R.W. Moreadith, Derivation and characterization of putative pluripotential embryonic stem cells from preimplantation rabbit embryos. *Mol. Reprod. Dev.,* 1993. 36(4): p. 424-33.

[9] Schoonjans, L., et al., Pluripotential rabbit embryonic stem (ES) cells are capable of forming overt coat color chimeras following injection into blastocysts. *Mol. Reprod. Dev.*, 1996. 45(4): p. 439-43.
[10] Iannaccone, P.M., et al., Pluripotent embryonic stem cells from the rat are capable of producing chimeras. *Dev. Biol.*, 1994. 163(1): p. 288-92.
[11] Brenin, D., et al., Rat embryonic stem cells: a progress report. *Transplant Proc.*, 1997. 29(3): p. 1761-5.
[12] Vassilieva, S., et al., Establishment of SSEA-1- and Oct-4-expressing rat embryonic stem-like cell lines and effects of cytokines of the IL-6 family on clonal growth. *Exp. Cell Res.*, 2000. 258(2): p. 361-73.
[13] Buehr, M., et al., Rapid loss of Oct-4 and pluripotency in cultured rodent blastocysts and derivative cell lines. *Biol. Reprod.*, 2003. 68(1): p. 222-9.
[14] Thomson, J.A., et al., Isolation of a primate embryonic stem cell line. *Proc. Natl. Acad. Sci. USA,* 1995. 92(17): p. 7844-8.
[15] Pau, K.Y. and D.P. Wolf, Derivation and characterization of monkey embryonic stem cells. *Reprod. Biol. Endocrinol.*, 2004. 2: p. 41.
[16] Thomson, J.A., et al., Pluripotent cell lines derived from common marmoset (Callithrix jacchus) blastocysts. *Biol. Reprod.*, 1996. 55(2): p. 254-9.
[17] Sucmori, H., et al., Establishment of embryonic stem cell lines from cynomolgus monkey blastocysts produced by IVF or ICSI. *Dev. Dyn*, 2001. 222(2): p. 273-9.
[18] Stevens, L.C., Origin of testicular teratomas from primordial germ cells in mice. *J. Natl. Cancer Inst*, 1967. 38(4): p. 549-52.
[19] Kahan, B.W. and B. Ephrussi, Developmental potentialities of clonal in vitro cultures of mouse testicular teratoma. *J. Natl. Cancer Inst.*, 1970. 44(5): p. 1015-36.
[20] Jacob, S.W. and R. Herschler, Pharmacology of DMSO. *Cryobiology*, 1986. 23(1): p. 14-27.
[21] Gearhart, J.D. and B. Mintz, Contact-mediated myogenesis and increased acetylcholinesterase activity in primary cultures of mouse teratocarcinoma cells. *Proc. Natl. Acad. Sci. USA*, 1974. 71(5): p. 1734-8.
[22] Stevens, L.C., The development of transplantable teratocarcinomas from intratesticular grafts of pre- and postimplantation mouse embryos. *Dev. Biol.*, 1970. 21(3): p. 364-82.
[23] Evans, M.J., The isolation and properties of a clonal tissue culture strain of pluripotent mouse teratoma cells. *J. Embryol. Exp. Morphol.*, 1972. 28(1): p. 163-76.
[24] Skarnes, W.C., et al., Capturing genes encoding membrane and secreted proteins important for mouse development. *Proc. Natl. Acad. Sci. USA*, 1995. 92(14): p. 6592-6.
[25] Papaioannou, V.E., et al., Fate of teratocarcinoma cells injected into early mouse embryos. *Nature,* 1975. 258(5530): p. 70-73.
[26] Berstine, E.G., et al., Alkaline phosphatase activity in mouse teratoma. *Proc. Natl. Acad. Sci. USA*, 1973. 70(12): p. 3899-903.
[27] Nicolas, J.F., et al., [Mouse teratocarcinoma: differentiation in cultures of a multipotential primitive cell line (author's transl)]. *Ann. Microbiol.* (Paris), 1975. 126(1): p. 3-22.
[28] McBurney, M.W., et al., Control of muscle and neuronal differentiation in a cultured embryonal carcinoma cell line. *Nature*, 1982. 299(5879): p. 165-7.

[29] Martin, G.R. and M.J. Evans, The morphology and growth of a pluripotent teratocarcinoma cell line and its derivatives in tissue culture. *Cell*, 1974. 2(3): p. 163-72.

[30] Mintz, B. and K. Illmensee, Normal genetically mosaic mice produced from malignant teratocarcinoma cells. *Proc. Natl. Acad. Sci. USA*, 1975. 72(9): p. 3585-9.

[31] Andrews, P.W., From teratocarcinomas to embryonic stem cells. *Philos. Trans R Soc. Lond B Biol. Sci.*, 2002. 357(1420): p. 405-17.

[32] Bradley, A., et al., Formation of germ-line chimaeras from embryo-derived teratocarcinoma cell lines. *Nature*, 1984. 309(5965): p. 255-6.

[33] Evans, M.J. and M.H. Kaufman, Establishment in culture of pluripotential cells from mouse embryos. *Nature,* 1981. 292(5819): p. 154-6.

[34] Wobus, A.M., et al., Characterization of a pluripotent stem cell line derived from a mouse embryo. *Exp. Cell Res.,* 1984. 152(1): p. 212-9.

[35] Doetschman, T.C., et al., The in vitro development of blastocyst-derived embryonic stem cell lines: formation of visceral yolk sac, blood islands and myocardium. *J. Embryol. Exp. Morphol.*, 1985. 87: p. 27-45.

[36] Hubner, K., et al., Derivation of oocytes from mouse embryonic stem cells. *Science*, 2003. 300(5623): p. 1251-6.

[37] Toyooka, Y., et al., Embryonic stem cells can form germ cells in vitro. *Proc. Natl. Acad. Sci. USA*, 2003. 100(20): p. 11457-62.

[38] Geijsen, N., et al., Derivation of embryonic germ cells and male gametes from embryonic stem cells. *Nature*, 2004. 427(6970): p. 148-54.

[39] Rohwedel, J., et al., Primordial germ cell-derived mouse embryonic germ (EG) cells in vitro resemble undifferentiated stem cells with respect to differentiation capacity and cell cycle distribution. *Cell Biol. Int.*, 1996. 20(8): p. 579-87.

[40] Labosky, P.A., D.P. Barlow, and B.L. Hogan, Embryonic germ cell lines and their derivation from mouse primordial germ cells. *Ciba Found Symp.*, 1994. 182: p. 157-68; discussion 168-78.

[41] Labosky, P.A., D.P. Barlow, and B.L. Hogan, Mouse embryonic germ (EG) cell lines: transmission through the germline and differences in the methylation imprint of insulin-like growth factor 2 receptor (Igf2r) gene compared with embryonic stem (ES) cell lines. *Development*, 1994. 120(11): p. 3197-204.

[42] Stewart, C.L., I. Gadi, and H. Bhatt, Stem cells from primordial germ cells can reenter the germ line. *Dev. Biol.*, 1994. 161(2): p. 626-8.

[43] Matsui, Y., K. Zsebo, and B.L. Hogan, Derivation of pluripotential embryonic stem cells from murine primordial germ cells in culture. *Cell*, 1992. 70(5): p. 841-7.

[44] Verfaillie, C.M., M.F. Pera, and P.M. Lansdorp, Stem cells: hype and reality. H*ematology* (Am Soc Hematol Educ Program), 2002: p. 369-91.

[45] Spangrude, G.J., S. Heimfeld, and I.L. Weissman, Purification and characterization of mouse hematopoietic stem cells. *Science*, 1988. 241(4861): p. 58-62.

[46] Weissman, I.L., Translating stem and progenitor cell biology to the clinic: barriers and opportunities. *Science,* 2000. 287(5457): p. 1442-6.

[47] Rheinwald, J.G. and H. Green, Serial cultivation of strains of human epidermal keratinocytes: the formation of keratinizing colonies from single cells. *Cell*, 1975. 6(3): p. 331-43.

[48] Asahara, T., et al., Isolation of putative progenitor endothelial cells for angiogenesis. *Science,* 1997. 275(5302): p. 964-7.
[49] Gage, F.H., Mammalian neural stem cells. *Science*, 2000. 287(5457): p. 1433-8.
[50] Gage, F.H., Structural plasticity: cause, result, or correlate of depression. *Biol. Psychiatry,* 2000. 48(8): p. 713-4.
[51] Schofield, R., The relationship between the spleen colony-forming cell and the haemopoietic stem cell. *Blood Cells*, 1978. 4(1-2): p. 7-25.
[52] Lin, H., The stem-cell niche theory: lessons from flies. *Nat. Rev. Genet*, 2002. 3(12): p. 931-40.
[53] Spradling, A., D. Drummond-Barbosa, and T. Kai, Stem cells find their niche. *Nature*, 2001. 414(6859): p. 98-104.
[54] Kopp, H.G., et al., The bone marrow vascular niche: home of HSC differentiation and mobilization. *Physiology* (Bethesda), 2005. 20: p. 349-56.
[55] Moore, K.A. and I.R. Lemischka, Stem cells and their niches. *Science*, 2006. 311(5769): p. 1880-5.
[56] Dazzi, F., et al., The role of mesenchymal stem cells in haemopoiesis. *Blood Rev.*, 2006. 20(3): p. 161-71.
[57] Friedenstein, A.J., et al., Precursors for fibroblasts in different populations of hematopoietic cells as detected by the in vitro colony assay method. *Exp. Hematol.*, 1974. 2(2): p. 83-92.
[58] Friedenstein, A.J., et al., Origin of bone marrow stromal mechanocytes in radiochimeras and heterotopic transplants. *Exp. Hematol.*, 1978. 6(5): p. 440-4.
[59] Caplan, A.I., Mesenchymal stem cells. *J. Orthop Res.*, 1991. 9(5): p. 641-50.
[60] Owen, M., Marrow stromal stem cells. *J. Cell Sci. Suppl.*, 1988. 10: p. 63-76.
[61] Owen, M. and A.J. Friedenstein, Stromal stem cells: marrow-derived osteogenic precursors. Ciba Found Symp, 1988. 136: p. 42-60.
[62] Prockop, D.J., Marrow stromal cells as stem cells for nonhematopoietic tissues. *Science,* 1997. 276(5309): p. 71-4.
[63] Dennis, J.E., et al., A quadripotential mesenchymal progenitor cell isolated from the marrow of an adult mouse. *J. Bone Miner Res.*, 1999. 14(5): p. 700-9.
[64] Bhagavati, S. and W. Xu, Isolation and enrichment of skeletal muscle progenitor cells from mouse bone marrow. *Biochem. Biophys. Res. Commun.*, 2004. 318(1): p. 119-24.
[65] Bianco, P. and P. Gehron Robey, Marrow stromal stem cells. *J. Clin. Invest,* 2000. 105(12): p. 1663-8.
[66] Bianco, P., et al., Bone marrow stromal stem cells: nature, biology, and potential applications. *Stem Cells,* 2001. 19(3): p. 180-92.
[67] Kuznetsov, S.A., et al., Circulating skeletal stem cells. *J. Cell Biol.*, 2001. 153(5): p. 1133-40.
[68] Reyes, M., et al., Purification and ex vivo expansion of postnatal human marrow mesodermal progenitor cells. *Blood,* 2001. 98(9): p. 2615-25.
[69] Jiang, Y., et al., Pluripotency of mesenchymal stem cells derived from adult marrow. *Nature*, 2002. 418(6893): p. 41-9.
[70] Pittenger, M.F., et al., Multilineage potential of adult human mesenchymal stem cells. *Science,* 1999. 284(5411): p. 143-7.
[71] Zvaifler, N.J., et al., Mesenchymal precursor cells in the blood of normal individuals. *Arthritis Res.*, 2000. 2(6): p. 477-88.

[72] Covas, D.T., et al., Isolation and culture of umbilical vein mesenchymal stem cells. *Braz. J. Med. Biol. Res.,* 2003. 36(9): p. 1179-83.

[73] In 't Anker, P.S., et al., Isolation of mesenchymal stem cells of fetal or maternal origin from human placenta. *Stem Cells*, 2004. 22(7): p. 1338-45.

[74] Zhang, Y., et al., Comparison of mesenchymal stem cells from human placenta and bone marrow. *Chin. Med. J.* (Engl), 2004. 117(6): p. 882-7.

[75] Miao, Z., et al., Isolation of mesenchymal stem cells from human placenta: Comparison with human bone marrow mesenchymal stem cells. *Cell Biol. Int.,* 2006. 30(9): p. 681-7.

[76] Phinney, D.G., et al., Plastic adherent stromal cells from the bone marrow of commonly used strains of inbred mice: variations in yield, growth, and differentiation. *J. Cell Biochem.,* 1999. 72(4): p. 570-85.

[77] Baddoo, M., et al., Characterization of mesenchymal stem cells isolated from murine bone marrow by negative selection. *J. Cell Biochem.*, 2003. 89(6): p. 1235-49.

[78] Tropel, P., et al., Isolation and characterisation of mesenchymal stem cells from adult mouse bone marrow. *Exp. Cell Res.*, 2004. 295(2): p. 395-406.

[79] Rochefort, G.Y., et al., Multipotential mesenchymal stem cells are mobilized into peripheral blood by hypoxia. *Stem Cells*, 2006. 24(10): p. 2202-8.

[80] Rochefort, G.Y., et al., Influence of hypoxia on the domiciliation of mesenchymal stem cells after infusion into rats: possibilities of targeting pulmonary artery remodeling via cells therapies? *Respir Res.*, 2005. 6: p. 125.

[81] Santa Maria, L., C.V. Rojas, and J.J. Minguell, Signals from damaged but not undamaged skeletal muscle induce myogenic differentiation of rat bone-marrow-derived mesenchymal stem cells. *Exp. Cell Res.*, 2004. 300(2): p. 418-26.

[82] Martin, D.R., et al., Isolation and characterization of multipotential mesenchymal stem cells from feline bone marrow. *Exp. Hematol.*, 2002. 30(8): p. 879-86.

[83] Devine, S.M., et al., Mesenchymal stem cells are capable of homing to the bone marrow of non-human primates following systemic infusion. *Exp. Hematol.*, 2001. 29(2): p. 244-55.

[84] Airey, J.A., et al., Human mesenchymal stem cells form Purkinje fibers in fetal sheep heart. *Circulation*, 2004. 109(11): p. 1401-7.

[85] Silva, G.V., et al., Mesenchymal stem cells differentiate into an endothelial phenotype, enhance vascular density, and improve heart function in a canine chronic ischemia model. *Circulation,* 2005. 111(2): p. 150-6.

[86] Moscoso, I., et al., Differentiation "in vitro" of primary and immortalized porcine mesenchymal stem cells into cardiomyocytes for cell transplantation. *Transplant Proc.*, 2005. 37(1): p. 481-2.

[87] Bosch, P., S.L. Pratt, and S.L. Stice, Isolation, characterization, gene modification, and nuclear reprogramming of porcine mesenchymal stem cells. *Biol. Reprod.*, 2006. 74(1): p. 46-57.

[88] Bosnakovski, D., et al., Isolation and multilineage differentiation of bovine bone marrow mesenchymal stem cells. *Cell Tissue Res.*, 2005. 319(2): p. 243-53.

[89] Worster, A.A., et al., Effect of transforming growth factor beta1 on chondrogenic differentiation of cultured equine mesenchymal stem cells. *Am. J. Vet. Res.*, 2000. 61(9): p. 1003-10.

[90] Ringe, J., T. Haupl, and M. Sittinger, [Mesenchymal stem cells for tissue engineering of bone and cartilage]. *Med. Klin.* (Munich), 2003. 98 Suppl 2: p. 35-40.
[91] Howell, J.C., et al., Pluripotent stem cells identified in multiple murine tissues. *Ann. NY Acad. Sci.,* 2003. 996: p. 158-73.
[92] da Silva Meirelles, L., P.C. Chagastelles, and N.B. Nardi, Mesenchymal stem cells reside in virtually all post-natal organs and tissues. *J. Cell Sci.*, 2006. 119(Pt 11): p. 2204-13.
[93] Herrera, M.B., et al., Isolation and Characterization of a Stem Cell Population from Adult Human Liver. *Stem Cells*, 2006.
[94] Seeberger, K.L., et al., Expansion of mesenchymal stem cells from human pancreatic ductal epithelium. *Lab. Invest,* 2006. 86(2): p. 141-53.
[95] Yoshimura, H., et al., Comparison of rat mesenchymal stem cells derived from bone marrow, synovium, periosteum, adipose tissue, and muscle. *Cell Tissue Res.*, 2006.
[96] Barry, F.P. and J.M. Murphy, Mesenchymal stem cells: clinical applications and biological characterization. *Int. J. Biochem. Cell Biol.*, 2004. 36(4): p. 568-84.
[97] Pierdomenico, L., et al., Multipotent mesenchymal stem cells with immunosuppressive activity can be easily isolated from dental pulp. *Transplantation,* 2005. 80(6): p. 836-42.
[98] Shih, D.T., et al., Isolation and characterization of neurogenic mesenchymal stem cells in human scalp tissue. *Stem Cells,* 2005. 23(7): p. 1012-20.
[99] Hoogduijn, M.J., E. Gorjup, and P.G. Genever, Comparative characterization of hair follicle dermal stem cells and bone marrow mesenchymal stem cells. *Stem Cells Dev.*, 2006. 15(1): p. 49-60.
[100] Moon, M.H., et al., Human adipose tissue-derived mesenchymal stem cells improve postnatal neovascularization in a mouse model of hindlimb ischemia. *Cell Physiol. Biochem.*, 2006. 17(5-6): p. 279-90.
[101] Dan, Y.Y., et al., Isolation of multipotent progenitor cells from human fetal liver capable of differentiating into liver and mesenchymal lineages. *Proc. Natl. Acad. Sci. USA,* 2006. 103(26): p. 9912-7.
[102] In 't Anker, P.S., et al., Mesenchymal stem cells in human second-trimester bone marrow, liver, lung, and spleen exhibit a similar immunophenotype but a heterogeneous multilineage differentiation potential. *Haematologica,* 2003. 88(8): p. 845-52.
[103] Campagnoli, C., et al., Identification of mesenchymal stem/progenitor cells in human first-trimester fetal blood, liver, and bone marrow. *Blood,* 2001. 98(8): p. 2396-402.
[104] Rzhaninova, A.A., S.N. Gornostaeva, and D.V. Goldshtein, Isolation and phenotypical characterization of mesenchymal stem cells from human fetal thymus. *Bull. Exp. Biol. Med.*, 2005. 139(1): p. 134-40.
[105] Hu, Y., et al., Isolation and identification of mesenchymal stem cells from human fetal pancreas. *J. Lab. Clin. Med.*, 2003. 141(5): p. 342-9.
[106] Igura, K., et al., Isolation and characterization of mesenchymal progenitor cells from chorionic villi of human placenta. *Cytotherapy,* 2004. 6(6): p. 543-53.
[107] Tsai, M.S., et al., Isolation of human multipotent mesenchymal stem cells from second-trimester amniotic fluid using a novel two-stage culture protocol. *Hum. Reprod.*, 2004. 19(6): p. 1450-6.
[108] Erices, A., P. Conget, and J.J. Minguell, Mesenchymal progenitor cells in human umbilical cord blood. *Br. J. Haematol.*, 2000. 109(1): p. 235-42.

[109] Kim, J.W., et al., Mesenchymal progenitor cells in the human umbilical cord. *Ann. Hematol.*, 2004. 83(12): p. 733-8.
[110] Villaron, E.M., et al., Mesenchymal stem cells are present in peripheral blood and can engraft after allogeneic hematopoietic stem cell transplantation. *Haematologica,* 2004. 89(12): p. 1421-7.
[111] O'Donoghue, K., et al., Identification of fetal mesenchymal stem cells in maternal blood: implications for non-invasive prenatal diagnosis. *Mol. Hum. Reprod.*, 2003. 9(8): p. 497-502.
[112] O'Donoghue, K., et al., Microchimerism in female bone marrow and bone decades after fetal mesenchymal stem-cell trafficking in pregnancy. *Lancet,* 2004. 364(9429): p. 179-82.
[113] Romanov, Y.A., V.A. Svintsitskaya, and V.N. Smirnov, Searching for alternative sources of postnatal human mesenchymal stem cells: candidate MSC-like cells from umbilical cord. *Stem Cells*, 2003. 21(1): p. 105-10.
[114] Lee, O.K., et al., Isolation of multipotent mesenchymal stem cells from umbilical cord blood. *Blood,* 2004. 103(5): p. 1669-75.
[115] Lee, M.W., et al., Mesenchymal stem cells from cryopreserved human umbilical cord blood. *Biochem. Biophys. Res. Commun.*, 2004. 320(1): p. 273-8.
[116] Kassis, I., et al., Isolation of mesenchymal stem cells from G-CSF-mobilized human peripheral blood using fibrin microbeads. *Bone Marrow Transplant*, 2006. 37(10): p. 967-76.
[117] Kucia, M., et al., Tissue-specific muscle, neural and liver stem/progenitor cells reside in the bone marrow, respond to an SDF-1 gradient and are mobilized into peripheral blood during stress and tissue injury. *Blood Cells Mol. Dis.*, 2004. 32(1): p. 52-7.
[118] Fernandez, M., et al., Detection of stromal cells in peripheral blood progenitor cell collections from breast cancer patients. *Bone Marrow Transplant*, 1997. 20(4): p. 265-71.
[119] Zyuz'kov, G.N., et al., Role of stem cells in adaptation to hypoxia and mechanisms of neuroprotective effect of granulocytic colony-stimulating factor. *Bull. Exp. Biol. Med.*, 2005. 140(5): p. 606-11.
[120] Kawada, H., et al., Nonhematopoietic mesenchymal stem cells can be mobilized and differentiate into cardiomyocytes after myocardial infarction. *Blood*, 2004. 104(12): p. 3581-7.
[121] Latsinik, N.V., et al., [The stromal colony-forming cell (CFUf) count in the bone marrow of mice and the clonal nature of the fibroblast colonies they form]. *Ontogenez,* 1986. 17(1): p. 27-36.
[122] Gronthos, S. and P.J. Simmons, The growth factor requirements of STRO-1-positive human bone marrow stromal precursors under serum-deprived conditions in vitro. *Blood,* 1995. 85(4): p. 929-40.
[123] Kuznetsov, S.A., A.J. Friedenstein, and P.G. Robey, Factors required for bone marrow stromal fibroblast colony formation in vitro. *Br. J. Haematol.*, 1997. 97(3): p. 561-70.
[124] Colter, D.C., et al., Rapid expansion of recycling stem cells in cultures of plastic-adherent cells from human bone marrow. *Proc. Natl. Acad. Sci. USA*, 2000. 97(7): p. 3213-8.

[125] Colter, D.C., I. Sekiya, and D.J. Prockop, Identification of a subpopulation of rapidly self-renewing and multipotential adult stem cells in colonies of human marrow stromal cells. *Proc. Natl. Acad. Sci. USA*, 2001. 98(14): p. 7841-5.

[126] Muraglia, A., R. Cancedda, and R. Quarto, Clonal mesenchymal progenitors from human bone marrow differentiate in vitro according to a hierarchical model. *J. Cell Sci.*, 2000. 113 (Pt 7): p. 1161-6.

[127] Okamoto, T., et al., Clonal heterogeneity in differentiation potential of immortalized human mesenchymal stem cells. *Biochem. Biophys. Res. Commun.*, 2002. 295(2): p. 354-61.

[128] Satomura, K., et al., Osteogenic imprinting upstream of marrow stromal cell differentiation. *J. Cell Biochem.*, 2000. 78(3): p. 391-403.

[129] Gronthos, S., et al., Differential cell surface expression of the STRO-1 and alkaline phosphatase antigens on discrete developmental stages in primary cultures of human bone cells. *J. Bone Miner Res.*, 1999. 14(1): p. 47-56.

[130] Bensidhoum, M., et al., Homing of in vitro expanded Stro-1- or Stro-1+ human mesenchymal stem cells into the NOD/SCID mouse and their role in supporting human CD34 cell engraftment. *Blood,* 2004. 103(9): p. 3313-9.

[131] Simmons, P.J., et al., Vascular cell adhesion molecule-1 expressed by bone marrow stromal cells mediates the binding of hematopoietic progenitor cells. *Blood,* 1992. 80(2): p. 388-95.

[132] Simmons, P.J. and B. Torok-Storb, Identification of stromal cell precursors in human bone marrow by a novel monoclonal antibody, STRO-1. *Blood,* 1991. 78(1): p. 55-62.

[133] Haynesworth, S.E., M.A. Baber, and A.I. Caplan, Cell surface antigens on human marrow-derived mesenchymal cells are detected by monoclonal antibodies. *Bone,* 1992. 13(1): p. 69-80.

[134] Barry, F., et al., The SH-3 and SH-4 antibodies recognize distinct epitopes on CD73 from human mesenchymal stem cells. *Biochem. Biophys. Res. Commun.*, 2001. 289(2): p. 519-24.

[135] De Ugarte, D.A., et al., Differential expression of stem cell mobilization-associated molecules on multi-lineage cells from adipose tissue and bone marrow. *Immunol. Lett.*, 2003. 89(2-3): p. 267-70.

[136] Vogel, G., Biotechnology. Stem cells lose market luster. *Science*, 2003. 299(5614): p. 1830-1.

[137] Vogel, W., et al., Heterogeneity among human bone marrow-derived mesenchymal stem cells and neural progenitor cells. *Haematologica,* 2003. 88(2): p. 126-33.

[138] Bruder, S.P., N. Jaiswal, and S.E. Haynesworth, Growth kinetics, self-renewal, and the osteogenic potential of purified human mesenchymal stem cells during extensive subcultivation and following cryopreservation. *J. Cell Biochem.*, 1997. 64(2): p. 278-94.

[139] Banfi, A., et al., Replicative aging and gene expression in long-term cultures of human bone marrow stromal cells. *Tissue Eng.*, 2002. 8(6): p. 901-10.

[140] Kawano, S., et al., Ca(2+) oscillations regulated by Na(+)-Ca(2+) exchanger and plasma membrane Ca(2+) pump induce fluctuations of membrane currents and potentials in human mesenchymal stem cells. *Cell Calcium.*, 2003. 34(2): p. 145-56.

[141] Pereira, R.F., et al., Cultured adherent cells from marrow can serve as long-lasting precursor cells for bone, cartilage, and lung in irradiated mice. *Proc. Natl. Acad. Sci. USA,* 1995. 92(11): p. 4857-61.
[142] Castro-Malaspina, H., et al., Characterization of human bone marrow fibroblast colony-forming cells (CFU-F) and their progeny. *Blood,* 1980. 56(2): p. 289-301.
[143] Bianchi, G., et al., Ex vivo enrichment of mesenchymal cell progenitors by fibroblast growth factor 2. *Exp. Cell Res.*, 2003. 287(1): p. 98-105.
[144] Bonyadi, M., et al., Mesenchymal progenitor self-renewal deficiency leads to age-dependent osteoporosis in Sca-1/Ly-6A null mice. *Proc. Natl. Acad. Sci. USA*, 2003. 100(10): p. 5840-5.
[145] Klein, A.K., et al., Characterization of canine fetal lymphohematopoiesis: studies of CFUGM, CFUL, and CFUF. *Exp. Hematol.*, 1983. 11(4): p. 263-74.
[146] Van den Heuvel, R.L., et al., Stromal stem cells (CFU-f) in yolk sac, liver, spleen and bone marrow of pre- and postnatal mice. *Br. J. Haematol.*, 1987. 66(1): p. 15-20.
[147] Charbord, P., et al., Early ontogeny of the human marrow from long bones: an immunohistochemical study of hematopoiesis and its microenvironment. *Blood*, 1996. 87(10): p. 4109-19.
[148] Mendes, S.C., C. Robin, and E. Dzierzak, Mesenchymal progenitor cells localize within hematopoietic sites throughout ontogeny. *Development*, 2005. 132(5): p. 1127-36.
[149] Friedenstein, A.J., S. Piatetzky, II, and K.V. Petrakova, Osteogenesis in transplants of bone marrow cells. *J. Embryol. Exp. Morphol.*, 1966. 16(3): p. 381-90.
[150] Dexter, T.M., T.D. Allen, and L.G. Lajtha, Conditions controlling the proliferation of haemopoietic stem cells in vitro. *J. Cell Physiol.*, 1977. 91(3): p. 335-44.
[151] Gupta, P., et al., Structurally specific heparan sulfates support primitive human hematopoiesis by formation of a multimolecular stem cell niche. *Blood*, 1998. 92(12): p. 4641-51.
[152] Calvi, L.M., et al., Osteoblastic cells regulate the haematopoietic stem cell niche. *Nature,* 2003. 425(6960): p. 841-6.
[153] Shi, S. and S. Gronthos, Perivascular niche of postnatal mesenchymal stem cells in human bone marrow and dental pulp. *J. Bone Miner Res.*, 2003. 18(4): p. 696-704.
[154] Moore, K.A., Recent advances in defining the hematopoietic stem cell niche. *Curr. Opin. Hematol.*, 2004. 11(2): p. 107-11.
[155] Arai, F., A. Hirao, and T. Suda, Regulation of hematopoietic stem cells by the niche. *Trends Cardiovasc. Med.,* 2005. 15(2): p. 75-9.
[156] Charbord, P., [The hematopoietic stem cell and the stromal microenvironment]. *Therapie,* 2001. 56(4): p. 383-4.
[157] Chagraoui, J., et al., Fetal liver stroma consists of cells in epithelial-to-mesenchymal transition. *Blood,* 2003. 101(8): p. 2973-82.
[158] Fuchs, E. and C. Byrne, The epidermis: rising to the surface. *Curr. Opin. Genet Dev.*, 1994. 4(5): p. 725-36.
[159] Lo, L., L. Sommer, and D.J. Anderson, MASH1 maintains competence for BMP2-induced neuronal differentiation in post-migratory neural crest cells. *Curr. Biol.*, 1997. 7(6): p. 440-50.
[160] Baron, M., Induction of embryonic hematopoietic and endothelial stem/progenitor cells by hedgehog-mediated signals. *Differentiation*, 2001. 68(4-5): p. 175-85.

[161] Soria, B., In-vitro differentiation of pancreatic beta-cells. *Differentiation*, 2001. 68(4-5): p. 205-19.

[162] Gupta, S., Hepatocyte transplantation. *J. Gastroenterol. Hepatol.*, 2002. 17 Suppl 3: p. S287-S293.

[163] Herzog, E.L., L. Chai, and D.S. Krause, Plasticity of marrow-derived stem cells. *Blood*, 2003. 102(10): p. 3483-93.

[164] Fridenshtein, A., [Stromal bone marrow cells and the hematopoietic microenvironment]. *Arkh Patol*, 1982. 44(10): p. 3-11.

[165] Gronthos, S. and P.J. Simmons, The biology and application of human bone marrow stromal cell precursors. *J. Hematother.*, 1996. 5(1): p. 15-23.

[166] Reyes, M., et al., Origin of endothelial progenitors in human postnatal bone marrow. J. *Clin. Invest.*, 2002. 109(3): p. 337-46.

[167] Brazelton, T.R., et al., From marrow to brain: expression of neuronal phenotypes in adult mice. Science, 2000. 290(5497): p. 1775-9.

[168] Sanchez-Ramos, J., et al., Adult bone marrow stromal cells differentiate into neural cells in vitro. *Exp. Neurol.,* 2000. 164(2): p. 247-56.

[169] Zhao, L.X., et al., Modification of the brain-derived neurotrophic factor gene: a portal to transform mesenchymal stem cells into advantageous engineering cells for neuroregeneration and neuroprotection. *Exp. Neurol.*, 2004. 190(2): p. 396-406.

[170] Schwartz, R.E., et al., Multipotent adult progenitor cells from bone marrow differentiate into functional hepatocyte-like cells. *J. Clin. Invest.*, 2002. 109(10): p. 1291-302.

[171] Sata, M., et al., The role of circulating precursors in vascular repair and lesion formation. *J. Cell Mol. Med.*, 2005. 9(3): p. 557-68.

[172] Liechty, K.W., et al., Human mesenchymal stem cells engraft and demonstrate site-specific differentiation after in utero transplantation in sheep. *Nat. Med.* 2000. 6(11): p. 1282-6.

[173] Sato, Y., et al., Human mesenchymal stem cells xenografted directly to rat liver are differentiated into human hepatocytes without fusion. *Blood*, 2005. 106(2): p. 756-63.

[174] Togel, F., et al., Administered mesenchymal stem cells protect against ischemic acute renal failure through differentiation-independent mechanisms. *Am. J. Physiol. Renal. Physiol*, 2005. 289(1): p. F31-42.

[175] Loeffler, M. and I. Roeder, Tissue stem cells: definition, plasticity, heterogeneity, self-organization and models--a conceptual approach. *Cells Tissues Organs*, 2002. 171(1): p. 8-26.

[176] Loeffler, M. and I. Roeder, Conceptual models to understand tissue stem cell organization. *Curr. Opin. Hematol.*, 2004. 11(2): p. 81-7.

[177] Roeder, I. and M. Loeffler, A novel dynamic model of hematopoietic stem cell organization based on the concept of within-tissue plasticity. *Exp. Hematol.*, 2002. 30(8): p. 853-61.

[178] Song, L. and R.S. Tuan, Transdifferentiation potential of human mesenchymal stem cells derived from bone marrow. *Faseb J.*, 2004. 18(9): p. 980-2.

[179] Park, S.R., R.O. Oreffo, and J.T. Triffitt, Interconversion potential of cloned human marrow adipocytes in vitro. *Bone*, 1999. 24(6): p. 549-54.

[180] Dennis, J.E., et al., The STRO-1+ marrow cell population is multipotential. *Cells Tissues Organs,* 2002. 170(2-3): p. 73-82.

[181] Terada, N., et al., Bone marrow cells adopt the phenotype of other cells by spontaneous cell fusion. *Nature*, 2002. 416(6880): p. 542-5.

[182] Spees, J.L., et al., Differentiation, cell fusion, and nuclear fusion during ex vivo repair of epithelium by human adult stem cells from bone marrow stroma. *Proc. Natl. Acad. Sci. USA*, 2003. 100(5): p. 2397-402.

[183] Wurmser, A.E., et al., Cell fusion-independent differentiation of neural stem cells to the endothelial lineage. *Nature,* 2004. 430(6997): p. 350-6.

[184] Saga, K., Structure and function of human sweat glands studied with histochemistry and cytochemistry. *Prog. Histochem. Cytochem*., 2002. 37(4): p. 323-86.

[185] Shikiji, T., et al., Keratinocytes can differentiate into eccrine sweat ducts in vitro: involvement of epidermal growth factor and fetal bovine serum. *J. Dermatol. Sci*., 2003. 33(3): p. 141-50.

[186] Li, H., et al., Adult bone-marrow-derived mesenchymal stem cells contribute to wound healing of skin appendages. *Cell Tissue Res*., 2006. 326(3): p. 725-736.

[187] Borue, X., et al., Bone marrow-derived cells contribute to epithelial engraftment during wound healing. *Am. J. Pathol*., 2004. 165(5): p. 1767-72.

[188] Wu, M., et al., Differentiation potential of human embryonic mesenchymal stem cells for skin-related tissue. *Br. J. Dermatol.,* 2006. 155(2): p. 282-91.

[189] Ronfard, V., et al., Long-term regeneration of human epidermis on third degree burns transplanted with autologous cultured epithelium grown on a fibrin matrix. *Transplantation*, 2000. 70(11): p. 1588-98.

[190] Shi, C., et al., Stem cells and their applications in skin-cell therapy. Trends Biotechnol, 2006. 24(1): p. 48-52.

[191] Gharzi, A., A.J. Reynolds, and C.A. Jahoda, Plasticity of hair follicle dermal cells in wound healing and induction. *Exp. Dermatol*., 2003. 12(2): p. 126-36.

[192] Chunmeng, S. and C. Tianmin, Effects of plastic-adherent dermal multipotent cells on peripheral blood leukocytes and CFU-GM in rats. *Transplant Proc*., 2004. 36(5): p. 1578-81.

[193] Deng, W., et al., Allogeneic bone marrow-derived flk-1+Sca-1- mesenchymal stem cells leads to stable mixed chimerism and donor-specific tolerance. *Exp. Hematol*., 2004. 32(9): p. 861-7.

[194] Heng, B.C., et al., Directing stem cells into the keratinocyte lineage in vitro. *Exp. Dermatol*., 2005. 14(1): p. 1-16.

[195] Reynolds, B.A. and S. Weiss, Generation of neurons and astrocytes from isolated cells of the adult mammalian central nervous system. *Science*, 1992. 255(5052): p. 1707-10.

[196] Woodbury, D., et al., Adult rat and human bone marrow stromal cells differentiate into neurons. *J. Neurosci. Res.,* 2000. 61(4): p. 364-70.

[197] Tondreau, T., et al., Bone marrow-derived mesenchymal stem cells already express specific neural proteins before any differentiation. *Differentiation*, 2004. 72(7): p. 319-26.

[198] Minguell, J.J., et al., Nonstimulated human uncommitted mesenchymal stem cells express cell markers of mesenchymal and neural lineages. *Stem Cells Dev*., 2005. 14(4): p. 408-14.

[199] Long, X., et al., Neural cell differentiation in vitro from adult human bone marrow mesenchymal stem cells. *Stem Cells Dev.,* 2005. 14(1): p. 65-9.

[200] Magaki, T., K. Kurisu, and T. Okazaki, Generation of bone marrow-derived neural cells in serum-free monolayer culture. *Neurosci. Lett.*, 2005. 384(3): p. 282-7.

[201] Tao, H., R. Rao, and D.D. Ma, Cytokine-induced stable neuronal differentiation of human bone marrow mesenchymal stem cells in a serum/feeder cell-free condition. *Dev. Growth Differ*, 2005. 47(6): p. 423-33.

[202] Azizi, S.A., et al., Engraftment and migration of human bone marrow stromal cells implanted in the brains of albino rats--similarities to astrocyte grafts. *Proc. Natl. Acad. Sci. USA,* 1998. 95(7): p. 3908-13.

[203] Munoz-Elias, G., et al., Adult bone marrow stromal cells in the embryonic brain: engraftment, migration, differentiation, and long-term survival. *J. Neurosci.*, 2004. 24(19): p. 4585-95.

[204] Deng, W., et al., In vitro differentiation of human marrow stromal cells into early progenitors of neural cells by conditions that increase intracellular cyclic AMP. *Biochem. Biophys. Res. Commun.*, 2001. 282(1): p. 148-52.

[205] Wehner, T., et al., Bone marrow-derived cells expressing green fluorescent protein under the control of the glial fibrillary acidic protein promoter do not differentiate into astrocytes in vitro and in vivo. *J. Neurosci.*, 2003. 23(12): p. 5004-11.

[206] Kim, B.J., et al., Differentiation of adult bone marrow stem cells into neuroprogenitor cells in vitro. *Neuroreport,* 2002. 13(9): p. 1185-8.

[207] Abouelfetouh, A., et al., Morphological differentiation of bone marrow stromal cells into neuron-like cells after co-culture with hippocampal slice. *Brain Res.*, 2004. 1029(1): p. 114-9.

[208] Mareschi, K., et al., Neural differentiation of human mesenchymal stem cells: Evidence for expression of neural markers and eag K+ channel types. *Exp. Hematol.*, 2006. 34(11): p. 1563-72.

[209] Mori, K., et al., Functional recovery of neuronal activity in rat whisker-barrel cortex sensory pathway from freezing injury after transplantation of adult bone marrow stromal cells. *J. Cereb. Blood Flow Metab.*, 2005. 25(7): p. 887-98.

[210] Zhao, L.R., et al., Human bone marrow stem cells exhibit neural phenotypes and ameliorate neurological deficits after grafting into the ischemic brain of rats. *Exp. Neurol.*, 2002. 174(1): p. 11-20.

[211] Dezawa, M., et al., Specific induction of neuronal cells from bone marrow stromal cells and application for autologous transplantation. *J. Clin. Invest*, 2004. 113(12): p. 1701-10.

[212] Chiou, S.H., et al., A novel in vitro retinal differentiation model by co-culturing adult human bone marrow stem cells with retinal pigmented epithelium cells. *Biochem. Biophys. Res. Commun.*, 2005. 326(3): p. 578-85.

[213] Kicic, A., et al., Differentiation of marrow stromal cells into photoreceptors in the rat eye. *J. Neurosci.*, 2003. 23(21): p. 7742-9.

[214] Arnhold, S., et al., Transplantation of bone marrow-derived mesenchymal stem cells rescue photoreceptor cells in the dystrophic retina of the rhodopsin knockout mouse. *Graefes Arch. Clin. Exp. Ophthalmol.*, 2006.

[215] Arnhold, S., et al., Adenovirally transduced bone marrow stromal cells differentiate into pigment epithelial cells and induce rescue effects in RCS rats. *Invest. Ophthalmol. Vis. Sci.,* 2006. 47(9): p. 4121-9.

[216] Tomita, M., et al., Bone marrow-derived stem cells can differentiate into retinal cells in injured rat retina. *Stem Cells*, 2002. 20(4): p. 279-83.
[217] Kershaw, E.E. and J.S. Flier, Adipose tissue as an endocrine organ. *J. Clin. Endocrinol. Metab.,* 2004. 89(6): p. 2548-56.
[218] Otto, T.C. and M.D. Lane, Adipose development: from stem cell to adipocyte. *Crit. Rev. Biochem. Mol. Biol.*, 2005. 40(4): p. 229-42.
[219] Rosen, E.D. and O.A. MacDougald, Adipocyte differentiation from the inside out. *Nat. Rev. Mol. Cell Biol.*, 2006. 7(12): p. 885-96.
[220] Neubauer, M., et al., Basic fibroblast growth factor enhances PPARgamma ligand-induced adipogenesis of mesenchymal stem cells. *FEBS Lett.*, 2004. 577(1-2): p. 277-83.
[221] Ogawa, R., et al., Adipogenic differentiation by adipose-derived stem cells harvested from GFP transgenic mice-including relationship of sex differences. *Biochem. Biophys. Res. Commun.*, 2004. 319(2): p. 511-7.
[222] Pakala, R., et al., Peroxisome proliferator-activated receptor gamma: its role in metabolic syndrome. *Cardiovasc. Radiat. Med.*, 2004. 5(2): p. 97-103.
[223] She, H., et al., Adipogenic transcriptional regulation of hepatic stellate cells. *J. Biol. Chem.*, 2005. 280(6): p. 4959-67.
[224] Tominaga, S., et al., Negative regulation of adipogenesis from human mesenchymal stem cells by Jun N-terminal kinase. *Biochem. Biophys. Res. Commun.*, 2005. 326(2): p. 499-504.
[225] Spinella-Jaegle, S., et al., Sonic hedgehog increases the commitment of pluripotent mesenchymal cells into the osteoblastic lineage and abolishes adipocytic differentiation. *J. Cell Sci.,* 2001. 114(Pt 11): p. 2085-94.
[226] Bennett, C.N., et al., Regulation of osteoblastogenesis and bone mass by Wnt10b. *Proc. Natl. Acad. Sci. USA,* 2005. 102(9): p. 3324-9.
[227] Suh, J.M., et al., Hedgehog signaling plays a conserved role in inhibiting fat formation. *Cell Metab.*, 2006. 3(1): p. 25-34.
[228] Jeon, M.J., et al., Activation of peroxisome proliferator-activated receptor-gamma inhibits the Runx2-mediated transcription of osteocalcin in osteoblasts. *J. Biol. Chem.*, 2003. 278(26): p. 23270-7.
[229] Akune, T., et al., PPARgamma insufficiency enhances osteogenesis through osteoblast formation from bone marrow progenitors. *J. Clin. Invest.*, 2004. 113(6): p. 846-55.
[230] Ali, A.A., et al., Rosiglitazone causes bone loss in mice by suppressing osteoblast differentiation and bone formation. *Endocrinology,* 2005. 146(3): p. 1226-35.
[231] Kawaguchi, H., et al., Distinct effects of PPARgamma insufficiency on bone marrow cells, osteoblasts, and osteoclastic cells. *J. Bone Miner Metab.*, 2005. 23(4): p. 275-9.
[232] Gimble, J.M., et al., Peroxisome proliferator-activated receptor-gamma activation by thiazolidinediones induces adipogenesis in bone marrow stromal cells. *Mol. Pharmacol.*, 1996. 50(5): p. 1087-94.
[233] Ahdjoudj, S., et al., Reciprocal control of osteoblast/chondroblast and osteoblast/adipocyte differentiation of multipotential clonal human marrow stromal F/STRO-1(+) cells. *J. Cell Biochem.*, 2001. 81(1): p. 23-38.
[234] Rosen, E.D. and B.M. Spiegelman, Molecular regulation of adipogenesis. *Annu. Rev. Cell Dev. Biol.*, 2000. 16: p. 145-71.

[235] Janderova, L., et al., Human mesenchymal stem cells as an in vitro model for human adipogenesis. *Obes. Res.*, 2003. 11(1): p. 65-74.
[236] Scavo, L.M., et al., Insulin-like growth factor-I stimulates both cell growth and lipogenesis during differentiation of human mesenchymal stem cells into adipocytes. *J. Clin. Endocrinol. Metab.*, 2004. 89(7): p. 3543-53.
[237] Kim, S.J., et al., Human adipose stromal cells expanded in human serum promote engraftment of human peripheral blood hematopoietic stem cells in NOD/SCID mice. *Biochem. Biophys. Res. Commun.*, 2005. 329(1): p. 25-31.
[238] Lin, T.M., et al., Accelerated growth and prolonged lifespan of adipose tissue-derived human mesenchymal stem cells in a medium using reduced calcium and antioxidants. *Stem Cells Dev.*, 2005. 14(1): p. 92-102.
[239] Olsen, B.R., A.M. Reginato, and W. Wang, Bone development. *Annu. Rev. Cell Dev. Biol.*, 2000. 16: p. 191-220.
[240] Long, M.W., Osteogenesis and bone-marrow-derived cells. *Blood Cells Mol. Dis.*, 2001. 27(3): p. 677-90.
[241] Fibbe, W.E., Mesenchymal stem cells. A potential source for skeletal repair. *Ann. Rheum. Dis.*, 2002. 61 Suppl 2: p. ii29-31.
[242] Ramoshebi, L.N., et al., Tissue engineering: TGF-beta superfamily members and delivery systems in bone regeneration. *Expert. Rev. Mol. Med.*, 2002. 2002: p. 1-11.
[243] Canalis, E., A.N. Economides, and E. Gazzerro, Bone morphogenetic proteins, their antagonists, and the skeleton. *Endocr. Rev.*, 2003. 24(2): p. 218-35.
[244] Rawadi, G., et al., BMP-2 controls alkaline phosphatase expression and osteoblast mineralization by a Wnt autocrine loop. *J. Bone Miner Res.*, 2003. 18(10): p. 1842-53.
[245] Sykaras, N. and L.A. Opperman, Bone morphogenetic proteins (BMPs): how do they function and what can they offer the clinician? *J. Oral Sci.*, 2003. 45(2): p. 57-73.
[246] Taguchi, Y., et al., Interleukin-6-type cytokines stimulate mesenchymal progenitor differentiation toward the osteoblastic lineage. *Proc. Assoc. Am. Physicians*, 1998. 110(6): p. 559-74.
[247] Kroger, H., E. Soppi, and N. Loveridge, Growth hormone, osteoblasts, and marrow adipocytes: a case report. *Calcif. Tissue Int.*, 1997. 61(1): p. 33-5.
[248] Thomas, T., et al., Leptin acts on human marrow stromal cells to enhance differentiation to osteoblasts and to inhibit differentiation to adipocytes. *Endocrinology*, 1999. 140(4): p. 1630-8.
[249] Maeda, S., et al., Sortilin is upregulated during osteoblastic differentiation of mesenchymal stem cells and promotes extracellular matrix mineralization. *J. Cell Physiol.*, 2002. 193(1): p. 73-9.
[250] Nurminskaya, M., et al., Chondrocyte-derived transglutaminase promotes maturation of preosteoblasts in periosteal bone. *Dev. Biol.*, 2003. 263(1): p. 139-52.
[251] Raisz, L.G., C.C. Pilbeam, and P.M. Fall, Prostaglandins: mechanisms of action and regulation of production in bone. *Osteoporos Int,* 1993. 3 Suppl 1: p. 136-40.
[252] Weinreb, M., A. Grosskopf, and N. Shir, The anabolic effect of PGE2 in rat bone marrow cultures is mediated via the EP4 receptor subtype. *Am. J. Physiol.*, 1999. 276(2 Pt 1): p. E376-83.
[253] van Leeuwen, J.P., et al., Vitamin D control of osteoblast function and bone extracellular matrix mineralization. *Crit. Rev. Eukaryot. Gene Expr.*, 2001. 11(1-3): p. 199-226.

[254] zur Nieden, N.I., G. Kempka, and H.J. Ahr, In vitro differentiation of embryonic stem cells into mineralized osteoblasts. *Differentiation*, 2003. 71(1): p. 18-27.

[255] Rogers, J.J., et al., Differentiation factors induce expression of muscle, fat, cartilage, and bone in a clone of mouse pluripotent mesenchymal stem cells. *Am. Surg.*, 1995. 61(3): p. 231-6.

[256] Buttery, L.D., et al., Differentiation of osteoblasts and in vitro bone formation from murine embryonic stem cells. *Tissue Eng,* 2001. 7(1): p. 89-99.

[257] Sottile, V., A. Thomson, and J. McWhir, In vitro osteogenic differentiation of human ES cells. *Cloning Stem Cells*, 2003. 5(2): p. 149-55.

[258] Notoya, K., et al., Enhancement of osteogenesis in vitro and in vivo by a novel osteoblast differentiation promoting compound, TAK-778. *J. Pharmacol. Exp. Ther.*, 1999. 290(3): p. 1054-64.

[259] Rosa, A.L. and M.M. Beloti, TAK-778 enhances osteoblast differentiation of human bone marrow cells. *J. Cell Biochem.*, 2003. 89(6): p. 1148-53.

[260] Sugiyama, M., et al., Compactin and simvastatin, but not pravastatin, induce bone morphogenetic protein-2 in human osteosarcoma cells. *Biochem. Biophys. Res. Commun.*, 2000. 271(3): p. 688-92.

[261] Ohnaka, K., et al., Pitavastatin enhanced BMP-2 and osteocalcin expression by inhibition of Rho-associated kinase in human osteoblasts. *Biochem. Biophys. Res. Commun.*, 2001. 287(2): p. 337-42.

[262] Phillips, B.W., et al., Compactin enhances osteogenesis in murine embryonic stem cells. *Biochem. Biophys. Res. Commun.*, 2001. 284(2): p. 478-84.

[263] Gerstenfeld, L.C., et al., Osteogenic differentiation is selectively promoted by morphogenetic signals from chondrocytes and synergized by a nutrient rich growth environment. *Connect. Tissue Res.*, 2003. 44 Suppl 1: p. 85-91.

[264] Gerstenfeld, L.C., et al., Chondrocytes provide morphogenic signals that selectively induce osteogenic differentiation of mesenchymal stem cells. *J. Bone Miner Res.*, 2002. 17(2): p. 221-30.

[265] Karadag, A., A.M. Scutt, and P.I. Croucher, Human myeloma cells promote the recruitment of osteoblast precursors: mediation by interleukin-6 and soluble interleukin-6 receptor. *J. Bone Miner Res.*, 2000. 15(10): p. 1935-43.

[266] Villars, F., et al., Effect of HUVEC on human osteoprogenitor cell differentiation needs heterotypic gap junction communication. *Am. J. Physiol. Cell Physiol.*, 2002. 282(4): p. C775-85.

[267] Zhou, J., et al., [Research in use of vascular endothelial cells to promote osteogenesis of marrow stromal cells]. *Sheng Wu Yi Xue Gong Cheng Xue Za Zhi*, 2003. 20(3): p. 447-50.

[268] Greenwald, J.A., et al., Biomolecular mechanisms of calvarial bone induction: immature versus mature dura mater. *Plast. Reconstr. Surg.*, 2000. 105(4): p. 1382-92.

[269] Spector, J.A., et al., Co-culture of osteoblasts with immature dural cells causes an increased rate and degree of osteoblast differentiation. *Plast. Reconstr. Surg.*, 2002. 109(2): p. 631-42; discussion 643-4.

[270] Aubin, J.E., Osteoprogenitor cell frequency in rat bone marrow stromal populations: role for heterotypic cell-cell interactions in osteoblast differentiation. *J. Cell Biochem.*, 1999. 72(3): p. 396-410.

[271] Bianco, P., et al., Expression of bone sialoprotein (BSP) in developing human tissues. *Calcif Tissue Int,* 1991. 49(6): p. 421-6.

[272] Helder, M.N., A.L. Bronckers, and J.H. Woltgens, Dissimilar expression patterns for the extracellular matrix proteins osteopontin (OPN) and collagen type I in dental tissues and alveolar bone of the neonatal rat. *Matrix,* 1993. 13(5): p. 415-25.

[273] Bronckers, A.L., et al., Developmental appearance of Gla proteins (osteocalcin) and alkaline phosphatase in tooth germs and bones of the rat. *Bone Miner*, 1987. 2(5): p. 361-73.

[274] Thomas, G., et al., Osteocrin, a novel bone-specific secreted protein that modulates the osteoblast phenotype. *J. Biol. Chem.*, 2003. 278(50): p. 50563-71.

[275] Krebsbach, P.H., et al., Bone formation in vivo: comparison of osteogenesis by transplanted mouse and human marrow stromal fibroblasts. *Transplantation*, 1997. 63(8): p. 1059-69.

[276] Kon, E., et al., Autologous bone marrow stromal cells loaded onto porous hydroxyapatite ceramic accelerate bone repair in critical-size defects of sheep long bones. *J. Biomed. Mater. Res.*, 2000. 49(3): p. 328-37.

[277] Petite, H., et al., Tissue-engineered bone regeneration. *Nat. Biotechnol.*, 2000. 18(9): p. 959-63.

[278] Chen, F., et al., Injectable bone. *Br. J. Oral. Maxillofac. Surg.*, 2003. 41(4): p. 240-3.

[279] Chang, S.C., et al., Cranial repair using BMP-2 gene engineered bone marrow stromal cells. *J. Surg. Res.*, 2004. 119(1): p. 85-91.

[280] Schantz, J.T., et al., Repair of calvarial defects with customised tissue-engineered bone grafts II. Evaluation of cellular efficiency and efficacy in vivo. *Tissue Eng*, 2003. 9 Suppl 1: p. S127-39.

[281] Dai, K.R., et al., Repairing of goat tibial bone defects with BMP-2 gene-modified tissue-engineered bone. *Calcif Tissue Int*, 2005. 77(1): p. 55-61.

[282] Li, Z., et al., Repair of sheep metatarsus defects by using tissue-engineering technique. *J. Huazhong Univ. Sci. Technolog. Med. Sci.,* 2005. 25(1): p. 62-7.

[283] Meinel, L., et al., Silk implants for the healing of critical size bone defects. *Bone*, 2005. 37(5): p. 688-98.

[284] Brodke, D., et al., Bone grafts prepared with selective cell retention technology heal canine segmental defects as effectively as autograft. *J. Orthop. Res.*, 2006. 24(5): p. 857-66.

[285] Yoon, E., et al., In Vivo Osteogenic Potential of Human Adipose-Derived Stem Cells/Poly Lactide-Co-Glycolic Acid Constructs for Bone Regeneration in a Rat Critical-Sized Calvarial Defect Model. *Tissue Eng*, 2006.

[286] Horwitz, E.M., et al., Transplantability and therapeutic effects of bone marrow-derived mesenchymal cells in children with osteogenesis imperfecta. *Nat. Med.*, 1999. 5(3): p. 309-13.

[287] Cancedda, R., et al., Tissue engineering and cell therapy of cartilage and bone. *Matrix Biol.*, 2003. 22(1): p. 81-91.

[288] Rose, F.R. and R.O. Oreffo, Bone tissue engineering: hope vs hype. *Biochem. Biophys. Res. Commun.,* 2002. 292(1): p. 1-7.

[289] Vats, A., et al., Scaffolds and biomaterials for tissue engineering: a review of clinical applications. *Clin. Otolaryngol. Allied Sci.*, 2003. 28(3): p. 165-72.

[290] Bruder, S.P., et al., Bone regeneration by implantation of purified, culture-expanded human mesenchymal stem cells. *J. Orthop. Res.*, 1998. 16(2): p. 155-62.

[291] El-Amin, S.F., et al., Integrin expression by human osteoblasts cultured on degradable polymeric materials applicable for tissue engineered bone. *J. Orthop. Res.*, 2002. 20(1): p. 20-8.

[292] Quarto, R., et al., Repair of large bone defects with the use of autologous bone marrow stromal cells. *N. Engl. J. Med.*, 2001. 344(5): p. 385-6.

[293] Vacanti, C.A., et al., Replacement of an avulsed phalanx with tissue-engineered bone. *N. Engl. J. Med.,* 2001. 344(20): p. 1511-4.

[294] Warnke, P.H., et al., Growth and transplantation of a custom vascularised bone graft in a man. *Lancet*, 2004. 364(9436): p. 766-70.

[295] Johnstone, B., et al., In vitro chondrogenesis of bone marrow-derived mesenchymal progenitor cells. *Exp. Cell Res.*, 1998. 238(1): p. 265-72.

[296] Yoo, J.U., et al., The chondrogenic potential of human bone-marrow-derived mesenchymal progenitor cells. *J. Bone Joint Surg. Am.*, 1998. 80(12): p. 1745-57.

[297] Kavalkovich, K.W., et al., Chondrogenic differentiation of human mesenchymal stem cells within an alginate layer culture system. *In Vitro Cell Dev. Biol. Anim.*, 2002. 38(8): p. 457-66.

[298] Lee, J.W., et al., Chondrogenic differentiation of mesenchymal stem cells and its clinical applications. *Yonsei Med. J.,* 2004. 45 Suppl: p. 41-7.

[299] Yang, I.H., et al., Comparison of phenotypic characterization between "alginate bead" and "pellet" culture systems as chondrogenic differentiation models for human mesenchymal stem cells. *Yonsei Med. J.,* 2004. 45(5): p. 891-900.

[300] Caplan, A.I., et al., Principles of cartilage repair and regeneration. *Clin. Orthop. Relat. Res.*, 1997(342): p. 254-69.

[301] Murphy, J.M., et al., Stem cell therapy in a caprine model of osteoarthritis. *Arthritis Rheum.,* 2003. 48(12): p. 3464-74.

[302] Wakitani, S., et al., Mesenchymal cell-based repair of large, full-thickness defects of articular cartilage. *J. Bone Joint Surg. Am.*, 1994. 76(4): p. 579-92.

[303] Wakitani, S., et al., Human autologous culture expanded bone marrow mesenchymal cell transplantation for repair of cartilage defects in osteoarthritic knees. *Osteoarthritis Cartilage*, 2002. 10(3): p. 199-206.

[304] Wakitani, S. and T. Yamamoto, Response of the donor and recipient cells in mesenchymal cell transplantation to cartilage defect. *Microsc. Res.Tech.*, 2002. 58(1): p. 14-8.

[305] Brittberg, M., et al., Treatment of deep cartilage defects in the knee with autologous chondrocyte transplantation. N Engl J Med, 1994. 331(14): p. 889-95.

[306] Jorgensen, C., et al., Stem cells for repair of cartilage and bone: the next challenge in osteoarthritis and rheumatoid arthritis. *Ann. Rheum. Dis.*, 2001. 60(4): p. 305-9.

[307] Schultz, O., et al., Emerging strategies of bone and joint repair. *Arthritis Res.*, 2000. 2(6): p. 433-6.

[308] Yamasaki, T., et al., Meniscal regeneration using tissue engineering with a scaffold derived from a rat meniscus and mesenchymal stromal cells derived from rat bone marrow. *J. Biomed. Mater. Res. A*, 2005. 75(1): p. 23-30.

[309] Gao, J., et al., Repair of osteochondral defect with tissue-engineered two-phase composite material of injectable calcium phosphate and hyaluronan sponge. *Tissue Eng.,* 2002. 8(5): p. 827-37.
[310] Caterson, E.J., et al., Three-dimensional cartilage formation by bone marrow-derived cells seeded in polylactide/alginate amalgam. *J. Biomed. Mater. Res.*, 2001. 57(3): p. 394-403.
[311] Tuan, R.S., G. Boland, and R. Tuli, Adult mesenchymal stem cells and cell-based tissue engineering. *Arthritis Res. Ther.*, 2003. 5(1): p. 32-45.
[312] Crevensten, G., et al., Intervertebral disc cell therapy for regeneration: mesenchymal stem cell implantation in rat intervertebral discs. *Ann. Biomed. Eng.*, 2004. 32(3): p. 430-4.
[313] Reddi, A.H., Role of morphogenetic proteins in skeletal tissue engineering and regeneration. *Nat. Biotechnol.*, 1998. 16(3): p. 247-52.
[314] van Beuningen, H.M., et al., Differential effects of local application of BMP-2 or TGF-beta 1 on both articular cartilage composition and osteophyte formation. *Osteoarthritis Cartilage*, 1998. 6(5): p. 306-17.
[315] Aung, T., et al., Chondroinduction of mouse mesenchymal stem cells in three-dimensional highly porous matrix scaffolds. *J. Biomed. Mater. Res.*, 2002. 61(1): p. 75-82.
[316] Ikeuchi, M., et al., Recombinant human bone morphogenetic protein-2 promotes osteogenesis within atelopeptide type I collagen solution by combination with rat cultured marrow cells. *J. Biomed. Mater. Res.*, 2002. 60(1): p. 61-9.
[317] Girotto, D., et al., Tissue-specific gene expression in chondrocytes grown on three-dimensional hyaluronic acid scaffolds. *Biomaterials*, 2003. 24(19): p. 3265-75.
[318] Awad, H.A., et al., Autologous mesenchymal stem cell-mediated repair of tendon. *Tissue Eng.*, 1999. 5(3): p. 267-77.
[319] Ringe, J., et al., Stem cells for regenerative medicine: advances in the engineering of tissues and organs. *Naturwissenschaften*, 2002. 89(8): p. 338-51.
[320] Awad, H.A., et al., Repair of patellar tendon injuries using a cell-collagen composite. *J. Orthop. Res.*, 2003. 21(3): p. 420-31.
[321] Young, R.G., et al., Use of mesenchymal stem cells in a collagen matrix for Achilles tendon repair. *J. Orthop. Res.,* 1998. 16(4): p. 406-13.
[322] Wolfman, N.M., et al., Ectopic induction of tendon and ligament in rats by growth and differentiation factors 5, 6, and 7, members of the TGF-beta gene family. *J. Clin. Invest.*, 1997. 100(2): p. 321-30.
[323] Ouyang, H.W., et al., The efficacy of bone marrow stromal cell-seeded knitted PLGA fiber scaffold for Achilles tendon repair. *Ann. NY Acad. Sci.*, 2002. 961: p. 126-9.
[324] Ouyang, H.W., et al., Knitted poly-lactide-co-glycolide scaffold loaded with bone marrow stromal cells in repair and regeneration of rabbit Achilles tendon. *Tissue Eng*, 2003. 9(3): p. 431-9.
[325] Juncosa-Melvin, N., et al., Effects of cell-to-collagen ratio in mesenchymal stem cell-seeded implants on tendon repair biomechanics and histology. *Tissue Eng*, 2005. 11(3-4): p. 448-57.
[326] Zammit, P. and J. Beauchamp, The skeletal muscle satellite cell: stem cell or son of stem cell? *Differentiation*, 2001. 68(4-5): p. 193-204.

[327] Charge, S.B. and M.A. Rudnicki, Cellular and molecular regulation of muscle regeneration. *Physiol. Rev.*, 2004. 84(1): p. 209-38.
[328] Gussoni, E., et al., Dystrophin expression in the mdx mouse restored by stem cell transplantation. *Nature*, 1999. 401(6751): p. 390-4.
[329] Polesskaya, A., P. Seale, and M.A. Rudnicki, Wnt signaling induces the myogenic specification of resident CD45+ adult stem cells during muscle regeneration. *Cell,* 2003. 113(7): p. 841-52.
[330] Majka, S.M., et al., Distinct progenitor populations in skeletal muscle are bone marrow derived and exhibit different cell fates during vascular regeneration. *J. Clin. Invest,* 2003. 111(1): p. 71-9.
[331] Williams, J.T., et al., Cells isolated from adult human skeletal muscle capable of differentiating into multiple mesodermal phenotypes. *Am. Surg.*, 1999. 65(1): p. 22-6.
[332] Young, H.E., et al., Human reserve pluripotent mesenchymal stem cells are present in the connective tissues of skeletal muscle and dermis derived from fetal, adult, and geriatric donors. *Anat Rec.*, 2001. 264(1): p. 51-62.
[333] Wakitani, S., T. Saito, and A.I. Caplan, Myogenic cells derived from rat bone marrow mesenchymal stem cells exposed to 5-azacytidine. *Muscle Nerve*, 1995. 18(12): p. 1417-26.
[334] Ferrari, G., et al., Muscle regeneration by bone marrow-derived myogenic progenitors. *Science*, 1998. 279(5356): p. 1528-30.
[335] Bittner, R.E., et al., Recruitment of bone-marrow-derived cells by skeletal and cardiac muscle in adult dystrophic mdx mice. *Anat. Embryol.* (Berl), 1999. 199(5): p. 391-6.
[336] LaBarge, M.A. and H.M. Blau, Biological progression from adult bone marrow to mononucleate muscle stem cell to multinucleate muscle fiber in response to injury. *Cell*, 2002. 111(4): p. 589-601.
[337] De Bari, C., et al., Skeletal muscle repair by adult human mesenchymal stem cells from synovial membrane. *J. Cell Biol.*, 2003. 160(6): p. 909-18.
[338] Muguruma, Y., et al., In vivo and in vitro differentiation of myocytes from human bone marrow-derived multipotent progenitor cells. *Exp. Hematol.*, 2003. 31(12): p. 1323-30.
[339] Dezawa, M., Insights into autotransplantation: the unexpected discovery of specific induction systems in bone marrow stromal cells. *Cell Mol. Life Sci.*, 2006. 63(23): p. 2764-72.
[340] Dezawa, M., et al., Bone marrow stromal cells generate muscle cells and repair muscle degeneration. *Science*, 2005. 309(5732): p. 314-7.
[341] Wu, G.D., et al., Migration of mesenchymal stem cells to heart allografts during chronic rejection. *Transplantation*, 2003. 75(5): p. 679-85.
[342] Toma, C., et al., Human mesenchymal stem cells differentiate to a cardiomyocyte phenotype in the adult murine heart. *Circulation*, 2002. 105(1): p. 93-8.
[343] Schulze, M., et al., Mesenchymal stem cells are recruited to striated muscle by NFAT/IL-4-mediated cell fusion. *Genes Dev.*, 2005. 19(15): p. 1787-98.
[344] Mizuno, H., et al., Myogenic differentiation by human processed lipoaspirate cells. *Plast Reconstr. Surg.*, 2002. 109(1): p. 199-209; discussion 210-1.
[345] Gang, E.J., et al., In vitro mesengenic potential of human umbilical cord blood-derived mesenchymal stem cells. *Biochem. Biophys. Res. Commun.*, 2004. 321(1): p. 102-8.

[346] Kinner, B., J.M. Zaleskas, and M. Spector, Regulation of smooth muscle actin expression and contraction in adult human mesenchymal stem cells. *Exp. Cell Res.*, 2002. 278(1): p. 72-83.

[347] Shi, D., et al., Myogenic fusion of human bone marrow stromal cells, but not hematopoietic cells. *Blood*, 2004. 104(1): p. 290-4.

[348] Goncalves, M.A., et al., Human mesenchymal stem cells ectopically expressing full-length dystrophin can complement Duchenne muscular dystrophy myotubes by cell fusion. *Hum. Mol. Genet.*, 2006. 15(2): p. 213-21.

[349] Mendell, J.R., et al., Myoblast transfer in the treatment of Duchenne's muscular dystrophy. *N. Engl. J. Med.*, 1995. 333(13): p. 832-8.

[350] Miller, R.G., et al., Myoblast implantation in Duchenne muscular dystrophy: the San Francisco study. *Muscle Nerve,* 1997. 20(4): p. 469-78.

[351] Neumeyer, A.M., et al., Pilot study of myoblast transfer in the treatment of Becker muscular dystrophy. *Neurology*, 1998. 51(2): p. 589-92.

[352] Sorrentino, V., Stem cells and muscle diseases. *J. Muscle. Res. Cell Motil.*, 2004. 25(3): p. 225-30.

[353] Makino, S., et al., Cardiomyocytes can be generated from marrow stromal cells in vitro. *J. Clin. Invest.,* 1999. 103(5): p. 697-705.

[354] Bittira, B., et al., In vitro preprogramming of marrow stromal cells for myocardial regeneration. *Ann. Thorac. Surg.,* 2002. 74(4): p. 1154-9; discussion 1159-60.

[355] Min, J.Y., et al., Transplantation of embryonic stem cells improves cardiac function in postinfarcted rats. *J. Appl. Physiol.*, 2002. 92(1): p. 288-96.

[356] Cheng, F., et al., Induced differentiation of human cord blood mesenchymal stem/progenitor cells into cardiomyocyte-like cells in vitro. *J. Huazhong Univ. Sci. Technolog Med. Sci.,* 2003. 23(2): p. 154-7.

[357] Erices, A.A., et al., Human cord blood-derived mesenchymal stem cells home and survive in the marrow of immunodeficient mice after systemic infusion. *Cell Transplant,* 2003. 12(6): p. 555-61.

[358] Fukuda, K., Application of mesenchymal stem cells for the regeneration of cardiomyocyte and its use for cell transplantation therapy. *Hum. Cell*, 2003. 16(3): p. 83-94.

[359] Rangappa, S., et al., Cardiomyocyte-mediated contact programs human mesenchymal stem cells to express cardiogenic phenotype. *J. Thorac. Cardiovasc. Surg.*, 2003. 126(1): p. 124-32.

[360] Vanelli, P., et al., Cardiac precursors in human bone marrow and cord blood: in vitro cell cardiogenesis. *Ital. Heart J.*, 2004. 5(5): p. 384-8.

[361] Xu, W., et al., Mesenchymal stem cells from adult human bone marrow differentiate into a cardiomyocyte phenotype in vitro. *Exp. Biol. Med.* (Maywood), 2004. 229(7): p. 623-31.

[362] Yoon, J., et al., Transdifferentiation of mesenchymal stem cells into cardiomyocytes by direct cell-to-cell contact with neonatal cardiomyocyte but not adult cardiomyocytes. *Ann. Hematol.*, 2005. 84(11): p. 715-21.

[363] Wang, T., et al., Cell-to-cell contact induces mesenchymal stem cell to differentiate into cardiomyocyte and smooth muscle cell. Int J Cardiol, 2005.

[364] Potapova, I., et al., Human mesenchymal stem cells as a gene delivery system to create cardiac pacemakers. *Circ. Res.,* 2004. 94(7): p. 952-9.

[365] Valiunas, V., et al., Human mesenchymal stem cells make cardiac connexins and form functional gap junctions. *J. Physiol.*, 2004. 555(Pt 3): p. 617-26.

[366] Min, J.J., et al., In vivo bioluminescence imaging of cord blood derived mesenchymal stem cell transplantation into rat myocardium. Ann Nucl Med, 2006. 20(3): p. 165-70.

[367] Min, J.Y., et al., Significant improvement of heart function by cotransplantation of human mesenchymal stem cells and fetal cardiomyocytes in postinfarcted pigs. *Ann. Thorac. Surg.*, 2002. 74(5): p. 1568-75.

[368] Shake, J.G., et al., Mesenchymal stem cell implantation in a swine myocardial infarct model: engraftment and functional effects. *Ann. Thorac. Surg.*, 2002. 73(6): p. 1919-25; discussion 1926.

[369] Dick, A.J., et al., Magnetic resonance fluoroscopy allows targeted delivery of mesenchymal stem cells to infarct borders in Swine. *Circulation*, 2003. 108(23): p. 2899-904.

[370] Kraitchman, D.L., et al., In vivo magnetic resonance imaging of mesenchymal stem cells in myocardial infarction. *Circulation,* 2003. 107(18): p. 2290-3.

[371] Wollert, K.C., et al., Intracoronary autologous bone-marrow cell transfer after myocardial infarction: the BOOST randomised controlled clinical trial. *Lancet,* 2004. 364(9429): p. 141-8.

[372] Chen, S.L., et al., Effect on left ventricular function of intracoronary transplantation of autologous bone marrow mesenchymal stem cell in patients with acute myocardial infarction. *Am. J. Cardiol.*, 2004. 94(1): p. 92-5.

[373] Miyahara, Y., et al., Monolayered mesenchymal stem cells repair scarred myocardium after myocardial infarction. *Nat. Med.*, 2006. 12(4): p. 459-65.

[374] Dennis, J.E. and P. Charbord, Origin and differentiation of human and murine stroma. *Stem Cells*, 2002. 20(3): p. 205-14.

[375] Charbord, P., et al., Analysis of the microenvironment necessary for engraftment: role of the vascular smooth muscle-like stromal cells. *J. Hematother. Stem Cell Res.*, 2000. 9(6): p. 935-43.

[376] Charbord, P., et al., The Hematopoietic Microenvironment: Phenotypic and Functional Characterization of Human Marrow Vascular Stromal Cells. *Hematol.*, 1999. 4(3): p. 257-282.

[377] Galmiche, M.C., et al., Stromal cells from human long-term marrow cultures are mesenchymal cells that differentiate following a vascular smooth muscle differentiation pathway. *Blood,* 1993. 82(1): p. 66-76.

[378] Lerat, H., et al., Role of stromal cells and macrophages in fibronectin biosynthesis and matrix assembly in human long-term marrow cultures. *Blood*, 1993. 82(5): p. 1480-92.

[379] Li, J., et al., Nontransformed colony-derived stromal cell lines from normal human marrows. II. Phenotypic characterization and differentiation pathway. *Exp. Hematol.*, 1995. 23(2): p. 133-41.

[380] Remy-Martin, J.P., et al., Vascular smooth muscle differentiation of murine stroma: a sequential model. *Exp. Hematol.*, 1999. 27(12): p. 1782-95.

[381] Glukhova, M.A., M.G. Frid, and V.E. Koteliansky, Developmental changes in expression of contractile and cytoskeletal proteins in human aortic smooth muscle. *J. Biol. Chem.*, 1990. 265(22): p. 13042-6.

[382] Glukhova, M.A., et al., Expression of fibronectin variants in vascular and visceral smooth muscle cells in development. *Dev. Biol.*, 1990. 141(1): p. 193-202.

[383] Slomp, J., et al., Differentiation, dedifferentiation, and apoptosis of smooth muscle cells during the development of the human ductus arteriosus. *Arterioscler. Thromb. Vasc. Biol.*, 1997. 17(5): p. 1003-9.
[384] Owens, G.K., Regulation of differentiation of vascular smooth muscle cells. *Physiol. Rev.*, 1995. 75(3): p. 487-517.
[385] Davies, J.A., The Kidney Development Database. *Dev. Genet.*, 1999. 24(3-4): p. 194-8.
[386] Imai, E. and T. Ito, Can bone marrow differentiate into renal cells? *Pediatr. Nephrol.*, 2002. 17(10): p. 790-4.
[387] Imasawa, T., et al., The potential of bone marrow-derived cells to differentiate to glomerular mesangial cells. *J. Am. Soc. Nephrol.*,. 2001. 12(7): p. 1401-9.
[388] Ito, T., et al., Bone marrow is a reservoir of repopulating mesangial cells during glomerular remodeling. *J. Am. Soc. Nephrol.*, 2001. 12(12): p. 2625-35.
[389] Poulsom, R., et al., Bone marrow contributes to renal parenchymal turnover and regeneration. *J. Pathol.*, 2001. 195(2): p. 229-35.
[390] Krause, D.S., et al., Multi-organ, multi-lineage engraftment by a single bone marrow-derived stem cell. *Cell*, 2001. 105(3): p. 369-77.
[391] Iwano, M., et al., Evidence that fibroblasts derive from epithelium during tissue fibrosis. *J. Clin. Invest.*, 2002. 110(3): p. 341-50.
[392] El Kossi, M.M. and A.M. El Nahas, Stem cell factor and crescentic glomerulonephritis. *Am. J. Kidney Dis.*, 2003. 41(4): p. 785-95.
[393] Gupta, S., et al., A role for extrarenal cells in the regeneration following acute renal failure. *Kidney Int*, 2002. 62(4): p. 1285-90.
[394] Bos, C., et al., In vivo MR imaging of intravascularly injected magnetically labeled mesenchymal stem cells in rat kidney and liver. *Radiology*, 2004. 233(3): p. 781-9.
[395] Semont, A., et al., Mesenchymal stem cells increase self-renewal of small intestinal epithelium and accelerate structural recovery after radiation injury. *Adv. Exp. Med. Biol.*, 2006. 585: p. 19-30.
[396] Morigi, M., et al., Mesenchymal stem cells are renotropic, helping to repair the kidney and improve function in acute renal failure. *J. Am. Soc. Nephrol.*, 2004. 15(7): p. 1794-804.
[397] Szczypka, M.S., et al., Rare incorporation of bone marrow-derived cells into kidney after folic acid-induced injury. *Stem Cells*, 2005. 23(1): p. 44-54.
[398] Brittan, M. and N.A. Wright, Gastrointestinal stem cells. *J. Pathol.*, 2002. 197(4): p. 492-509.
[399] Brittan, M., et al., Bone marrow derivation of pericryptal myofibroblasts in the mouse and human small intestine and colon. *Gut,* 2002. 50(6): p. 752-7.
[400] Matsumoto, T., et al., Increase of bone marrow-derived secretory lineage epithelial cells during regeneration in the human intestine. *Gastroenterology,* 2005. 128(7): p. 1851-67.
[401] Okamoto, R., et al., Damaged epithelia regenerated by bone marrow-derived cells in the human gastrointestinal tract. *Nat. Med.,* 2002. 8(9): p. 1011-7.
[402] Brittan, M., et al., A regenerative role for bone marrow following experimental colitis: contribution to neovasculogenesis and myofibroblasts. *Gastroenterology*, 2005. 128(7): p. 1984-95.
[403] Rizvi, A.Z., et al., Bone marrow-derived cells fuse with normal and transformed intestinal stem cells. *Proc. Natl. Acad. Sci. USA*, 2006. 103(16): p. 6321-5.

[404] Komori, M., et al., Efficiency of bone marrow-derived cells in regeneration of the stomach after induction of ethanol-induced ulcers in rats. *J. Gastroenterol.*, 2005. 40(6): p. 591-9.
[405] Oh, S.H., et al., Hepatocyte growth factor induces differentiation of adult rat bone marrow cells into a hepatocyte lineage in vitro. *Biochem. Biophys. Res. Commun.*, 2000. 279(2): p. 500-4.
[406] Avital, I., et al., Isolation, characterization, and transplantation of bone marrow-derived hepatocyte stem cells. *Biochem. Biophys. Res. Commun.*, 2001. 288(1): p. 156-64.
[407] Miyazaki, M., et al., Improved conditions to induce hepatocytes from rat bone marrow cells in culture. *Biochem. Biophys. Res. Commun.*, 2002. 298(1): p. 24-30.
[408] Okumoto, K., et al., Differentiation of bone marrow cells into cells that express liver-specific genes in vitro: implication of the Notch signals in differentiation. *Biochem. Biophys. Res. Commun.*, 2003. 304(4): p. 691-5.
[409] Lee, K.D., et al., In vitro hepatic differentiation of human mesenchymal stem cells. *Hepatology*, 2004. 40(6): p. 1275-84.
[410] Kang, X.Q., et al., Rat bone marrow mesenchymal stem cells differentiate into hepatocytes in vitro. *World J. Gastroenterol.*, 2005. 11(22): p. 3479-84.
[411] Lange, C., et al., Hepatocytic gene expression in cultured rat mesenchymal stem cells. *Transplant Proc.*, 2005. 37(1): p. 276-9.
[412] Moriscot, C., et al., Human bone marrow mesenchymal stem cells can express insulin and key transcription factors of the endocrine pancreas developmental pathway upon genetic and/or microenvironmental manipulation in vitro. *Stem Cells*, 2005. 23(4): p. 594-603.
[413] Theise, N.D., et al., Liver from bone marrow in humans. *Hepatology*, 2000. 32(1): p. 11-6.
[414] Fiegel, H.C., et al., Liver-specific gene expression in cultured human hematopoietic stem cells. *Stem Cells*, 2003. 21(1): p. 98-104.
[415] Lange, C., et al., Liver-specific gene expression in mesenchymal stem cells is induced by liver cells. *World J. Gastroenterol*, 2005. 11(29): p. 4497-504.
[416] Seo, M.J., et al., Differentiation of human adipose stromal cells into hepatic lineage in vitro and in vivo. *Biochem. Biophys. Res. Commun.*, 2005. 328(1): p. 258-64.
[417] Petersen, B.E., et al., Bone marrow as a potential source of hepatic oval cells. *Science,* 1999. 284(5417): p. 1168-70.
[418] Shapiro, A.M., et al., Islet transplantation in seven patients with type 1 diabetes mellitus using a glucocorticoid-free immunosuppressive regimen. *N. Engl. J. Med.*, 2000. 343(4): p. 230-8.
[419] Shapiro, A.M., C. Ricordi, and B. Hering, Edmonton's islet success has indeed been replicated elsewhere. *Lancet,* 2003. 362(9391): p. 1242.
[420] Schwitzgebel, V.M., et al., Expression of neurogenin3 reveals an islet cell precursor population in the pancreas. *Development,* 2000. 127(16): p. 3533-42.
[421] Eberhardt, M., et al., Multipotential nestin and Isl-1 positive mesenchymal stem cells isolated from human pancreatic islets. *Biochem. Biophys. Res. Commun.*, 2006. 345(3): p. 1167-76.
[422] Zulewski, H., et al., Multipotential nestin-positive stem cells isolated from adult pancreatic islets differentiate ex vivo into pancreatic endocrine, exocrine, and hepatic phenotypes. *Diabetes*, 2001. 50(3): p. 521-33.

[423] Zulewski, H., Stem cells with potential to generate insulin producing cells in man. *Swiss Med Wkly*, 2006. 136(41-42): p. 647-54.
[424] Bonner-Weir, S. and A. Sharma, Pancreatic stem cells. *J. Pathol.*, 2002. 197(4): p. 519-26.
[425] D'Amour, K.A., et al., Efficient differentiation of human embryonic stem cells to definitive endoderm. *Nat. Biotechnol.*, 2005. 23(12): p. 1534-41.
[426] Zalzman, M., et al., Reversal of hyperglycemia in mice by using human expandable insulin-producing cells differentiated from fetal liver progenitor cells. *Proc. Natl. Acad. Sci. USA*, 2003. 100(12): p. 7253-8.
[427] Sapir, T., et al., Cell-replacement therapy for diabetes: Generating functional insulin-producing tissue from adult human liver cells. *Proc. Natl. Acad. Sci. USA*, 2005. 102(22): p. 7964-9.
[428] Kodama, S., et al., Islet regeneration during the reversal of autoimmune diabetes in NOD mice. *Science*, 2003. 302(5648): p. 1223-7.
[429] Hori, Y., et al., Differentiation of insulin-producing cells from human neural progenitor cells. *PLoS Med.*, 2005. 2(4): p. e103.
[430] Hess, D., et al., Bone marrow-derived stem cells initiate pancreatic regeneration. *Nat. Biotechnol.*, 2003. 21(7): p. 763-70.
[431] Oh, S.H., et al., Adult bone marrow-derived cells trans-differentiating into insulin-producing cells for the treatment of type I diabetes. *Lab. Invest.*, 2004. 84(5): p. 607-17.
[432] Timper, K., et al., Human adipose tissue-derived mesenchymal stem cells differentiate into insulin, somatostatin, and glucagon expressing cells. *Biochem. Biophys. Res. Commun.*, 2006. 341(4): p. 1135-40.
[433] Gomi, T., et al., Stages in the development of the rat lung: morphometric, light and electron microscopic studies. *Kaibogaku Zasshi,* 1994. 69(4): p. 392-405.
[434] Yamada, Y., et al., Bone regeneration following injection of mesenchymal stem cells and fibrin glue with a biodegradable scaffold. *J. Craniomaxillofac. Surg.*, 2003. 31(1): p. 27-33.
[435] Engelhardt, J.F., Stem cell niches in the mouse airway. *Am. J. Respir. Cell Mol. Biol.*, 2001. 24(6): p. 649-52.
[436] Cardoso, W.V., Molecular regulation of lung development. *Annu. Rev. Physiol.*, 2001. 63: p. 471-94.
[437] in 't Anker, P.S., et al., Nonexpanded primary lung and bone marrow-derived mesenchymal cells promote the engraftment of umbilical cord blood-derived CD34(+) cells in NOD/SCID mice. *Exp. Hematol.*, 2003. 31(10): p. 881-9.
[438] Reddy, R., et al., Isolation of a putative progenitor subpopulation of alveolar epithelial type 2 cells. *Am. J. Physiol. Lung Cell Mol. Physiol.*, 2004. 286(4): p. L658-67.
[439] Kim, C.F., et al., Identification of bronchioalveolar stem cells in normal lung and lung cancer. *Cell*, 2005. 121(6): p. 823-35.
[440] Summer, R., et al., Embryonic lung side population cells are hematopoietic and vascular precursors. *Am. J. Respir. Cell Mol. Biol.*, 2005. 33(1): p. 32-40.
[441] Boers, J.E., A.W. Ambergen, and F.B. Thunnissen, Number and proliferation of basal and parabasal cells in normal human airway epithelium. *Am. J. Respir. Crit. Care Med.*, 1998. 157(6 Pt 1): p. 2000-6.

[442] Duan, D., et al., Lef1 transcription factor expression defines airway progenitor cell targets for in utero gene therapy of submucosal gland in cystic fibrosis. *Am. J. Respir. Cell Mol. Biol.*, 1998. 18(6): p. 750-8.
[443] Danto, S.I., et al., Reversible transdifferentiation of alveolar epithelial cells. *Am. J. Respir. Cell Mol. Biol.*, 1995. 12(5): p. 497-502.
[444] Rippon, H.J., et al., Derivation of distal lung epithelial progenitors from murine embryonic stem cells using a novel three-step differentiation protocol. *Stem Cells,* 2006. 24(5): p. 1389-98.
[445] Wang, G., et al., Adult stem cells from bone marrow stroma differentiate into airway epithelial cells: potential therapy for cystic fibrosis. *Proc. Natl. Acad. Sci. USA*, 2005. 102(1): p. 186-91.
[446] Kotton, D.N., et al., Bone marrow-derived cells as progenitors of lung alveolar epithelium. *Development,* 2001. 128(24): p. 5181-8.
[447] Ortiz, L.A., et al., Mesenchymal stem cell engraftment in lung is enhanced in response to bleomycin exposure and ameliorates its fibrotic effects. *Proc. Natl. Acad. Sci. USA*, 2003. 100(14): p. 8407-11.
[448] Di Nicola, M., et al., Human bone marrow stromal cells suppress T-lymphocyte proliferation induced by cellular or nonspecific mitogenic stimuli. *Blood,* 2002. 99(10): p. 3838-43.
[449] Krampera, M., et al., Bone marrow mesenchymal stem cells inhibit the response of naive and memory antigen-specific T cells to their cognate peptide. *Blood*, 2003. 101(9): p. 3722-9.
[450] Glennie, S., et al., Bone marrow mesenchymal stem cells induce division arrest anergy of activated T cells. Blood, 2005. 105(7): p. 2821-7.
[451] Tintut, Y., et al., Multilineage potential of cells from the artery wall. *Circulation*, 2003. 108(20): p. 2505-10.
[452] Eliopoulos, N., et al., Allogeneic marrow stromal cells are immune rejected by MHC class I- and class II-mismatched recipient mice. *Blood,* 2005. 106(13): p. 4057-65.
[453] Ildstad, S.T. and D.H. Sachs, Reconstitution with syngeneic plus allogeneic or xenogeneic bone marrow leads to specific acceptance of allografts or xenografts. *Nature*, 1984. 307(5947): p. 168-70.
[454] Bartholomew, A., et al., Mesenchymal stem cells suppress lymphocyte proliferation in vitro and prolong skin graft survival in vivo. *Exp. Hematol.* 2002. 30(1): p. 42-8.
[455] Potian, J.A., et al., Veto-like activity of mesenchymal stem cells: functional discrimination between cellular responses to alloantigens and recall antigens. *J. Immunol.*, 2003. 171(7): p. 3426-34.
[456] Aggarwal, S. and M.F. Pittenger, Human mesenchymal stem cells modulate allogeneic immune cell responses. *Blood*, 2005. 105(4): p. 1815-22.
[457] Augello, A., et al., Bone marrow mesenchymal progenitor cells inhibit lymphocyte proliferation by activation of the programmed death 1 pathway. *Eur. J. Immunol.*, 2005. 35(5): p. 1482-90.
[458] Meisel, R., et al., Human bone marrow stromal cells inhibit allogeneic T-cell responses by indoleamine 2,3-dioxygenase-mediated tryptophan degradation. *Blood,* 2004. 103(12): p. 4619-21.
[459] Barry, F.P., et al., Immunogenicity of adult mesenchymal stem cells: lessons from the fetal allograft. Stem Cells Dev., 2005. 14(3): p. 252-65.

[460] Plumas, J., et al., Mesenchymal stem cells induce apoptosis of activated T cells. *Leukemia*, 2005. 19(9): p. 1597-604.
[461] Ryan, J.M., et al., Mesenchymal stem cells avoid allogeneic rejection. *J. Inflamm.* (Lond), 2005. 2: p. 8.
[462] Deng, W., et al., Effects of allogeneic bone marrow-derived mesenchymal stem cells on T and B lymphocytes from BXSB mice. *DNA Cell Biol.*, 2005. 24(7): p. 458-63.
[463] Corcione, A., et al., Human mesenchymal stem cells modulate B-cell functions. *Blood,* 2006. 107(1): p. 367-72.
[464] Krampera, M., et al., Role for interferon-gamma in the immunomodulatory activity of human bone marrow mesenchymal stem cells. *Stem Cells,* 2006. 24(2): p. 386-98.
[465] Spaggiari, G.M., et al., Mesenchymal stem cell-natural killer cell interactions: evidence that activated NK cells are capable of killing MSCs, whereas MSCs can inhibit IL-2-induced NK-cell proliferation. *Blood*, 2006. 107(4): p. 1484-90.
[466] Sotiropoulou, P.A., et al., Interactions between human mesenchymal stem cells and natural killer cells. *Stem Cells,* 2006. 24(1): p. 74-85.
[467] Zhang, W., et al., Effects of mesenchymal stem cells on differentiation, maturation, and function of human monocyte-derived dendritic cells. *Stem Cells Dev.,* 2004. 13(3): p. 263-71.
[468] Jiang, X.X., et al., Human mesenchymal stem cells inhibit differentiation and function of monocyte-derived dendritic cells. *Blood,* 2005. 105(10): p. 4120-6.
[469] Beyth, S., et al., Human mesenchymal stem cells alter antigen-presenting cell maturation and induce T-cell unresponsiveness. *Blood*, 2005. 105(5): p. 2214-9.
[470] Zappia, E., et al., Mesenchymal stem cells ameliorate experimental autoimmune encephalomyelitis inducing T-cell anergy. *Blood,* 2005. 106(5): p. 1755-61.
[471] Horwitz, E.M., et al., Isolated allogeneic bone marrow-derived mesenchymal cells engraft and stimulate growth in children with osteogenesis imperfecta: Implications for cell therapy of bone. *Proc. Natl. Acad. Sci. USA*, 2002. 99(13): p. 8932-7.
[472] Koc, O.N., et al., Allogeneic mesenchymal stem cell infusion for treatment of metachromatic leukodystrophy (MLD) and Hurler syndrome (MPS-IH). *Bone Marrow Transplant*, 2002. 30(4): p. 215-22.
[473] Koc, O.N., et al., Rapid hematopoietic recovery after coinfusion of autologous-blood stem cells and culture-expanded marrow mesenchymal stem cells in advanced breast cancer patients receiving high-dose chemotherapy. *J. Clin. Oncol.*, 2000. 18(2): p. 307-16.
[474] Lazarus, H.M., et al., Cotransplantation of HLA-identical sibling culture-expanded mesenchymal stem cells and hematopoietic stem cells in hematologic malignancy patients. *Biol. Blood Marrow Transplant*, 2005. 11(5): p. 389-98.
[475] Nauta, A.J., et al., Donor-derived mesenchymal stem cells are immunogenic in an allogeneic host and stimulate donor graft rejection in a nonmyeloablative setting. *Blood*, 2006. 108(6): p. 2114-20.
[476] Le Blanc, K., et al., Treatment of severe acute graft-versus-host disease with third party haploidentical mesenchymal stem cells. *Lancet,* 2004. 363(9419): p. 1439-41.
[477] Sudres, M., et al., Bone marrow mesenchymal stem cells suppress lymphocyte proliferation in vitro but fail to prevent graft-versus-host disease in mice. *J. Immunol.*, 2006. 176(12): p. 7761-7.

[478] Gao, J., et al., The dynamic in vivo distribution of bone marrow-derived mesenchymal stem cells after infusion. *Cells Tissues Organs,* 2001. 169(1): p. 12-20.

[479] Barbash, I.M., et al., Systemic delivery of bone marrow-derived mesenchymal stem cells to the infarcted myocardium: feasibility, cell migration, and body distribution. *Circulation*, 2003. 108(7): p. 863-8.

[480] Francois, S., et al., Local irradiation not only induces homing of human mesenchymal stem cells at exposed sites but promotes their widespread engraftment to multiple organs: a study of their quantitative distribution after irradiation damage. *Stem Cells*, 2006. 24(4): p. 1020-9.

[481] Dahir, G.A., et al., Pluripotential mesenchymal cells repopulate bone marrow and retain osteogenic properties. *Clin. Orthop. Relat. Res.*, 2000(379 Suppl): p. S134-45.

[482] Mahmud, N., et al., Studies of the route of administration and role of conditioning with radiation on unrelated allogeneic mismatched mesenchymal stem cell engraftment in a nonhuman primate model. *Exp. Hematol.*, 2004. 32(5): p. 494-501.

[483] Javazon, E.H., K.J. Beggs, and A.W. Flake, Mesenchymal stem cells: paradoxes of passaging. *Exp. Hematol.*, 2004. 32(5): p. 414-25.

[484] Alvarez-Dolado, M., et al., Fusion of bone-marrow-derived cells with Purkinje neurons, cardiomyocytes and hepatocytes. *Nature*, 2003. 425(6961): p. 968-73.

[485] Pereira, R.F., et al., Marrow stromal cells as a source of progenitor cells for nonhematopoietic tissues in transgenic mice with a phenotype of osteogenesis imperfecta. *Proc. Natl. Acad. Sci. USA*, 1998. 95(3): p. 1142-7.

[486] Horwitz, E.M., et al., Clinical responses to bone marrow transplantation in children with severe osteogenesis imperfecta. *Blood,* 2001. 97(5): p. 1227-31.

[487] Genbacev, O. and R.K. Miller, Post-implantation differentiation and proliferation of cytotrophoblast cells: in vitro models--a review. Placenta, 2000. 21 Suppl A: p. S45-9.

[488] Jauniaux, E., et al., In-vivo measurement of intrauterine gases and acid-base values early in human pregnancy. *Hum. Reprod.*, 1999. 14(11): p. 2901-4.

[489] Kiserud, T., Physiology of the fetal circulation. *Semin. Fetal. Neonatal. Med.*, 2005. 10(6): p. 493-503.

[490] Ishikawa, Y. and T. Ito, Kinetics of hemopoietic stem cells in a hypoxic culture. *Eur. J. Haematol.*, 1988. 40(2): p. 126-9.

[491] Chow, D.C., et al., Modeling pO(2) distributions in the bone marrow hematopoietic compartment. I. Krogh's model. *Biophys. J.,* 2001. 81(2): p. 675-84.

[492] Cipolleschi, M.G., P. Dello Sbarba, and M. Olivotto, The role of hypoxia in the maintenance of hematopoietic stem cells. *Blood*, 1993. 82(7): p. 2031-7.

[493] Danet, G.H., et al., Expansion of human SCID-repopulating cells under hypoxic conditions. *J. Clin. Invest.*, 2003. 112(1): p. 126-35.

[494] Taneja, R., et al., Effects of hypoxia on granulocytic-monocytic progenitors in rats. Role of bone marrow stroma. *Am. J. Hematol.*, 2000. 64(1): p. 20-5.

[495] Lennon, D.P., J.M. Edmison, and A.I. Caplan, Cultivation of rat marrow-derived mesenchymal stem cells in reduced oxygen tension: effects on in vitro and in vivo osteochondrogenesis. *J. Cell Physiol.*, 2001. 187(3): p. 345-55.

[496] Fink, T., et al., Induction of adipocyte-like phenotype in human mesenchymal stem cells by hypoxia. *Stem Cells*, 2004. 22(7): p. 1346-55.

[497] Honczarenko, M., et al., Human bone marrow stromal cells express a distinct set of biologically functional chemokine receptors. *Stem Cells*, 2006. 24(4): p. 1030-41.

[498] Moussavi-Harami, F., et al., Oxygen effects on senescence in chondrocytes and mesenchymal stem cells: consequences for tissue engineering. *Iowa Orthop J.*, 2004. 24: p. 15-20.

[499] Robins, J.C., et al., Hypoxia induces chondrocyte-specific gene expression in mesenchymal cells in association with transcriptional activation of Sox9. *Bone*, 2005. 37(3): p. 313-22.

[500] Malladi, P., et al., Effect of reduced oxygen tension on chondrogenesis and osteogenesis in adipose-derived mesenchymal cells. *Am. J. Physiol. Cell Ph*ysiol., 2006. 290(4): p. C1139-46.

[501] Zhu, W., et al., Hypoxia and serum deprivation-induced apoptosis in mesenchymal stem cells. *Stem Cells,* 2006. 24(2): p. 416-25.

[502] Grayson, W.L., et al., Effects of hypoxia on human mesenchymal stem cell expansion and plasticity in 3D constructs. *J. Cell Physiol.*, 2006. 207(2): p. 331-9.

[503] Martin-Rendon, E., et al., Transcriptional profiling of human cord blood CD133+ and cultured bone marrow mesenchymal stem cells in response to hypoxia. *Stem Cells,* 2006.

[504] Gojo, S., et al., In vivo cardiovasculogenesis by direct injection of isolated adult mesenchymal stem cells. *Exp. Cell Res.*, 2003. 288(1): p. 51-9.

[505] Mangi, A.A., et al., Mesenchymal stem cells modified with Akt prevent remodeling and restore performance of infarcted hearts. *Nat. Med.*,. 2003. 9(9): p. 1195-201.

[506] Massas, R. and D. Benayahu, Parathyroid hormone effect on cell-to-cell communication in stromal and osteoblastic cells. *J. Cell Biochem.*, 1998. 69(1): p. 81-6.

[507] Bleul, C.C., et al., A highly efficacious lymphocyte chemoattractant, stromal cell-derived factor 1 (SDF-1). *J. Exp. Med.*, 1996. 184(3): p. 1101-9.

[508] Thayer, J.M., et al., Formation of the arterial media during vascular development. *Cell Mol. Biol. Res.*, 1995. 41(4): p. 251-62.

[509] Owens, G.K., S.M. Vernon, and C.S. Madsen, Molecular regulation of smooth muscle cell differentiation. *J. Hypertens. Suppl.*, 1996. 14(5): p. S55-64.

[510] Hungerford, J.E. and C.D. Little, Developmental biology of the vascular smooth muscle cell: building a multilayered vessel wall. *J. Vasc. Res.*, 1999. 36(1): p. 2-27.

[511] Li, D.Y., et al., Defective angiogenesis in mice lacking endoglin. *Science,* 1999. 284(5419): p. 1534-7.

[512] Lin, Q., et al., Requirement of the MADS-box transcription factor MEF2C for vascular development. *Development,* 1998. 125(22): p. 4565-74.

[513] Yang, Y., et al., Embryonic mesenchymal cells share the potential for smooth muscle differentiation: myogenesis is controlled by the cell's shape. *Development,* 1999. 126(13): p. 3027-33.

[514] Arakawa, E., et al., A mouse bone marrow stromal cell line, TBR-B, shows inducible expression of smooth muscle-specific genes. *FEBS Lett,* 2000. 481(2): p. 193-6.

[515] Hegner, B., et al., Differential regulation of smooth muscle markers in human bone marrow-derived mesenchymal stem cells. *J. Hypertens,* 2005. 23(6): p. 1191-202.

[516] Andrades, J.A., et al., A recombinant human TGF-beta1 fusion protein with collagen-binding domain promotes migration, growth, and differentiation of bone marrow mesenchymal cells. *Exp. Cell Res.*, 1999. 250(2): p. 485-98.

[517] Sensebe, L., et al., Cytokines active on granulomonopoiesis: release and consumption by human marrow myoid [corrected] stromal cells. *Br. J. Haematol.*, 1997. 98(2): p. 274-82.
[518] Jeon, E.S., et al., Sphingosylphosphorylcholine induces differentiation of human mesenchymal stem cells into smooth-muscle-like cells through a TGF-beta-dependent mechanism. *J. Cell Sci.*, 2006. 119(Pt 23): p. 4994-5005.
[519] Cai, D., et al., Lapine and canine bone marrow stromal cells contain smooth muscle actin and contract a collagen-glycosaminoglycan matrix. *Tissue Eng,* 2001. 7(6): p. 829-41.
[520] Kawano, S., et al., ATP autocrine/paracrine signaling induces calcium oscillations and NFAT activation in human mesenchymal stem cells. *Cell Calcium*, 2006.
[521] Kawano, S., et al., Characterization of Ca(2+) signaling pathways in human mesenchymal stem cells. *Cell Calcium*, 2002. 32(4): p. 165-74.
[522] Zahanich, I., et al., Molecular and functional expression of voltage-operated calcium channels during osteogenic differentiation of human mesenchymal stem cells. *J. Bone Miner Res.,* 2005. 20(9): p. 1637-46.
[523] Heubach, J.F., et al., Electrophysiological properties of human mesenchymal stem cells. *J. Physiol.*, 2004. 554(Pt 3): p. 659-72.
[524] Li, G.R., et al., Characterization of ionic currents in human mesenchymal stem cells from bone marrow. *Stem Cells,* 2005. 23(3): p. 371-82.
[525] Amberger, A., et al., Reversible expression of sm alpha-actin protein and sm alpha-actin mRNA in cloned cerebral endothelial cells. *FEBS Lett,* 1991. 287(1-2): p. 223-5.
[526] Arciniegas, E., et al., Transforming growth factor beta 1 promotes the differentiation of endothelial cells into smooth muscle-like cells in vitro. *J. Cell Sci.*, 1992. 103 (Pt 2): p. 521-9.
[527] DeRuiter, M.C., et al., Embryonic endothelial cells transdifferentiate into mesenchymal cells expressing smooth muscle actins in vivo and in vitro. *Circ. Res.*, 1997. 80(4): p. 444-51.
[528] Oswald, J., et al., Mesenchymal stem cells can be differentiated into endothelial cells in vitro. *Stem Cells*, 2004. 22(3): p. 377-84.
[529] Gang, E.J., et al., In vitro endothelial potential of human UC blood-derived mesenchymal stem cells. *Cytotherapy,* 2006. 8(3): p. 215-27.
[530] Frid, M.G., V.A. Kale, and K.R. Stenmark, Mature vascular endothelium can give rise to smooth muscle cells via endothelial-mesenchymal transdifferentiation: in vitro analysis. *Circ. Res.,* 2002. 90(11): p. 1189-96.
[531] Yamashita, J., et al., Flk1-positive cells derived from embryonic stem cells serve as vascular progenitors. *Nature,* 2000. 408(6808): p. 92-6.
[532] Haynesworth, S.E., M.A. Baber, and A.I. Caplan, Cytokine expression by human marrow-derived mesenchymal progenitor cells in vitro: effects of dexamethasone and IL-1 alpha. *J. Cell Physiol.*, 1996. 166(3): p. 585-92.
[533] Majumdar, M.K., et al., Human marrow-derived mesenchymal stem cells (MSCs) express hematopoietic cytokines and support long-term hematopoiesis when differentiated toward stromal and osteogenic lineages. *J. Hematother. Stem. Cell Res.*, 2000. 9(6): p. 841-8.

[534] Majumdar, M.K., et al., Phenotypic and functional comparison of cultures of marrow-derived mesenchymal stem cells (MSCs) and stromal cells. *J. Cell Physiol.*, 1998. 176(1): p. 57-66.

[535] Ahmed, N., et al., Effect of bone morphogenetic protein-6 on haemopoietic stem cells and cytokine production in normal human bone marrow stroma. *Cell Biol. Int.*, 2001. 25(5): p. 429-35.

[536] Petit, I., et al., G-CSF induces stem cell mobilization by decreasing bone marrow SDF-1 and up-regulating CXCR4. *Nat. Immunol.*, 2002. 3(7): p. 687-94.

[537] Taichman, R.S., et al., Augmented production of interleukin-6 by normal human osteoblasts in response to CD34+ hematopoietic bone marrow cells in vitro. *Blood*, 1997. 89(4): p. 1165-72.

[538] Kinnaird, T., et al., Marrow-derived stromal cells express genes encoding a broad spectrum of arteriogenic cytokines and promote in vitro and in vivo arteriogenesis through paracrine mechanisms. *Circ. Res.*, 2004. 94(5): p. 678-85.

[539] Kinnaird, T., et al., Local delivery of marrow-derived stromal cells augments collateral perfusion through paracrine mechanisms. *Circulation*, 2004. 109(12): p. 1543-9.

[540] Tang, Y.L., et al., Paracrine action enhances the effects of autologous mesenchymal stem cell transplantation on vascular regeneration in rat model of myocardial infarction. *Ann. Thorac. Surg.*, 2005. 80(1): p. 229-36; discussion 236-7.

[541] Tang, Y.L., et al., Autologous mesenchymal stem cell transplantation induce VEGF and neovascularization in ischemic myocardium. *Regul. Pept.*, 2004. 117(1): p. 3-10.

[542] Caplan, A.I. and J.E. Dennis, Mesenchymal stem cells as trophic mediators. *J. Cell Biochem.*, 2006. 98(5): p. 1076-84.

[543] Wakelee, H.A. and J.H. Schiller, Targeting angiogenesis with vascular endothelial growth factor receptor small-molecule inhibitors: novel agents with potential in lung cancer. *Clin. Lung Cancer,* 2005. 7 Suppl 1: p. S31-8.

[544] Thebaud, B., et al., Vascular endothelial growth factor gene therapy increases survival, promotes lung angiogenesis, and prevents alveolar damage in hyperoxia-induced lung injury: evidence that angiogenesis participates in alveolarization. *Circulation*, 2005. 112(16): p. 2477-86.

[545] deMello, D.E., et al., Early fetal development of lung vasculature. *Am. J. Respir. Cell Mol. Biol.*, 1997. 16(5): p. 568-81.

[546] Anderson-Berry, A., et al., Vasculogenesis drives pulmonary vascular growth in the developing chick embryo. *Dev. Dyn.*, 2005. 233(1): p. 145-53.

[547] Mitani, Y., et al., Vascular smooth muscle cell phenotypes in primary pulmonary hypertension. *Eur. Respir. J.*, 2001. 17(2): p. 316-20.

[548] Ghamra, Z.W. and R.A. Dweik, Primary pulmonary hypertension: an overview of epidemiology and pathogenesis. *Cleve Clin. J. Med.*, 2003. 70 Suppl 1: p. S2-8.

[549] Tuder, R.M., et al., Exuberant endothelial cell growth and elements of inflammation are present in plexiform lesions of pulmonary hypertension. *Am. J. Pathol*, 1994. 144(2): p. 275-85.

[550] Tuder, R.M., et al., Expression of angiogenesis-related molecules in plexiform lesions in severe pulmonary hypertension: evidence for a process of disordered angiogenesis. *J. Pathol.*, 2001. 195(3): p. 367-74.

[551] Hyvelin, J.M., et al., Inhibition of Rho-kinase attenuates hypoxia-induced angiogenesis in the pulmonary circulation. *Circ. Res.*, 2005. 97(2): p. 185-91.

[552] Akeson, A.L., et al., Embryonic vasculogenesis by endothelial precursor cells derived from lung mesenchyme. *Dev. Dyn.*, 2000. 217(1): p. 11-23.

[553] Sata, M., Role of circulating vascular progenitors in angiogenesis, vascular healing, and pulmonary hypertension: lessons from animal models. *Arterioscler. Thromb. Vasc. Biol.*, 2006. 26(5): p. 1008-14.

[554] Hashimoto, N., et al., Bone marrow-derived progenitor cells in pulmonary fibrosis. *J. Clin. Invest.*, 2004. 113(2): p. 243-52.

[555] Davie, N.J., et al., Hypoxia-induced pulmonary artery adventitial remodeling and neovascularization: contribution of progenitor cells. *Am. J. Physiol. Lung Cell Mol. Physiol.*, 2004. 286(4): p. L668-78.

[556] Hu, Y., et al., Abundant progenitor cells in the adventitia contribute to atherosclerosis of vein grafts in ApoE-deficient mice. *J. Clin. Invest.*, 2004. 113(9): p. 1258-65.

[557] Hayashida, K., et al., Bone marrow-derived cells contribute to pulmonary vascular remodeling in hypoxia-induced pulmonary hypertension. *Chest,* 2005. 127(5): p. 1793-8.

[558] Kanki-Horimoto, S., et al., Implantation of mesenchymal stem cells overexpressing endothelial nitric oxide synthase improves right ventricular impairments caused by pulmonary hypertension. *Circulation*, 2006. 114(1 Suppl): p. I181-5.

[559] Zhao, Y.D., et al., Rescue of monocrotaline-induced pulmonary arterial hypertension using bone marrow-derived endothelial-like progenitor cells: efficacy of combined cell and eNOS gene therapy in established disease. *Circ. Res.,* 2005. 96(4): p. 442-50.

[560] Li, X. and J.W. Wilson, Increased vascularity of the bronchial mucosa in mild asthma. *Am. J. Respir. Crit. Care Med.*, 1997. 156(1): p. 229-33.

[561] Hoshino, M., Y. Nakamura, and Q.A. Hamid, Gene expression of vascular endothelial growth factor and its receptors and angiogenesis in bronchial asthma. *J. Allergy Clin. Immunol.*, 2001. 107(6): p. 1034-8.

[562] Favre, C.J., et al., Expression of genes involved in vascular development and angiogenesis in endothelial cells of adult lung. *Am. J. Physiol. Heart Circ Physiol.*, 2003. 285(5): p. H1917-38.

[563] Salvato, G., Quantitative and morphological analysis of the vascular bed in bronchial biopsy specimens from asthmatic and non-asthmatic subjects. *Thorax*, 2001. 56(12): p. 902-6.

[564] McDonald, D.M., Angiogenesis and remodeling of airway vasculature in chronic inflammation. *Am. J. Respir. Crit. Care Med.*, 2001. 164(10 Pt 2): p. S39-45.

[565] Roberts, W.G. and G.E. Palade, Neovasculature induced by vascular endothelial growth factor is fenestrated. *Cancer Res.*, 1997. 57(4): p. 765-72.

[566] Denburg, J.A., et al., Systemic aspects of allergic disease: bone marrow responses. *J. Allergy Clin. Immunol.*, 2000. 106(5 Suppl): p. S242-6.

[567] Delplanque, A., et al., Epithelial stem cell-mediated development of the human respiratory mucosa in SCID mice. *J. Cell Sci.*, 2000. 113 (Pt 5): p. 767-78.

[568] Kamihata, H., et al., Improvement of collateral perfusion and regional function by implantation of peripheral blood mononuclear cells into ischemic hibernating myocardium. *Arterioscler. Thromb. Vasc. Biol.*, 2002. 22(11): p. 1804-10.

[569] Yeh, E.T., et al., Transdifferentiation of human peripheral blood CD34+-enriched cell population into cardiomyocytes, endothelial cells, and smooth muscle cells in vivo. *Circulation*, 2003. 108(17): p. 2070-3.

[570] Crystal, R.G., et al., Future research directions in idiopathic pulmonary fibrosis: summary of a National Heart, Lung, and Blood Institute working group. *Am. J. Respir. Crit. Care Med.*, 2002. 166(2): p. 236-46.

[571] Selman, M., et al., Idiopathic pulmonary fibrosis: pathogenesis and therapeutic approaches. *Drugs*, 2004. 64(4): p. 405-30.

[572] Cosgrove, G.P., et al., Pigment epithelium-derived factor in idiopathic pulmonary fibrosis: a role in aberrant angiogenesis. *Am. J. Respir. Crit. Care Med.*, 2004. 170(3): p. 242-51.

[573] Ebina, M., et al., Heterogeneous increase in CD34-positive alveolar capillaries in idiopathic pulmonary fibrosis. *Am. J. Respir. Crit Care Med.*, 2004. 169(11): p. 1203-8.

[574] Epperly, M.W., et al., Bone marrow origin of myofibroblasts in irradiation pulmonary fibrosis. *Am. J. Respir. Cell Mol. Biol.*, 2003. 29(2): p. 213-24.

[575] Voelkel, N.F. and R.M. Tuder, Hypoxia-induced pulmonary vascular remodeling: a model for what human disease? *J. Clin. Invest.*, 2000. 106(6): p. 733-8.

[576] Wiebe, B.M. and H. Laursen, Lung morphometry by unbiased methods in emphysema: bronchial and blood vessel volume, alveolar surface area and capillary length. *Apmis*, 1998. 106(6): p. 651-6.

[577] Taraseviciene-Stewart, L., et al., Is alveolar destruction and emphysema in chronic obstructive pulmonary disease an immune disease? *Proc. Am. Thorac. Soc.*, 2006. 3(8): p. 687-90.

[578] Abe, S., et al., Lung cells transplanted to irradiated recipients generate lymphohematopoietic progeny. *Am. J. Respir. Cell Mol. Biol.*, 2004. 30(4): p. 491-9.

[579] Dunsmore, S.E. and S.D. Shapiro, The bone marrow leaves its scar: new concepts in pulmonary fibrosis. *J. Clin. Invest.*, 2004. 113(2): p. 180-2.

[580] Ambrose, J.A., Myocardial ischemia and infarction. *J. Am. Coll Cardiol.*, 2006. 47(11 Suppl): p. D13-7.

[581] Soonpaa, M.H., et al., Formation of nascent intercalated disks between grafted fetal cardiomyocytes and host myocardium. *Science*, 1994. 264(5155): p. 98-101.

[582] Murry, C.E., et al., Skeletal myoblast transplantation for repair of myocardial necrosis. *J. Clin. Invest.,* 1996. 98(11): p. 2512-23.

[583] Taylor, D.A., et al., Regenerating functional myocardium: improved performance after skeletal myoblast transplantation. *Nat. Med.*, 1998. 4(8): p. 929-33.

[584] Tomita, S., et al., Autologous transplantation of bone marrow cells improves damaged heart function. *Circulation*, 1999. 100(19 Suppl): p. II247-56.

[585] Strauer, B.E., et al., Repair of infarcted myocardium by autologous intracoronary mononuclear bone marrow cell transplantation in humans. *Circulation,* 2002. 106(15): p. 1913-8.

[586] Menasche, P., Stem cells for clinical use in cardiovascular medicine: current limitations and future perspectives. *Thromb. Haemost*, 2005. 94(4): p. 697-701.

[587] Assmus, B., et al., Transplantation of Progenitor Cells and Regeneration Enhancement in Acute Myocardial Infarction (TOPCARE-AMI). *Circulation*, 2002. 106(24): p. 3009-17.

[588] Stamm, C., et al., Autologous bone-marrow stem-cell transplantation for myocardial regeneration. *Lancet*, 2003. 361(9351): p. 45-6.

[589] Katritsis, D.G., et al., Transcoronary transplantation of autologous mesenchymal stem cells and endothelial progenitors into infarcted human myocardium. *Catheter Cardiovasc. Interv.*, 2005. 65(3): p. 321-9.

[590] Perin, E.C., et al., Transendocardial, autologous bone marrow cell transplantation for severe, chronic ischemic heart failure. *Circulation*, 2003. 107(18): p. 2294-302.

[591] Perin, E.C., et al., Improved exercise capacity and ischemia 6 and 12 months after transendocardial injection of autologous bone marrow mononuclear cells for ischemic cardiomyopathy. *Circulation,* 2004. 110(11 Suppl 1): p. II213-8.

[592] Mc, D.D. and J.M. Potter, A method for the study of arterial anastomoses. *J. Anat,.* 1950. 84(4): p. 327-8.

[593] Urschel, H.C., Jr. and E.J. Roth, Small arterial anastomoses: I. Nonsuture. *Ann. Surg.*, 1961. 153: p. 599-610.

[594] Urschel, H.C., Jr. and E.J. Roth, Small arterial anastomoses: II. Suture. *Ann. Surg.*, 1961. 153: p. 611-6.

[595] Fulton, W.F., The Dynamic Factor in Enlargement of Coronary Arterial Anastomoses, and Paradoxical Changes in the Subendocardial Plexus. *Br. Heart J.*, 1964. 26: p. 39-50.

[596] Fulton, W.F., The Time Factor in the Enlargement of Anastomoses in Coronary Artery *Disease. Scott .Med. J.*, 1964. 9: p. 18-23.

[597] Risau, W., Mechanisms of angiogenesis. *Nature,* 1997. 386(6626): p. 671-4.

[598] Heil, M. and W. Schaper, Influence of mechanical, cellular, and molecular factors on collateral artery growth (arteriogenesis). *Circ. Res.*, 2004. 95(5): p. 449-58.

[599] Ross, R., The pathogenesis of atherosclerosis: a perspective for the 1990s. *Nature,* 1993. 362(6423): p. 801-9.

[600] Simper, D., et al., Smooth muscle progenitor cells in human blood. *Circulation,* 2002. 106(10): p. 1199-204.

[601] Sata, M., et al., Hematopoietic stem cells differentiate into vascular cells that participate in the pathogenesis of atherosclerosis. *Nat. Med.*, 2002. 8(4): p. 403-9.

[602] Campbell, J.H., J.L. Efendy, and G.R. Campbell, Novel vascular graft grown within recipient's own peritoneal cavity. *Circ. Res.*, 1999. 85(12): p. 1173-8.

[603] Montfort, M.J., et al., Adult blood vessels restore host hematopoiesis following lethal irradiation. *Exp. Hematol.*, 2002. 30(8): p. 950-6.

[604] Covas, D.T., et al., Mesenchymal stem cells can be obtained from the human saphena vein. *Exp. Cell Res.*, 2005. 309(2): p. 340-4.

[605] Wu, X., et al., Mesenchymal stem cells participating in ex vivo endothelium repair and its effect on vascular smooth muscle cells growth. *Int. J. Cardiol.*, 2005. 105(3): p. 274-82.

[606] Caplice, N.M., et al., Smooth muscle cells in human coronary atherosclerosis can originate from cells administered at marrow transplantation. *Proc. Natl. Acad. Sci. USA*, 2003. 100(8): p. 4754-9.

[607] Shimizu, K., et al., Host bone-marrow cells are a source of donor intimal smooth-muscle-like cells in murine aortic transplant arteriopathy. *Nat. Med.*, 2001. 7(6): p. 738-41.

[608] Forte, A., et al., Molecular analysis of arterial stenosis in rat carotids. *J. Cell Physiol.*, 2001. 186(2): p. 307-13.

[609] Xu, Y., et al., Role of bone marrow-derived progenitor cells in cuff-induced vascular injury in mice. *Arterioscler. Thromb. Vasc. Biol.*, 2004. 24(3): p. 477-82.

[610] Tanaka, K., et al., Diverse contribution of bone marrow cells to neointimal hyperplasia after mechanical vascular injuries. *Circ. Res.*, 2003. 93(8): p. 783-90.

[611] Aoki, J., et al., Endothelial progenitor cell capture by stents coated with antibody against CD34: the HEALING-FIM (Healthy Endothelial Accelerated Lining Inhibits Neointimal Growth-First In Man) Registry. *J. Am. Coll Cardiol.*, 2005. 45(10): p. 1574-9.

[612] Silber, S., Capturing circulating endothelial progenitor cells: a new concept tested in the HEALING studies. *Minerva Cardioangiol.*, 2006. 54(1): p. 1-3.

[613] Han, C.I., G.R. Campbell, and J.H. Campbell, Circulating bone marrow cells can contribute to neointimal formation. *J. Vasc. Res.*, 2001. 38(2): p. 113-9.

[614] Folkman, J., et al., Isolation of a tumor factor responsible for angiogenesis. *J. Exp. Med.*, 1971. 133(2): p. 275-88.

[615] Hanahan, D. and R.A. Weinberg, The hallmarks of cancer. *Cell,* 2000. 100(1): p. 57-70.

[616] Vakkila, J. and M.T. Lotze, Inflammation and necrosis promote tumour growth. *Nat. Rev. Immunol.*, 2004. 4(8): p. 641-8.

[617] Mueller, M.M. and N.E. Fusenig, Friends or foes - bipolar effects of the tumour stroma in cancer. *Nat. Rev. Cancer,* 2004. 4(11): p. 839-49.

[618] Bergers, G. and L.E. Benjamin, Tumorigenesis and the angiogenic switch. *Nat. Rev. Cancer,* 2003. 3(6): p. 401-10.

[619] Condeelis, J. and J.W. Pollard, Macrophages: obligate partners for tumor cell migration, invasion, and metastasis. *Cell*, 2006. 124(2): p. 263-6.

[620] de Visser, K.E., A. Eichten, and L.M. Coussens, Paradoxical roles of the immune system during cancer development. *Nat. Rev. Cancer,* 2006. 6(1): p. 24-37.

[621] Carmeliet, P., Angiogenesis in life, disease and medicine. *Nature*, 2005. 438(7070): p. 932-6.

[622] Ferrara, N. and R.S. Kerbel, Angiogenesis as a therapeutic target. *Nature,* 2005. 438(7070): p. 967-74.

[623] Lyden, D., et al., Impaired recruitment of bone-marrow-derived endothelial and hematopoietic precursor cells blocks tumor angiogenesis and growth. *Nat. Med.*, 2001. 7(11): p. 1194-201.

[624] Heissig, B., et al., Recruitment of stem and progenitor cells from the bone marrow niche requires MMP-9 mediated release of kit-ligand. *Cell,* 2002. 109(5): p. 625-37.

[625] De Palma, M., et al., Targeting exogenous genes to tumor angiogenesis by transplantation of genetically modified hematopoietic stem cells. *Nat. Med.*, 2003. 9(6): p. 789-95.

[626] Peters, B.A., et al., Contribution of bone marrow-derived endothelial cells to human tumor vasculature. *Nat. Med.*, 2005. 11(3): p. 261-2.

[627] Sun, B., et al., Correlation between melanoma angiogenesis and the mesenchymal stem cells and endothelial progenitor cells derived from bone marrow. *Stem. Cells Dev.*, 2005. 14(3): p. 292-8.

[628] Zhu, W., et al., Mesenchymal stem cells derived from bone marrow favor tumor cell growth in vivo. *Exp. Mol. Pathol.*, 2006. 80(3): p. 267-74.

[629] Campbell, C.D., D. Goldfarb, and R. Roe, A small arterial substitute: expanded microporous polytetrafluoroethylene: patency versus porosity. *Ann. Surg.*, 1975. 182(2): p. 138-43.
[630] Lepidi, S., et al., In vivo regeneration of small-diameter (2 mm) arteries using a polymer scaffold. *Faseb J.*, 2006. 20(1): p. 103-5.
[631] Jarrell, B.E., et al., Use of an endothelial monolayer on a vascular graft prior to implantation. Temporal dynamics and compatibility with the operating room. *Ann. Surg.,* 1986. 203(6): p. 671-8.
[632] Herring, M.B., et al., Seeding arterial prostheses with vascular endothelium. The nature of the lining. *Ann. Surg.*, 1979. 190(1): p. 84-90.
[633] Niklason, L.E., et al., Functional arteries grown in vitro. *Science,* 1999. 284(5413): p. 489-93.
[634] Yu, H., et al., Smooth muscle cells improve endothelial cell retention on polytetrafluoroethylene grafts in vivo. *J. Vasc. Surg.*, 2003. 38(3): p. 557-63.
[635] L'Heureux, N., et al., A completely biological tissue-engineered human blood vessel. *Faseb J.,* 1998. 12(1): p. 47-56.
[636] Kaushal, S., et al., Functional small-diameter neovessels created using endothelial progenitor cells expanded ex vivo. *Nat. Med,.* 2001. 7(9): p. 1035-40.
[637] Cho, S.W., et al., Small-diameter blood vessels engineered with bone marrow-derived cells. *Ann. Surg.*, 2005. 241(3): p. 506-15.
[638] Cho, S.W., et al., Vascular patches tissue-engineered with autologous bone marrow-derived cells and decellularized tissue matrices. *Biomaterials,* 2005. 26(14): p. 1915-24.
[639] Kanki-Horimoto, S., et al., Synthetic vascular prosthesis impregnated with genetically modified bone marrow cells produced recombinant proteins. *Artif. Organs*, 2005. 29(10): p. 815-9.
[640] Zhang, J., et al., Engineering of vascular grafts with genetically modified bone marrow mesenchymal stem cells on poly (propylene carbonate) graft. *Artif. Organs*, 2006. 30(12): p. 898-905.
[641] Chisholm, M.H., D. Navarro-Llobet, and Z. Zhou, Poly(propylene carbonate). 1. More about Poly(propylene carbonate) Formed from the Copolymerization of Propylene Oxide and Carbon Dioxide Employing a Zinc Glutarate Catalyst. *Macromolecules,* 2002. 35(17): p. 6494-6504.
[642] Kadner, A., et al., A new source for cardiovascular tissue engineering: human bone marrow stromal cells. *Eur. J. Cardiothorac. Surg.*, 2002. 21(6): p. 1055-60.
[643] Matsumura, G., et al., First evidence that bone marrow cells contribute to the construction of tissue-engineered vascular autografts in vivo. *Circulation,* 2003. 108(14): p. 1729-34.
[644] Cho, S.W., et al., Smooth muscle-like tissues engineered with bone marrow stromal cells. *Biomaterials,* 2004. 25(15): p. 2979-86.
[645] Cassell, O.C., et al., The influence of extracellular matrix on the generation of vascularized, engineered, transplantable tissue. *Ann. NY Acad. Sci*, 2001. 944: p. 429-42.
[646] Stock, U.A., et al., Patch augmentation of the pulmonary artery with bioabsorbable polymers and autologous cell seeding. *J. Thorac. Cardiovasc. Surg.*, 2000. 120(6): p. 1158-67; discussion 1168.

[647] Wilson, G.J., et al., Acellular matrix: a biomaterials approach for coronary artery bypass and heart valve replacement. *Ann. Thorac. Surg.*, 1995. 60(2 Suppl): p. S353-8.
[648] Kim, B.S. and D.J. Mooney, Scaffolds for engineering smooth muscle under cyclic mechanical strain conditions. *J. Biomech. Eng.*, 2000. 122(3): p. 210-5.
[649] Dartsch, P.C. and H. Hammerle, Orientation response of arterial smooth muscle cells to mechanical stimulation. *Eur. J. Cell Biol.*, 1986. 41(2): p. 339-46.
[650] Dartsch, P.C., H. Hammerle, and E. Betz, Orientation of cultured arterial smooth muscle cells growing on cyclically stretched substrates. *Acta Anat* (Basel), 1986. 125(2): p. 108-13.
[651] Thyberg, J., Differentiated properties and proliferation of arterial smooth muscle cells in culture. *Int. Rev. Cytol.*, 1996. 169: p. 183-265.
[652] Osol, G., Mechanotransduction by vascular smooth muscle. *J. Vasc. Res.*, 1995. 32(5): p. 275-92.
[653] Baskin, L., P.S. Howard, and E. Macarak, Effect of physical forces on bladder smooth muscle and urothelium. *J. Urol.*, 1993. 150(2 Pt 2): p. 601-7.
[654] Birukov, K.G., et al., Stretch affects phenotype and proliferation of vascular smooth muscle cells. *Mol. Cell Biochem.*, 1995. 144(2): p. 131-9.
[655] Reusch, P., et al., Mechanical strain increases smooth muscle and decreases nonmuscle myosin expression in rat vascular smooth muscle cells. *Circ. Res.*, 1996. 79(5): p. 1046-53.
[656] Niklason, L.E., et al., Morphologic and mechanical characteristics of engineered bovine arteries. *J. Vasc. Surg.*, 2001. 33(3): p. 628-38.
[657] Niklason, L.E. and R.S. Langer, Advances in tissue engineering of blood vessels and other tissues. *Transpl. Immunol.*, 1997. 5(4): p. 303-6.
[658] Kim, B.S., et al., Cyclic mechanical strain regulates the development of engineered smooth muscle tissue. *Nat. Biotechnol.*, 1999. 17(10): p. 979-83.
[659] Kobayashi, N., et al., Mechanical stress promotes the expression of smooth muscle-like properties in marrow stromal cells. *Exp. Hematol.*, 2004. 32(12): p. 1238-45.
[660] Kurpinski, K., et al., Regulation of vascular smooth muscle cells and mesenchymal stem cells by mechanical strain. *Mol. Cell Biomech.*, 2006. 3(1): p. 21-34.
[661] Weinberg, C.B. and E. Bell, A blood vessel model constructed from collagen and cultured vascular cells. *Science*, 1986. 231(4736): p. 397-400.
[662] Hoerstrup, S.P., et al., Tissue engineering of small caliber vascular grafts. *Eur. J. Cardiothorac. Surg.*, 2001. 20(1): p. 164-9.
[663] Hoerstrup, S.P., et al., Living, autologous pulmonary artery conduits tissue engineered from human umbilical cord cells. *Ann. Thorac. Surg.*, 2002. 74(1): p. 46-52; discussion 52.

In: Perspectives in Stem Cell Research
Editors: Brenda M. Davis and Christopher B. Halton
ISBN: 978-1-61122-985-1

Chapter V

NEURAL STEM CELLS AND TAURINE

Eulalia Bazán[1*], Antonio S. Herranz[1], Diana Reimers[1], Maria V.T. Lobo[1,2], Carolina Redondo[1], Miguel A. López-Toledano[1,3], Rafael Gonzalo-Gobernado[1], Maria J. Asensio[1] and Raquel Alonso[1]

[1]Servicio de Neurobiología-Investigación, Hospital Ramón y Cajal, Madrid and
[2]Departamento de Biología Celular y Genética, Universidad de Alcalá, Madrid, Spain
[3]Miguel A. López-Toledano present address: Department of Pathology, Columbia-Presbyterian Medical Center, Columbia University, 630w, 168th Street. New York, New York, 10032, USA

ABSTRACT

Taurine is a β-amino acid that serves important functions in mammalian brain development. However, no data are available about its distribution and possible roles in neural precursors from a non-retinal origin. Neural stem cells (NSC) with self-renewal and multilineage potential are an important tool to study the signals involved in the regulation of brain development. The aim of this study was to investigate the role played by taurine during the differentiation of NSC from fetal rat striatum. Taurine content was analyzed in the cultures by HPLC at different times post-plating. Between 2 and 24 hours taurine was detected at a basal value of 7 nmol/mg protein. As cells were maintained in culture, this value increased to reach 40 nmol/mg protein at 10 days post-plating. Taurine immunoreactivity was found in nestin, A2B5, β-tubulin III and O1 positive cells. The addition for 1 to 3 days of 2 mM taurine to recently seeded neurospheres increased its intracellular content by 28 fold, and high taurine levels were maintained even 7 days after taurine withdrawal. By contrast, cultures treated with 2 mM of the high-affinity taurine transporter inhibitor guanidinoethanesulfonic acid (GES) showed a sharp decrease in taurine content. When taurine was applied in combination with GES, taurine levels were significantly higher than those observed after GES treatment. Taurine treatment did not

[*] Corresponding author: Dr. Eulalia Bazán, Servico de Neurobiologia-Investigación, Hospital Ramón y Cajal, Carretera de Colmenar Km. 9,1,28034 Madrid, España. Phone: 34-913368384. Fax: 34-913369016. E-mail: eulalia.bazan@hrc.es

affect the relative amount of neurons and oligodendrocytes in the cultures, but promoted the differentiation of O1-positive cells that showed an increase in the length and number of their processes. We conclude that NSC develop specific taurine uptake mechanisms at early stages differentiation. Since taurine was not present in the feeding medium, we suggest that NSC and their progeny have the machinery for taurine synthesis. Present results also indicate that taurine might influence the development of NSC oligodendroglial progeny.

Keywords: neural stem cells, neurospheres, development, taurine, guanidine-oethanesulfonic acid, trophic factors

INTRODUCTION

Taurine (2-aminoethanesulfonic acid), an end-product of sulphur amino acid catabolism, is a β-amino acid found at high concentrations in several cell types (reviewed in: Huxtable, 1989, 1992; Sturman, 1993). Its zwitterionic nature, at physiological pH, gives high water solubility and low lipophilicity. Thus, the diffusion of taurine across cell membranes does not account for the intracellular levels of this amino acid, which are maintained high from biosynthesis and/or the specific uptake from the extracellular space (Huxtable, 1992). Because taurine does not incorporate into proteins, the greatest proportion of both extracellular and intracellular taurine is in the free form. Several functions have been proposed for this amino acid, such as osmoregulation, membrane stabilization, detoxification, antioxidation, modulation of ion flux, and as a neurotransmitter or neuromodulator and its roles in the control of synaptic transmission have been explored (Thurston et al., 1980; Solís et al., 1988, 1990; Huxtable, 1989, 1992; Galarreta et al., 1996; Schuller-Levis and Park, 2003). Immunohistochemical studies have clarified the cellular localization of taurine in the Central Nervous System (Ottersen et al,. 1985; Lake and Verdone-Smith, 1989; Lee et al. 1992; Nagelhus et al., 1993). It has been demonstrated that taurine is essential during retinal development in mammals and potentiates the production of rod photoreceptors by signaling through the glycine receptor GlyRα2 (Renteria et al., 2004; Young and Cepko, 2004). In addition, taurine is the most abundant neurotransmitter in the developing neocortex. During the development of the visual cortex and the cerebellum, it is required for normal ontogeny of neurons. Taurine depletion impairs the migration of cerebellar granule cells in co-cultures of dissociated cerebellum from neonatal mice and neuronal cells (Maar et al., 1995). Sustained taurine deficits during the prenatal and immediate postnatal period result in permanent abnormalities. Taurine-deficient cats have defects that include retinal degeneration, abnormalities of the brain cortex and delayed cerebellar granule cells migration and growth (Strurman et al., 1985; Palackal et al., 1986). All these observations support the notion that taurine is determinant for neural development. However, the moment in which taurine becomes essential for brain development has not been determined, since its possible roles in neural stem/progenitor cells biology is unknown, except for retinal precursor cells.

Neural stem cells are defined as clonogenic cells with self-renewal capacity and the ability to generate all neural lineages. Cells with these characteristics have been isolated from the embryonic and adult Central Nervous System. Under specific conditions, these cells proliferate in cultures as cell clusters called "neurospheres" and differentiate into neurons, glia, and non-neural cell types (reviewed in: Gage, 2000; Kennea and Mehmet, 2002; Bazan et al., 2004). NSC cultures represent a useful model for neurodevelopment studies. Different growth factors, cytokines, extracellular matrix proteins, and neurotransmitters have been implicated in the epigenetic regulation of proliferation and differentiation processes of these cells (Burrows et al., 1997; Arsenijevic and Weiss, 1998; Edlund and Jessell, 1999). Several studies have determined in vitro conditions for promoting the differentiation of NSC into specific cellular phenotypes (Daadi and Weiss, 1999; Reimers et al., 2001; Lopez-Toledano et al., 2004). Here we explore the possibility that taurine could influence the fate determination of neural progenitors in vitro.

Materials and Methods

Differentiation of EGF-Expanded Neural Stem Cells

Striatal primordia from E15 Sprage-Dawley rat embryos were dissected and mechanically dissociated. Cell suspensions were grown in a defined medium (DF12) composed of Dulbecco's modified Eagle's medium and Ham's F-12 (1:1), 2 mM L-glutamine, 1 mM sodium piruvate (all from Gibco BRL, Life Technologies Inc, Grand Island, New York), 0.6% glucose, 25 μg/ml insulin, 20 nM progesterone, 60 μM putrescine, and 30 nM sodium selenite (all from Sigma Chemical Co, St Louis, MO), 100 μg/ml human transferrin and 20 ng/ml human recombinant epidermal growth factor (EGF) (both from Boehringer Mannheim GmbH, Germany). The cells grew as floating neurospheres, and were passaged by mechanical dissociation every 2-3 days.

After a minimum of four passages, EGF-expanded NSC (EGF-NSC) were plated at a density of 20,000 to 30,000 cells/cm^2 on 15 μg/ml poly-l-ornithine (Sigma Chemical Co) coated glass coverslips (ø 12 mm) or plastic dishes (Ø 35 mm). Cultures were maintained in DF12 and 20 ng/ml EGF for 3 days and then switched to DF12 without EGF for longer culture periods (untreated group). At 2 hours post-plating, parallel cultures were treated with 2 mM taurine (TAU), or 2 mM GES (Toronto Research Chemicals Inc., Ontario, Canada), or both (TAU+GES). Immunocytochemical and biochemical analysis were performed at 1, 3, 4 and 10 days post plating (dpp).

Indirect Immunocytochemistry

Rabbit polyclonal antibodies and mouse monoclonal antibodies directed against neural antigens, taurine and taurine transporter (TauT) were used as primary antibodies for indirect immunocytochemistry. Polyclonal antibodies against taurine and TauT were purchased from Chemicon International (Temecula, CA) and GFAP from Dakopatts a/s, (Glostrup, Denmark). Monoclonal antibodies against β-tubulin III were obtained from Sigma Chemical Co. (St. Louis, MO), and anti-nestin (clone Rat 401) and anti-A2B5, O4 and O1 from Developmental Studies Hybridoma Bank (University of Iowa). Secondary antibodies raised in goat against rabbit and in sheep against mouse immunoglobulins, conjugated to lisamine rhodamine

(1:100) and fluorescein isothiocyanate (1:100), were purchased from Jackson Immunoresearch Laboratories Inc, (West Grove, PA), and Boehringer Mannheim GmbH, respectively.

For immunocytochemical studies cells were fixed with 4% paraformaldehyde for 10 min and immunostained for A2B5 (1:10), O4 (1:10), O1 (1:10), GFAP (1:500) and β-tubulin III (1:200). For taurine immunostaining, cells were fixed with 2% paraformaldehyde and 0.5% glutaraldehyde. Coverslips were mounted in a medium containing p-phenylenediamine and bisBenzimide (Hoechst 33342, Sigma Chemical Co).

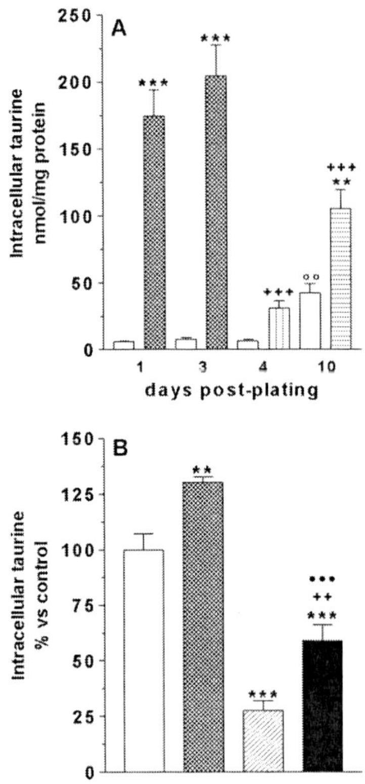

Figure 1. Taurine levels during the differentiation in vitro of neural stem cells. EGF-expanded neurospheres were plated on plastic dishes in DF12 and 20 ng/ml EGF. In A, 2 hours post-plating neurospheres were treated with vehicle (control) or 2 mM taurine (TAU). Three days later, the medium was switched to DF12 without EGF and cultures were maintained in the absence of any treatment for 1 or 7 additional days. The intracellular content of taurine was measured by HPLC at 1, 3, 4 or 10 days post-plating (dpp). Note the increase in intracellular taurine observed in control cultures at 10 dpp (A, white bars). The intracellular content of the amino acid was significantly increased in those cultures treated for 1 to 3 days with taurine (A, dot bars). Moreover, the intracellular taurine content remained higher than their respective controls after 1 (A, vertical lines bar) or 7 (A, horizontal lines bar) days of taurine withdrawal. In B, 2 hours post-plating neurospheres were treated with vehicle (control) (white bar), or 2 mM taurine (TAU) (dot bar), or 2 mM guanidinoethyl sulphonate (GES) (lined bar), or both (TAU+GES) (black bar) and the intracellular taurine content was measured 3 days later by HPLC. Note the decrease in the intracellular content of taurine observed in GES treated cultures (B, lined bar) and the inhibition in taurine uptake observed after 3 days of TAU+GES treatment (B, black bar). Results represent the mean ± ESM of 8 to 12 plates from 3 independent experiments. ** $p \leq 0.01$, *** $p \leq 0.001$ vs their respective controls. OO $p \leq 0.01$ vs control at 1 dpp. ++ $p \leq 0.01$, +++ $p \leq 0.001$ vs 3 dpp TAU treated cultures. ●●● $p \leq 0.001$ vs 3 dpp GES treated cultures.

Taurine Content Determination

Cells on plastic dishes were washed three times in 2 ml of PBS and scraped at 4 °C in 250 μl of 0.2 N perchloric acid - 0.2 mM EDTA - 0.5 mM sodium meta-bisulphite ($Na2S2O5$). Cell suspensions were sonicated three times for 15 sec and centrifuged at 7200 g x 5 min. The supernatants were frozen at -80 °C until they were analyzed. The pellets were used for protein evaluation. The samples were analyzed for taurine content using the reverse-phase high performance liquid chromatography (HPLC) procedure with O-phthaldialdehide (OPA) precolumn derivatization and fluorimetric detection. This method coincides essentially with that described by Jones and Stein (1981) except that 3-mercaptopropionic acid was used instead of 2-mercaptoethanol in the derivatization reaction. This change improved the sensitivity of the analysis as much as two-fold (Herranz et al., 1985).

Data Analysis and Cell Counting

Results are expressed as the mean ± SEM from 3 independent experiments done in triplicates or quadruplicates. Where indicated, data represent the mean ± SEM of several coverslips. In each coverslip stereological sampling of 25 visual fields (magnification of 200 or 400x) was performed under fluorescence microscopy. The number of cells was corrected for coverslip area. Statistical analyses were performed using Student's t test, or one way ANOVA followed by Bonferoni multiple comparison test and the difference was considered significant when $p \leq 0.05$.

RESULTS

EGF- Expanded Neural Stem Cells Synthesize Taurine During Their Differentiation In Vitro

EGF-expanded neurospheres were seeded onto adherent substrate and treated with EGF during the first 3 days in culture, in order to enhance the expansion of precursor cells. After this period the mitogen was withdrawn, and cells grew in defined medium. Between 2 hours and 3 dpp cultures comprised mainly nestin-positive undifferentiated precursors (Lobo et al., 2003). As cells are maintained in culture, there is a gradual loss of nestin expression and an increase in the relative content of neurons, oligodendrocytes and astrocytes, as described previously (Bazan et al. 1998; Reimers et al. 2001).

The intracellular content of taurine was analyzed by HPLC at different times post-plating. At 1 dpp, taurine was detectable at a basal value of 7 nmol/mg protein. This basal value was maintained up to day 4 post-plating, but as cells were further maintained in culture, the intracellular taurine content increased to reach an average value of 40 nmol/mg protein at 10 dpp (Fig. 1A).

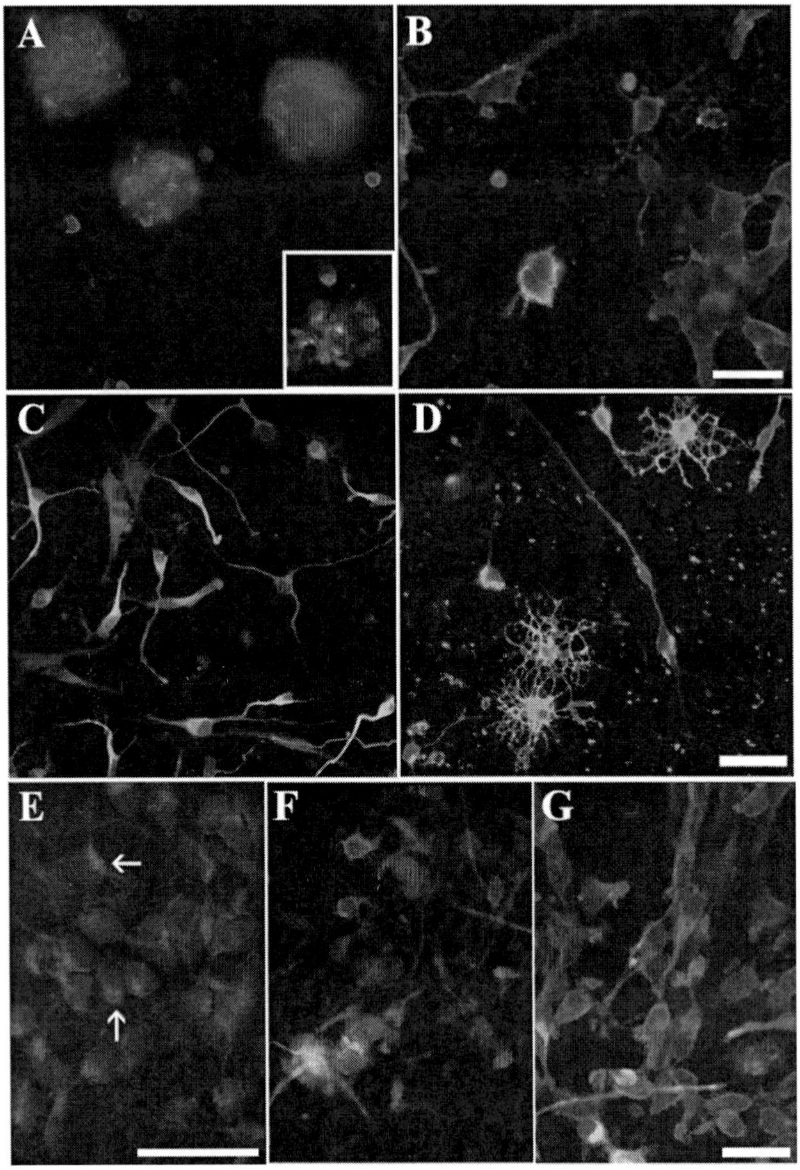

Figure 2.- Taurine immunoreactivity during the differentiation in vitro of neural stem cells. EGF-expanded neurospheres were plated on poly-l-ornithine coated coverslips in DF12 and 20 ng/ml EGF for 3 days. Then, the medium was switched to DF12 without EGF and cultures were maintained for 3 additional days. Double immunostaining for taurine (A-D and F-G, red) and neural antigens was performed at different times post-plating. Taurine-positive cells were observed in recently seeded neurospheres (A, red). Inside the neurospheres some nestin-positive cells (A, green) co-expressed taurine, but taurine and nestin compartments were different (A, insert). At 3 days post-plating (dpp), some A2B5-positive progenitors (B, green) were taurine immuno-positive (B, yellow). At 6 dpp, a subset of β tubulin III-positive (C, green) and O1-positive (D, green) cells co-expressed taurine (C and D, yellow). At 1dpp, EGF-expanded neural stem cells showed taurine transporter immunoreactivity (E, arrows). In F and G, nestin (green) and taurine (red) immunolabeling was analyzed in cultures treated with vehicle (F) or 2 mM taurine (G) for 24 hours. Note the increase in taurine immunoreactivity promoted by the treatment with the amino acid (G, red). Scale bars, 30 μm.

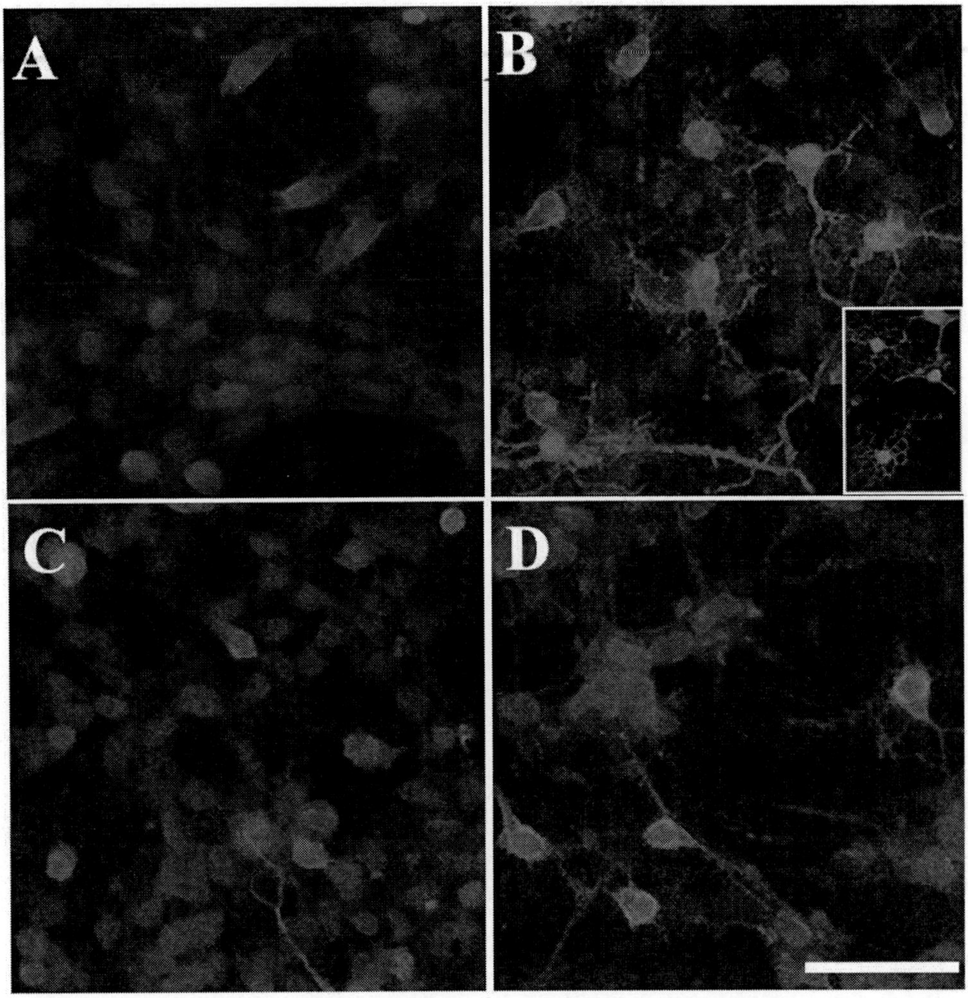

Figure 3.- Neural stem cells express functional taurine transporter in vitro. EGF-expanded neurospheres were plated on poly-l-ornithine coated coverslips in DF12 and 20 ng/ml EGF. At 2 hours post-plating, cultures were treated with vehicle (A), or 2 mM taurine (TAU) (B), or 2 mM guanidinoethyl sulphonate (GES) (C), or both (TAU+GES) (D). Three days later, cultures were fixed and taurine immunoreactivy was analyzed. Taurine imunolabeling was increased in those cultures treated with the amino acid (B, red). Note the increase in taurine immunoreactivity in the cell processes (B, insert). By contrast, the treatment with GES decreased the number of taurine-positive cells (C, red) as compared with vehicle (A) or TAU treated cultures (B). When taurine was applied in the presence of GES (D, red), taurine immunopositivity was lower than in TAU treated cultures. In blue, cell nuclei labeled with Hoechst. Scale bar, 50 μm.

When the extracellular content of taurine was analyzed, levels from 2 to 5 nmol/plate were detected between 1 to 10 dpp (data not shown). To determine the cell source for taurine in the cultures double-immunostaning studies were performed using specific antibodies directed against neural antigens and taurine. In recently seeded neurospheres (2 hours post-plating), some nestin-positive/taurine-positive cells were observed (Fig. 2A). Between 1 and 3 dpp taurine was detected in nestin-positive and A2B5-positive progenitors (Fig. 2B, F). After 5 dpp, taurine was observed in neurons (Fig. 2C) and oligodendrocytes (Fig. 2D). However,

GFAP-positive cells present in the cultures were immunonegative for taurine at any time analyzed (Fig. 4B).

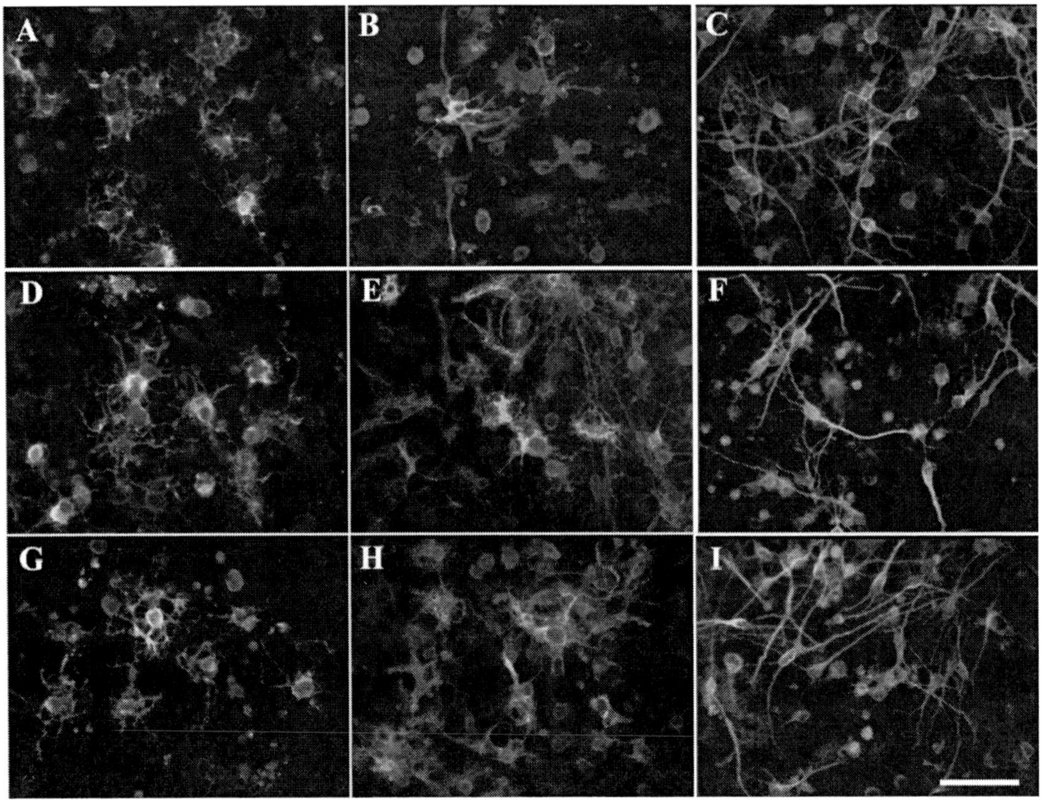

Figure 4.- Effects of taurine and GES treatment in EGF-expanded neural stem cells progeny. At 2 hours post-plating, cultures were treated with vehicle (A, B, C), or 2 mM taurine (D, E, F), or 2 mM guanidinoethyl sulphonate (GES) (G, H, I). Three days later, the medium was switched to DF12 without EGF and cultures were maintained in the absence of any treatment for 7 additional days and double immunostaining analysis for taurine (A-I, red) and O1 (A, D, G, green), GFAP (B, E, H, green) and β tubulin III (C, F, I, green) was performed. Under all experimental conditions, taurine immunoreactivity was observed in O1-positive (A, D, G, yellow) and β tubulin III-positive cells (C, F, I, yellow) while GFAP-positive cells did not co labeled with taurine (B, E, H). Note that after 7 days of taurine withdrawal oligodendrocytes show a more mature aspect with an increase in their size, and in the length and number of their cellular processes (D). Scale bar, 50 μm.

EGF-Expanded Neural Stem Cells Express Functional Taurine Transporter During Their Differentiation In Vitro

During the expansive phase (2 hours to 3 dpp), cultures of EGF-NSC showed TauT immunoreactivity (Fig. 2E). To determine whether the addition of exogenous taurine in the culture medium can change its intracellular content, 2 mM taurine was added for 3 days and the cultures were analyzed after 1 and 3 days of treatment, and 1 or 7 days after taurine withdrawal. Taurine immunoreactivity was increased in the cultures after 1or 3 days of treatment with the amino acid (Fig. 2G and Fig. 3B). These results were confirmed when the intracellular taurine content was measured by HPLC (Fig. 1A). One or 7 days after taurine withdrawal, the number of taurine-positive cells in the cultures remained 1.3 to 1.6 fold above controls. At these later experimental times, the intracellular taurine content was lower than during the treatment period (0-3 days), but remained higher than their respective controls (Fig. 1A) confirming the immunocytochemical data. To asses if a mature active taurine transport mechanism is present in these cells, some cultures were treated for the first 3 days with the inhibitor of taurine transporter GES (2 mM) in the absence or presence of 2 mM taurine. The intracellular taurine content was reduced in the cultures after 3 days of GES treatment (Fig. 1B). Taurine-positive cells were also reduced after 3 days of treatment with the inhibitor (Fig. 3C). When taurine was added to EGF-NSC cultures in combination with GES, taurine content was higher than with GES alone, but lower than in control or taurine treated cells (Fig. 1B). Similarly, taurine immunoreactivity was increased in TAU+GES treated cultures as compared with those cultures treated with GES for 3 days (Fig. 3C, D).

Role Of Taurine In The Maturation Of Oligodendrocytes Derived From EGF-Neural Stem Cells

To determine if changes in the intracellular levels of taurine may affect the in vitro differentiation of EGF-NSC, cultures were treated with taurine or GES for 3 days. Double-immunostaning studies were performed 7 days later using specific antibodies directed against neural antigens and taurine. Under all experimental conditions, taurine immunoreactivity was observed in O1-positive (Fig. 4A, D, G) and β tubulin III-positive cells (Fig. 4C, F, I), while no GFAP-positive cells co-labeled with taurine in the cultures (Fig. 4B, E, H). Although no changes in the relative amount of β tubulin III-positive and O1-positive cells were observed (data not shown), the morphology of oligodendrocytes changed in those cultures treated with taurine showing a more mature aspect, with an increase in their size and in the length and number of their cellular processes (Fig. 4D). Interestingly, our immunocytochemical studies performed at 3 dpp showed intense taurine immunoreactivity in cells with the morphology of oligodendrocytes after taurine treatment (Fig. 3B, insert), and this effect was partially prevented by the concomitant treatment with GES (Fig. 3D).

Discussion

Taurine is one of the most abundant amino acid in the brain of mammals, where it is thought to play important roles during development (reviewed in: Sturman, 1993). However, poorly is known about the source of endogenous derived taurine and its transport during the development of neural progenitors. Here we show that taurine can be detected in neural progenitor cells and that active transport mechanisms and biosynthesis of taurine must exist in these cells in vitro. We also show that taurine promotes the maturation of the oligodendrocytes derived from EGF-NSC.

Previously, we reported that recently seeded neurospheres contain detectable levels of taurine (Bazán et al., 1996). Present results show that EGF-NSC maintain relatively high levels of the amino acid during their in vitro differentiation. These result are in agreement with other studies that suggest that taurine is necessary for growth and migration of neural precursors (Maar et al., 1995; Benitez-Diaz e al., 2003). In fact, high levels of taurine were detected in the mouse cerebral cortex during the proliferative stage of neurogenesis, consistent with a possible role as a trophic factor of this amino acid during cortical development. Besides, a protective role for taurine against postnatal excitatory neurotoxicity has been postulated (Benitez-Diaz et al., 2003). Interestingly, the highest levels of intracellular taurine were observed at 10 dpp, a time point when high levels of glutamate are detected in the cultures (Bazan et al., 1996, 1998), as well as the maximal number of neurons and glial cells (Reimers et al., 2001).

In the adult brain, both a glial and a neuronal origin for taurine has been postulated (Dominy et al., 2004). In EGF-NSC, taurine was immunodetected in nestin-positive and A2B5-positive progenitor cells. Because taurine was absent in the feeding medium, the presence of its biosynthetic machinery in neural precursors can be concluded. In our cultures, taurine immunoreactivity was also detected in β tubulin III-positive and O1-positive cells, indicating that neurons and oligodendrocytes derived from these cells are able to synthesize the amino acid. Co- localization of taurine and cysteine sulfinate decarboxylase (CSD), the enzyme that mediates the synthesis of hypotaurine from cysteine, has been described in Purkinje cerebellar neurons (Magnusson et al., 1988). Moreover, in the cerebellum CDS-positive cells were found in the white matter that were typically arranged in rows like oligodendrocytes (Almarghini et al., 1991). Other studies suggest that astrocytes are capable of taurine synthesis (Tappaz et al., 1994; Reymond et al., 1996; Brand et al., 1998). Astrocytes derived from EGF-NSC did not co-labeled with taurine at any time analyzed. The lack of taurine detection could be explained if astrocytes derived from EGF-NSC are only a source for hypotaurine, or if taurine levels in these cells are so low that could not be detected by immunocytochemistry. In addition, it is possible that only mature astrocytes will develop the machinery needed to synthesize hypotaurine and taurine. The use of antibodies to CSD, when commercially available, will be of great value to clarify these observations.

The intracellular taurine concentration is controlled by taurine biosynthetic enzymes and taurine transporters (reviewed in: Lambert, 2004; Tapaz, 2004). Intracellular accumulation of taurine was observed when the amino acid was added to recently seeded EGF-expanded neurospheres indicating that taurine transport mechanisms are present in these cells. High-affinity taurine transportes have been described in different brain areas (Smith et al., 1992; Pow et al., 2002). In EGF-NSC, TauT immunoreactivity was observed at early stages of their differentiation in vitro, and the intracellular taurine content was significantly decreased after the chronic administration of the competitive inhibitor of high-affinity taurine transporter GES (Huxtable et al., 1979; Huxtable and Lippincott, 1981). Moreover, taurine uptake was partially inhibited by the inhibitor. Altogether these results indicate that EGF-NSC must express a high-affinity taurine transporter. Other studies reported that 100 μM GES is sufficient for a 70% inhibition of the TauT activity in cultures of Bergmann glial cells (Barakat et al., 2002) and 2mM GES completely inhibit the taurine transport in astrocytes and neurons from the mouse cerebellum (Moran and Pasantes-Morales, 1991). We used 2 mM GES, so a nearly complete inhibition of TauT was expected. However, as we already mentioned, taurine uptake was significantly reduced but not completely abolished by GES. These results suggest that additional taurine transport mechanisms might be present in the cultures. Taurine can activate equally TauT and GABA transporter (GABAT) but high concentrations (1.3 to 2.9 mM) are required for 50% of taurine uptake via GABAT (Sivakami et al., 1992; Liu et al., 1993; Borden., 1996; Seergeva et al., 2003). Since we use taurine at a concentration of 2 mM, a GABAT mediated transport can not be excluded. Taurine can be also transported by low-affinity transport systems in the brain and retina (Saransaari and Oja, 1992, Sanchez-Olea et al., 1993, Martin del Rio and Solis, 1998, Militante and Lombardini, 1999). It is plausible that a low-affinity transport system might serve to accumulate taurine in EGF-NSC. In the future, the presence and identity of this low-affinity transport system will be studied.

Taurine uptake has been identified in mature neurons and glial cells including oligodendrocytes (Reynolds and Herschkowithz 1986; Walz and Allen, 1987; Della Corte et al., 1990; Kritzer et al., 1992; Pow et al., 2002; Walz, 2002). According to our immunocytochemical results, nestin-positive neural precursors also have the ability to accumulate taurine when the amino acid was added to the culture medium. On the other hand, high levels of the amino acid were observed in the neuronal and oligodendroglial progeny after taurine treatment. Because no mature neurons and oligodendrocytes are present in the cultures at the time point when taurine is applied, we may argue that taurine transport mechanisms must be expressed by their progenitors. It is noteworthy that changes in the intracellular taurine content increase the size of the oligodendrocytes derived from EGF-NSC and the length and number of their cellular processes. Although taurine stimulates neurite outgrowth in neurons (Chen et al., 1998; Lima, 1999), to our knowledge this is the first study showing a trophic effect of taurine in oligodendrocytes. The fact that these effects were partially prevented by the concomitant treatment of taurine with GES (Fig. 3D) suggest that the high-affinity taurine transporter mediates, at least in part, this action of the amino acid. On the other hand, taurine could stimulate the differentiation of oligodendrocytes by acting on Glycine receptors (GlyRs). Taurine is a ligand of GABA receptors (GABAR) and GlyRs (Haas and Hosli, 1973; Hussy et al., 1997; Sergeeva and Haas, 2001; Barakat et al., 2002), and GlyRs have been proposed as mediators for the functions of taurine during brain development (Flint et al., 1998). GlyRs have been described in cultured oligodendrocyte progenitors (Belachew et al., 1998) and high levels of Glycine were detected in EGF-NSC during their differentiation in vitro (Bazan et al., 1996, 1998). Moreover, similarly than taurine GES is able to interact with GlyRs and $GABA_AR$ in cultures of neurons (Sergeeva et al., 2002; Herranz et al., 1990).

We conclude that NSC develop specific taurine uptake mechanisms at early stages of their differentiation in vitro. Moreover, NSC and their neuronal and oligodendroglial progeny have the machinery needed for taurine synthesis. The present study also indicates that taurine probably acts as a trophic factor on oligodendrocytes derived from NSC. While these findings suggest a role of taurine on the development of NSC, further experiments are needed to better understand the functions of this factor.

ACKNOWLEDGMENTS

This work was supported by Fondo de Investigaciones Sanitarias (FIS 97/0269 and FIS 02/0853). and Raquel Alonso by Fundación MAPFRE Medicina. We are grateful to Dr. Rafael Martín del Río (Servicio de Neurolobiología-Invetigación, Hospital Ramón y Cajal, Madrid, Spain) for comments and critical reading of this manuscript.

REFERENCES

Almarghini K, Remy A, Tappaz M. *Immunocytochemistry of the taurine biosynthesis enzyme, cysteine sulfinate decarboxylase, in the cerebellum: evidence for a glial localization.*

Arsenijevic Y, Weiss S. Insulin-like growth factor-I is a differentiation factor for postmitotic CNS stem cell-derived neuronal precursors: distinct actions from those of brain-derived neurotrophic factor. *J Neurosci.* 1998, 18:2118-2128.

Barakat L, Wang D, Bordey A. Carrier-mediated uptake and release of taurine from Bergmann glia in rat cerebellar slices. *J Physiol.* 2002, 541:753-67.

Bazan E, Alonso FJ, Redondo C et al. In vitro and in vivo characterization of neural stem cells. *Histol Histopathol.* 2004, 19:1261-75.

Bazan E, Lopez-Toledano MA, Mena MA, Martín del Rio R, Paino CL and Herranz A S. Endogenous Amino Acid Profile During In Vitro Differentiation of Neural Stem Cells. *In Fiskum G, ed. Neurodegenerative Diseases. New York, Plenum Press, 1996, 225-234.*

Bazan E, Lopez-Toledano MA, Redondo C, Alcazar A, Paino CL, Herranz AS. Characterization of rat neural stem cells from embryonic striatum and mesencephalon during in vitro differentiation. In Castellano B, González B, Nieto-Sampedro M, eds. *Understanding Glial Cells*. Dordrecht, Kluwer Academic Publishers, 1998, 133-147.

Belachew S, Rogister B, Rigo JM, Malgrange B, Mazy-Servais C, Xhauflaire G, Coucke P, Moonen G. Cultured oligodendrocyte progenitors derived from cerebral cortex express a glycine receptor which is pharmacologically distinct from the neuronal isoform. *Eur J Neurosci.* 1998; 10:3556-64.

Benitez-Diaz P, Miranda-Contreras L, Mendoza-Briceno RV, Pena-Contreras Z, Palacios-Pru E. Prenatal and postnatal contents of amino acid neurotransmitters in mouse parietal cortex. *Dev Neurosci.* 2003, 25:366-374.

Borden LA. GABA transporter heterogeneity: pharmacology and cellular localization. *Neurochem Int.* 1996, 29:335-356.

Brand A, Leibfritz D, Hamprecht B, Dringen R. Metabolism of cysteine in astroglial cells: synthesis of hypotaurine and taurine. *J Neurochem.* 1998, 71:827-32.

Burrows RC, Wancio D, Levitt P, Lillien L. Response diversity and the timing of progenitor cell maturation are regulated by developmental changes in EGFR expression in the cortex. *Neuron* 1997, 19:251-267.

Chen XC, Pan ZL, Liu DS, Han X. Effect of taurine on human fetal neuron cells: proliferation and differentiation. *Adv Exp Med Biol.* 1998; 442:397-403.

Daadi MM, Weiss S. Generation of tyrosine hydroxylase-producing neurons from precursors of the embryonic and adult forebrain. *J Neurosci.* 1999, 19:4484-4497.

Della Corte L, Bolam JP, Clarke DJ, Parry DM, Smith AD. Sites of [3H]taurine Uptake in the Rat Substantia Nigra in Relation to the Release of Taurine from the Striatonigral Pathway. *Eur J Neurosci.* 1990, 2:50-61.

Dominy J, Eller S, Dawson R Jr. Building biosynthetic schools: reviewing compartmentation of CNS taurine synthesis. *Neurochem Res.* 2004, 29:97-103.

Edlund T, Jessell TM. Progression from extrinsic to intrinsic signaling in cell fate specification: a view from the nervous system. *Cell* 1999, 96:211-224.

Flint AC, Liu X, Kriegstein AR. Nonsynaptic glycine receptor activation during early neocortical development. *Neuron* 1998, 20: 43-53.

Gage. Mammalian neural stem cells. *Science* 2000; 287:1433-8.

Galarreta M, Bustamante J, Martin del Rio R, Solis JM. Taurine induces a long-lasting increase of synaptic efficacy and axon excitability in the hippocampus. *J Neurosci.* 1996, 16: 92-102.

Haas HL, Hosli L. The depression of brain stem neurones by taurine and its interaction with strychnine and bicuculline. *Brain Res.* 1973, 52:399-402.

Herranz , A.S., Cristín, J. L., Lerma, J. and Martín del Rio, R.. Incremento de sensibilidad en los análisis por CLAE de los OPA-amioácidos usando como reactivo de derivación el ácido 3-mercapto-propiónico. Resúmenes de la Reunión Científica anual del grupo de Cromatografía y Tecnicas afines, *RSEQ.* 1985, 58-59.

Herranz AS, Solis JM, Herreras O, Menendez N, Ambrosio E, Orensanz LM, Martin del Rio R. The epileptogenic action of the taurine analogue guanidinoethane sulfonate may be caused by a blockade of GABA receptors. *J Neurosci Res.* 1990, 26:98-104.

Hussy N, Deleuze C, Pantaloni A, Desarmenien MG, Moos F. Agonist action of taurine on glycine receptors in rat supraoptic magnocellular neurones: possible role in osmoregulation. *J Physiol.* 1997, 502:609-621.

Huxtable RJ. Taurine in the central nervous system and the mammalian actions of taurine. *Prog Neurobiol.* 1989, 32:471-533.

Huxtable RJ. Physiological actions of taurine. *Physiol Rev.* 1992, 72:101-163.

Huxtable RJ, Laird HE, Lippincott SE. The transport of taurine in the heart and the rapid depletion of tissue taurine content by guanidinoethyl sulfonate. *J Pharmacol Exp Ther.* 1979; 211:465-71.

Huxtable RJ, Lippincott SE. Sources and turnover rates of taurine in newborn, weanling, and mature rats. *Adv Exp Med Biol.* 1981;139:23-45.

Jones B N, Stein S. Amino acid analysis and enzymatic sequence determination of peptides by an improved O-phthaldialdehyde precolumn lavelling procedure. *J. Liquid Chromatogr.* 1981, 4: 565-586.

Kennea NL, Mehmet H. Neural stem cells. *J Pathol.* 2002 Jul;197(4):536-50.

Kritzer MF, Cowey A, Ottersen OP, Streit P, Somogyi P. Immunoreactivity for Taurine Characterizes Subsets of Glia, GABAergic and non-GABAergic Neurons in the Neo- and Archicortex of the Rat, Cat and Rhesus Monkey: Comparison with Immunoreactivity for Homocysteic Acid. *Eur J Neurosci.* 1992; 4:251-270.

Lake N, Verdone-Smith C. Immunocytochemical localization of taurine in the mammalian retina. *Curr Eye Res.* 1989, 8:163-173.

Lambert IH. Regulation of the cellular content of the organic osmolyte taurine in mammalian cells. *Neurochem Res.* 2004; 29:27-63.

Lee IS, Renno WM, Beitz AJ. A quantitative light and electron microscopic analysis of taurine-like immunoreactivity in the dorsal horn of the rat spinal cord. *J Comp Neurol.* 1992, 321:65-82.

Lima L. Taurine and its trophic effects in the retina. *Neurochem Res.* 1999; 24:1333-8.

Liu QR, Lopez-Corcuera B, Mandiyan S, Nelson H, Nelson N.Molecular characterization of four pharmacologically distinct gamma-aminobutyric acid transporters in mouse brain. *J Biol Chem.* 1993, 268:2106-2112.

Lobo MV, Alonso FJ, Redondo C, Lopez-Toledano MA, Caso E, Herranz AS, Paino CL, Reimers D, Bazan E. Cellular characterization of epidermal growth factor-expanded free-floating neurospheres. *J Histochem Cytochem.* 2003, 51: 89-103.

Lopez-Toledano MA, Redondo C, Lobo MV, Reimers D, Herranz AS, Paino CL, Bazan E.Tyrosine hydroxylase induction by basic fibroblast growth factor and cyclic AMP analogs in striatal neural stem cells: role of ERK1/ERK2 mitogen-activated protein kinase and protein kinase C. *J Histochem Cytochem.* 2004, 52:1177-1189.

Maar T, Moran J, Schousboe A, Pasantes-Morales H. Taurine deficiency in dissociated mouse cerebellar cultures affects neuronal migration. *Int J Dev Neurosci.* 1995, 13:491-502

Magnusson KR, Madl JE, Clements JR, Wu JY, Larson, Beitz AJ. Colocalization of taurine- and cysteine sulfinic acid decarboxylase-like immunoreactivity in the cerebellum of the rat with monoclonal antibodies against taurine. *J Neurosci.* 1988, 8:4551-4564.

Martin del Rio R, Solis JM. The anion-exchanger AE1 is a diffusion pathway for taurine transport in rat erythrocytes. *Adv Exp Med Biol.* 1998; 442:255-60.

Militante JD, Lombardini JB. Taurine uptake activity in the rat retina: protein kinase C-independent inhibition by chelerythrine. *Brain Res.* 1999; 818:368-74.

Moran J, Pasantes-Morales H. Taurine-deficient cultured cerebellar astrocytes and granule neurons obtained by treatment with guanidinoethane sulfonate. *J Neurosci Res.* 1991, 29:533-537.

Nagelhus EA, Lehmann A, Ottersen OP.Neuronal-glial exchange of taurine during hypo-osmotic stress: a combined immunocytochemical and biochemical analysis in rat cerebellar cortex. *Neuroscience* 1993, 54:615-631.

Ottersen OP, Madsen S, Meldrum BS, Storm-Mathisen J. Taurine in the hippocampal formation of the Senegalese baboon, Papio papio: an immunocytochemical study with an antiserum against conjugated taurine. *Exp Brain Res.* 1985, 59:457-462.

Palackal T, Moretz R, Wisniewski H, Sturman J. Abnormal visual cortex development in the kitten associated with maternal dietary taurine deprivation. *J Neurosci Res.* 1986, 15:223-239.

Pow DV, Sullivan R, Reye P, Hermanussen S. Localization of taurine transporters, taurine, and (3)H taurine accumulation in the rat retina, pituitary, and brain. *Glia.* 2002, 37:153-168.

Reimers D, Lopez-Toledano MA, Mason I, Cuevas P, Redondo C, Herranz AS, Lobo MV, Bazan E. Developmental expression of fibroblast growth factor (FGF) receptors in neural stem cell progeny. Modulation of neuronal and glial lineages by basic FGF treatment. *Neurol Res.* 2001, 23:612-621.

Renteria RC, Johnson J, Copenhagen DR. Need rods? Get glycine receptors and taurine. *Neuron* 2004, 41:839-41.

Reymond I; Almarghini K, Tappaz M. Immunocytochemical localization of cysteine sulfinate decarboxylase in astrocytes in the cerebellum and hippocampus: a quantitative double immunofluorescence study with glial fibrillary acidic protein and S-100 protein. *Neuroscience* 1996, 75:619-33.

Reynolds R, Herschkowitz N. Selective uptake of neuroactive amino acids by both oligodendrocytes and astrocytes in primary dissociated culture: a possible role for oligodendrocytes in neurotransmitter metabolism. *Brain Res.* 1986, 371:253-66.

Sanchez-Olea R, Pena C, Moran J, Pasantes-Morales H. Inhibition of volume regulation and efflux of osmoregulatory amino acids by blockers of Cl- transport in cultured astrocytes. *Neurosci Lett.* 1993, 156:141-144.

Saransaari P, Oja SS. Taurine transport in the mouse cerebral cortex during development and ageing. *Adv Exp Med Biol.* 1992;315:215-20.

Schuller-Levis GB, Park E. Taurine: new implications for an old amino acid. *FEMS Microbiol Lett.* 2003;226:195-202.

Sergeeva OA, Chepkova AN, Doreulee N, Eriksson KS, Poelchen W, Monnighoff I, Heller-Stilb B, Warskulat U, Haussinger D, Haas HL. Taurine-induced long-lasting enhancement of synaptic transmission in mice: role of transporters. *J Physiol.* 2003, 550:911-919.

Sergeeva OA, Chepkova AN, Haas HL.Guanidinoethyl sulphonate is a glycine receptor antagonist in striatum. *Br J Pharmacol.* 2002, 137:855-60.

Sergeeva OA, Haas HL. Expression and function of glycine receptors in striatal cholinergic interneurons from rat and mouse. *Neuroscience* 2001, 104:1043-1055.

Sivakami S, Ganapathy V, Leibach FH, Miyamoto Y. The gamma-aminobutyric acid transporter and its interaction with taurine in the apical membrane of the bovine retinal pigment epithelium. *Biochem J.* 1992, 283:391-397.

Smith KE, Borden LA, Wang CH, Hartig PR, Branchek TA, Weinshank RL. Cloning and expression of a high affinity taurine transporter from rat brain. *Mol Pharmacol.* 1992, 42:563-569.

Solis JM, Herranz AS, Herreras O, Lerma J, Martin del Rio R. Does taurine act as an osmoregulatory substance in the rat brain? *Neurosci Lett.* 1988, 91:53-58.

Solis JM, Herranz AS, Herreras O, Menendez N, del Rio RM. Weak organic acids induce taurine release through an osmotic-sensitive process in in vivo rat hippocampus. *J Neurosci Res.* 1990, 26:159-167.

Sturman J A. Taurine in development. *Physiol Rev.* 1993, 73:119-47.

Sturman JA, Moretz RC, French JH, Wisniewski HM. Taurine deficiency in the developing cat: persistence of the cerebellar external granule cell layer. *J Neurosci Res.* 1985; 13:405-416.

Tappaz M, Almarghini K, Do K. Cysteine sulfinate decarboxylase in brain: identification, characterization and immunocytochemical location in astrocytes. *Adv Exp Med Biol.* 1994, 359:257-268.

Tappaz ML. Taurine biosynthetic enzymes and taurine transporter: molecular identification and regulations. *Neurochem Res.* 2004;29:83-96.

Thurston JH, Hauhart RE, Dirgo JA. Taurine: a role in osmotic regulation of mammalian brain and possible clinical significance. *Life Sci.* 1980, 26:1561-1568.

Young, TL, Cepko CL. A role for ligand-gated ion channels in rod photoreceptor development. *Neuron* 2004, 41:867-879.

Walz W. Chloride/anion channels in glial cell membranes. Glia. 2002; 40:1-10.

Walz W, Allen AF. Evaluation of the osmoregulatory function of taurine in brain cells. *Exp Brain Res.* 1987; 68:290-8.

In: Perspectives in Stem Cell Research ISBN: 978-1-61122-985-1
Editors: Brenda M. Davis and Christopher B. Halton

Chapter VI

CIRCULATING ENDOTHELIAL PROGENITOR CELLS: RELEVANT IN PHYSIOPATHOLOGY, A PROMISE FOR CLINICAL APPLICATIONS, AND YET SO DIFFICULT TO BE CHARACTERIZED

***Margherita Massa*[1,*], *Rita Campanelli*[2] *and Vittorio Rosti*[2]**
[1]Biotechnology Laboratory, [2]Organ Transplantation Laboratory, Istituto di Ricovero e Cura a Carattere Scientifico (IRCCS) Policlinico San Matteo, Pavia, Italy.

ABSTRACT

The recent identification of endothelial progenitor cells (EPCs) in the peripheral blood of adult individuals has highlighted the possibility that vasculogenesis can take place in the postnatal life. It has been reported that circulating EPCs can be recruited and incorporated into sites of active neovascularization but they can also play a role in replacing lost endothelial cells on the vessel wall mediating a mechanism of maintenance of the normal vascular homeostasis. An accurate and unique phenotypical and functional characterization of circulating EPC subsets is still matter of debate; infact, neither a precise and unique panel of cell surface markers nor universally accepted protocols are available up to now for their in vitro growth.

Methods for the identification and characterization of circulating endothelial cells able to participate to postnatal vasculogenesis and endothelial repair will be part of our review, that will be focused mainly on physiological and pathological conditions characterized by a spontaneous increase of the number of circulating EPCs. The possible role of a number of soluble factors able to induce the mobilization of EPCs from the bone marrow into the peripheral blood will be also discussed.

Keywords: Endothelial progenitor cells, mobilization, vascular repair

* Correspondence concerning this article should be addressed to Dr. Margherita Massa, IRCCS Policlinico San Matteo, Laboratorio Clinica Pediatrica, 19, P.le Golgi; 27100 Pavia, Italy. Fax: +39 0382 527976; telephone: +39 0382 502703; e-mail: m.massa@smatteo.pv.it.

INTRODUCTION

The first evidence that human adult circulating cells contain elements able to give rise to colonies of cells with an endothelial-like phenotype *in vitro*, and to incorporate into new vessels *in vivo* was reported in 1997 by Asahara and coll. in a seminal paper published in Science [1]. As a matter of fact, the presence of cells circulating in the peripheral blood with an endothelial-like phenotype was already known; however, these cells were shown to be mature, terminally differentiated endothelial cells, which are shed off from the vessel wall possibly because of senescence and/or following vessel wall injuries [2,3,4,5]. On the contrary, the cell population identified by Asahara and coll showed features that are typical of progenitor cells, namely the capability to proliferate, to form colonies of differentiated endothelial cells in vitro, and to migrate to sites of active vasculogenesis in vivo. These cells were referred to as circulating endothelial progenitor cells (EPCs) in order to distinguish them from their mature counterpart (circulating mature endothelial cells, ECs) and their importance was soon highlighted by several experiments which confirmed their involvement in neoangiogenetic processes associated with limb ischemia, myocardial infarction, atherosclerosis, wound healing, retinal neovascularization, and a possible use for therapeutic strategies [6,7].

This review will focus on some aspects of EPCs, by summarizing how they can be identified and enumerated in the peripheral blood (PB) of adult individuals and by discussing their involvement in human adult vessel wall homeostasis and in different pathological conditions. Finally, attention will be paid to the possible therapeutic role of these EPCs.

The existence of cells with the potential of proliferation and differentiation into mature endothelial cells was believed to pertain only to the embryonic development where the differentiation of mesodermal cells to angioblasts and subsequently to maturing endothelial cells is well known [8]. This principle was challenged by the experiments of Asahara and coll which showed that human adult circulating $CD34^+$ cells can differentiate into cells expressing some endothelial markers in vitro and have the functional capability to partecipate to neovessel formation at sites of ischemia in a murine model [1]. Following this report many efforts have been made in order to better identify and enumerate these cells, to understand their origin and to define "standard" conditions for their in vitro growth and differentiation (in an attempt similar to what has been done in the last 30 years with hematopoietic progenitor cells). This task quickly revealed to be quite hard because it emerged soon that an unique phenotypic marker for the EPCs able to differentiate them from mature endothelial cells and from other type of hematopoietic progenitor cells (HPCs) did not exist [6]. In addition, also from a functional point of view, it became evident that different culture conditions were able to allow the in vitro growth of different types of EPCs. Last but not least, things were further complicated by the low frequency of these cells in the human adult PB and bone marrow (BM).

PHENOTYPIC CHARACTERIZATION OF EPC

Often, EPCs have been phenotipically characterized by the presence on their membrane of the CD34 antigen and of the type 2 receptor of the vascular endothelial growth factor

(VEGFR-2) [1]. However, this couple of markers does not identify exclusively EPCs because they are also expressed by at least some mature ECs [9] and HPCs [10]. In 2000 Peichev and coll convincingly showed that EPCs, but not mature ECs, did express the early hematopoietic antigen CD133, thus suggesting that EPC should be regarded as a cell co-expressing the CD34 and the CD133 antigens, and the VEGFR-2, and that such kind of cell can be identified by flow cytometry at very low frequency in the adult PB, and at a higher frequency in the adult BM, adult mobilized PB, and umbilical cord blood [11]. In the same year, Gehling and coll confirmed at thc functional level the importance of CD133 as a marker of EPCs by showing that purified $CD133^+$ cells were able to differentiate into endothelial cells in vitro [12]. Things however, turned out to be more complex because it was suggested [11,12] that this $CD34^+CD133^+VEGFR\text{-}2^+$ EPC could rather represent a multipotent progenitor cell capable of differentiating towards both the hematopoietic and the endothelial lineage, called hemangioblast [13,14,15,16]. The existence in the adult PB of a progenitor cell with a bi-potential hematopoietic and endothelial capability of differentiation such as the hemangioblast was regarded as a surprise but did not appear completely incomprehensible. In fact, an intimate association between endothelial and hematopoietic lineages is well described in the yolk sack of the developing embryo [17,18] and by experiments of gene knocking out in the animal model [19].

To further increase the list of surface antigens associated to the endothelial lineage, it has been reported that the CD117 antigen, the receptor of the hematopoietic cytokine stem cell factor (SCF), can identify cells able to participate to neovascularization of the injured myocardium of the mouse [20,21]. Indeed, in that experimental setting, only cells expressing at a high level the CD117 antigen could have part in this process. Subsequent experiments, again in the mouse model, confirmed the functional endothelial capacity of $CD117^+$ cells [22]. Unfortunately, as for CD133, also CD117 is expressed both on hematopoietic [23] and EPCs [24] and can not be regarderd as an unique marker of the endothelial lineage, neither when associated to other antigens such as CD34 and VEGFR-2. Besides these antigens, a number of other markers have been and are currently used to identify EPCs [6]. However, none of these is *per se* useful to identify EPCs because either they are also expressed on mature endothelial cells or they also belong to the hematopoietic lineage or both. For example Tie-2, VE-cadherin, CD146 and E-selectin are mainly or only expressed on mature or maturing endothelial cells, whereas CD31 (PECAM), von Willebrand factor (vWf), VEGFR-1 and Tie-2 (in addition to CD34, VEGFR-2, CD133 and CD117) are expressed on both endothelial and hematopoietic cells. Also the ability to incorporate 1,1'-dioctadecyl-3,3,3',3'-tetramet-hylindocarbocyanine-labeledacetylated low density lipoprotein (Di-LDL) and to bind lectins such as Ulex europeus or Bandeira semplicifolia, a combination of markers frequently used in the last years to identify EPCs, falls among these aspecific lineage markers [6]. Therefore, as it appears from the aforementioned considerations, the precise phenotype of the EPCs remains substantially indefinable. The assessment of the co-expression of multiple antigens seems to be an absolute requirement for the detection and consequently for the enumeration of circulating EPCs, and in keeping with this assumption, the assessment of the co-expression of CD34, VEGFR-2, and CD133 seems to be the more precise way for the identification, at the phenotype level, of at least a subset of "true" EPCs [25,26].

In Vitro Growth of EPCs

If the immuno-phenotypic characterization of the EPCs is still far from being exactly defined, the in vitro growth of EPCs is actually a matter of debate and controversy. In fact, in vitro attempts of growing EPCs made in these years have given different results suggesting that, at a functional level, different types of circulating cells can assume an endothelial phenotype. Moreover, in vivo studies have confirmed that these different type of putative EPCs can actively participate in effective neovascularization.

Asahara and coll [1] cultivated PB-derived $CD34^+$ cells on collagen or fibronectin coated dishes in the presence of Fetal Calf Serum and VEGF and after 7 days of culture obtained colonies of spindle shaped cells which were positive for a number of endothelial antigens, including CD31, Tie-2, E selectin, CD34 and Flk-1, and expressed endothelial nitric oxide synthase (eNOS) and VEGFR-2. Although this experiment remains a milestone in the history of circulating EPCs it was soon evident that this type of in vitro EPC derived colonies did not explained completely the proliferating and differentiating potential of the circulating EPCs. In fact, the purified $CD34^+$ cell population used was partially contaminated by mononuclear cells, thus leaving open the question of the precise identification and origin of the circulating EPCs, and the short term culture conditions suggested that other possible long term culture progenitors, endowed with a higher proliferative potential, could exist. These questions could be addressed by using different culture conditions including a more defined starting cell population, different culture medium favouring endothelial differentiation, and longer time of incubation. This turned out into a number of newly designed experiments for the in vitro growth of EPCs. A first evidence that more than one kind of EPC could exist came from the experiments of Lin and coll who showed that morphological and functional distinct type of EPCs can be grown in vitro starting from PB mononuclear cells [27]. They found that besides the small colonies of spindle-like cells obtained after 7 days of culture and endowed with a low proliferative potential, it was possible to obtain "late outgrowing cells" which appeared in culture after 3-4 weeks, had high proliferative potential, were able to form typical cobblestone areas, were positive for VE-cadherin, Flk-1, vWF, and CD36 and negative for some hematopoietic antigens such as CD45 and CD14. The Authors regarded these cells as true EPCs or angioblasts [27], probably derived directly from the putative hemangioblast. This experimental approach found a great success and was the starting point on which other experimental settings for the in vitro growth of EPCs were designed. In particular, Ingram and coll recently developed a culture system which basically stems from the work of Lin in which the Authors precisely identify both in the PB of adult individuals (at a very low frequency) and in the umbilical cord blood (at a 10 fold higher frequency than in PB) diverse sorts of EPCs able to form at different times of culture different types of colonies in a hierarchical model very similar to the well known hierarchical model of hematopoiesis [28,29]. It should be noted that in all these types of protocols for the in vitro growth of EPCs, PB mononuclear cells were plated as a whole population and non-adherent cells were discarded after the first days of culture. In this way, however, contaminating adherent cells such as monocytes and mature ECs remain in the culture dish and cause a certain degree of heterogeneity of the cultivated cells, although it is likely that monocytes and mature ECs do not survive after the 4 weeks when the late outgrowing ECs emerge from the cultures. In this respect, some researchers have used the pre-plating of the mononuclear cells as a way for getting rid of adherent cells of monocytic origin [30,31]. However, yet again this method can eliminate some contaminating cells of myeloid origin, mainly monocytes, but not other not adherent cells of hematopoietic and non-hematopoietic origin which may participate to the *in vitro* growth and differentiation of cells with an endothelial phenotype and function. In fact, there is increasing evidence that also cells expressing mature hematopoietic antigens such as CD14 (a typical monocytic marker) can give rise to endothelial-like cells in vitro. In particular $CD14^{+}CD34^{-}$ PB derived cells can co-express endothelial markers, secrete angiogenic factors, and form tubular structures in matrigel [32,33,34] and when properly expanded ex-vivo, they can be incorporated in new vessels in an animal model [35]. Interestingly and in line with these observations, a subset of human PB monocytes has been reported to act as a pluripotent stem cell, *in vitro* [36,37]. In addition to all these points, few studies suggest that other cells which are not of hematopoietic origin (neither immature, i.e. the hemangioblast, nor mature such as the aforementioned $CD14^{+}CD34^{-}$ cell population) can give rise to endothelial cells *in vitro* and *in vivo*. For instance, Hillebrands and coll reported that cells other than BM derived were responsible of the endothelial cell replacement in a mouse model of transplant arteriosclerosis [38]. In another *in vivo* experimental setting Verfaille's group showed that the so called MAPC (multipotent adult progenitor cell) which are circulating BM-derived cells different from hematopoietic stem cells (being $CD34^{-}$, $CD117^{-}$) can differentiate into distinct lineages, including endothelium [39]. Finally, cells belonging to the "side population" (a small circulating subset of $CD34^{-}$ stem cells, selected on the basis of Hoechst dye staining), are able to differentiate into various lineages including hematopoiesis, skeletal muscle, and endothelium [40].

These data suggest that a search for an unique definition of the real EPC is very difficult, at least at the functional level. It rather seems that a sort of heterogeneity of circulating EPCs exist and more in general, different subsets of circulating cells which are capable of assuming an endothelial phenotype and function are responsible for the different behaviour observed *in vitro.*

MECHANISMS OF MOBILIZATION FROM BONE MARROW TO PERIPHERAL BLOOD

As reported in the previous paragraphs, EPCs have been mainly detected in the adult PB and in the umbilical cord blood. However, there are evidences that circulating EPCs derive from the BM [1,30,41], even when cells of non-hematopoietic origin are considered (see previous paragraph). How do EPCs leave the BM and mobilize to the PB? And how is possible to increase their otherwise very low frequency in the PB?

The spontaneous (not pharmacologically induced) mobilization of EPCs from the BM to the PB is a complex process regulated by a variety of factors, including growth factors and chemokines, receptors of adhesion molecules and enzymes [42].

A crucial step in the mobilization process is the loosening of the interactions between stromal cells (which are the main constituent of the bone marrow niche, the microenvironment where stem/progenitor cells are located) and EPCs which determines the recruitment of the progenitor cells from the BM to the PB. Activation of matrix metalloproteinase-9 (MMP-9) and of other proteinases (MMP-2, cathepsin G, elastases) mediates the cleavage of adhesion molecules and of the membrane bound form of Kit ligand (CD117) to its soluble form (s-Kit) [43]. These events are followed by the release of early $CD117^+$ progenitor cells (among which both hematopoietic and EPCs are included) from the niche to the vascular zone of the BM. In addition, also the BM derived e-NOS can play a role in EPCs mobilization since mice deficient in e-NOS showed reduced MMP-9 activity and impaired mobilization [44]. The most effective factor in inducing mobilization of EPCs from the BM to the PB is ischemia [45] which, by means of the Hypoxia Inducible Factor-1α-mediated up-regulation of VEGF and/or Stromal Derived Factor-1α (SDF-1α) [46] activates the cascade of events which causes proteinase activation and in turn EPC release from the marrow niches. A number of physiological and pathological conditions can affect the number of circulating EPCs, and these will be discussed below. Here, we will consider the effect of some pharmacological substances that can influence the EPC number in humans, namely Granulocyte-Colony Stimulating Factor (G-CSF), erythropoietin, VEGF, and statins. G-CSF is a cytokine commonly used for mobilization of $CD34^+$ cells in patients for HPC transplantation. It was shown that after G-CSF administration the proportion of circulating $CD34^+$ cells co-expressing VEGFR-2 and CD133 increased from a median of 0.4% to a median of 2.0% [11]. Another hematopoietic growth factor, erythropoietin, which is a well known modulator of erythroid progenitor and precursors proliferation and differentiation is also a potent mobilizer of EPCs from BM into PB [47,48]. VEGF, administered via gene therapy in patients with critical limb ischemia, determined an increase in circulating EPCs up to 30 folds [49]. Last but not least, statins (the inhibitors of 3-hydroxy-3-methylglutaryl coenzyme A –HMG-CoA reductase) were shown to increase the number and functional activity of EPCs in vitro [50,51] and in patients with coronary artery disease [52]. This latter effect on EPC mobilization might further shed light onto the well known beneficial effects of statins as a medication against atherosclerotic vascular disease in addition to the already known effectiveness in lowering cholesterol levels.

Human EPCs in Healthy Subjects

The number of circulating EPCs in healthy subjects is rather low (0.01%) [6]. However, this number is not constant but it can change consistently. In fact, a variation in the number of circulating EPCs have been described in a number of physiological conditions, where pharmacologic interventions were absent. This phenomenon could have important consequences because circulating EPCs have been shown to participate in maintaining the vessel wall homeostasis, providing a circulating pool of cells that can take part in replacing dysfunctional endothelium or in repairing sites where a denuding injury occurred. This is quite relevant considering that endothelial injury leads to the loss of the anti-thrombotic properties of the vessel wall, and acts as a critical initial step in the development of atherosclerotic plaques [53]. The complete regeneration of injured endothelium may also occur by migration and proliferation of surrounding mature ECs as in adult angiogenesis; however, mature ECs are terminally differentiated cells with a low proliferative potential and their capacity to substitute damaged ECs and to create new vessels is relatively limited [54]. On the contrary, a role in vessel integrity could be played, rather than by mature ECs, by a functionally active population of EPCs, that has been recently described by Ingram and coll

[55]. These EPCs are resident in the vessel wall and are able to proliferate and to differentiate in vitro.

Pregnancy

Evidences have been presented that circulating EPCs able to form late-outgrowth colonies are present in women during pregnancy, while in non pregnant women and in men the circulating ECs observed have the characteristic morphology of mature cells, uniform staining for vWF, and are unable to form this type of colonies [56]. The number of EPCs increases with gestation in normal pregnancies, and is directly correlated with both the gestational age and the plasma estradiol levels, suggesting that EPCs may play an important role in the regulation and maintenance of placental development and vascular integrity during pregnancy [57]. Previous reports have shown that in animal models of experimentally induced tissue injury estrogens increase the mobilization and influence the kinetics of EPCs that, leaving the bone marrow, incorporate into the neoendothelium contributing to the reendothelization process. This effect has been shown to be mainly dependent on eNOS expression, since both EPC mobilization and acceleration of reendothelization are absent in estradiol-treated eNOS null mice; in addition, both a mitogenic activity and an anti-apoptotic effect of estradiol on EPCs has been documented [58,59].

Vascular Trauma

The normal menstrual cycle in women represents a physiological condition in which the endometrium undergoes shedding of the upper zone; this in turn induces a mechanism of cyclical repair, regeneration, and tissue remodelling that involves the growth of the vasculature [60]. Angiogenesis in the human uterus is required to support the reconstruction of endometrium and to provide a vascularized, receptive tissue for implantation and placentation three weeks later. By using the chick embryo chorioallantoic membrane in vivo assay for angiogenesis [61], it has been reported that human endometrial fragments, obtained at different phases of the menstrual cycle, have angiogenic potential, with a nadir in the late proliferative phase and significantly higher potential in the early proliferative, early secretory and late secretory phases [62]. VEGF and VEGFR-2 seem to play a role in the menstrual cycle, although data on their actual function are confusing both in animal models [63] and in humans [62,64,65]. Indeed, it has been suggested that during the premenstrual phase of the cycle there is an up-regulation of both the production of VEGF, and of the expression of its receptor VEGFR-2 on the stromal cells of the endometrium; however, at this stage of the cycle the physiologic role of this cytokine would be non angiogenic due to the fact that stromal cells expressing VEGFR-2 up-regulate the production of MMPs and induce the tissue expressing these factors to be eventually sloughed. Alternatively, the increase in VEGF levels in the early proliferative endometrium may be responsible for the elongation of the existing vessels, essential for tissue reconstruction [61].

There are no data regarding the possible recruitment of EPCs from the BM to the endometrium in order to support a vasculogenesis rather than an angiogenesis during the different phases of the physiological menstrual cycle. By both cytofluorimetric analysis and *in vitro* functional assay, we studied the percentage of circulating EPCs in a number of fertile women 24-48 hours before the beginning of the menstrual cycle, and 12, 24 hours, 15, and 23 days after the beginning of the menstrual cycle. Preliminary data suggest that fertile women, 24-48 hours before and 12 hours after the menstrual cycle, had a number of circulating EPCs, evaluated as $CD34^{+}VEGR\text{-}2^{+}$ cells, significantly higher than that found in a control group of age matched males; similarly, the percentage of circulating $CD34^{+}CD133^{+}VEGFR\text{-}2^{+}$ cells at 24-48 hours before and 15 days after the beginning of the menstrual cycle was significantly higher than that found in the control group (personal observations). No difference was found in the number of endothelial colonies obtained after 7 day culture assay of PB mononuclear cells, drawn from subjects of the control group or from fertile women tested at the defined different time points. In addition, no correlation was found between the number of circulating EPCs and plasma VEGF levels (personal observation). The possibility exists that the lack of correspondence between the increased number of circulating EPCs and the number of in vitro colonies during the different phases of the physiological menstrual cycle is due to the fact that we performed a culture assay which favours the growth of EPCs with a low proliferative potential and not the late-outgrowing EPCs. This, however, do not exclude their ability to participate in vascular repair processes or new vessel formation at the site of vascular injury (i.e. the endometrium). In a previous study, the number of circulating $34^{+}VEGFR\text{-}2^{+}$ EPCs was found increased in women with increased estrogen plasma levels due to ovarian hyperstimulation in the context of planned in vitro fertilization, and these cells also appeared to be resistant to *in vitro* induced apoptosis [58]. We did not find correlations between the increased number of circulating EPCs and plasma hormone levels (i.e. estrogens); this phenomenon may be less evident in physiological conditions, where both the variability between subjects that do not undergo any defined pharmacological treatment may be relevant, and the plasma levels are lower than those reached during hyperstimulation protocols. However, although further investigations are needed to understand the mechanisms underlying this finding, a physiological monthly amplification of EPC population may have a role in explaining the low rate of cardiovascular adverse events documented in fertile women with respect to men and to women that reached the menopause. In this regard, we found that the number of circulating $CD34^{+}CD133^{+}VEGFR\text{-}2^{+}$ EPCs was significantly higher in fertile women 24-48 hours before the beginning of the menstrual cycle than in women who met the criteria defining the menopause (personal observations).

Other less physiological vascular trauma induced by burn or by mechanical disruption, such as during surgical procedures, has been shown to lead to a cascade of events that results in an early increase of VEGF plasma levels promoting an increase in the number of circulating EPCs ($VEGFR\text{-}2^{+}CD133^{+}$) within 6-12 hours; these data further support the hypothesis that EPCs may enhance the re-endothelization of denuded prothrombotic injured vasculature [66].

Physical Activity

Physical activity is associated with an improvement of blood pressure, insulin sensitivity, and hemostatic and inflammatory parameters [67,68]. However, despite the wealth of evidence derived from epidemiological and interventional trials, there is limited understanding of the underlying molecular mechanisms. Notably, physical training reduces vascular oxidative stress at least in part via increased activity of eNOS and extracellular superoxide dismutase, which in turn may exert beneficial vascular effects [69,70]. Exercise is a non pharmacologic intervention that can acutely mobilize specific mononuclear cell subsets into circulation (i.e T suppressor/cytotoxic cells) [71,72], and it has been recently observed that in voluntarily running mice there was an increase in the EPC number in BM, PB and spleen, which was mediated by a NO-dependent increase of VEGF plasma levels. Moreover, a decreased rate of EPC apoptosis, diminished neointima formation after vascular injury, and enhanced neoangiogenesis were also reported [73]. The effect of exercise (bicycle exercise test) on circulating EPCs in humans has been recently investigated [74]. In this study, an acute (within 5 to 10 minutes after the exercise was completed) increase of circulating $CD133^{+}$VE-$Cadherin^{+}$ cells (known to be involved in angiogenesis) was observed. In addition, after a 4 day culture period of PB-derived mononuclear cells, the Authors found that "angiogenic cells" able to bind Ulex lectin, and showing the typical uptake of Di-LDL, were increased compared with those grown in culture performed with blood obtained before the bicycle test. While the increase of EPCs, within 5 to 10 minutes after completion of exercise may indicate a mobilization either from BM or from the marginal pool, via beta adrenergic mechanisms similar to those of lymphocytes [71], the increase of EPCs after 4 days of culture seems to reflect a slower but more effective mobilization of functionally active progenitor cells. Interestingly, supernatants from these cultured cells were richer of endothelial growth factors such as VEGF, hepatocyte growth factors, G-CSF, and GM-CSF than those from cultured cells obtained from PB before the exercise was performed. According to these data, circulating EPCs may therefore be mobilized by exercise, possibly contributing to endothelial repair by homing to areas of dysfunctional endothelium and differentiate in new ECs or secreting vasculoprotective growth factors [74]. Alternatively but not exclusively, the beneficial effects of exercise can be at least in part attributed to an increase in blood flow. In fact, an increased flow enhances endothelium dependent vasodilatation by increasing the vascular expression of NO synthase and increases the release of NO inhibiting multiple processes involved in atherogenesis [75]. Another interesting finding of this study [74] was that exercise was also associated to an increase of $CD133^{+}$VE-$cadherin^{-}$ cells, which is likely to represent hematopoietic stem/progenitor cells. The increase of HPCs after exercise is reminiscent of a previous finding [76] obtained evaluating the number of circulating $CD34^{+}$ HPCs in healthy subjects trained to perform a marathon, half marathon, or sedentary controls. The runners had increased number of $CD34^{+}CD38^{-}$, $CD34^{+}CD33^{-}$ cell subsets with respect to the sedentary controls; however, no significant variation was noted, between the values obtained before and after they run the marathon or half marathon. Interestingly, there was a decrease of the number of circulating $CD34^{+}$ cells the morning after the race with respect to the values found before and immediately after the race. The physiological role of increased circulating HPCs is quite difficult to explain. It is possible that an increased turn over of polymorfonuclear (PMN) cells associated with exercise and the consequent inflammatory state may stimulate the HPC mobilization; in this case, the decrease of the HPCs after the race might reflect simply a maturation and replenishment of the peripheral PMN compartment. Alternatively, the HPC population may include cells with angioblastic potential having phenotypic markers in common with HPCs. Further supporting the role of exercise in EPC mobilization, it has been reported that a 44-year old healthy subject tested before, 1 day, and

45 days after a trek in the Himalayas, showed a significant increase of the number of both circulating EPCs ($CD45^-CD146^+CD144^+$) and of endothelial colonies ($CD31^+CD105^+CD144^+CD146^{low}CD133^-vWf^{low}$) 1 day after the exercise with respect to that found before and 45 days after the trek, and that found in a group of healthy controls [77]. According to these data, it is likely that the association of the effects of a higher oxygen demand induced by exercise, and of the hypoxia occurring at high altitude and determining a low oxygen saturation are strong stimuli for a rapid EPC mobilization. On the other hand, it has been shown that there was no significant change in the number of circulating $CD34^+VEGFR\text{-}2^+$ EPCs, in a group of healthy subjects undergoing a maximal exercise test on a calibrated electronically braked bicycle evaluated before and 2, 4, 6, 8, 24, and 48 hours after the test [78]. According with this finding, we also have unpublished data obtained in a group of healthy subjects and in a group of athletes who trained since at least 3 months, 3 times per week for a minimum of one hour. They all underwent the maximal test on a calibrated electronically braked bicycle, and the circulating EPCs were evaluated before the exercise and within 1 hour from the end of the exercise. No difference was found in the percentage of EPCs evaluated either as $CD34^+VEGFR\text{-}2^+$ or $CD34^+CD133^+VEGFR\text{-}2^+$ cells in healthy subjects or in athletes tested before and after the exercise; however, in athletes, the number of endothelial colonies obtained from 7 day culture of PB drawn before the exercise was higher than that found with PB from healthy sedentary controls. Similarly, the number of HPCs, tested by ISHAGE [79], were higher in athletes than in healthy sedentary controls evaluated before the test was performed. Taken together, these results suggest an influence of physical exercise in mobilization of progenitor cells (EPCs and/or HPCs) although they can not be considered conclusive. Further experiments are needed to define the relation between exercise and EPC mobilization. In fact, it has been suggested that EPC mobilization may in part explain the significant cardiovascular benefits of exercise; however, it is still a matter of debate whether healthy subjects and specific subsets of patients (i.e. patients with coronary artery disease) would demonstrate similar pattern of cell mobilization after acute/long lasting exercise.

AGING

Whereas pregnancy, menstrual cycle, and physical exercise seem to be able to increase the number of circulating EPCs, other factors have been described to negatively influence the number and function of these cells in healthy subjects. The most physiological of them, with no doubt, is the aging, that has been suggested to be associated with a decrease in the number and function of vascular stem and progenitor cells. Preliminary results from animal models indicated that transplantation of BM from old mice into young mice led to minimal neo-vascularization when compared to transplantation of young BM [80]. It was also demonstrated that EPCs from older patients with clinical ischemia had a significantly less therapeutic effect in rescuing ischemic hind limb of a nude mouse compared with those obtained from younger ischemic patients [80,81], providing evidence that an age dependent impairment in neo-vascularization may be heavenly influenced by the EPC phenotype. The mechanisms for this age-dependent impairment are largely unknown, and may be in part explained by the presence of a number of risk factors that are often associated to the older age and may constitute additional elements to be considered in studying the mechanisms that induce EPC impairment. Indeed, Hill et al [72] evaluated, by the Framingham risk factor score, the total burden of risk factors for cardiovascular disease, in a population of relatively healthy subjects, with a mean age of 50 years, who never had symptomatic cardiovascular diseases, or any condition in which angiogenesis may be present. Women were excluded from the study because of the possible confounding effects of the angiogenetic processes occurring during the menstrual cycle. The results showed that the EPCs, evaluated as number of colony forming units, in high-risk subjects were both fewer in number and become senescent more rapidly than those in low-risk subjects.

In addition, a decrease in VEGF plasma levels and the number of circulating EPCs has been found in subjects of advanced age (>62 years) compared with those with a younger age (<62 years) [83]. Recently, a comprehensive analysis of the association between age-related endothelial dysfunction and the number and function of EPCs, defined by the expression of $CD34^{+}VEGFR\text{-}2^{+}$ and $CD133^{+}VEGFR\text{-}2^{+}$, has been published [84]. No quantitative differences in EPCs were observed; however, culture-enriched EPCs from old but healthy subjects resulted impaired in terms of functional features like proliferation, migration, and survival. Changes in stem and progenitor cells may be of great importance for the aging process, potentially leading to progressive deterioration of functional and proliferative homeostasis in organs [85].

Recent studies support the notion that one possible mechanism for the vascular changes in advancing aging is the exhaustion of progenitor cells, in particular BM cells, that are capable of vascular repair. Exhaustion of this component of BM in number, function, or both, could produce disequilibrium between vascular injury and vascular repair [82].

SMOKING

Smoking is another factor, although not a physiological one, that have been described to negatively influence the number of circulating EPCs in healthy subjects. Almost ten years ago, it was reported that long-term cigarette smoking might be involved in inducing an impairment in basal nitric oxide mediated vasodilation [86]. More recently, the number of circulating EPCs has been evaluated in chronic smokers and in non smoking subjects by both culture assay and cytofluorimetric analysis [87]. Interestingly, while the viability of mononuclear cells, assessed in an *in vitro* culture, from heavy smokers was similar to that of mononuclear cells derived from non smokers, the number of circulating EPCs (assessed by cytofluorimetric analysis as $CD45^{low}CD34^{+}CD133^{+}VEGFR\text{-}2^{+}$) from smokers was significantly lower than that of non smoking subjects. To be noted, the effect of smoking cessation was appreciable after two weeks, induced significant increase of circulating EPCs in chronic smokers in four weeks, and the phenomenon was more evident in light than in heavy smokers. The quick recovery of EPCs after quitting smoking rapidly disappeared when smoking was resumed.

The possibility exists that the rapid change in circulating EPC number associated with smoking status is related to an actual endothelial dysfunction in smokers. Injured vessels in smokers may benefit from EPCs for maintaining endothelial function, and their number may increase quitting smoking due to a decreased number of injured vessels; on the other hand, smoking may affect BM environment and EPC mobilization could be decreased by smoking.

EPCs in Human Pathological Conditions

Cardiovascular Diseases

Age, hyperlipidemia, hyperglycemia, hypertension, familiarity for cardiovascular diseases, and smoking impair the function of the vascular endothelium and are considered cardiovascular risk factors. The number of circulating EPCs, that are involved in endothelial repair, have been negatively associated to risk factors, and it has recently been shown that the evaluation of their number in the PB may be a surrogate marker of vascular function, but also of cumulative cardiovascular risk, evaluated in term of Framingham risk score [88,82]. More importantly in a 2 year follow up study it has been shown that patients suffering from one cardiovascular event during the time of observation had significantly lower EPC number at the time of admission in the study than that of subjects who had an event free course, strongly suggesting that these cells contribute to ongoing vascular repair and their number may predict a disease progression [89]. In this study the evaluation of EPCs was performed by cytofluorimetric analysis and their phenotype was characterized by antibodies recognizing the CD34 antigen and the VEGFR-2 on the membrane; however, this is still one of the many ways used to count circulating EPCs, it may include a number of mature ECs, and it does not allow any conclusion about the functionality of these cells. So far, these limitations may give only a potential clinical value to this finding.

The number of circulating EPCs has been widely studied in patients with coronary artery disease (CAD) with a particular attention to verify the possible effect of ischemic or non ischemic condition. In the most of the studies patients were divided according with the presence of an angiografically documented stenotic, non stenotic, or ricanalized coronary artery. Actually, the number of EPCs evaluated the most of the time by cytofluorimetric analysis as $CD34^{+}VEGFR\text{-}2^{+}$ cells was decreased, although not significantly, in patients with CAD with respect to healthy controls, irrespectively of the presence of a stenotic coronary [78,90,89]. Low levels of circulating EPCs in patients with coronary artery disease could be the consequence of a number of mechanisms. It is possible that risk factors, by modulating the levels of oxidative stress, nitric oxide activity, or other physiologic processes, directly influence the mobilization or half life of EPCs. An alternative explanation supported by the data from Schmidt-Licke and coll [89] is that continuous endothelial damage or dysfunction leads to an eventual depletion or exhaustion of a presumable finite supply of EPCs.

To evaluate whether a single reversible episode of ischemia is sufficient to induce any measurable change in the number of circulating EPCs, additional investigations were performed in patients with CAD who underwent single symptom-limited exercise stress test. In the most of the studies the maximal exercise test was performed on a calibrated electronically braked-bicycle, and the workload was increased progressively. Myocardial ischemia, when present, was evidenced by typical angina pectoris or a significant exercise induced ST-segment depression. Exercise was terminated when patients experienced chest pain, exhaustion, or when 3mm horizontal ST segment depression was reached. The results of these studies demonstrate that after the single exercise test a detectable increase of circulating EPCs is evident at 24-48 hours only in those patients that experienced a myocardial ischemia during the test; this was associated also to increased VEGF plasma levels [78]. Similarly, patients with documented peripheral arterial occlusive disease that reported an ischemic leg pain during the exercise showed a significantly increased number of circulating EPCs, with respect to patients who were enrolled after revascularization, or those with stable CAD [90]. On the other hand, Schmidt-Lucke et al evaluated the number of circulating EPCs in patients with CAD without acute coronary syndrome, and in patients with acute coronary syndrome and troponin T levels indicative of myocardial necrosis. The results showed that the number of circulating EPCs was significantly lower than that found in healthy controls in all the groups of patients, irrespectively of the presence of the acute coronary syndrome; however, it has to be pointed out that this finding may be influenced by the enrolment of patients with acute coronary syndrome who had a higher incidence of risk factors (i.e. smoking, CRP serum levels, LDL serum cholesterol levels) than patients with stable CAD, and were less likely to be treated with statins. Although it is difficult to compare the results obtained in this last study to those previously mentioned, it appears that the association between ischemia and EPCs mobilization is an actual finding.

An important question with respect to potential therapeutic approaches is whether the EPC pool can be increased in vivo in patients with CAD. Exercise training has evolved as an accepted therapy to improve endothelial cell number and function. To this regard, a number of studies have been performed in animal models [73] and humans with respect to exercise training and its effects on endothelial function and EPC number in different clinical contexts, especially in the presence of cardiovascular risk factors. In patients with CAD the endothelial dysfunction, documented by abnormal acetylcholine induced coronary vasoconstriction, resulted significantly improved after 4 weeks of intensive physical training, showing a coronary-artery constriction in response to acetylcholine reduced by 54% [91]; in addition, in a recently published trial [92] patients with CAD were randomly assigned to 12 months of exercise training or to percutaneous coronary intervention. Patients trained had a significantly higher event-free survival than those undergoing the standard intervention procedure. Further supporting the beneficial effects of training, Laufs and coll [73] described a significant increase of circulating EPCs after a 4 week rehabilitation training program in patients with stable CAD.

Acute Myocardial Infarction (AMI)

Differently from angina pectoris, AMI is characterized by the presence of the necrosis of the cardiac tissue. The combination of ischemia and necrosis can exert sinergistic effect on EPC mobilization and in turn in inducing reparative processes. The first report in this field [93] described an increased concentration of $CD34^+$ cells and increased VEGF plasma levels after AMI with a peak on the seventh day after the acute event. Culture assays of PB mononuclear cells showed also an increased number of attaching cells expressing endothelial lineage markers on day 7. These data were partially confirmed and extended by us [94]. We found that the highest mobilization of $CD34^+$ cells was evident at time of admission of patients with AMI (within 6 hours from the first symptoms), together with the highest number of endothelial colonies, and highest VEGF plasma levels. On day 7, the number of circulating $CD34^+$ cells was already reduced, but still higher than that found in healthy controls. The increased $CD34^+$ cells in patients with AMI at admission included an increase both in hematopoietic $CD34^+$ cells (defined by the International Society of Hematotherapy and Graft

Engineering – ISHAGE- guidelines) [79], and an increase in circulating CD34^{+}VEGFR-2^{+} cells. This last subset was shown to include increased percentages of CD34^{+}CD133^{+}VEGFR-2^{+} and CD34^{+}CD117^{+}VEGFR-2^{+} "true" EPCs. It seems intriguing to think that in the early phase of AMI HPCs and EPCs could play different roles, if any, in tissue repair, with EPCs devoted to neoangiogenesis, and HPCs, due to their "plasticity", to new myocardium generation.

So far, data suggesting that spontaneous mobilization of CD34^{+} cells might contribute to determine a more favourable post-AMI remodelling are lacking. Recently, Leone and coll [95], in a limited number of patients tested at time of AMI and after 1 year follow up, showed a significant and favourable correlation between the number of circulating CD34^{+} cells and changes of the left ventricular ejection fraction, the wall motion score index, and the left ventricular end-systolic volume. Further supporting the hypothesis of a "regeneration role" of the increased number of circulating CD34^{+} cells at the onset of AMI, Wojakowski and coll [96] found a simultaneous increase in expression of mRNA for specific early cardiac, muscle, and endothelial markers in the population of PB mononuclear cells in patients after AMI. Although this finding is still a matter of debate mainly because the evaluation of the mRNA expression should have been performed on purified CD34^{+} cells [97], all these data may contribute to a better understanding of the repairing processes spontaneously occurring after AMI, and in turn may help in identifying the best strategy for the use of a cell-based therapy in the regeneration of human myocardium.

Diabetes Mellitus

A decreased number and/or function of circulating EPCs have been described in diabetic patients [98,99], where they could be involved in the pathogenesis of the typical vascular complications of the disease. These observations were confirmed in a recent report [100] that showed that the number of circulating EPCs, evaluated by cytofluorimetric analysis as CD34^{+}VEGFR-2^{+} cells, was reduced in diabetic patients with respect to healthy controls. However, the reduction was larger when the number of circulating EPCs of healthy subjects was compared either with that of patients with diabetes associated with peripheral vascular disease or of patients suffering from ischemic foot lesions complicating end-stage obstructive vascular disease. More importantly, a significant inverse correlation was found between the values of glucose and the absolute number of EPCs. It was suggested that the lower number of EPCs in diabetic patients may reflect a shortened peripheral survival of these cells rather than a weak BM mobilization. Supporting this hypothesis, it has been reported that high glucose concentration is able to induce apoptosis of cultured ECs in vitro [101].

Hematological Diseases

Myelofibrosis with Myeloid Metaplasia (MMM)

Myelofibrosis with myeloid metaplasia (MMM) is a clonal Philadelphia-negative chronic myeloproliferative disorder (Ph^{-} CMPD) characterized by a variable degree of BM fibrosis, extramedullary haematopoiesis, and presence of immature myeloid cells in the PB. [102,103]. Recently, it has been reported that an increased number of circulating $CD34^+$ HPCs is a diagnostic marker of the disease and that it is related to the progression of the disease [104]. Neoangiogenesis has been documented in the BM of patients with MMM, where microvessel density has been reported to be higher than in other CMPDs [105]. This finding was successively extended also to the spleen [106]. Indeed, in patients with MMM, spleen sectional area occupied by capillary vascular structures was found to be up to three times larger than the upper value of normal subjects; in addition, patients with the highest extent of spleen localization of $CD34^+$ cells had the highest extent of capillary vascular density [106]. These results, together with data showing that the number of spleen $CD34^+$ HPCs paralleled that of PB $CD34^+$ HPCs, are in keeping with the concept that a tight equilibrium exists between blood and spleen haematopoietic cell compartments and that spleen myeloid metaplasia and capillary neoangiogenesis are correlated mechanisms. Supporting this finding, $CD34^+CD133^+VEGFR\text{-}2^+$ EPCs were found in the spleen of patients with MMM, constituting up to 13% of $CD34^+$ cells, and were associated with a sustained spleen neoangiogenesis [106]. The frequency of $CD34^+CD133^+VEGFR\text{-}2^+$ EPCs was also increased in the PB of patients with MMM compared with healthy subjects [107]. Interestingly, a higher number of these cells resulted significantly associated with a younger age, a diagnosis of prefibrotic MMM and a reduced number of immature myeloid cells and blasts in PB. These observations support the hypothesis that increased trafficking of EPCs characterizes those patients with a mild clinical phenotype. In addition, circulating $CD34^+$ cells from MMM patients were able to form colonies whose cells were $CD31^+$VE-cadherin$^+$vWF$^+$CD45$^-$, confirming the presence of increased number of EPCs in the PB. The fact that both HPCs and EPCs are increased in the PB of MMM patients opens new perspectives in the interpretation of the pathogenesis of this disease. In fact, by assuming the same BM origin for EPCs and HPCs, high levels of circulating EPCs and HPCs in MMM could be the result of a common aberration of BM stem and progenitor cells or of BM microenvironment that could directly influence their mobilization. The finding of decreasing levels of circulating EPCs observed in patients with greater numbers of circulating HPCs [107] may be due to a competitive relationship between EPCs and HPCs mobilization or to an eventual depletion of a presumably limited supply of EPCs, caused by the continuous stimulation of the marrow compartment, or may be due to the progressive trapping of EPCs in extramedullary organs.

Multiple Myeloma (MM)

Neoangiogenesis has also been thought to have a governing role in multiple myeloma (MM) pathogenesis and progression. This has been indicated by the presence of an increased BM microvascular density that was positively correlated with disease activity, and by increased expression of angiogenic factors such as VEGF [108,109,110,111,112]. More recently, Hong Zhang and coll were the first to evaluate the number of circulating endothelial cells (CEC) in MM [113]. By cytofluorimetric analysis and culture assays they found that both the number of CEC and that of EPCs is elevated in patients with MM. In addition, as already shown for EPCs derived from the BM of patients with MM [114], also circulating EPCs were able to grow on matrigel and display a capillary network formation in vitro. The clinical relevance of this finding was due to the direct relation of both CEC and EPCs with β2 globulin and the monoclonal component, markers that reflect tumor mass and prognosis; in addition, the demonstration of a suppressive effect of thalidomide on circulating EPCs may represent the key mechanism by which the drug affects angiogenesis in MM, indicating that patients in whom thalidomide is ineffective can be identified by high colony growth and high monoclonal protein levels.

Clinical Applications of Endothelial Progenitor Cells

Several small–scale feasibility and safety clinical trials have been recently performed in humans to evaluate the use of BM cell transplantation for the treatment of myocardial infarction and peripheral limb ischemia. With the exception of the study by Stamm and coll [115] where autologous purified $CD133^+$ BM cells were injected into the infarct border zone, in the most of the other published studies the transplantation procedure, either by intracoronary delivery or by injection into the myocardial tissue, was performed with unfractioned autologous BM mononuclear cells [116,117]. Alternatively, unfractioned BM and *ex vivo* expanded PB derived mononuclear cells were intracoronary infused into a randomized group of patients with riperfused AMI [118,119]. The recently published 1 year follow up of this study showed sustained improvement in left ventricular function, and smaller infarct sizes in the 2 groups of patients receiving cell therapy [120]. Wollert and coll [121] reported recently the results of BOOST randomized controlled trial in two groups of patients treated with standard medical therapy for AMI alone, or in association with intracoronary infusion of autologous BM cells [121]. Similarly, in a small number of patients Fernandez-Aviles and coll used intracoronary delivery of BM cells that were injected about 13 days after AMI [122]. All the results obtained in these studies indicate that such therapeutic approach is feasible and safe. Moreover, an improvement in ventricular function and enhancement of coronary perfusion was reported after cell therapy in the BOOST study [121]. Autologous BM mononuclear cells were delivered also into the gastrocnemius muscle of patients with unilateral or bilateral leg ischemia caused by severe peripheral artery disease [123]. In this protocol, the BM mononuclear cell transplantation resulted a safe and an effective strategy for treatment of peripheral ischemic diseases. All these trials have a number of limitations. They consisted of a limited number of patients, were single center, and almost all of them were uncontrolled. Moreover, in the most of these studies there was not a pre-selection of a single cell population to be injected. Therefore, the encouraging results reported should be considered preliminary although of potential clinical interest and, due to the use of unselected cells, can not be attributed only to EPCs.

Pharmacological Mobilization of EPCs

An important question for designing potential therapeutic approaches based on the use of EPCs is whether the BM EPC pool can be mobilized in vivo by treatment with pharmacologic agents or cytokines [124]. Several studies performed in animal models have shown that treatment with hematopoietic and endothelial growth factors (SCF, G-CSF, SDF-1α, VEGF) can induce the recruitment of progenitor cells from the BM to the infarcted myocardium

[125,126,49]. However, the principal concern in applying this strategy in humans is represented by the possible recruitment of EPCs not only to sites of vessel injuries but also to sites of occult neoplasia, leading to vascularization of dormant tumors. In addition, in a recent clinical trail that used G-CSF for the mobilization of EPCs in patients with AMI, the potential beneficial effects of EPC mobilization on damaged myocardium was counteracted by an increased rate of in-stent restenosis that led to the cancellation of the trial [127]. Besides this discouraging result, a number of studies have shown a possible role for erythropoietin (EPO) as EPC mobilizer. It has been reported that EPO treated mice showed an increased number of both BM and PB EPCs. In addition, in *in vivo* models of post natal vascularization, EPO significantly increased ischemia induced neovascularization [47]. In keeping with these data, Parsa and coll [128] described that EPO treatment leads to significant improvement of cardiac function in animal models of myocardial infarction; this protection, however, was mainly associated with a decreased apoptosis of cardiomyocytes. Preliminary studies in humans described an increased endogenous production of EPO in patients with unstable CAD with respect to patients with stable CAD, suggesting that ischemia may induce a spontaneous release of this cytokine acting on cell subsets different from those involved in erythropoiesis; interestingly, in patients with unstable CAD, EPO serum levels were correlated with both the number of $CD34^{+}VEGFR\text{-}2^{+}$ cells and the number of endothelial colonies [47]. The hypothesis that EPO stimulates EPCs in humans was further investigated in patients with renal anemia who received therapeutic standard doses of recombinant human EPO. The treatment induced an increase in the number of functionally active EPCs assessed in cell culture and in tube formation assays in patients treated with respect to those not treated [48], suggesting that patients with renal failure, often dying for cardiovascular complication such as AMI and stroke possibly caused by impaired vascular repair mechanisms, may gain some additional benefits in addition to the amelioration of anemia when treated with EPO. Moreover, a safety and efficacy trial has been performed in patients who received high doses of recombinant EPO intravenously ($3.3x10^{4}$ IU/day) for the first 3 days after cerebral ischemic stroke [129]: the results obtained indicated that high doses of recombinant EPO were well tolerated, and no safety concerns were identified. The treatment was associated with an improvement during the 1 month follow up, mainly sustained by a strong reduction in infarct size observed by magnetic resonance imaging. Longer follow up and larger scale controlled studies are needed to confirm these preliminary findings. In fact, the use of Epo outside the usual indication of correcting anemia, could be limited by a number of adverse effects such as an excessive increase of hematocrit and the appearance of anti-Epo auto-antibodies leading to serious pure red cell aplasia [130]. It has to be considered that regarding the possibility of an increase in hematocrit values, it is well known that the efficacy of infused EPO is reduced if the supplementation of Fe is lacking [131]; in addition, Ehrenreich and coll [129], although testing high doses of EPO, did not report significant changing of either the hematocrit or the red blood cell count during a 30 day follow up of the patients enrolled in the study. According to the possible appearance of anti-EPO antibodies, this side effect has been previously described in patients with chronic renal failure undergoing a chronic clinical treatment with EPO. This appeared to be mainly due to the use of an EPO formulation that has now been withdrawn; this resulted in an actual documented frequency of this event of 1 out of 100.000 [132]. However, the possibility to completely avoid these complications may be EPO derivatives, that have been recently described [133]. EPO derivatives are carbamylated EPO (CEPO), or certain EPO mutants that do not bind to the classical EPO receptor and lack hematopoietic activity, yet retain full tissue protection (i.e. anti apoptotic function). It has been well documented that there is a physical association [134] and functional interaction of EPO receptor with the common β receptor (βcR) subunit, which provides increased ligand-binding affinity to the receptor complex and it is also the signal-transducing component common to the GM-CSF, IL-3, and IL-5 receptors [135]. The hematopoietic and tissue protective activities of EPO are distinct and separate, implicating the existence of different receptors. In fact, EPO receptor exhibits no affinity for CEPO, while the βcR subunit binds this EPO derivative; in addition, CEPO has no cytoprotective effects on tissues from βcR knockout mice, that exhibit normal hematopoiesis [136]. These data demonstrate that CEPO exherts a protective function through the βcR subunit, and shows no effects on erythropoiesis. Therefore, CEPO may represent a new therapeutic approach for patients who may have benefits from the use of EPO either as anti-apoptotic agent or as mobilizer of EPCs, avoiding the side effects that may derive from the hematopoietic function of the natural molecule.

CONCLUSION

At present, no exclusive surface antigen, or combination of antigens, that could characterize the endothelial progenitor cell subset has been defined. Therefore, EPCs should still be considered as a pool of cells that, although sharing surface markers with different cell subsets of the HPCs, or deriving from a unique hemoangioblast, or from monocytes, are able to form endothelial colonies or vascular structures once seeded on the appropriate substrate or infused in *in vivo* models of vascular injury. Despite the lack of a definitive characterization of EPCs, in the last years many studies have investigated their role both in physiological and pathological conditions. In this last setting, EPCs have acquired a great relevance since they have been shown to be part of mechanisms of vascular repair, including both angiogenesis and vasculogenesis processes.

These findings have highlighted the possible use of EPCs for therapeutic approaches. Looking from this point of view to the past, the first pilot studies in which un-separated BM derived cells were injected in the infarcted zone of patients with AMI, have possibly been a solution to the alternative, still lacking, of properly characterize the actual EPC subset and than inject it. It is possible that the, although modest, clinical improvements obtained following injection of "EPCs" in the heart of patients with AMI is due to additional effects of different bone marrow cell subsets secreting factors helping the repairing function EPC mediated. To this regard, the most promising approach in the clinical practice may be the evaluation of the administration of mobilizing factors (ie EPO) in order to induce an increase in the number of circulating EPCs and possible "accessory cells" that will home to the site of the vascular injury. On the other hand, further studies aimed to identify EPCs may allow to discover soluble factors exclusively produced by these cells, paving the way for new therapeutic approaches.

ACKNOWLEDGMENT

The contribution of Dott. Maurizio Ferrario, Cardiology Department, IRCCS Policlinico San Matteo, and of Dott. Giovanni Barosi, head of the Laboratory of Clinical Epidemiology, IRCCS Policlinico San Matteo, is warmly acknowledged. We also thank Dott. Valentina Meli for the excellent technical assistance.

This work was supported by grants from IRCCS Policlinico San Matteo (Ricerca Corrente #80520 and #80545).

REFERENCES

[1] Asahara T, Murohara T, Sullivan A, Silver M, van der Zee R, Li T, Witzenbichler B, Schatteman G, Isner JM. Isolation of putative progenitor endothelial cells for angiogenesis. *Science 275*:964-967, 1997.

[2] Stump MM, Jordan GL Jr, Debakey ME, Halpert B. Endothelium grown from circulating blood on isolated intravascular Dacron hub. *Am J Pathol 43*:361-367, 1963.

[3] Hladovec J, Prerovsky I, Stanek V, Fabian J. Circulating endothelial cells in acute myocardial infarction and angina pectoris. *Klin Wochenschr 56*: 1033- 1036, 1978.

[4] George F, Poncelet P, Laurent JC, Massot O, Arnoux D, Lequeux N, Ambrosi P, Chicheportiche C, Sampol J. Cytofluorometric detection of human endothelial cells in whole blood using S-Endo 1 monoclonal antibody. *J Immunol Methods 139(1*):65-75, 1991.

[5] George F, Brisson C, Poncelet P, Laurent JC, Massot O, Arnoux D, Ambrosi P, Klein-Soyer C, Cazenave JP, Sampol J . Rapid isolation of human endothelial cells from whole blood using S-Endo1 monoclonal antibody coupled to immuno-magnetic beads: demonstration of endothelial injury after angioplasty. *Thromb Haemost 67(1):*147-153,1992.

[6] Rafii S, Lyden D. Therapeutic stem and progenitor cell transplantation for organ vascularization and regeneration. *Nat Med 9*:702-712, 2003.

[7] Carmeliet P. Angiogenesis in health and disease. *Nat Med 9(6):*653-660, 2003.

[8] Coffin JD, Harrison J, Schwartz S, Heimark R. Angioblast differentiation and morphogenesis of the vascular endothelium in the mouse embryo. *Dev Biol 148(1):*51-62, 1991.

[9] Flamme I, Breier G, Risau W. Vascular endothelial growth factor (VEGF) and VEGF receptor 2 (flk-1) are expressed during vasculogenesis and vascular differentiation in the quail embryo. *Dev Biol 169(2):*699-712, 1995.

[10] Ziegler BL, Valtieri M, Porada GA, De Maria R, Muller R, Masella B, Gabbianelli M, Caszella I, Pelosi E, Bock T, Zanjani ED, Peschle C. KDR receptor: a key marker definig hematopoietic stem cells. *Science 285:*1553-1558, 1999.

[11] Peichev M, Nayer AJ, Pereira D, Zhu Z, Lane WJ, Williams M, Oz MC, Hicklin DJ, Witte L, Moore MA, Rafii S. Expression of VEGFR-2 and AC133 by circulating human CD34(+) cells identifies a population of functional endothelial precursors. *Blood 95(3):*952-958, 2000.

[12] Gehling UM, Ergun S, Schumacher U, Wagener C, Pantel K, Otte M, Schuch G, Schafhausen P, Mende T, Kilic N, Kluge K, Schafer B, Hossfeld DK, Fielder W. In vitro differentiation of endothelial cells from AC133-positive progenitor cells. *Blood 95(10)*:3106-3112, 2000.

[13] Pelosi E, Valtieri M, Coppola S, Botta R, Gabbianelli M, Lulli V, Marziali G, Masella B, Muller R, Sgadari C, Testa U, Bonanno G, Peschle C. Identification of the hemangioblast in postnatal life. *Blood 100(9)*:3203-3208, 2002.

[14] Choi K, Kennedy M, Kazarov A, Papadimitriou JC, Keller G. A common precursor for hematopoietic and endothelial cells. *Development (4)*:725-732, 1998.

[15] Cogle CR, Wainman DA, Jorgensen ML, Guthrie SM, Mames RN, Scott EW. Adult human hematopoietic cells provide functional hemangioblast activity. *Blood 103(1)*:133-135, 2004.

[16] Mikkola HK, Orkin SH. The search for the hemangioblast. *J Hematother Stem Cell Res 11(1)*:9-17, 2002.

[17] Auerbach R, Huang H, Lu L. Hematopoietic stem cells in the mouse embryonic yolk sac. *Stem Cells 14(3):*269-280, 1996.

[18] Eichmann A, Corbel C, Nataf V, Vaigot P, breant C, Le Douarin NM. Ligand-dependent development of the endothelial and hematopoietic lineages from embryonic mesodermal cells expressing vascular endothclail growth factor receptor 2. *Proc Natl Acad Sci USA 94*: 5141-5146, 1997.

[19] Shalaby F, Rossant J, Yamaguchi TP, Gertsenstein M, Wu XF, Breitman ML, Schuh AC. Failure of blood-island formation and vasculogenesis in Flk-1-deficient mice. *Nature 376*:62-66, 1995.

[20] Orlic D, Kajstura J, Chimenti S, Jakoniuk I, Anderson SM, Li B, Pickel J, McKay R, Nadal-Ginard B, Bodine DM, Leri A, Anversa P. Bone marrow cells regenerate infarcted myocardium. *Nature 410*:701-705, 2001.

[21] Orlic D, Kajstura J, Chimenti S, Limana F, Jakoniuk I, Quaini F, Nadal-Ginard B, Bodine DM, Leri A, Anversa P. Mobilized bone marrow cells repair the infarcted heart, improving function and survival. *Proc Natl Acad Sci U S A 410*:701-705, 2001.

[22] Li TS, Hamano K, Nishida M, Hayashi M, Ito H, Mikamo A, Matsuzaki M. CD117+ stem cells play a key role in therapeutic angiogenesis induced by bone marrow cell implantation. *Am J Physiol Heart Circ Physiol 285(3)*:H931-H937, 2003.

[23] Orlic D, Fischer R, Nishikawa S, Nienhuis AW, Bodine DM. Purification and characterization of heterogeneous pluripotent hematopoietic stem cell populations expressing high levels of c-kit receptor. *Blood 82(3)*:762-770, 1993.

[24] Kocher AA, Schuster MD, Szabolcs MJ, Takuma S, Burkhoff D, Wang J, Homma S, Edwards NM, Itescu S. Neovascularization of ischemic myocardium by human bone-marrow-derived angioblasts prevents cardiomyocyte apoptosis, reduces remodeling and improves cardiac function. *Nat Med 7(4)*:430-436, 2001.

[25] Urbich C, Dimmeler S. Endothelial progenitor cells: characterization and role in vascular biology. *Circ Res 95(4):*343-353, 2004.

[26] Hristov M, Weber C. Endothelial progenitor cells:characterization, pathophysiology, and possible clinical relevance. *J Cell Mol Med 8;4*:498-508, 2004.

[27] Lin Y, Weisdorf DJ, Solovey A, Hebbel RP. Origins of circulating endothelial cells and endothgelail outgrowth from blood. *J Clin Invest 105*:71-77, 2000.

[28] Ingram DA, Mead LE, Tanaka H, Meade V, Fenoglio A, Mortell K, Pollok K, Ferkowicz MJ, Gilley D, Yoder MC. Identification of a novel hierarchy of endothelial progenitor cells using human peripheral and umbilical cord blood. *Blood 104(9)*:2752-2760, 2004.

[29] Bessler M. Endothelial progenitor cells: reporting for duty. *Blood 104*: 2616-2617, 2004.

[30] Shi Q, Rafii S, Wu MH, Wijelath ES, Yu C, Ishida A, Fujita Y, Kothari S, Mohle R, Sauvage LR, Moore MA, Storb RF, Hammond WP. Evidence for circulating bone marrow-derived endothelial cells. *Blood 92(2)*:362-367, 1998.

[31] Ito H, Rovira II, Bloom ML, Takeda K, Ferrans VJ, Quyyumi AA, Finkel T. Endothelial progenitor cells as putative targets for angiostatin. *Cancer Res 59(23)*:5875-5877, 1999.

[32] Schmeisser A, Garlichs CD, Zhang H, Eskafi S, Graffy C, Ludwig J, Strasser RH, Daniel WG. Monocytes coexpress endothelial and macrophagocytic lineage markers and form cord-like structures in Matrigel under angiogenic conditions. *Cardiovasc Res 49(3)*:671-680, 2001.

[33] Rehman J, Li J, Orschell CM, March KL. Peripheral blood "endothelial progenitor cells"are derived from monocyte/macrophages and secrete angiogenic growth factors. *Circulation 107*:1164-1169, 2003.

[34] Gulati R, Jevremovic D, Peterson TE, Chatterjee S, Shah V, Vile RG, Simari RD. Diverse origin and function of cells with endothelial phenotype obtained from adult human blood. *Circ Res 93(11)*:1023-1025, 2003.

[35] Urbich C, Heeschen C, Aicher A, Dernbach E, Zeiher AM, Dimmeler S. Relevance of monocytic features for neovascularization capacity of circulating endothelial progenitor cells. *Circulation 108(20)*:2511-2516, 2003.

[36] Zhao Y, Glesne D, Huberman E,. A human peripheral blood monocyte subset acts as pluripotent stem cell. *Proc Natl Acad Sci USA 100*:2426-2431, 2003.

[37] Romagnani P, Annunziato F, Liotta F, Lazzeri E, Mazzinghi B, Frosali F, Cosmi L, Maggi L, Lasagni L, Scheffold A, Kruger M, Dimmeler S, Marra F, Gensini G, Maggi E, Romagnani S. CD14+CD34low Cells With Stem Cell Phenotypic and Functional Features Are the Major Source of Circulating Endothelial Progenitors. *Circ Res 97*:0-0, 2005.

[38] Hillebrands JL, Klatter FA, van Dijk WD, Rozing J. Bone marrow does not contribute substantially to endothelial-cell replacement in transplant arteriosclerosis. *Nat Med 8(3)*:194-195, 2002.

[39] Reyes M, Dudek A, Jahagirdar B, Koodie L, Marker PH, Verfaillie CM. Origin of endothelial progenitors in human postnatal bone marrow. *J Clin Invest 109(3)*:337-346, 2002.

[40] Jackson KA, Majka SM, Wang H, Pocius J, Hartley CJ, Majesky MW, Entman ML, Michael LH, Hirschi KK, Goodell MA. Regeneration of ischemic cardiac muscle and vascular endothelium by adult stem cells. *J Clin Invest 107(11)*:1395-1402, 2001.

[41] Quirici N, Soligo D, Caneva L, Servida F, Bossolasco P, Deliliers GL. Differentiation and expansion of endothelial cells from human bone marrow CD133(+) cells. *Br J Haematol 115(1)*:186-194, 2001.

[42] Lapidot T, Petit I. Current understanding of stem cell mobilization: the roles of chemokines, proteolytic enzymes, adhesion molecules, cytokines, and stromal cells. *Exp Hematol 30(9):*973-981, 2002.

[43] Heissig B, Hattori K, Dias S, Friedrich M, Ferris B, Hackett NR, Crystal RG, Besmer P, Lyden D, Moore MA, Werb Z, Rafii S. Recruitment of stem and progenitor cells from the bone marrow niche requires MMP-9 mediated release of kit-ligand. *Cell 109(5)*:625-637, 2002.

[44] Aicher A, Heeschen C, Mildner-Rihm C, Urbich C, Ihling C, Technau-Ihling K, Zeiher AM, Dimmeler S. Essential role of endothelial nitric oxide synthase for mobilization of stem and progenitor cells. *Nat Med 9(11):*1370-1376, 2003.

[45] Lee SH, Wolf PL, Escudero R, Deutsch R, Jamieson SW, Thistlethwaite PA. Early expression of angiogenesis factors in acute myocardial ischemia and infarction. *N Eng J Med 342*:626-633, 2000.

[46] Ceradini DJ, Kulkarni AR, Callaghan MJ, Tepper OM, Bastidas N, Kleinman ME, Capla JM, Galiano RD, Levine JP, Gurtner GC. Progenitor cell trafficking is regulated by hypoxic gradients through HIF-1 induction of SDF-1. *Nat Med 10(8)*:858-864, 2004.

[47] Heeschen C, Aicher A, Lehmann R, Fichtlscherer S, Vasa M, Urbich C, Mildner-Rihm C, Martin H, Zeiher AM, Dimmeler S. Erythropoietin is a potent physiologic stimulus for endothelial progenitor cell mobilization. *Blood 102(4)*:1340-1346, 2003.

[48] Bahlmann FH, De Groot K, Spandau JM, Landry AL, Hertel B, Duckert T, Boehm SM, Menne J, Haller H, Fliser D. Erythropoietin regulates endothelial progenitor cells. *Blood 103(3)*:921-926, 2004.

[49] Kalka C, Masuda H, Takahashi T, Gordon R, Tepper O, Gravereaux E, Pieczek A, Iwaguro H, Hayashi SI, Isner JM, Asahara T. Vascular endothelial growth factor(165) gene transfer augments circulating endothelial progenitor cells in human subjects. *Circ Res 86(12)*:1198-1202, 2000.

[50] Llevadot J, Murasawa S, Kureishi Y, Uchida S, Masuda H, Kawamoto A, Walsh K, Isner JM, Asahara T. HMG-CoA reductase inhibitor mobilizes bone marrow--derived endothelial progenitor cells. *J Clin Invest 108(3):*399-405, 2001.

[51] Dimmeler S, Aicher A, Vasa M, Mildner-Rihm C, Adler K, Tiemann M, Rutten H, Fichtlscherer S, Martin H, Zeiher AM. HMG-CoA reductase inhibitors (statins) increase endothelial progenitor cells via the PI 3-kinase/Akt pathway. *J Clin Invest 108(3)*:391-397, 2001.

[52] Vasa M, Fichtlscherer S, Adler K, Aicher A, Martin H, Zeiher AM, Dimmeler S. Increase in circulating endothelial progenitor cells by statin therapy in patients with stable coronary artery disease. *Circulation 103(24)*:2885-2890, 2001.

[53] Davignon J, Ganz P. Role of endothelial dysfunction in atherosclerosis. *Circulation 109(23 Suppl 1)*:III27-32, 2004.

[54] Hristov M, Weber C Endothelial progenitor cells:characterization, pathophysiology, and possible clinical relevance. *J Cell Mol Med 8;4*:498-508, 2004.

[55] Ingram DA, Caplice NM, Yoder MC. Unresolved questions, changing definitions, and novel paradigms for defining endothelial progenitor cells. *Blood* 2005.

[56] Gussin HAE, Bischoff FZ, Hoffman R, Elias S. Endothelial precursor cells in the peripheral blood of pregnant women. *J Soc Gynecol Investig 9*:357-361, 2002.

[57] Sugawara J, Mitsui-Saito M, Hoshiai T, Hayashi C, Kimura Y, Okamura K. Circulating endotheial progenitor cells during human pregnancy. *J Clin Endocrinol Metab 90*:1845-1848, 2005.

[58] Strehlow K, Werner N, Berweiler J, Link A, Dirnagl U, Priller J, Laufs K, Ghaeni L, Milosevic M, Bohm M, Nickenig G. Estrogen increases bone marrow derived endothelial progenitor cell production and diminishes neointima formation. *Circulation 107*:3059-3065, 2003.

[59] Iwakura A, Luedemann C, Shastry S, Hanley A, Kearney M, Aikawa R, Isner JM, Asahara T, Losordo DW. Estrogen-mediated, endothelial nitric oxide synthase-dependent mobilization of bone marrow- derived endothelial progenitor cells contributes to reendothelization after arterial injury. *Circulation 108*:3115-3121, 2003.

[60] Gordon JD, Shifren JL, Foulk RA, Taylor RN, Jaffe RB. Angiogenesis in the human female reproductive tract. *Obset Gynecol Surv 50*:688-697, 1995.

[61] Maas JWM, Groothuis PG, Dunselman GAJ, de Goeij AFPM, Struyker Boudier HAJ, Evers JLH. Endometrial angiogenesis throughout the human menstrual cycle. *Hum Reprod 16(8)*:1557-1561, 2001.

[62] Brenner RM, Nayak NR, Slayden OD, Critchley HO, Kelly RW. Premenstrual and menstrual changes in the macaque and human endometrium: relevance to endometriosis. *Ann N Y Acad Sci 955*:60-74, 2002.

[63] Nayak NR, Brenner RM. Vascular proliferation and vascular endothelial growth factor expression in the rhesus macaque endometrium. *J Clin Endocrinol Metab 87(4)*:1845-1855, 2002.

[64] McIlhenny C, George WD, Doughty JC. A comparison of serum and plasma levels of vascular endothelial growth factor during the menstrual cycle in healthy female volunteers. *Br J Cancer 86(11)*:1786-1789, 2002.

[65] Print C, Valtola R, Evans A, Lessan K, Malik S, Smith S. Soluble factors from human endometrium promote angiogenesis and regulate the endothelial cell transcriptome. *Hum Reprod 19(10)*:2356-2366, 2004.

[66] Gill M, Dias S, Hattori K, Rivera ML, Hicklin D, Witte L, Girardi L, Yurt R, Himel H, Rafii S. Vascular trauma induces rapid but transient mobilization of VEGFR-2(+)AC133(+) endothelial precursor cells. *Circ Res 88*:167-174, 2001.

[67] Stewart KJ. Exercise training and the cardiovascular consequence of type 2 diabetes and hypertension: plausible mechanisms for improving cardiovascular health. *JAMA 288*:1622-1631, 2002.

[68] Wannamethee SG, Lowe GD, Whincup PH, Rumley A, Walker M, Lennon L. Physical activity and hemostatic and inflammatory variables in elderly men. *Circulation 105*:1785-1790, 2002.

[69] Kojda G, Cheng YC, Burchfield J, Harrison DG. Dysfunctional regulation of endothelial nitric oxide synthase (eNOS) expression in response to exercise in mice lacking one eNOS gene. *Circulation 103*:2839-2844, 2001.

[70] Fukai T, Siegfried MR, Ushio-Fukai M, Cheng Y, Kojda G, Harrison DG. Regulation of the vascular extracellular superoxide dismutase by nitric oxide and exercise training. *J Clin Invest 105*:1631-1639, 2000.

[71] Maisel AS, Knowlton KU, Fowler P, Rearden A, Ziegler MG, Motulsky HJ, Insel PA, Michel MC. Adrenergic control of circulating lymphocyte subpopulations. Effects of

congestive heart failure, dynamic exercise, and terbutaline treatment. *J Clin Invest 85*:462-467, 1990.

[72] Barret AJ, Longhurst P, Sneath P, Watson JG. Mobilization of CFU-C by exercise and ACTH induced stress in man. *Exp Hematol 6*:590-594, 1978.

[73] Laufs U, Werner N, Link A, Endres M, Wassmann S, Jurgens K, Miche E, Bohm M, Nickenig G. Physical training increases endothelial progenitor cells, inhibits neointima formation, and enhances angiogenesis. *Circulation 109(2)*:220-226, 2004.

[74] Rehman J, Li J, Parvathaneni L, Karlsson G, Panchal VR, Temm CJ, Mahenthiran J, March KL. Exercise acutely increases circulating endothelial progenitor cells and monocyte-/macrophage-derived angiogenic cells. *J Am Coll Cardiol 43(12)*:2314-2318, 2004.

[75] Niebauer J, Cooke JP. Cardiovascular effects of exercise: role of endothelial shear stress. *J Am coll Cardiol 28*:1652-1660, 1996.

[76] Bonsignore MR, Morici G, Santoro A, Pagano M, Cascio L, Bonanno A, Abate P, Mirabella F, Profita M, Insalaco G, Gioia M, Vignola AM, Majolino I, Testa U, Hogg JC. Circulating hematopoietic progenitor cells in runners. *J Appl Physiol 93(5)*:1691-1697, 2002.

[77] Ciulla MM, Giorgetti A, Lazzari L, Cortiana M, Silvestris I, Annoni G, De Asmundis C, Fiore AV, Montelatici E, Paliotti R, Magrini F, Rebulla P, Cortelezzi A. High-altitude trekking in the Himalayas increases the activity of circulating endothelial cells. *Am J Hematol 79(1)*:76-78, 2005.

[78] Adams V, Lenk K, Linke A, Lenz D, Erbs S, Sandri M, Tarnok A, Gielen S, Emmrich F, Schuler G, Hambrecht R. Increase of circulating endothelial progenitor cells in patients with coronary artery disease after exercise-induced ischemia. *Arterioscler Thromb Vasc Biol 24(4)*:684-690, 2004.

[79] Sutherland DR, Anderson L, Keeney M, Nayar R, Chin-Yee I. The ISHAGE guidelines for CD34+ cell determination by flow cytometry. International Society of Hematotherapy and Graft Engineering. *J Hematother 5(3)*:213-226, 1996.

[80] Edelberg JM, Tang L, Hattori K, Lyden D, Rafii S. Young adult bone marrow-derived endothelial precursor cells restore aging-impaired cardiac angiogenic function. *Circ Res 90(10)*:E89-93, 2002.

[81] Murayama T, Kalka C, Silver M, Ma H, Asahara T. Aging impairs therapeutic contribution of human endothelial progenitor cells to postnatal neovascularization. *Circulation 104 Suppl II*:II68, 2001.

[82] Hill JM, Zalos G, Halcox JPJ, Schenke WH, Waclawiw MA, Quyyumi AA, Finkel T. Circulating endothelial progenitor cells, vascular function, and cardiovascular risk. *NEJM 7*:593-600, 2003.

[83] Scheubel RJ, Zorn H, Silber RE, Kuss O, Morawietz H, Holtz J, Simm A. Age-dependent depression in circulating endothelial progenitor cells in patients undergoing coronary artery bypass grafting. *J Am Coll Cardiol 42(12)*:2073-2080, 2003.

[84] Heiss C, Keymel S, Niesler U, Ziemann J, Kelm M, Kalka C. Impaired progenitor cell activity in age-related endothelial dysfunction. *J Am Coll Cardiol 45(9)*:1441-1448, 2005.

[85] Van Zant G, Liang Y. The role of stem cells in aging. *Exp Hematol 31*:659-672, 2003.

[86] Mc Veigh GE, Lemay L, Morgan D, Cohn JN. Effects of long-term cigarette smoking on endothelium-dependent responses in humans. *Am J Cardiol 78(6)*:668-72, 1996.

[87] Kondo T, Hayashi M, Takeshita K, Numaguchi Y, Kobayashi K, Iino S, Inden Y, Murohara T. Smoking cessation rapidly increases circulating progenitor cells in peripheral blood in chronic smokers. *Arterioscler Thromb Vasc Biol 24(8)*:1442-1447, 2004.

[88] Vasa M, Fichtlscherer S, Aicher A, Adler K, Urbich C, Martin H, Zeiher AM, Dimmeler S. Number and migratory activity of circulating endothelial progenitor cells inversely correlate with risk factors for coronary artery disease. *Circ Res 89(1)*:E1-E7, 2001.

[89] Schmidt-Lucke C, Rossig L, Fichtlscherer S, Vasa M, Britten M, Kamper U, Dimmeler S, Zeiher AM. Reduced number of circulating endothelial progenitor cells predicts future cardiovascular events: proof of concept for the clinical importance of endogenous vascular repair. *Circulation 111(22)*:2981-2987, 2005.

[90] Sandri M, Adams V, Gielen S, Linke A, Lenk K, Krankel N, Lenz D, Erbs S, Scheinert D, Wilhelm Mohr F, Schuler G, Hambrecht R . Effects of exercise and ischemia on mobilization and functional activation of blood-derived progenitor cells in patients with ischemic syndromes: results of 3 randomized studies. *Circulation 111(25)*:3391-3399, 2005.

[91] Hambrecht R, Wolf S, Gielen S, Linke A, Hofer J, Erbs S, Schoene N, Schuler G. Effect of exercise on coronary endothelial function in patients with coronary artery disease. *N Engl J Med 342(7)*:454-460, 2000.

[92] Hambrecht R, Walther C, Mobius-Winkler S, Gielen S, Linke A, Conradi K, Erbs S, Kluge R, Kendziorra K, Sabri O, Sick P, Schuler G. Percutaneous coronary angioplasty compared with exercise training in patients with stable coronary artery disease: a randomized trial. *Circulation 109(11)*:1371-1378, 2004.

[93] Shintani S, Murohara T, Ikeda H, Ueno T, Honma T, Katoh A, Sasaki K, Shimada T, Oike Y, Imaizumi T. Mobilization of endothelial progenitor cells in patients with acute myocardial infarction. *Circulation 103(23)*:2776-2779, 2001.

[94] Massa M, Rosti V, Ferrario M, Campanelli R, Ramajoli I, Rosso R, De Ferrari GM, Ferlini M, Goffredo L, Bertoletti A, Klersy C, Pecci A, Moratti R, Tavazzi L. Increased circulating hematopoietic and endothelial progenitor cells in the early phase of acute myocardial infarction. *Blood 105(1)*:199-206, 2005.

[95] Leone AM, Rutella S, Bonanno G, Abbate A, Rebuzzi AG, Giovannini S, Lombardi M, Galiuto L, Liuzzo G, Andreotti F, Lanza GA, Contemi AM, Leone G, Crea F. Mobilization of bone marrow-derived stem cells after myocardial infarction and left ventricular function. *Eur Heart J 26(12)*:1196-1204, 2005.

[96] Wojakowski W, Tendera M, Michalowska A, Majka M, Kucia M, Maslankiewicz K, Wyderka R, Ochala A, Ratajczak MZ. Mobilization of CD34/CXCR4+, CD34 /CD117+, c-met+ stem cells, and mononuclear cells expressing early cardiac, muscle, and endothelial markers into peripheral blood in patients with acute myocardial infarction. *Circulation 110(20)*:3213-3220, 2004.

[97] Wolf D, Rumpold H, Gunsilius E. Correspondence. Circulation 111:e307-e308, 2005.

[98] Tepper OM, Galiano RD, Capla JM, Kalka C, Gagne PJ, Jacobowitz GR, Levine JP, Gurtner GC. Human endothelial progenitor cells from type II diabetics exhibit impaired proliferation, adhesion, and incorporation into vascular structures. *Circulation 106(22)*:2781-2786, 2002.

[99] Loomans CJ, de Koning EJ, Staal FJ, Rookmaaker MB, Verseyden C, de Boer HC, Verhaar MC, Braam B, Rabelink TJ, van Zonneveld AJ. Endothelial progenitor cell dysfunction: a novel concept in the pathogenesis of vascular complications of type 1 diabetes. *Diabetes 53(1)*:195-199, 2004.

[100] Fadini GP, Miorin M, Facco M, Bonamico S, Baesso I, Grego F, Menegolo M, de Kreutzenberg SV, Tiengo A, Agostini C, Avogaro A. Circulating endothelial progenitor cells are reduced in peripheral vascular complications of type 2 diabetes mellitus. *J Am Coll Cardiol 45(9)*:1449-1457, 2005.

[101] Baumgartner-Parzer SM, Wagner L, Pettermann M, Grillari J, Gessl A, Waldhausl W. Hight glucose-triggered apoptosis in cultured endothelial cells. *Diabetes 44*:1323-1327, 1995.

[102] Barosi G. Myelofibrosis with myeloid metaplasia: diagnostic definition and prognostic classification for clinical studies and treatment guidelines. *J Clin Oncol (7)*: 2954-2970, 1999.

[103] Tefferi A. Myelofibrosis with myeloid metaplasia. *N Engl J Med 342(17)*:1255-1265, 2000.

[104] Barosi G, Viarengo G, Pecci A, Rosti V, Piaggio G, Marchetti M, Frassoni F. Diagnostic and clinical relevance of the number of circulating CD34(+) cells in myelofibrosis with myeloid metaplasia. *Blood 98(12)*:3249-3255, 2001.

[105] Mesa RA, Hanson CA, Rajkumar SV, Schroeder G, Tefferi A. Evaluation and clinical correlations of bone marrow angiogenesis in myelofibrosis with myeloid metaplasia. *Blood (96)*: 3374-3380, 2000.

[106] Barosi G, Rosti V, Massa M, Viarengo GL, Pecci A, Necchi V, Ramajoli I, Campanelli R, Marchetti M, Bazzan M, Magrini U. Spleen neoangiogenesis in patients with myelofibrosis with myeloid metaplasia. *Br J Haematol (124)*: 618-625, 2004.

[107] Massa M, Rosti V, Ramajoli I, Campanelli R, Pecci A, Viarengo G, Meli V, Marchetti M, Hoffman R, Barosi G. Circulating CD34+,CD133+, and vascular endothelial growth factor receptor 2-positive endothelial progenitor cells in myelofibrosis with myeloid metaplasia. *J Clin Oncol (24)*:5688-5695, 2005.

[108] Vacca A, Ribatti D, Roncali l, Ranieri G, Serio G, Silvestris F, Dammacco F. Bone marrow angiogenesis and progression in multiple myeloma. *Br J Haematol 87(3)*:503-8, 1994.

[109] Rajkumar SV, Mesa RA, Fonseca R, Schroeder G, Plevak MF, Dispenzieri A, Lacy MQ, Lust JA, Witzig TE, Gertz MA, Kyle RA, Russell SJ, Greipp PR. Bone marrow angiogenesis in 400 patients with monoclonal gammopathy of undetermined significance, multiple myeloma, and primary amyloidosis. *Clin Cancer Res 8(7)*:2210-2216, 2002.

[110] Pruneri G, Ponzoni M, Ferreri AJ, Decarli N, Tresoldi M, Raggi F, Baldessari C, Freschi M, Baldini L, Goldaniga M, Neri A, Carboni N, Bertolini F, Viale G. Microvessel density, a surrogate marker of angiogenesis, is significantly related to survival in multiple myeloma patients. *Br J Haematol 118(3)*:817-820, 2002.

[111] Sezer O, Niemoller K, Kaufmann O, Eucker J, Jakob C, Zavrski I, Possinger K. Decrease of bone marrow angiogenesis in myeloma patients achieving a remission after chemotherapy. *Eur J Haematol 66(4)*:238-244, 2001.

[112] Rajkumar SV, Fonseca R, Witzig TE, Gertz MA, Greipp PR. Bone marrow angiogenesis in patients achieving complete response after stem cell transplantation for multiple myeloma. *Leukemia 13(3)*:469-472, 1999.

[113] Zhang H, Vakil V, Braunstein M, Smith EL, Maroney J, Chen L, Dai K, Berenson JR, Hussain MM, Klueppelberg U, Norin AJ, Akman HO, Ozcelik T, Batuman OA. Circulating endothelial progenitor cells in multiple myeloma: implications and significance. *Blood 105(8)*:3286-3294, 2005.

[114] Vacca A, Ria R, Semeraro F, Marchionne F, Coluccia M, Boccarelli A, Scavelli C, Nico B, Gernone A, Battelli F, Tabilio A, Guidolin D, Petrucci MT, Ribatti D Dammacco F. Endothelial cells in the bone marrow of patients with multiple myeloma. *Blood 102(9)*:3340-3348, 2003.

[115] Stamm C, Westphal B, Kleine HD, Petzsch M, Kittner C, Klinge H, Schumichen C, Nienaber CA, Freund M, Steinhoff G. Autologous bone-marrow stem-cell transplantation for myocardial regeneration. *Lancet 361(9351)*:45-46, 2003.

[116] Strauer BE, Brehm M, Zeus T, Kostering M, Hernandez A, Sorg RV, Kogler G, Wernet P. Repair of infarcted myocardium by autologous intracoronary mononuclear bone marrow cell transplantation in humans. *Circulation 106(15)*:1913-1918, 2002.

[117] Tse HF, Kwong YL, Chan JK, Lo G, Ho CL, Lau CP. Angiogenesis in ischaemic myocardium by intramyocardial autologous bone marrow mononuclear cell implantation. *Lancet 361(9351)*:47-49, 2003.

[118] Assmus B, Schachinger V, Teupe C, Britten M, Lehmann R, Dobert N, Grunwald F, Aicher A, Urbich C, Martin H, Hoelzer D, Dimmeler S, Zeiher AM. Transplantation of Progenitor Cells and Regeneration Enhancement in Acute Myocardial Infarction (TOPCARE-AMI). *Circulation 106(24)*:3009-3017, 2002.

[119] Britten MB, Abolmaali ND, Assmus B, Lehmann R, Honold J, Schmitt J, Vogl TJ, Martin H, Schachinger V, Dimmeler S, Zeiher AM. Infarct remodeling after intracoronary progenitor cell treatment in patients with acute myocardial infarction (TOPCARE-AMI): mechanistic insights from serial contrast-enhanced magnetic resonance imaging. *Circulation 108(18)*:2212-2218, 2003.

[120] Schachinger V, Assmus B, Britten MB, Honold J, Lehmann R, Teupe C, Abolmaali ND, Vogl TJ, Hofmann WK, Martin H, Dimmeler S, Zeiher AM. Transplantation of progenitor cells and regeneration enhancement in acute myocardial infarction: final one-year results of the TOPCARE-AMI Trial. *J Am Coll Cardiol 44(8)*:1690-1699, 2004.

[121] Wollert KC, Meyer GP, Lotz J, Ringes-Lichtenberg S, Lippolt P, Breidenbach C, Fichtner S, Korte T, Horning B, Messinger D, Arseniev L, Hertenstein B, Ganser A, Drexler H. Intracoronary autologous bone-marrow cell transfer after myocardial infarction: the BOOST randomised controlled clinical trial. *Lancet 364(9429)*:141-148, 2004.

[122] Fernandez-Aviles F, San Roman JA, Garcia-Frade J, Fernandez ME, Penarrubia MJ, de la Fuente L, Gomez-Bueno M, Cantalapiedra A, Fernandez J, Gutierrez O, Sanchez PL, Hernandez C, Sanz R, Garcia-Sancho J, Sanchez A. Experimental and clinical regenerative capability of human bone marrow cells after myocardial infarction. *Circ Res 95(7)*:742-748, 2004.

[123] Tateishi-YuyamaE, Matsubara H, Murohara T, Ikeda U, Shintani S, Masaki H, Amano K, Kishimoto Y, Yoshimoto K, Akashi H, Shimada K, Iwasaka T, Imaizumi T.

Therapeutic angiogenesis using cell transplantation (TACT) study investigators. Therapeutic angiogenesis for patients with limb ischaemia by autologous transplantation of bone-marrow cells: a pilot study and a randomised controlled trial. *Lancet 360(9331)*:427-435, 2002.

[124] Dimmeler S, Vasa-Nicotera M. Aging of progenitor cells: limitation for regenerative capacity? *J Am Coll Cardiol 42(12)*:2081-2082, 2003.

[125] Orlic D, Kajstura J, Chimenti S, Limana F, Jakoniuk I, Quaini F, Nadal-Ginard B, Bodine DM, Leri A, Anversa P. Mobilized bone marrow cells repair the infarcted heart, improving function and survival. *Proc Natl Acad Sci U S A 410*:701-705, 2001.

[126] De Falco E, Porcelli D, Torella AR, Straino S, Iachininoto MG, Orlandi A, Truffa S, Biglioli P, Napolitano M, Capogrossi MC, Pesce M. SDF-1 involvement in endothelial phenotype and ischemia-induced recruitment of bone marrow progenitor cells. *Blood 104(12)*:3472-3482, 2004.

[127] Kang HJ, Kim HS, Zhang SY, Park KW, Cho HJ, Koo BK, Kim YJ, Soo Lee D, Sohn DW, Han KS, Oh BH, Lee MM, Park YB. Effects of intracoronary infusion of peripheral blood stem-cells mobilised with granulocyte-colony stimulating factor on left ventricular systolic function and restenosis after coronary stenting in myocardial infarction: the MAGIC cell randomised clinical trial. *Lancet 363(9411)*:751-6, 2004.

[128] Parsa CJ, Matsumoto A, Kim J, Riel RU, Pascal LS, Walton GB, Thompson RB, Petrofski JA, Annex BH, Stamler JS, Koch WJ. A novel protective effect of erythropoietin in the infarcted heart. *J Clin Invest 2003 112(7)*:999-1007.

[129] Ehrenreich H, Hasselblatt M, Dembowski C, Cepek L, Lewczuk P, Stiefel M, Rustenbeck HH, Breiter N, Jacob S, Knerlich F, Bohn M, Poser W, Ruther E, Kochen M, Geffeler O, Gleiter C, Wessel TC, De Ryck M, Itri L, Prange H, Cerami A, Brines M, Siren AL. Erythropoietin therapy for acute stroke is both safe and beneficial. *Mol Med 8(8)*:495-505, 2002.

[130] Casadevall N, Nataf J, Viron B, Kolta A, Kiladjian JJ, Martin-Dupont P, Michaud P, Papo t, Ugo V, Teyssandier I, Varet B, Mayeux P. Pure red-cell aplasia and antierythropoietin antibodies in patients treated with recombinant erythropoietin. *N Engl J Med 346(7)*:469-475, 2002.

[131] Macdougall IC, Hutton RD, Cavill I, Coles GA, Williams JD. Poor response to treatment of renal anaemia with erythropoietin corrected by iron given intravenously. *BMJ 299(6692)*:157-158, 1989.

[132] Bennet CL, Luminari S, Nissenson AR, Tallman MS, Klinge SA, McWilliams N, McKoy JM, Kim B, Lyons EA, Trifilio SM, Raisch DW, Evens AM, Kuzel TM, Schumock GT, Belknap SM, Locatelli F, Rosset J, Casadevall N. Pure red-cell aplasia and epoetin therapy. *N Engl J Med 351(14)*:1403-1408, 2004.

[133] Leist M, Ghezzi P, Grasso G, Bianchi R, Villa P, Fratelli M, Savino C, Bianchi M, Nielsen J, Gerwien J, Kallunki P, Larsen AK, Helboe L, Christensen S, Pedersen LO, Nielsen M, Torup L, Sager T, Sfacteria A, Erbayraktar S, Erbayraktar Z, Gokmen N, Yilmaz O, Cerami-Hand C, Xie QW, Coleman T, Cerami A, Brines M. Derivatives of erythropoietin that are tissue protective but not erythropoietic. *Science 305(5681)*: 239-242, 2004.

[134] Jubinsky PT, Krijanovski OI, Nathan DG, Tavernier J, Sieff CA. The beta chain of the interleukin-3 receptor functionally associates with the erythropoietin receptor. *Blood 90*:1867-1873, 1997.

[135] D'Andrea RJ, Gonda TJ. A model for assembly and activation of the GM-CSF, IL-3 and IL-5 receptors: insights from activated mutants of the common beta subunit. *Exp Hematol 28*:231-243, 2000.

[136] Brines M, Grasso G, Fiordaliso F, Sfacteria A, Ghezzi P, Fratelli M, Latini R, Xie QW, Smart J, Su-Rick CJ, Pobre E, Diaz D, Gomez D, Hand C, Coleman T, Cerami A. Erythropoietin mediates tissue protection through an erythropoietin and common beta-subunit heteroreceptor. *Proc Natl Acad Sci U S A 101(41)*:14907-1412, 2004.

In: Perspectives in Stem Cell Research ISBN: 978-1-61122-985-1
Editors: Brenda M. Davis and Christopher B. Halton © 2011 Nova Science Publishers, Inc.

Chapter VII

RED BLOOD CELL TRANSFUSIONS IN THE ERA OF REDUCED INTENSITY CONDITIONING ALLOGENEIC STEM CELL TRANSPLANTATION

***Vadim Ivanov*[1,2], *Mohamad Mohty*[1,2] *and Didier Blaise*[1,2,*]**

[1]Unit of Transplantation and Cellular Therapy, Institut Paoli-Calmettes;
[2]Department of Hematology, Institut Paoli-Calmettes; Marseille, France

ABSTRACT

Among main toxicities of standard myeloablative conditioning (MAC) regimens for allogeneic stem cell transplantation (allo-SCT), anemia is a well recognised complication, and virtually every patient would require red blood cells support. In the last few years, in an attempt to reduce treatment-related morbidity and mortality associated with standard MAC allo-SCT, different reduced intensity and less ablative conditioning regimens (RIC) have been developed with encouraging results in regards to feasibility and engraftment. In the RIC setting, the burden of disease eradication is shifted towards the graft-versus-tumor effect, while reduced myelosuppression creates a different pattern of post-transplant hemopoeitic reconstitution. Although RIC regimens are usually highly immunosuppressive, the toxicity profile may still vary from one regimen to another because of variability in the degree of myeloablation. The aim of this work is to analyse the available research evidence related to red blood cell transfusions (RBCT) in the era of RIC allo-SCT. An ever-growing body of data suggests that RIC allo-SCT is associated with decreased transfusion requirements and a different pattern of RBC recovery in comparison to MAC allo-SCT. Recently, we demonstrated that the intensity of the conditioning (RIC vs. MAC; P=.0005) and graft source (PBSC vs. BM; P<.0001) independently predicted RBCT requirements. Hb recovery was accelerated after RIC when compared to MAC allo-SCT (P=0.02). In RIC patients the number of RBCTs was

* Correspondence concerning this article should be addressed to Didier Blaise, Unité de Transplantation et de Thérapie Cellulaire (UTTC), Institut Paoli-Calmettes and Université de la Méditerranée, 232 Bd. Ste Marguerite, 13273 Marseille Cedex 09, France. Phone: +33 491 223754; Fax: +33 491 223579; Email: uttc@marseille.fnclcc.fr

inversely correlated with Hb level prior to conditioning (P<.0001) and the dose of anti-thymocyte globulin used as a part of the RIC preparative regimen (P=.009). Moreover, Hb level prior to allo-SCT significantly influenced Hb recovery kinetics after RIC but had no impact on RBCT requirements and Hb recovery after MAC. This data suggests that Hb recovery pattern is different after RIC and may represent a setting for the use of rHuEPO, even if its use after MAC allo-SCT has been associated with only marginal effects on Hb recovery and the number of RBCTs.

In this perspective, we initiated a pilot trial of rHuEPO administration early after matched sibling RIC allo-SCT. RHuEPO treatment was analyzed in terms of toxicity, impact on the frequency of RBCTs and kinetic of Hb recovery within the 60 days post-allo-SCT. Results were compared with a matched population who did not receive EPO. In the first 2 months after allo-SCT, all patients with rHuEPO (100%) achieved an Hb level>11 g/dL at a median of 30 (15-35) days post-allo-SCT, as compared to only 63% of the patients without rHuEPO (P=.007) at a median of 35 (20-55) days (P=.03). Seventy percent (95% CI, 50-90%) of rHuEPO patients maintained an Hb over 11 g/dL for the second month as compared to only 19% (95% CI, 4-34) in the other group (P=.0004). In patients receiving RBCTs, the use of rHuEPO was associated with a trend towards reduced RBCT requirements, highlighting the potential benefit of early administration of rHuEPO after RIC allo-SCT on early erythropoietic recovery.

Overall, the use of RIC regimens creates a different pattern of erythropoietic recovery as compared with standard regimens warranting further studies aimed at a further reduction of RBCT requirements and acceleration of Hb recovery.

Keywords: Red blood cell transfusions, allogeneic stem cell transplantation, hemoglobin, erythropoietin

INTRODUCTION

Historically, the strategy of conventional allogeneic stem cell transplantation (allo-SCT) was based on high-dose, myeloablative chemoradiotherapy to eradicate underlying disease, create marrow space and suppress the immune system of recipient to prevent the rejection of donor stem cell graft. The effect of the highly myeloablative conditioning regimen results in the complete oblation of patients' hemopoiesis, and leading to acute and profound pancytopenia. The allograft then serve to rescue the hemopoietic system and reconstitute the recipient's immune system [1]. It was later shown that: 1) some hematological malignancies cannot be cured despite the use of very intensive conditioning regiments [2,3] and 2) the allogeneic grafts can not only rescue hemopoiesis in a myeloablated patient, but also exert an anti-tumor effect, the so-called "graft-versus-tumor" effect through the recognition of tumor cell antigens by initiating immune allogeneic reaction [4]. Over the last 20 years several pre-clinical and clinical studies documented that this effect is responsible for patients' long term cure [5].

However, though conventional allogeneic transplantation has led to long-term cures for otherwise incurable patients, wide application of this approach has been limited by the toxicity associated with the myeloablative conditioning regimens. The severity of post-transplant complications has limited this type of procedure to relatively young patients (usually less that 50 to 55 years) and to patients without important co-morbidities or previous medical history [1].

More recently, in an attempt to reduce the high rate of treatment-related morbidity and mortality (TRM) associated with standard myeloablative allo-SCT, different reduced intensity and less ablative conditioning regimens (RIC) have been developed with encouraging results in regards to feasibility, engraftment and early toxicity [6-9]. In the setting of RIC, immunosuppression of the host has become the major goal for allowing transferred donor immunocompetent effectors to engraft, while significantly decreasing toxicity. Thus, the application of RIC transplantation could reduce the frequency of several transplant-related toxicities, at least in the early period after transplantation, and the use of RIC has rapidly increased over the past few years [10].

Among important toxicities and adverse effects of intensive myeloablative regimens, anemia is a well recognized complication that is associated with a higher rate of fatigue and altered quality of life. During aplasia, virtually every transplanted patient would require transfusion support with platelets and donor red blood cell concentrates. Also, transfusion requirements are responsible for increasing both costs of transplant procedure and infectious risk due to exposure to human blood derivates.

The reduction or even elimination of post-transplant RBC requirements and shortening of anemia duration would obviously of important benefit. Although, all RIC regimens have been shown to be highly immunosuppressive, the toxicity profile might still vary from one regimen to another because of the variability in degree of myelotoxicity: from truly non-myeloablative fludarabine, and low dose TBI-based regimens to the reduced-intensity regimens including several combinations of chemotherapy and/or low dose irradiation. It is not yet well-defined whether the modification of conditioning-related toxicity profile accompanying the different RIC regimens can be translated into the improvement of erythroid recovery and reduction of RBC requirements in the posttransplant period.

I. Is Favorable Pattern of Erythropoiesis Recovery the Common Feature of RIC Conditioning Regimens?

The first data in this field has come from the Seattle group: Weissinger et al. [11] compared the red blood cell transfusion requirements in 40 patients with hematological malignancies given nonmyeloablative allo-SCT with a control group of 67 patients allotransplanted after standard conventional allo-SCT. Nonmyeloablative transplantation was applied to elderly or medically infirm patients who were ineligible for conventional transplantation. The nonmyeloablative regimen consisted of either 2 Gy Total Body Irradiation (TBI) alone (n=30) or TBI preceded by Fludarabine 30 mg/m^2/d on days –4, –3 and –2 (n=10) with postgraft immunosuppression with mycophenolate mophetil (MMF) and cyclosporine A (CSA). The conditioning regimens of the control group included myeloablative combinations of TBI (12 – 14 Gy) with busulfan or cyclophosphamide, or busulfan plus cyclophosphamide. All patients were given PBSC grafts from genotypically HLA-identical siblings, collected after granulocyte colony-stimulating factor mobilisation. The number of CD34+ cells transplanted and number of ABO-incompatible transplants were not significantly different between the two groups.

Only sixty-three percent of non-myeloablative recipients required RBC transfusions compared with 96% of those with conventional grafts (P=.0001). The number of RBC units transfused was also reduced significantly, with a median of 2 (range, 0 to 50) compared with a median of 6 units (range, 0 to 34) after conventional transplantation (P=.0002). High transfusion requirements before transplantation and donor-recipient ABO incompatibility increased transfusion requirements in both groups of patients. Neither patient age, splenomegaly at transplantation, or GVHD development, nor posttransplantation cytomegalovirus antigenemia or cytomegalovirus disease had statistically significant influences on posttransplantation transfusions.

According to these authors, there are at least three possible reasons for the decreased transfusion requirements in patients receiving low dose TBI-based nonmyeloablative transplants:

1. In animal models [12], the single dose 2 Gy TBI delivered at the low exposure rate of 0.07 Gy/min, while causing moderate pancytopenia, did not lead to irreversible marrow damage. The decline in peripheral blood counts in dogs given 2 Gy TBI and no subsequent marrow rescue was slow, and granulocyte and platelet nadirs were not reached until 14 to 20 days after TBI. Virtually all animals showed complete hematopoietic recoveries within a few weeks of irradiation. In line with these observations, in a group of comparable 45 nonmyeloablative patients described by McSweeney et al. [13], the median granulocyte nadir was 750/mm^3 and the platelet nadir 75000/mm^3. Typically, conventional allogeneic PBSC recipients remain profoundly neutropenic (PNN < 500/mm3) for a median of 16 (range, 11- 29) days and thrombocytopenic (platelets < 20.000/mm3) for a median of 13 (range, 5 – 41) days [14]. Recovery of RBC production and RBC independence are usually later, with medians around 60 to 70 days.
2. The low dose TBI conditioning was delivered just hours before transplantation. This led to a considerable reduction of the period of pancytopenia compared with conventional 7-days high-dose conditioning busulfan-cyclophosphamide therapy. Interestingly, extending the regimen for several days by the addition of fludarabine to low dose TBI increased the transfusion requirements.
3. The major complications of conventional conditioning, such as gastrointestinal damage, veno-occlusive liver disease, hemorrhagic cystitis and bacterial sepsis were either completely absent or significantly reduced (bacterial sepsis) in nonmyeloablative patients.

In a retrospective, non comparative analysis, Ruiz-Arguelles et al. [15] used a more myelotoxic nonmyeloablative conditioning regimen, including oral busulfan 4 mg/kg delivered on days – 6 and – 5; i.v. cyclophosphomide, 350 mg/m^2 on days – 4, – 3 and – 2; i.v. fludarabine 30 mg/m^2; oral CSA 5mg/kg started on day – 1 and i.v. methotrexate 5 mg/m^2 on days +1, +3, +5 and + 11, in 73 recipients of PBSC allografts. The transfusion requirements were analyzed till day+100. In 45 % of the procedures no RBC transfusions were used. The median of transfused RBC units was 1 (range, 0 – 9). The correlation between the number of CD34+ cells infused and the RBC transfusion requirements was analyzed and was not found statistically significant. The methodological difficulty for comparison of this study with other studies, is the transfusion policy of this center, situated in the city of Puebla, 2220 m above sea level. Consequently, patients were transfused if significant symptoms of anemia coexisted with hemoglobin levels below 12.5 g/dL, the normal range in Puebla.

Authors specify that the triggers for RBC transfusions were the symptoms (tachycardia, dyspnea, dizziness, hyposthenia, hypodynamia) and not the Hb level.

RBC Transfusions After ATG-Based RIC Transplantation

Antithymocyte globulin (ATG)-based RIC is another widely used conditioning platform suitable for many patients regardless of diagnosis. However, specific data on the potential impact of ATG-based RIC on RBCTs is still sparse and poorly defined.

Recently, we have compared RBCT requirements and predictive factors for transfusions in the first 2 months after allo-SCT in two series of patients: the RIC group, receiving a RIC regimen combining fludarabine, intermediate doses of busulfan (8 mg/Kg total dose), and ATG as initially described by Slavin et al. [6], vs. a group of patients who underwent a standard myeloablative conditioning regimens (MACs).

Between 1997 and 2002, one hundred and twenty five consecutive patients with an HLA-identical sibling donor received an allo-SCT at the Institut Paoli-Calmettes (Marseille, France) [16]. Among these 125 patients, 15 were excluded from this analysis either because they were treated with post graft recombinant EPO (n = 10) in a research program or died before Day 60 early after allo-SCT (n = 5) of nontransfusion or RBC-related causes. Of the remaining 110 patients, 64 patients (58%) received a RIC regimen, while 46 (42%) were prepared with standard dosed MAC. Patients were treated with a RIC regimen because of high-risk clinical features that made them ineligible for our standard transplant program. "High-risk" was defined by the presence of one or more of the following features: 1) patient age older than 50 years; 2) patients with diagnoses known to be high risk for allo-SCT, such as malignant lymphoma and multiple myeloma; 3) heavily pretreated patients with more than two lines of chemotherapy before allo-SCT, including patients with metastatic solid tumors; and 4) patients with poor performance status due to significant medical comorbidities. All protocols were approved by the Institut Paoli-Calmettes Institutional Review Board, the local ethical committee of Marseille II (Comité Consultatif de Protection des Personnes dans la Recherche Biomédicale), and the French agency for health products security (Agence Française de Sécurité Sanitaire des Produits de Santé (AFSSAPS) whenever applicable [17-20]. All patients and donors gave their informed consent before participation.

Conditioning Regimens

The RIC regimen was adapted from that reported by Slavin et al. [6]. It included fludarabine (Fludara; Schering AG, Lys-Lez-Lannoy, France) with a daily dose of 30 mg/m^2 for 6 consecutive days (administered intravenously over 30 minutes), oral busulfan (BU) (4 mg/Kg/d for 2 consecutive days) (Glaxo-Smith-Kline, Marly-le-Roi, France) and various doses of anti-thymocyte globulin (ATG) (Thymoglobulin ®, Genzyme, Lyon, France) as indicated hereinafter. Per protocol, the ATG dose was decreased step-wise from 10 to 2.5 mg/kg/day. Twenty-one and 13 patients received 10 and 7.5 mg/kg/day respectively, while 3 patients received 5 mg/kg/day and 27 patients received 2.5 mg/kg/day in an attempt to optimize the procedure [20]. The majority of patients treated with MAC (n=43; 93%) received cyclophosphamide (120 mg/kg) and total-body irradiation (TBI) [21] (median dose,12 (range, 11-13.5) Gy with a median of six fractions (range, 5-6)) for a median time of 3 days (range, 3-5). Four patients (9%) treated for acute lymphocytic leukemia (ALL) received etoposide (60 mg/kg) in addition to cyclophosphamide-TBI [22]. The 3 remaining patients received busulfan (16 mg/kg) instead of TBI and Cyclophosphamide (200 mg/kg) (n=2) or melphalan (140 mg/kg) (n=1). Twenty of these 46 patients (43%) were also treated with ATG for 2 consecutive days (2.5 mg/kg/day) to increase the immunosuppression of recipients receiving T cell depleted grafts [17,18].

PBSC Collection and Infusion

All donors and patients were HLA-A-, HLA-B- identical by serological typing and HLA-DR-identical by molecular typing. Sixty four patients (58%) received a marrow (BM) graft while 46 (42%) were infused with mobilized allogeneic PBSC. The day of cell infusion was designated as day 0. In the PBSC group, mobilization consisted of daily subcutaneous administration of lenograstim at the dose of 10 μg/Kg. Treatment started on day – 5 and ended on day – 1. Per protocol, the collection of at least 4 x 10^6 CD34+ cells per kg in one, two or three (maximum) apheresis was sought. In the BMT group, a collection of at least 2 x 10^8 nucleated cells per kg was requested [19]. In 26 patients treated with MAC (marrow, n=20; PBSC, n=6), grafts were in vitro positively selected for $CD34^+$ as a mean to T lymphocyte depletion [17,18]. The remaining 20 MAC patients received unmanipulated grafts. The final PBSC product was analyzed in terms of stem cells content ($CD34^+$ cells) and lymphocyte ($CD3^+$ cell) content using standard flow cytometry procedures [20].

Graft Versus Host Disease (GVHD)

CSA was started intravenously on Day – 2 in all patients, at the dose of 2 mg per kg, and switched to oral formulation as soon as patients were able to resume oral intake. The dosage was adapted to blood levels and renal function [21,22]. In addition to CSA, 28 patients treated with MAC received a short course of methotrexate (on Days 1 (15 mg/m²), 3 and 6 (10 mg/m²)) [23]. Acute GVHD (aGVHD) was graded according to standard criteria [24,25]. None of the patients included in this study received donor lymphocyte infusion during the first 60 days after allo-SCT.

Supportive Care

Supportive care was provided according to standard procedures and was similar for patients treated with MAC or RIC. It included antibacterial prophylaxis with intravenous vancomycin at 2 g daily starting at day – 2 (vancomycin was stopped as soon as the absolute neutrophil count (ANC) exceeded 0.5x10^9 per L). *Pneumocystis carinii* prophylaxis included trimethoprim/sulfamethoxazole administered before transplantation and as soon as ANC exceeded 0.5x10^9/L twice weekly. Prophylaxis against herpes simplex virus included intravenous acyclovir or oral valacyclovir. Empiric broad-spectrum antibiotics were begun for temperature more than 38.5°C or clinical signs of infection. During the whole study period, RBCT policy remained unchanged and was identical between the two study groups. For the purpose of this study, data related to RBCTs was carefully reviewed and assessed for each individual patient. Each transfusion event included two irradiated and WBC-filtered RBC packs and was performed when Hb level reached below 8 g/dL or when the patient had symptomatic anemia. RBCs were of the same ABO group when donor and patient were ABO compatible, of recipient or donor type in case of major (presence of alloantibodies in recipient against RBC antigens of the donor) or minor (presence of alloantibodies in the donor against RBC antigens of the recipient) incompatibility and always of type O in case of bidirectional incompatibility respectively. All patients received RBCTs of donor-type rhesus and Kell factor. All patients received intravenous heparin (100 UI/kg) until ANC reached $0.5x10^9/L$, to prevent veno-occlusive disease (VOD) [19,20].

Study Design and Statistics

The primary endpoints of the study were to analyze RBCs, transfusion requirements, and Hb kinetics from the start of the conditioning until Day 60 after transplant and to investigate potential pregraft prognostic factors for RBCT. Day 60 was chosen as a relatively early endpoint to essentially evaluate the direct impact of conditioning regimen . Descriptive statistics are reported as frequencies, percentage, median, and range. Distributions of categorical variables were compared using standard chi-squared tests. Continuous variables were compared between groups using t-test or ANOVA where applicable and the Mann-Whitney test otherwise. The following factors were tested for a potential predictive impact on RBCT: patient and donor age, patient and donor gender, ABO compatibility, diagnosis, Hb level before conditioning, graft source, in vitro CD34+ cell selection, ATG dose, and the presence of aGVHD. To account for the differences in variables related to RBCT requirements between the two groups, a multiple linear regression model was used to identify factors associated with the number of RBCTs within 60 days of conditioning [26]. Significant variables in the univariate analysis were included in the first model. We then used a selection procedure based on the adjusted r^2. The best model identified was the model with the largest adjusted r^2, whether or not the variables included were significant. The model assumptions were assessed from the residual plot. We assessed the co-linearity between the different covariates using the variance inflation factor for each variable. To identify outliers that could influence the model, cook's distances were calculated [26]. We reran the model after removing observations identified as outliers (n = 4). We used the same methodology to identify factors associated with the number of RBCTs for the RIC population (outliers, n = 3). All analyses were performed using the SAS software (SAS 8.2, SAS Institute, Cary, NC; or SEM, SILEX, Mirefleurs, France).

Results

The median age was 45 years (range, 16-60) and sex ratio (M/F) was 63/47. Patients were treated for hematologic (myeloid, n = 53 (48%); lymphoid, n = 44 (40%)) or non-hematologic malignancies (n = 13 (12%)). Age, diagnoses, and clinical status determined the choice of conditioning between RIC and MAC. Thus, populations between the two groups differed significantly based on these variables (age, P<.0001; diagnosis, P=.01), as well as for some aspects of allo-SCT procedures as determined by the type of transplantation (use of pregraft ATG, P<.0001, graft CD34+ selection, P<.0001; postgraft immunosuppression, P<.0001). A total of 64 patients were prepared with RIC regimen (Table 1). All patients became neutropenic and achieved neutrophil engraftment, reaching an absolute neutrophil count (ANC) of $0.5 \times 10^9/L$ at a median of 14 days (range, 6-23). Sixty-one patients (95%) reached

a self-sustaining platelets (PLT) count > $20 \times 10^9/L$ before Day 60, at a median of 15 (range, 1-45) days. Twenty patients (31%) developed Grade 2 or higher aGVHD (Grade 2, n = 9; Grades 3-4, n = 11) within the first 60 days after allo-SCT. The characteristics of the 46 patients treated with MAC are shown in Table 1. All patients achieved neutrophil engraftment reaching an ANC of $0.5 \times 10^9/L$ at a median of 19 days (range, 9-43). Twenty-three patients (50%) reached a self-sustaining PLT count of higher than $20 \times 10^9/L$ before Day 60, at a median of 22 days (range, 11-48). In this group, 13 patients (28%) developed Grade 2 or higher aGVHD (Grade 2, n = 6; Grades 3-4, n = 7) within the first 60 days of transplant.

Table 1. Patient characteristics.

	RIC N (%)	**MAC N (%)**
N	64	46
Age years, median (range)	48 (40-56)	36 (27-45)
Donor age, years, median (range)	46 (35-57)	37 (25-49)
Patient gender: Male: N (%)	35 (55)	28 (61)
Donor gender: Male: N (%)	31 (48)	25 (54)
ABO compatibility		
Compatible	46 (72)	33 (72)
Major incompatibility	8 (13)	6 (13)
A → O	5	3
B → O	3	1
AB → O		1
AB → A		1
Minor incompatibility	8 (13)	6 (13)
O→ A	8	6
Bidirectional incompatibility	2 (3)	1(2)
B → A	2	1
Diagnosis N (%)		
Myeloid malignancies	25 (39)	28 (61)
Acute myeloid leukemia	16	18
Chronic myeloid leukemia	5	10
Myelodysplasic syndrome	3	
Myeloproliferative syndrome	1	
Lymphoid malignancies	27 (42)	17 (36)
Acute lymphoid leukemia	3	11
Non Hodgkin lymphoma	11	2
Multiple Myeloma	7	2
Chronic lymphocytic leukemia	6	2
Solid tumors	12 (19)	1 (2)
Breast carcinoma	5	1
Malignant Melanoma	4	
Renal Cell Carcinoma	2	
Colorectal carcinoma	1	
Hb level prior to conditioning		
Hb < 10g/dL	27 (42)	17 (37)
10g/dL ≤ Hb <12g/dL	24 (38)	16 (35)
Hb ≥ 12 g/dL	13 (20)	13 (28)
ATG dose		
none	-	26 (57)
5-10 mg/kg	37 (58)	20 (43)
2.5 mg/kg	27 (42)	–
Stem cell source		
Bone Marrow	34 (53)	30 (65)
PBSC	30 (47)	16 (35)
CD34+ cell dose (x106/Kg recipient body weight; mean ± sd)	5.2 ± 4.5	3.7 ± 3.8
GVHD prophylaxis		
CSA	61 (95)	18 (39)
CSA+MMF	3 (5)	–
CSA+MTX	–	28 (61)

Abbreviations: ATG, anti-thymocyte globulin; GVHD, graft-versus-host disease; Hb, hemoglobin; CSA, cyclosporine; MTX, Methotrexate

RBC Transfusions

At the start of conditioning, 20 (18%) patients (RIC, n = 10 (16%); MAC, n = 10 (22%)]) (P = NS) were transfusion-dependent according to our transfusion criteria. The 110 patients received a median of 8 RBC units (range, 0-56) from the start of conditioning until Day 60 after transplant. Overall, the 64 RIC patients received a median of 4 (range, 0-28) RBC units as compared to a median of 12 (range, 2-56) for the MAC patients (P<.0001). The latter translated into an earlier Hb recovery early after RIC allo-SCT (Figure 1) with 9 of the 64 (14%) patients reaching a self-sustained Hb level higher than 12 g/dL by Day 60, as compared to none of the patients in the MAC group (p = 0.02). For patients treated with RIC, the first transfusion occurred at a median of day + 4 (range, – 9 - +28). Seven (11%) patients were never transfused and nine (14%) were still transfusion dependent at Day 60 after allo-SCT. The 48 other patients (75%) became RBCT independent at a median of 15 (range, –1 - +47) days after allo-SCT. Forty-two patients (66%) received more than 2 RBC units. All patients treated with MAC received at least one transfusion with 2 RBC units. Forty-four patients (96%) received more than 2 RBC units. The first transfusion occurred by Day + 3 (range, –6 - +19). Twenty two patients (48%) were still transfusion dependent on Day 60. The 24 others reached transfusion independence by Day +29 (range, 6-48) after allo-SCT.

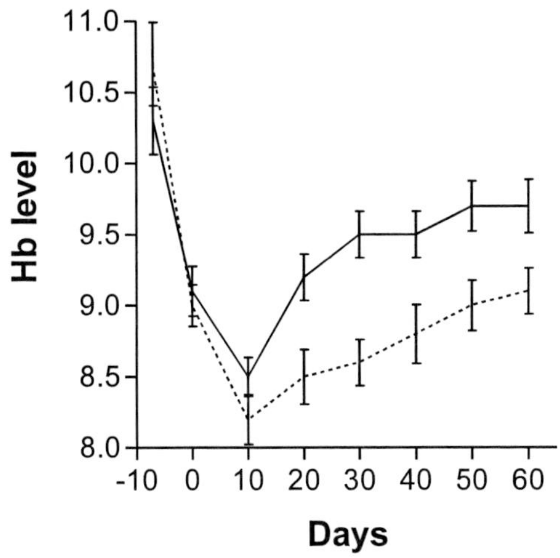

Figure 1. Post graft Hb level evolution after RIC or MAC regimen. Hb (g/dL) level (mean ± SEM) every 10 days are presented after RIC (plain curve) or MAC (dashed curve).

Prognostic Factors for RBC Transfusions

Univariate analysis of potential predictive factors for RBCT is shown in Table 2. Stem cell source was the only variable associated with a significant effect on RBCTs in both groups. Therefore, it was the only variable entered in the multivariate model for the whole study population along with the type of conditioning regimen (MAC vs. RIC) (Table 3). MAC was associated with an increase of 3.65 RBCTs as compared to RIC. Marrow graft was associated with an increase of 2.72 RBCTs as compared to PBSC graft. These two variables remained significant after controlling for the four identified outliers, which were characterized by a large number of RBCTs (range, 13- 28) and a low Hb level (range, 7.4-9.1), with all of them receiving a marrow graft. Four factors appeared to impact on the number of transfusions in the RIC population: diagnosis, stem cell source, ATG dose, and Hb level before allo-SCT (Table 2). In a multiple linear regression, the two last variables (ATG dose and Hb level) were the only ones to remain significantly associated with the number of RBCTs (Table 3). These two variables remained significant after controlling for the three identified outliers (Model 2, Table 3). The three outliers were each characterized by requiring a large number of RBCTs (range, 11-14), a low Hb level before allo-SCT (range, 7.1-8.3), and receiving an ATG dose of 10 mg/kg. For most of the studied endpoints, pre-graft Hb level influenced characteristics of RBCTs (Table 4). In addition, the highest levels were also associated with a better Hb recovery kinetic (Figure 2A). In the MAC setting, the use of PBSCs compared to marrow was the only factor predicting RBC needs in a univariate analysis (Table 2). This remained true when the analysis was restricted to unmanipulated graft (PBSC: n = 10; median, 6; range, 2-22; mean ± SD, 4.5 ± 3.1; BM: n = 10; median, 15; range, 4-56; mean ± SD, 10.7 ± 7.8; p = 0.037). Graft manipulation with positive CD34+ cell selection did not influence postgraft transfusions. Interestingly and conversely to the RIC setting, Hb count before conditioning had no significant impact on RBCTs (Table 2) or Hb recovery after allo-SCT (Figure 2B).

In this study, we investigated RBCT requirements after allo-SCT in patients treated either with a MAC or with a RIC regimen. Patients treated with RIC required less RBCTs in comparison to those treated with a MAC regimen, and transfusion independence was reached earlier in the RIC group, that is in line with similar differences, reported by the Seattle group [11]. Written RBCT policies in the two institutions seem to be relatively similar: At the Fred Hutchinson Cancer Research Center (FHCRC), RBCs were transfused when Hct was less than 26 percent (0.26) or when patients were symptomatic [11] compared to our criteria of having a Hb value under 8 g/dL or for patients being symptomatic. However, quality of RBC products may be different in the two institutions and account for the different results. On the other hand, it is more likely that differences in the transplant regimen account for this discrepancy. When comparing our RIC and MAC groups, the use of cyclosporine alone for GVHD prophylaxis in the RIC population, in contrast to the MAC patients, who received a short course of methotrexate and cyclosporine, adds another layer to the complexity of the analysis. But because this was part of the design of the RIC regimen itself, it can hardly be assessed in this study. Furthermore, the combination of high doses of fludarabine and intermediate doses of busulfan cannot be considered completely 'nonmyeloablative'. Thus, one might expect higher RBCT requirements in our group of patients in comparison to a truly nonmyeloablative regimen as the one used in Seattle. In addition, we found that the use of ATG in the RIC regimen may be associated with increased posttransplant RBCTs: in this study, we observed that higher doses of ATG were associated with more RBCT requirements. Little information is currently available to explain a relationship between the ATG dose and RBCT needs. Furthermore, a substantial proportion of our patients were transplanted with marrow rather than PBSCs. Therefore, when considering only the 26 patients treated with the lower ATG dose and reinfused with PBSCs, 15 (58%) received no or a maximum of 2 RBC units of transfusions, a figure quite comparable to the one reported by Weissinger et al. [11].

Table 2. Univariate analysis of risk factors for red blood cell transfusion in patients prepared with RIC or MAC regimen.

		RIC			MAC		
	No. of cases	RBC units	P	No. of cases	RBC units		F
Patient age			NS		14.5 ± 10.5		N
Younger than 50 y	32	7.6 ± 7.1		41	13.6 ± 4.1	S	
50 y or older	32	5.2 ± 4.3		5			
Donor gender			NS				N
Female	33	6.2 ± 5.7		21	12.8 ± 6.4	S	
Male	31	6.7 ± 6.2		25	15.8 ± 12.1		
ABO			NS		14.1 ± 11.1		N
Compatible	46	6.3 ± 6.0		33	15.0 ± 7.9	S	
Major mismatch	8	7.3 ± 4.7		6	17.0 ± 3.2		
Minor mismatch	8	7.0 ± 7.6		6	6		
Bidirectional mismatch	2	4.0		1			
Diagnosis			0.04				N
Myeloid malignancies	25	7.9 ± 5.6		28	7.1 ± 4.5	S	
Lymphoid malignancies	27	4.8 ± 5.3		17	7.1 ± 5.7		
Solid tumors	12	7.0 ± 7.2		1	11		
Hb level prior to conditioning			0.0001				N
Hb < 10g/dL	27	9.9 ± 6.6		17	17.5 ± 13.5	S	
10g/dL ≤ Hb <12g/dL	24	4.8 ± 4.1		16	13.0 ± 7.1		
Hb ≥ 12 g/dL	13	2.3 ± 3.1		13	12.0 ± 5.7		
ATG dose			0.0002		14.6 ± 9.0		N
5-10 mg/kg	37	8.5 ± 6.5		20	–	S	
2.5 mg/kg	27	3.6 ± 3.5		–	14.2 ± 10.6		
No	–	–		26			
Stem cell source			0.002		16.8 ± 10.9		.
Bone marrow	34	8.5 ± 6.7		30	9.9 ± 5.8	02	
PBSC	30	4.1 ± 3.7		16			

Abbreviations: ATG, anti-thymocyte globulin; Hb, hemoglobin; PBSC, peripheral blood stem cells.

Table 3. Multivariate analysis of risk factors for red blood cell transfusions prior to day 60 post allo-SCT.

A) Total population: Model 1: 110 patients; Model 2: 106 patients, after exclusion of 4 outlier patients (RIC: reduced intensity conditioning; MAC: myeloablative conditioning; Ref.: group of reference)

	Model 1		Model 2	
variables	**parameters**	**p-value**	**parameters**	**p-value**
Graft				
PBSC	Ref.		Ref.	
Bone Marrow	2.72	0.0003	1,92	.0005
Group				
RIC	Ref.		Ref.	
MAC	3.65	<0.0001	3.29	<.0001
Adjusted R-square	0.30		0.36	

B) RIC population: Model 1: 64 patients; Model 2: 61 patients, after exclusion of 3 outlier patients (Hb: hemoglobin; Ref.: group of reference)

	Model 1		Model 2	
variables	**parameters**	**p-value**	**parameters**	**p-value**
ATG dose 2.5 mg/kg 5-10 mg/kg	 Ref. 2.28	 0.05	 Ref. 2.26	 .009
Hb level prior to conditioning Hb ≥ 12 g/dL 10 g/dL ≤ Hb < 12 g/dL Hb < 10 g/dL	 Ref. 0.90 3.26	 0.0005	 Ref. 1.12 2.46	 .005
Diagnosis Lymphoid malignancies Myeloid malignancies Solid tumors	 Ref. 0.61 0.88	 0.37	 Ref. 0.89 0.23	 0.42
Graft Bone marrow PBSC	 Ref. 0.04	 0.98	 Ref. 0.78	 0.37
Adjusted R-square	0.35		0.36	

Abbreviations: ATG, anti-thymocyte globuline; Hb, hemoglobin; PBSC, peripheral blood stem cells.

Table 4. Red blood cell transfusion features after RIC allo-SCT according to pre-conditioning Hb level.

Hemoglobin level (g/dL) prior to RIC	**Hb < 10**	**10 ≤ Hb < 12**	**Hb ≥ 12**	
N	27	24	13	
Untransfused patients	0	2 (8%)	5 (36%)	.003
Patients transfused with more than 2 RBC units	26 (96%)	13 (54%)	3 (23%)	< .0001
Transfusion independence on day 60	20 (74%)	22 (92%)	12 (92%)	NS
Day of first transfusion	- 1 ± 4	6 ± 5	11 ± 7	< .0001
Day of last transfusion	22 ± 13	17 ± 11	15 ± 8	0.10

It is more difficult to compare our results with the results of the Mexican group, because of differences in conditioning regimens, but also in RBC transfusion policies, but it clearly appears from our study and from other studies that the use of a reduced intensity or nonmyeloablative conditioning regimen is associated with lower RBCT requirements when compared to MAC, irrespective of the composition of the so-called RIC regimen.

This study also showed that Hb level before allo-SCT is a major predictive factor for RBCT needs in the RIC setting but not for the control group of patients transplanted with MAC regimen. This factor also influenced Hb recovery kinetics after RIC but not after MAC conditioning (Figure 2). This observation is different from those reported by Xenocostas et al. [27] reporting a significant predictive impact of a pregraft Hb level for transfusions in a series of 519 consecutive patients undergoing MAC allo-SCT and receiving a marrow graft.

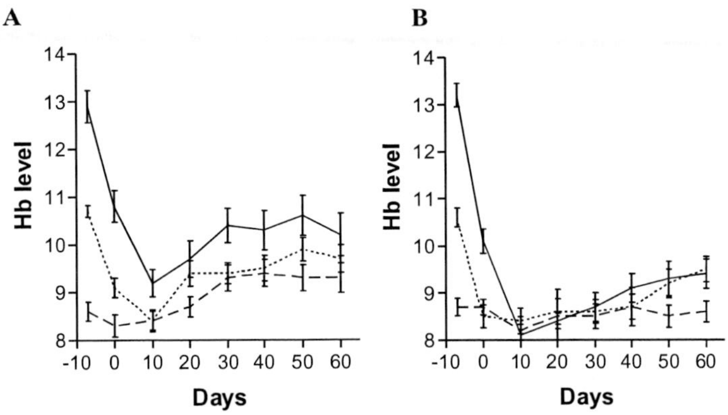

Figure 2. Post graft Hb level evolution according to pre-graft Hb level after RIC or MAC regimen. Hb (g/dL) level (mean ± SEM) every 10 days are presented according to pre-graft Hb level after RIC (upper panel: A) or MAC (bottom panel: B) (plain line: Hb ≥ 12g/dL; Small dotted line: 10 g/dL ≤ Hb < 12 g/dL; Large dotted line: Hb < 10 g/dL) (mean ± SEM).

The Xenocostas report analyzed transfusions over a longer period: 180 days, a difference that may account for this discrepancy. The relatively low number of patients in the control MAC group from our series could also contribute to this discrepancy. In addition, our study could not document a significant effect of major ABO incompatibility on RBCT requirement. The latter is usually contrary to general expectations in allogeneic SCT where immune pure RBC aplasia can be seen and lasts many months. Furthermore Weissinger et al. [11] showed that this was also the case after RIC/F-TBI (fludarabine-total body irradiation). Obviously, the relatively small number of patients in this subgroup (n = 8) might explain the absence of significance. However, one cannot definitely exclude that the use of ATG itself might play an important role in this setting. Diagnoses and graft source presented a strong colinearity association with pregraft Hb level and ATG dose, respectively (diagnoses and pregraft Hb level, p=.02; graft source and ATG dose, p<.0001). With a relatively low number of patients, this may explain that our study has not the statistical power to really assess the role of these two factors as independent predictive factors of RBCTs in the patients treated with RIC. Besides the economical and safety benefits of lower RBCT requirements, our data suggest that the Hb level before RIC allo-SCT might represent a simple and predictive variable for patient peritransplant RBCT requirements. Anemia, defined as an unsupported Hb value below 12 g/dL, is often associated with a higher rate of fatigue in cancer patients [28,29]. Although this study did not focus on patient quality of life after RIC allo-SCT, the quicker Hb recovery observed after RIC might account for the better clinical status of the patients within the first 2 months after allo-SCT, allowing most of them to be maintained in an ambulatory care setting. In cancer patients, this fatigue may be prevented by administration of recombinant EPO, especially in elderly patients [30]. So far, treatment of patients undergoing MAC allo-SCT with recombinant EPO has been associated with contradictory results. Some authors even recommended delaying its use after transplantation [31]. The data from this study suggests that Hb recovery after RIC is different and may represent a setting to the use of recombinant EPO early.

II. Is EPO Administration Effective Early after RIC Allotransplantation?

Over the last decade recombinant human erythropoietin (rHuEPO) has become a well-established treatment for anemia in different hematological malignancies and solid tumors [28]. However, the use of rHuEPO after allo-SCT is still to be defined [32]. Low EPO levels have been documented in patients with low Hb levels after allo-SCT giving a rationale for its clinical use [33,34]. Until recently, the rHuEPO experience in the standard myeloablative allo-SCT remains controversial. When given early after allo-SCT, rHuEPO only marginally decreased transfusion requirements and improved Hb levels without a significant impact on quality of life and was not cost effective [6,35-37]. Recent EORTC guidelines for the use of erythropoietic proteins in anemic patients with cancer are cautious in the allotransplant setting and precise that for patients undergoing standard allo-SCT the clinical impact of erythropoietic proteins is limited and they can only be recommended on an individual basis [38].

Recently, a prospective randomized trial from the German group including 48% of patients receiving RIC, reported that the reconstitution of erythropoiesis seems to be accelerated by early treatment with RHuEPO and reduces number of RBC transfusions in ABO minor incompatibility situations after allo PBSCT [39].

With this background, and our experience confirming a different pattern of erythropoiesis reconstitution after RIC and MAC, we hypothesized that RIC allo-SCT may represent an attractive setting for the use of rHuEPO as opposed to standard highly myelotoxic and myeloablative conditioning regimens. To test this hypothesis, we conducted a pilot study evaluating the efficacy and safety of early administration of rHuEPO after RIC allo-SCT [40].

Twenty patients with hematological malignancies or metastatic solid tumors received a RIC allo-SCT from an HLA identical sibling in a pilot study assessing the impact of early administration of rHuEPO after RIC allo-SCT. These patients were matched and compared to a historical control group of 27 patients receiving the same preparative RIC regimen, but not receiving rHuEPO post-allo-SCT. The same above-mentioned criteria were applied for the choice of reduced-intensity conditioning for the patients who were not eligible for conventional transplantation.

Transplantation Characteristics

The RIC preparative regimen was identical into both groups of patients and included fludarabine with a daily dose of 30 mg/m^2 for 6 or 5 consecutive days (administered intravenously over 30 minutes), oral busulfan (4 mg/kg/d for 2 consecutive days) and a single dose 2.5 mg/kg of ATG, all medications from the same manufacturers cited above. PBSC harvest, stem cell product control, supportive care, aGVHD grading and transfusion policies remain unchangeable (see above). None of the patients included in this series received either donor lymphocyte infusion or G-CSF stimulation during the first 60 days post-allo-SCT. GVHD prophylaxis was performed in all patients by CSA alone using the same scheme.

RHuEPO Treatment

Twenty patients eligible for RIC allo-SCT with a pre-transplant Hb level less than 14 g/dL and no history of thrombotic complications were included in this study over a period of

14 months. For all patients the day of the first intravenous (i.v.) injection of rHuEPO was the day after the last donor PBPC infusion. Nine patients received epoetine-beta (Neorecormon, Roche, Neuilly-sur-Seine, France) at the dose of 10.000 IU thrice weekly. The remaining 11 patients received darbopoetine alpha (Aranesp, Amgen, Neuilly-sur-Seine, France) 150 mg per week when approval for its use in hematological malignancies was obtained in France. Both erythropoetins were given as the IV infusion during hospitalization and than as subcutaneous injections in an ambulatory setting. Treatment was continued until Hb level reached 14 g/dL or day +60. All EPO+ patients received iron supplementation at the dose of 150 – 250 mg of elemental iron per day p.o. Patients from the matched control group were treated in the period immediately prior to or immediately after the end of this pilot study. They were treated identically in every way except for rHuEPO and iron administration.

Study Design and Statistics

In this study we analyzed the impact of early rHuEPO on both Hb recovery and RBC requirements during the first 60 days after transplantation in patients treated with rHuEPO as compared with patients who have not received EPO treatment. For this purpose, only patients surviving beyond day 60 were considered. During the study period two patients died before day 60: one on day 5 (cerebral hemorrhage) and the other on day 59 (severe acute GVHD IV). Both patients did not receive EPO and were excluded from this analysis. Descriptive statistics are reported as frequencies and percentage, median and range. Distributions of categorical variables were compared using standard chi-squared tests. Continuous variables were compared between groups using t-test, Wilcoxon or Kruskal-Wallis when applicable, the Mann-Whitney test otherwise.

Results

Patients, donors and transplant characteristics are summarized in Table 1 and did not differ between the 2 groups (Table 5). Two patients from the EPO+ group and 3 patients from the EPO– group were transfused at least once in the month preceding the conditioning regimen. Median Hb level prior to conditioning was 10.8 (range, 6.8-15.2) g/dL. Twenty-five of the 47 patients (53%) had an Hb level < 11 g/dL prior to the beginning of conditioning without any significant difference between the 2 groups. The Hb level cut off of 11 g/dL was chosen for further subgroup analysis following the WHO grading system for anemia and to differentiate grade 0 anemia (Hb≥11 g/dL) vs. more advanced anemia grades [41]. After transplantation, 26 patients experienced grade II-IV aGVHD at a median of 30 (range, 15-60) days post allo-SCT, with no significant differences between the 2 groups. A total of 9 patients (Group EPO+: 3 (15%); Group EPO-: 6 (22%); P=NS)) had severe gut GVHD. No significant differences in GVHD characteristics could be documented between patients receiving epoetine-beta or darbopoetine-alpha. In this series no serious unexpected adverse events, notably thromboembolic episodes or signs of pure red-cell aplasia [42] were attributed to rHuEPO administration. RHuEPO was withdrawn at a median of +42 (range, 1-56) days after allo-SCT, without any difference between the 2 products.

Times to achieve an absolute neutrophil count (ANC) above 0.5 x 10^9/L and a platelet count > 20 x 10^9/L, were respectively 17 (range, 0-24) and 13 (range, 0-23) days without a significant difference between patients treated with rHuEPO or not (Table 5). Accordingly, PLT transfusion requirements appeared to be identical between both patient groups. Thirteen patients in the EPO+ group (65%) and 12 patients in the control (EPO-) group (44%) did not receive any platelet transfusion during the study period (P=NS). For transfused patients, platelet requirements were minimal in both groups: 1 (range, 1-2) unit for EPO+ and 1 (range, 2-3) unit for EPO –.

Table 5. Patients, Donor And Transplant Characteristics Of Patients.

	EPO+	EPO –	P
N	20	27	NS
Age years, median (range)	48 (27-61)	49 (27-60)	NS
Donor age, years, median (range)	51 (24-62)	44 (26-76)	NS
Donor female gender, n (%)	7 (35)	14 (52)	NS
ABO compatibility, n (%)			
Compatible	18 (90)	20 (74)	NS
Major incompatibility	2 (10)	2 (7.5)	
Minor incompatibility	0	4 (15)	
Bi-directional incompatibility	0	1 (3.5)	
Diagnosis, n (%)			
Hematological malignancies	15 (75)	21(78)	NS
Solid tumors	5 (25)	6 (22)	
$CD34^+$ cell dose ($x10^6$/kg recipient body weight, median, (range))	5.3 (2.9-11.4)	6.4 (1.4-11)	NS
Transfusion-dependent patients before allo-SCT, n (%)	2 (10)	3 (11)	NS
Hb prior to conditioning, g/dL, median, (range)	11 (7 – 13.6)	10.3 (6.8 –15.2)	NS
Patients with pre-conditioning Hb, n (%)			
< 11 g/dL	10 (50)	15 (56)	NS
≥ 11 g/dL	10 (50)	12 (44)	
Median day (range) to reach ANC above 0.5 x 10^9/L	16 (0 –20)	18 (10 – 24)	NS
Median day (range) to reach platelet count above 20 x 10^9/L	11 (6-15)	14 (0-23)	NS
Patients with Grade II-IV aGVHD before day +60, n (%)	10 (50)	16 (59)	NS

Abbreviations: allo-SCT – allogenic stem cell transplantation; ANC - absolute neutrophil count; aGVHD – acute graft-versus-host disease

Table 6. RBC Transfusion Features After RIC Allo-SCT.

	EPO + (n=20)	EPO – (n=27)	P
Hb level on day 20, g/dL, median, (range)	10.4 (8.7-13.3)	9.2 (7.4-13.3)	.03
Hb level on day 30, g/dL, median, (range)	11.6 (9.8-14.1)	10.0 (8.0-12.9)	.0001
Hb level on day 60, g/dL, median, (range)	12.8 (9.0-14.9)	9.9 (7.9-14.3)	.0000
Patients achieving Hb level ≥ 11 g/dL over the first 60 days, n (%)	20 (100%)	17 (63%)	.007
Time to reach Hb level ≥ 11 g/dL, days	30 (15-35)	35 (20-55)	.03

Abbreviations: RIC – reduced intensity conditioning; allo-SCT – allogenic stem cell transplantation.

Overall, RBCT requirements were relatively low: 12 patients (6 in each group, P= NS) were never transfused, while 35 patients received a median of 2 (range, 2-12) RBC units with a trend towards less transfusions for patients treated with rHuEPO (Group EPO+: 2 (2-4); group EPO– : 4 (2-12); P=.07). There were two patients in EPO+ (10%) and 7 patients in EPO- group (26%, P=NS) with ABO blood group donor/recipient incompatibility. There was no case of hemolysis in ABO mismatch recipients during posttransplant period. The highest number of RBC units transfused (12 from day 0 till day+60) was found in three ABO-compatible patients from EPO- group.

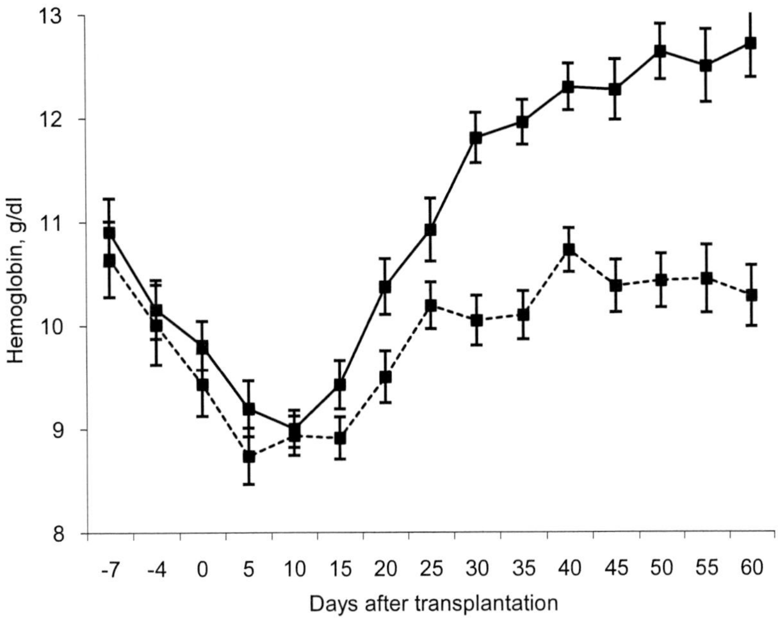

Figure 3. Post graft Hb level evolution (mean ± SEM) after RIC regimen according to rHuEPO treatment (group EPO+ (plain curve) vs. group EPO – (dashed curve).

The major difference between the 2 groups consisted in a hastened Hb recovery after day 15 (Table 6; Figures 3 and 4). In addition, after discontinuation of rHuEPO, this difference remained and continued to be evident during the second month after allo-SCT (figure 3): at any time point during the second month, 14 patients in the EPO group (70%, 95%CI: 50-90) had an Hb above 11 g/dL as compared to 5 patients (19% (95%CI, 4-34)) in the EPO- group (P=.0004) (Figure 2).

Hb level prior to transplantation was predictive of RBCT requirements. Of the 22 patients with a Hb level >= to 11 g/dL, 10 were never transfused while 12 received 1 transfusion of 2 RBC units as compared to the 25 patients presenting with a Hb level < 11 g/dL: 2 patients were never transfused (P=.003) while 23 received a median of 4 (range, 2-12) RBC units (P<.001).

Patients presenting with a low Hb count before conditioning were likely to benefit more from the rHuEPO treatment (Figures 5 A and B). The difference in Hb recovery between the two groups (EPO+ vs. EPO-) was achieved earlier in patients with lower pre-transplant Hb level. It was also the only situation were RBCT requirements was different between the two groups: patients with low pre-transplant Hb level treated with rHuEPO received significantly less RBC units than the ones without rHuEPO (Group EPO+: 2 (range, 0-4); Group EPO-: 4 (range, 2-12); P=.01).

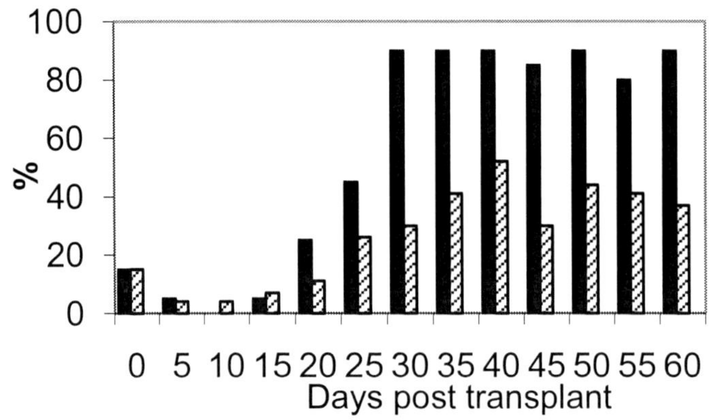

Figure 4. Percentage of patients with Hb level above 11 g/dL (group EPO+ (black columns) vs. group EPO – (dashed columns)). (all P< .005 after day 25).

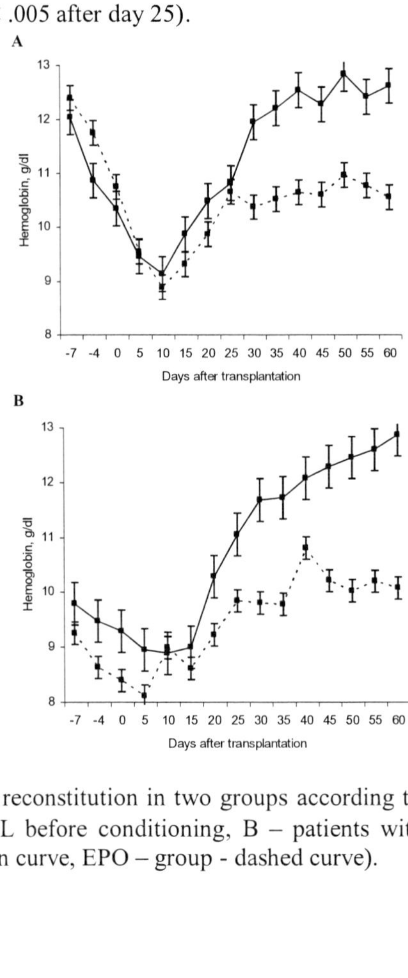

Figure 5. A and B. Hemoglobin reconstitution in two groups according to the pre-graft Hb level (A – patients with Hb level ≥11 g/dL before conditioning, B – patients with Hb level <11 g/dL before conditioning, EPO + group - plain curve, EPO – group - dashed curve).

Median follow-up of surviving patients was 16 (range, 11-43) months. The two years survival was not different between the 2 groups (Group EPO+: 57 % (44-69); group EPO-: 51% (41-62)).

In the first part of our work we showed that the use of Fludarabin, Busulfan and ATG-based RIC regimen was associated with lower RBCT requirements and quicker Hb recovery kinetics as compared to standard myeloablative conditioning in the allogeneic setting. These results suggested that the pattern of erythroid reconstitution after RIC could leave a place for efficacious use of rHuEPO in the early posttransplant period. The use of rHuEPO after myeloablative allo-SCT has been widely reported and has been rather disappointing. Although low levels of serum erythropoietin were documented after standard myeloablative allo-SCT, the use of rHuEPO did not translate towards a substantial improvement of erythropoietic recovery or major reduction of RBCT requirements[35],[43,44]. Profound myeloablation delivered by a standard conditioning is likely to induce elimination of progenitor cells targeted by rHuEPO. This might explain, at least in part, these poor results. The latter hypothesis is in line with previous data showing that a delayed administration of rHuEPO, i.e. after bone marrow repopulation, is associated with reduction of RBCTs [31]. RIC regimens are by definition less myeloablative than standard regimens. This means that a substantial number of EPO-responsive erythroid progenitors of recipient origin might persist after allo-SCT, before being gradually replaced by the expansion of equivalent donor-derived cells. In this regard, the presence of relatively high and adequate endogenous erythropoietin levels reported after RIC-allo-SCT suggests that rHuEPO might exert its stimulatory effect early after allo-SCT [45]. This is in accordance with the quicker Hb recovery we previously described after RIC allo-SCT as compared to myeloablative standard allo-SCT. However, one could argue that the detection of adequate levels of endogenous erythropoietin cannot justify the use of rHuEPO in this setting [45]. The latter can be partially true, but we can also hypothesize that the maintenance of erythropoietic progenitor cells early after allo-SCT can be an attractive situation to benefit from post-graft rHuEPO stimulation.

The source of the graft could also contributes into the greater efficiency of EPO in the PBSCT settings: it was shown that PB-derived stem cells contain a larger amount of EPO-susceptible progenitor cells as compared to the bone marrow cells used in the older trials [46].

In this study, we initially used rHuEPO thrice a week. However, when darbopoetin became available in France we switched to this product in order to administer a weekly and more practical treatment. The use of long-term acting rHuEPO derivatives every other or third week is likely to be even more attractive, being fully compatible with an ambulatory patients' management that is increasingly used in the RIC allo-SCT setting.

From a statistical point of view, our analysis included a relatively small number of patients. Only a fully powered and randomized study would allow definitive conclusions. However, results from this pilot study might pave the way for such a randomized large scale study. Moreover, both patient groups were similar in terms of major factors influencing Hb recovery. They all received PBSC transplantation, a similar dose of $CD34^+$ cells and the same dose of ATG. The proportions of RBCT dependant patients and patients with a low initial Hb count were also not different, allowing a certain level of confidence as for the interpretation of the results.

The use of rHuEPO was clearly associated with a quicker Hb kinetics, with 80% of the patients achieving a level above 12 g/dL in the second months post allo-SCT in sharp contrast with patients not treated with rHuEPO. This effect started as soon as day 20, probably allowing patients to experience less fatigue [47]. Evaluation of quality of life (QOL) was not part of this pilot study. Nonetheless, the effect on QOL can be expected to be even greater in patients presenting with a low Hb levels prior to transplantation. Surprisingly, more rapid Hb recovery after early administration of rHuEPO was associated only with the trend towards decrease of RBCT requirements (P=.07). This apparent discrepancy is probably related to two parameters: (i) the relatively low patient number in this study cannot provide sufficient statistical power to detect such difference; (ii) the group of patients starting transplantation with the higher Hb level, already required only a few RBCT, if any, contributing to the absence of difference. Finally, one should keep in mind that RBCT requirement is only a surrogate and incomplete marker of patient anemia and QOL.

Despite its obvious limitations, this pilot study strongly suggests that the early use of rHuEPO can hasten Hb recovery and potentially lower transfusion requirements after ATG-based RIC allo-SCT. Better results can even be expected in situations combining both a high Hb level prior to allo-SCT transplant and post-transplant rHuEPO treatment, giving a rationale for the use of rHuEPO in the weeks preceding allo-SCT. In such studies, prospective assessment of QOL and economic evaluation would obviously be major determinants for the ultimate outcome.

CONCLUSION

In conclusion, our observations of fewer RBCTs and a quicker kinetics of Hb recovery after RIC allo-SCT, further support the early benefits of RIC strategy as compared to MAC. Increasing knowledge of different clinical and biological features of RIC allo-SCT, allows us to aim for a further reduction in procedure-related toxicity and improvement in patients' quality of life as obvious targets in order to improve the safety and outcomes of low intensity or nonmyeloablative allo-SCT. On the assumption of: (1) the Hb level prior to conditioning is an independent predictive factor for both RBCT requirement and Hb level recovery after the ATG-based RIC regimen and (2) early EPO utilization after ATG-based RIC could show it's efficacy starting from the day +20, it is logical to suggest, that an ideal candidate for RIC transplantation with minimal or no posttransplantation RBC transfusion requirements ("Bloodless RIC") must be a patient who:

- has a normal pre-transplant level of Hb (that can be provided by pre-transplant EPO administration);
- received adequate early EPO support (started on the day after the last PBSC infusion), that was continued during the period long enough to allow for stable allogeneic reconstitution of erythropoiesis (Figure 6).

It is not unreasonable to suggest that by using this approach we could move one step closer towards the "Bloodless transplantation – transplantation without transfusions" with potential benefits of avoidance of various hazards of human blood products use: transfusion transmitted infections, alloimmunisation, adverse reactions as well as higher costs of. This strategy might also lead to improvement of patient's QOL by reducing the length of posttransplant in-patient stay, aiming eventually at mainly out-patient-based transplantation in the foreseeable future.

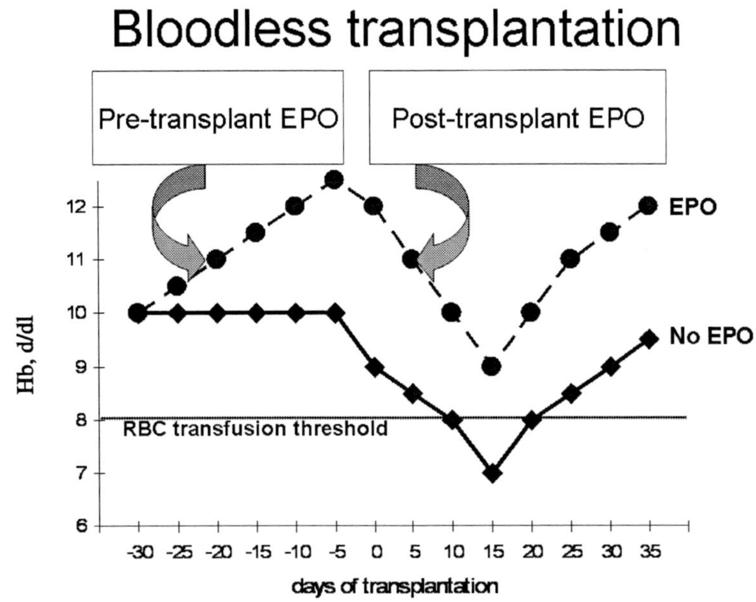

Figure 6. Bloodless – transfusion-free - transplants: combined utilization of pre- and posttransplantation EPO could permit to avoid RBC transfusion requirements in the early posttransplant period.

References

[1] Georges, G.E. and R. Storb, Review of "minitransplantation": nonmyeloablative allogeneic hematopoietic stem cell transplantation. *Int J Hematol*, 2003. 77(1): p. 3-14.

[2] Thomas, E., et al., Bone-marrow transplantation (first of two parts). *N Engl J Med*, 1975. 292(16): p. 832-43.

[3] Thomas, E.D., et al., Bone-marrow transplantation (second of two parts). *N Engl J Med*, 1975. 292(17): p. 895-902.

[4] Appelbaum, F.R., Haematopoietic cell transplantation as immunotherapy. *Nature,* 2001. 411(17 May): p. 385-389.

[5] Thomas, E.D. and K.G. Blume, Historical markers in the development of allogeneic hematopoietic cell transplantation. *Biol Blood Marrow Transplant*, 1999. 5(6): p. 341-6.

[6] Link, H., et al., A controlled trial of recombinant human erythropoietin after bone marrow transplantation. *Blood*, 1994. 84(10): p. 3327-35.

[7] Giralt, S., et al., Engrafment of allogeneic hematopoietic progenitor cells ith purine analog-containing chemotherapy : harnessing graft-versus-leukemia without myeloablative therapy. *Blood*, 1997. 89(12): p. 4531-4536.

[8] Storb, R., Non-myeloablative preparative regimens : experimental data and clinical practice. *J Clin Oncol*, 1998: p. 241-249.

[9] Djulbegovic, B., et al., Nonmyeloablative allogeneic stem-cell transplantation for hematologic malignancies: a systematic review. *Cancer Control*, 2003. 10(1): p. 17-41.

[10] Gratwohl, A., et al., Increasing use of reduced intensity conditioning transplants: report of the 2001 EBMT activity survey. *Bone Marrow Transplant*, 2002. 30(12): p. 813-31.

[11] Weissinger, F., et al., Decreased transfusion requirements for patients receiving nonmyeloablative compared with conventional peripheral blood stem cell transplants from HLA-identical siblings. *Blood*, 2001. 98(13): p. 3584-8.

[12] Storb, R., et al., Marrow toxicity of fractionated vs. single dose total body irradiation is identical in a canine model. *Int J Radiat Oncol Biol Phys*, 1993. 26(2): p. 275-83.

[13] McSweeney, P.A., et al., Hematopoietic cell transplantation in older patients with hematologic malignancies: replacing high-dose cytotoxic therapy with graft-versus-tumor effects. *Blood*, 2001. 97(11): p. 3390-400.

[14] Bensinger, W.I., et al., Transplantation of bone marrow as compared with peripheral-blood cells from HLA-identical relatives in patients with hematologic cancers. *N Engl J Med*, 2001. 344(3): p. 175-81.

[15] Ruiz-Arguelles, G.J., et al., Bloodless (transfusion-free) hematopoietic stem cell transplants: the Mexican experience. *Bone Marrow Transplant*, 2005. 36(8): p. 715-20.

[16] Ivanov, V., et al., Decreased RBCTs after reduced intensity conditioning allogeneic stem cell transplantation: predictive value of prior Hb level. *Transfusion*, 2004. 44(4): p. 501-8.

[17] Viret, F., et al., Transplantation of allogeneic CD34+ blood cells in leukemia or lymphoma patients at high risk of GVHD [letter]. *Bone Marrow Transplant*, 1999. 24(2): p. 225-7.

[18] Stoppa, A.M., et al., Feasibility of CD34 selected allogeneic bone marrow transplantation (ABMT) followed after 3 months by prophylactic donor lymphocytes infusion (DLI) in hematologic malignacies. *Blood*, 2000. 96(11): p. 790a.

[19] Blaise, D., et al., Randomized trial of bone marrow versus lenograstim-primed blood cell allogeneic transplantation in patients with early-stage leukemia: a report from the Societe Francaise de Greffe de Moelle. *J Clin Oncol*, 2000. 18(3): p. 537-46.

[20] Mohty, M., et al., Graft-versus-host disease following allogeneic HLA-identical sibling transplantation with anti-thymocyte globulin-based reduced intensity preparative regimen. *Blood*, 2003. prepublished online March 20, 2003; DOI 10.1182/blood-2002-12-3629.

[21] Blaise, D., et al., Long term follow-up of a randomized trial comparing the combination ofcyclophosphamide with total body irradiation or busulfan as conditioning regimen for patients receiving HLA -identical marrow grafts for acute myeloid leukemia in first complete remission;. *Blood*, 2001. 97(11): p. 3669-3671.

[22] Blume, K., et al., Total body irradiation and high-dose etoposide : a new preparatory regimen for bone marrow transplantation in patients with advanced hematologic malignancies. *Blood*, 1987. 69(4): p. 1015-1020.

[23] Storb, R., et al., Methotrexate and cyclosporine compared with cyclosporin alone prophylaxis of acute graft versus host disease after marrow transplantation for leukemia. *The New England Journal of Medicine*, 1986. 314: p. 729-735.

[24] Glucksberg, H., et al., Clinical manifestations of graft-versus-host disease in human recipients from HL-A-matched sibling donors. *Transplantation*, 1974. 18(4): p. 295-304.

[25] Przepiorka, D., et al., 1994 Consensus Conference on Acute GVHD Grading. *Bone Marrow Transplant*, 1995. 15(6): p. 825-8.

[26] Kleinbaum, D., L. Kupper, and K. Muller, eds. *Applied Regression Analysis and other Multivariable Methods*., ed. S. Edition. 1988, PWS-KENT.

[27] Xenocostas, A., et al., RBC transfusion requirements after allogeneic marrow transplantation: impact of the before-transplant Hb level on transfusion and early survival. *Transfusion*, 2003. 43(3): p. 373-82.

[28] Ludwig, H., Epoetin in cancer-related anaemia. *Nephrol Dial Transplant*, 1999. 14 Suppl 2: p. 85-92.

[29] Given, C.W., et al., Predictors of pain and fatigue in the year following diagnosis among elderly cancer patients. *J Pain Symptom Manage*, 2001. 21(6): p. 456-66.

[30] Jilani, S.M. and J.A. Glaspy, Impact of epoetin alfa in chemotherapy-associated anemia. *Semin Oncol*, 1998. 25(5): p. 571-6.

[31] Baron, F., et al., Optimization of recombinant human erythropoietin therapy after allogeneic hematopoietic stem cell transplantation. *Exp Hematol*, 2002. 30(6): p. 546-54.

[32] Kasper, C., Recombinant human erythropoietin in the treatment of anemic patients with hematological malignancies. *Ann Hematol*, 2001. 80(6): p. 319-29.

[33] Bosi, A., et al., Inadequate erythropoietin production in allogeneic bone marrow transplant patients. *Haematologica*, 1991. 76(4): p. 280-4.

[34] Miller, C.B., et al., Impaired erythropoietin response to anemia after bone marrow transplantation. *Blood*, 1992. 80(10): p. 2677-82.

[35] Steegmann, J.L., et al., Erythropoietin treatment in allogeneic BMT accelerates erythroid reconstitution: results of a prospective controlled randomized trial. *Bone Marrow Transplant*, 1992. 10(6): p. 541-6.

[36] Klaesson, S., et al., Treatment with erythropoietin after allogeneic bone marrow transplantation: a randomized, double-blind study. *Transplant Proc*, 1994. 26(3): p. 1827-8.

[37] Biggs, J.C., et al., Prospective randomised double-blind trial of the in vivo use of recombinant human erythropoietin in bone marrow transplantation from HLA-identical sibling donors. The Australian Bone Marrow Transplant Study Group. *Bone Marrow Transplant*, 1995. 15(1): p. 129-34.

[38] Bokemeyer, C., et al., EORTC guidelines for the use of erythropoietic proteins in anaemic patients with cancer. *Eur J Cancer*, 2004. 40(15): p. 2201-16.

[39] Klink A, K.C., Scholl S et al. First report of a prospective randomised controlled trial of recombinant human erythropoietin after allogenic blood stem cell transplantation. *in Blood*. 2004.

[40] Ivanov, V., et al., Early administration of recombinant erythropoietin improves hemoglobin recovery after reduced intensity conditioned allogeneic stem cell transplantation. *Bone Marrow Transplant*, 2005.

[41] Crawford, J., et al., Relationship between changes in hemoglobin level and quality of life during chemotherapy in anemic cancer patients receiving epoetin alfa therapy. *Cancer*, 2002. 95(4): p. 888-95.

[42] Bennett, C.L., et al., Pure red-cell aplasia and epoetin therapy. *N Engl J Med*, 2004. 351(14): p. 1403-8.

[43] Beguin, Y., et al., Circulating erythropoietin levels after bone marrow transplantation: inappropriate response to anemia in allogeneic transplants. *Blood,* 1991. 77(4): p. 868-73.

[44] Beguin, Y., R. Oris, and G. Fillet, Dynamics of erythropoietic recovery following bone marrow transplantation: role of marrow proliferative capacity and erythropoietin production in autologous versus allogeneic transplants. *Bone Marrow Transplant*, 1993. 11(4): p. 285-92.

[45] Baron, F., G. Fillet, and Y. Beguin, Erythropoiesis after nonmyeloablative stem-cell transplantation is not impaired by inadequate erythropoietin production as observed after conventional allogeneic transplantation. *Transplantation*, 2002. 74(12): p. 1692-6.

[46] Lemoli, R.M., et al., Cycling status of CD34+ cells mobilized into peripheral blood of healthy donors by recombinant human granulocyte colony-stimulating factor. *Blood*, 1997. 89(4): p. 1189-96.

[47] Groopman, J.E. and L.M. Itri, Chemotherapy-induced anemia in adults: incidence and treatment. *J Natl Cancer Inst*, 1999. 91(19): p. 1616-34.

In: Perspectives in Stem Cell Research ISBN: 978-1-61122-985-1
Editors: Brenda M. Davis and Christopher B. Halton

Chapter VIII

Interactions between Transplanted Neural Stem Cells and Host Tissue: A Two-Way Street

Teresita L. Briones*
Department of Medical-Surgical Nursing
University of Illinois at Chicago, IL, USA

Abstract

Research on stem cell transplantation as potential therapy for neurodegenerative disorders has increased dramatically in the last 5 years. However, the mechanism whereby transplanted cells might integrate 'appropriately' throughout the mammalian nervous system is still poorly understood. Recent studies have demonstrated that transplanted neural stem cells are capable of engrafting in a cytoarchitecturally and developmentally appropriate manner within the normal and abnormal central nervous system (CNS) following transplantation. Furthermore, studies have shown that the transplanted neural stem cells are capable of migrating to areas of the CNS affected by disease or injury; that is, these transplanted cells have the ability to 'hone in' on pathology, even over great distances. Given these recent reports, discussion on this chapter will include the phenomenon of how the host CNS environment instructs and influence the fate of transplanted neural stem cells migrating to areas of pathology and assuming the phenotype(s) of host cells that are affected by disease or injury. Moreover, the emerging data on the capability of transplanted cells to instruct and alter the fate of host CNS tissue will also be covered in this chapter. The growing evidence to support the notion that donor neural stem cells and host tissue communicate in a reciprocal fashion will also be discussed. For example, while it has been demonstrated that a given host CNS environment is instructive of donor stem cells, influencing their migration and differentiation patterns, the donor neural stem cells are apparently equally capable of manipulating their milieu. However, the signals generated by neural stem cells to

* Correspondence: Teresita L. Briones, Ph.D., University of Illinois at Chicago, 845 S. Damen Avenue, M/C 802, Rm. 750, Chicago, IL 60612. Phone: (312)355-3142. Gsc: (312) 996-4979. E-mail: tbriones@uic.edu

communicate with the host tissue have yet to be identified but it is speculated that molecules such as growth factors, cell adhesion molecules, cytokines and chemokines are involved. This continuously evolving understanding of how the donor neural stem cells are interacting with host tissue in a regenerative or restorative manner will be the main focus of this chapter.

INTRODUCTION

The mammalian central nervous system (CNS) is incredibly complex and possesses only a limited ability to recover from injury. These characteristics of the CNS have made therapeutic management of neurological disorders very difficult. The limited inherent capability of the CNS to recover from insult is also the main reason why most research into brain and spinal cord injuries primarily focused on promoting axonal regeneration and reducing neuronal degeneration. Fortunately, the discovery of self-renewing stem cell populations within the fetal and adult brain has opened promising lines of investigation into the treatment of CNS disorders [1,2]. More recently, the potential of using stem cells as a tool to treat CNS disorders has gained increased attention because of encouraging results in neural transplantation research. The original intent to use neural grafts for CNS repair was to take advantage of the highly plastic characteristics of dividing cells residing in the germinal zones of the developing brain and spinal cord, and at the same time of the relatively higher immunologic tolerance of the CNS [3]. The possibility that the immature donor tissue might replace dysfunctional host cells or deliver missing substances into the impaired host tissue has generated new hope in developing therapies for the management of CNS disorders. Yet the current data, although promising still present some doubts on the effectiveness of cell replacement therapy as a cure for neurodegeneration or CNS injury. Some of the difficulties encountered in cell replacement therapy (e.g. poor cell survival and limited differentiation) may be attributed to the topographic maps in the CNS that are interrelated to one another in very specific ways. Thus, to replace damaged neural cells presents a problem that cannot be easily solved by 'just' delivering suitable cells that would survive and differentiate in the host environment – the common experimental approach used in cell replacement therapy. For grafted cells to become functional, it is necessary for the donor cells to establish appropriate afferent and efferent connections to maintain the specificity of the CNS topographic map. Consequently, it is important to understand the reciprocal signals generated by the donor and host cells to communicate with each other - the main focus of this review - so that successful regeneration can be facilitated.

SOURCES OF CELLS FOR TRANSPLANATION

Depending on the donor material, neural grafts have been proposed to facilitate morphologic and functional recovery of the recipient CNS by either: (1) replacing affected cell populations (or its structural components like myelin) and their connections, which can then lead to functional recovery, (2) delivering missing neuroactive molecules, such as enzymes and neurotransmitters, (3) providing a growth-permissive tissue "bridges" for host axonal regeneration and target-oriented guidance of growing axons, and (4) enhancing secretion of neurotrophic and other regeneration-promoting substances that supports the survival and growth of both graft and host cells. There are four main sources of cells for transplantation: neural tissue stem cells, embryonic stem cells, non-neuronal tissue cells, and immortalized cell lines.

Neural Tissue Stem Cells. Neural tissue cells (NSCs) have been identified in many areas of the developing mammalian brain, and also in specific regions of the adult CNS [1,4]. Such cells are easy to expand and have been demonstrated to differentiate into all three neural cell types - neurons, oligodendrocytes and astrocytes [5,6]. For instance, murine NSCs isolated from developing brain and spinal cord generated neurospheres, self-renewed and differentiated into neurons and glia. Subsequent transplantation of these neurospheres into the lateral ventricles of immunodeficient newborn NOD/SCID mice then showed engraftment, migration and region-specific neuronal differentiation on examination up to 7 months later [7]. When considering NSCs for cell replacement therapies, it is important to be cognizant of the fact that cells from different brain regions are not identical, displaying different growth characteristics, trophic factor requirements and restricted patterns of differentiation. In addition, these multipotent cells clearly differ in their potential according to the developmental stage at which they were isolated and the specific brain region from which they were isolated. Although the bulk of experimental data has been obtained using rodent NSCs, similar multipotent cells have been identified in humans.

The presence of NSCs are not exclusive to the developing or fetal brain as demonstrated by numerous pioneering studies that identified two distinct regions of the adult mammalian CNS that contain populations of NSCs [1,2,8]. The identified sites where NSCs are present in the adult brain are the: subgranular zone of the dentate gyrus [1] and the subventricular zone (SVZ) of the lateral ventricles [9]. It has also been shown that NSCs in the adult brain are not only present in the SVZ but also in the entire rostral extension, including the distal portion within the olfactory bulb [10]. Although these endogenous adult NSCs have been shown to proliferate, migrate to the olfactory bulb and hippocampus, and ultimately differentiate into mature neurons, their functionality is not clear. In an elegant study done that used a virus-based trans-synaptic neuronal tracing and *c-fos* mapping it was demonstrated that the endogenous NSCs upregulated the expression of *c-fos* proto-oncogene in the olfactory bulb in response to an odor-induced signal [6,11]. These results indicate that adult NSCs can differentiate into newly formed adult neurons and functionally integrate into the synaptic circuitry of the mature brain.

Adult NSCs can also be isolated from the adult human brain. Indeed, such cells have now been cultured from human cadavers up to 20 days after death [12]. Although adult NSCs demonstrate a high degree of plasticity, they are difficult to isolate, found in smaller numbers, have a more limited proliferative capacity and seem to have a more restricted differentiation potential than their fetal counterparts [13].

Embryonic Stem Cells. Embryonic stem (ES) cells are obtained from the inner cell mass of the blastocyst of fetuses and can give rise to all tissues in the body, including those of the nervous system. ES cells are also multipotent, can be propagated *in vitro* and can be engineered to express therapeutic genes thus, provide the most promising alternative source of cells for transplant. When used for transplant, ES cells can migrate and differentiate into regionally appropriate cell types, and did not appear to interfere with normal brain development [14]. Initially, it has been reported that murine ES cells can be induced to express multiple neural phenotypes in culture using retinoic acid as the trigger for differentiation [15]. Following differentiation, it was found that the newly formed neurons were capable of generating action potentials and expressed numerous ion channels. In addition, others have reported that the ES cells expanded and differentiated into oligodendrocyte precursors were able to effectively myelinate host axons in animal models of human myelin disease [16,17].

Other studies have demonstrated that ES cells transplanted following focal forebrain ischaemic injury in adult rats not only survived in the infarct area but also established connections to the surrounding brain regions, with a resulting improvement in motor function [18-20], spatial learning, and memory [21,22]. Moreover, clinical trials of patients with Parkinson's disease that received ES cell grafts into the striatum showed that the grafted cells were spontaneously active and was able to restore dopamine release to near-normal levels with symptomatic improvement [23,24]. However, cell-based therapy in humans using ES cells has mixed results since in a recent clinical trial in Denver and New York, 15% of grafted patients developed unacceptable dyskinesias [23]. Immune rejection and subsequent failure of the graft can also be a problem associated with ES cell therapy, particularly in human clinical trials.

The major concern in using ES cells is its limited supply and the small number of neurons that can be generated and become available for transplant [13]. However, this problem may be partially overcome by *in vitro* expansion as demonstrated in a study wherein human ES cell isolated from the forebrain were expanded for up to a year in culture using epithelial growth factor (EGF), fibroblast growth factor (FGF), and leukemia inhibitory factor (LIF) [25]. Additionally, prolonged culture did not profoundly affect the potential of these expanded ES cells, and indeed injection of these cell lines into the developing rat brain showed extensive migration and integration [26]. Others have confirmed these findings and have shown that enriched neural precursors from human ES cells can incorporate into brain tissue and differentiate *in vivo* [27,28]. When these expanded human ES cells were transplanted into the lateral ventricles of newborn mice, migration to multiple brain regions was observed, followed by differentiation into cells with mature neuronal and astrocytic phenotypes but no mature oligodendrocytes were seen. In addition, embryonic day 12 (E12) cells propagated in culture have also been shown to retain the capacity to differentiate into dopaminergic neurons and to improve outcome in a rat model of Parkinson's disease [29]. These studies demonstrating the success of ES cell grafts *in vivo* has led to further work in other injury models to see whether transplanted cells can integrate and functionally improve outcome in different CNS injuries. Although present results on neural grafting using ES cells are encouraging, it is clear that challenges remain notwithstanding the highly controversial nature of the source of these cells.

Non-neuronal Tissue Cells. To circumvent the ethical issues concerning the use of ES cells for transplantation, a growing number of studies suggest that non-neural cell types (e.g. bone marrow cells) can be propagated and differentiated into neural lineages. Much of this work is controversial but if useful neural cells could be obtained from this source, it would avoid the ethical problems associated with the use of ES cells, and the practical issues of deriving cells from post-mortem brains. The early *in vivo* experimental data using non-neuronal cells was based on bone marrow transplantation (BMT) studies in lethally irradiated mice [30]. More recently, it has been shown that bone marrow-derived cells transplanted into the adult rat striatum after cerebral ischemia resulted in the amelioration of ischemia-induced neurological deficits [31]. There are now several published protocols for directing bone marrow stromal cells to neural lineages using different approaches that can range from using chemical demethylating or reducing agents, to retinoids to more physiological growth factors [32]. The successful generation of neural cells from blood could either be due to the presence of a minute subpopulation of highly pluripotent cells in the marrow, or explained by the reprogramming (trans- or dedifferentiation) of an already committed blood progenitor. Blood or bone marrow would be an ethically acceptable and easily accessible source of cells for neural replacement, although research in this area is still at an early stage and the findings are controversial.

Immortalized Cell Lines. Another alternative to ES cells comes in the form of immortalized cell lines. A pioneering study that used an exogenous cell line for regeneration in areas of the CNS was done in a rat model of stroke [33]. The cells used in that study was derived from a teratocarcinoma cell line, Ntera 2/cl.D1 (NT2), expanded in cell culture, and differentiated into pure postmitotic human neuronal cells following treatment with retinoic acid. Specifically, using the middle cerebral artery (MCA) occlusion model of stroke in rats, injection of the immortalized cells into the area of ischemia resulted in a partial restoration of behavioral and motor function [34]. Furthermore, follow-up study at 14 months showed no toxicity or tumor formation in the animals that received the graft [33]. Thereafter, a clinical trial that included 12 patients with basal ganglia stroke onset ranging from 6 months to 6 years received stereotactic injections of human teratocarcinoma (hNT) cells into their ischemic brain regions [35]. Results of this clinical trial showed an increase in the European Stroke Scale scores in patients that received the graft, thereby demonstrating that neuronal cell transplantation may be a therapeutic option for stroke patients with motor deficits. Further, using serial metabolic brain imaging with [^{18}F]fluorodeoxyglucose positron emission tomography that was obtained both before and after neural transplantation, patients that received the graft showed a 10% increase in functional activity at 6 months, with a return to baseline at 12 months. Although the immortalized cell lines showed promise as evident in these studies, they are not true stem cells and have been criticized for the difficulty in generating them especially for large-scale clinical use. Another criticism involving immortalized cell lines is that the initial reports lack convincing evidence on whether these cells actually integrated into the damaged parenchyma to form functionally significant neural network connections within the existing cytoarchitecture or how they might have contributed to behavioral recovery. Though a recent report using hNT cell lines transplanted into a rat model of complete spinal cord contusion with loss of motor evoked potentials addressed this concern [36]. In this spinal cord study, rats that underwent immediate and delayed (2 weeks after injury) transplantation of hNT showed significant functional recovery demonstrated by the return of motor evoked potentials and some degree of improvement in motor function.

Other cells lines that has been developed and tested are: C17.2 and CG4. The C17.2 immortalized cell line is derived from murine cerebellar external granular layer progenitor cells and transduced with a v-*myc* oncogene [37]. When transplanted into a targeted area of apoptotic neurodegeneration in the adult mouse neocortex, approximately 5% of the C17.2 cells differentiated into neurons and graft survival was seen up to 22 months [38]. In contrast, the CG4 immortalized cell line is an oligodendrocyte progenitor cells that has been used successfully for demyelinating diseases. For instance, a number of studies have demonstrated that CG4 transplantation into the spinal cord of rats with experimental autoimmune encephalomyelitis (EAE) survived for long periods of time, migrated as far as 6 cm from the site of injection, and repopulated areas of demyelination [39,40]. These studies suggest that immortalized cell lines may represent an additional source of exogenous cells to participate in neural repair involving CNS disorders. There are, however, considerable fears that immortalized cell lines may be prone to tumorigenesis and that they may not be able to replace the wide variety of cell types lost after CNS injury which makes their clinical use limited.

Evidence of Graft/Host Communication Following Neural Transplantation

Over a decade ago, it was demonstrated that grafting fetal neural tissue induce plasticity in the host brain resulting in the repair of damaged neurons in a manner that was different from that seen in spontaneous CNS recovery [41]. This was evident in an earlier study in neural transplantation wherein primary neural tissue from the fetal mouse (embryonic day 14, E14) neopallium was transplanted into the mechanically damaged barrel field area of primary somatosensory cortex of juvenile mice [42]. In this study, two co-isogenic mouse strains were used so that donor cells could be easily and unambiguously identified from host cells by allelic differences in their Thy-1 antigen (cell surface marker for neural cells). Results from this study showed that one month after transplantation the lesion cavity in 70-80% of mice that received the grafted cells appeared to become "filled" by relatively well-organized cortical tissue that even presented cellular arrangements reminiscent of barrels and displayed some degree of electrical activity. In comparison, the barrel field lesion in mice that did not receive the grafted cells remained unaltered or in some instances grew even larger. Surprisingly, anti Thy-1 immunohistochemistry demonstrated that virtually all transplant-induced regenerated tissue was of host origin in over 50% animals. These results were later validated using a xenotransplantation paradigm (transplantation between different species) wherein mouse tissue was transplanted into lesioned cat CNS [43]. Specifically, neural tissue from fetal embryonic (E14) mouse neopallium was transplanted into the primary visual cortical lesion of 1-month-old kittens and results similar to the earlier study were seen. However, the percentage of successful xenografting was lower than that of the previous allografts (grafts between individuals within the same species). To examine whether de novo neurogenesis could explain the results seen in these studies, barrel field lesioned mice received either tritiated thymidine ([^{3}H]T) or bromodeoxyuridine (BrdU) which are nucleotide analogs that label dividing cells during the S-phase of the cell cycle [43]. The investigators found that the majority of ([^{3}H]T)- and BrdU-labeled host cells to be of glial and endothelial origin, although no significant gliosis or glial scar was evident . Because limited endogenous neurogenesis was seen in this study, it was not sufficient to account for the substantial tissue recovery seen. Thus, other mechanisms such as "remodeling" of surrounding tissue by existing postmitotic cells as well as prevention of necrosis and secondary host cell death in the vicinity of the cavity may explain the graft/host interaction that led to the enhanced plasticity seen in the previous studies [44].

Others have also reported a similar graft-dependent regeneration in the injured brain. Using bilateral parietal cortex lesion in rats, others have found that primary fetal neural tissue grafted unilaterally influenced neuronal regeneration in the contralateral non-transplanted cavity wherein the lesion became smaller as compared to the non-grafted lesioned controls [45]. More recently, graft/host interactions during brain development were examined where human NSCs were grafted *in utero* into the ventricles of a midgestation non-human primate brain [8]. Results from this study showed that the donor cells not only survived the xenotransplantation, but also integrated into the host brain. Evidence of this integration was seen when the grafted cells entered the subventricular zone, interdigitated with the endogenous NSCs, and together both host and donor cells subdivided into different phenotype in the developing brain. This "teamwork" of donor and host NSCs seen during brain development was reflected in a prevalent morphogenetic scenario. That is, many of the NSCs migrated out of the subventricular zone and started to differentiate into various types of neural cells, while other subpopulations of donor and host NSCs remained undifferentiated and formed quiescent pools of multipotent cells, possibly for later use during ontogeny or maintenance of CNS homeostasis. Based on the observations of graft-induced host plasticity in the developing and injured brain, it is likely that reciprocal communication between graft and host cells is multifaceted [44]. Other indications of graft/host communication have been demonstrated in the aged brain and in CNS pathologies due to trauma or genetic disorders.

Graft/host Communication in the Aged Brain. The slow disintegration of neural function associated with aging provides an ideal opportunity to examine the reciprocal communication between the graft and host brain in an environment *not* confounded by excessive necrosis, excitotoxicity, anoxia, or trauma. Since dopaminergic neurons are typically compromised in advanced age, the study used systemic injection of MPTP (1-methyl-4-phenyl-1,2,3,6-tetrahydropyridine), a toxin selectively affecting dopaminergic neurons [46]. This model simulates the pathological processes known to accompany Parkinson's disease. In the study, rats received unilateral implantation of murine NSCs above the right ventral tegmental area at 1 and 4 weeks following systemic injection of MPTP. Extensive migration of donor cells was seen in both hemispheres of the aged MPTP-treated host brain compared to the young or intact aged brains. Neural transplantation resulted in a gradual reconstruction of the damaged mesostriatal system that was first seen unilaterally followed by bilateral regeneration. On the contrary, no regeneration was seen in MPTP-treated animals that did not receive NSC transplant. When immunohistochemical analysis was done, it showed that the newly formed cells express dopamine, the key neurotransmitter in the striatum. Further analysis showed that even though the restoration of the mesostriatal system was graft-dependent, it was not primarily due to differentiation of the donor NSCs into dopaminergic neurons. While a random and unstructured conversion of NSCs to become mature dopaminergic neurons was seen that contributed to the reconstruction of the mesostrital system, the majority of mesencephalic neurons involved in the recovery process were actually *"rescued" host cells*. These data suggest that the injured host CNS benefited from transplanted NSCs not because the grafted cells replaced the dysfunctional cells, but mainly because the donor cells were able to rescue the damaged neurons. This often ignored new possibility of saving damaged host circuitry and increasing the endogenous regenerative capacity of an adult injured CNS by a plasticity-promoting dialogue between graft and host has now been corroborated in several other studies [21,47-49].

Graft/host Communication in Head Injury. Communication between grafted and host cells have also been documented to occur in an excitotoxic environment. In an adult rat model of experimentally-induced apoptosis where pyramidal neurons in the neocortex were selectively targeted, NSCs were transplanted into this neurodegenerative environment [50].

Investigators found that 15% of the grafted cells differentiated into pyramidal neurons partially replacing the neuronal population lost due to apoptosis. In addition, it was demonstrated that some 'replacement' neurons were able to form axons that send projections across the corpus callosum to appropriate targets in the contralateral brain hemisphere. These data suggest that even in the presence of a neurodegenerative environment, cues generated by donor and host tissue may be able to direct migration, proliferation, and differentiation of NSCs.

Graft/host communication in injury was also seen during brain development. Using the hypoxic-ischemic injury model, newborn mice were subjected to unilateral carotid ligation combined with reduced ambient oxygen. This model results in extensive hypoxic–ischemic brain (HI) injury throughout the ipsilateral cerebral hemisphere. In this study, the immortalized cells C17.2 were grafted prior to HI injury to a subgroup of animals so that they can integrate into the cytoarchitecture of the host brain during development creating a virtual chimeric brain of host and donor stem cells [51,52] while another subgroup of animals received the C17.2 donor stem cell graft at different intervals following HI injury. The movements and responses of the donor stem cells to HI injury were tracked by its *lacZ* reporter gene expression. The investigators reported that a subpopulation of donor stem cells and host cells transiently re-entered the cell cycle and migrated preferentially to the ischemic site in response to HI injury. Also, it was reported that grafted cells integrated extensively in the injured areas of the brain and even cells transplanted in the intact contralateral hemisphere migrated toward regions of injury. Additionally, a subpopulation of both donor- and host-derived cells differentiated into new neurons and oligodendrocytes, particularly in the penumbral area. Interestingly, a 5-fold increase in donor-derived oligodendrocytes was seen in the injured brain as compared with the intact neocortex. The findings of increased oligodendrocyte production are important because this neural cell type is least likely to regenerate spontaneously following injury to the postnatal CNS. Parallel results were reported in the postnatal spinal cord (SC) injury model using sciatic axotomy resulting in segmental α-motorneuron (MN) degeneration [53]. Following NSC transplantation, a significant portion of the grafted cells migrated toward the injured area and 'repopulated' the ventral horn of the spinal cord. It was reported that approximately 20% of the grafted cells in the ventral horn then differentiated into cells that resemble the lost α-MNs. Again, the importance of these findings must be re-emphasized because α-MNs are normally formed only during fetal development. Taken together, these data suggest the possibility that grafted NSCs whether engineered or not can differentiate, enhance neurite outgrowth and form proper connectivity into the host brain even in a neurodegenerative milieu.

Graft/host Communication in Genetic Disorders. In verifying that graft/host communication also occurs in CNS disorders with genetic origin, mice with a variety of genetic mutations were tested. These mouse mutants are suitable for conducting well-controlled and well-defined models of complex CNS dysfunctions. For instance, in the *meander tail* (*mea*) mutant, a model characterized by the failure of sufficient granule neurons to develop in certain regions of the cerebellum, NSCs were implanted at birth via the intracerebroventricular method [54]. In this study, the investigators found that the transplanted cells were able to 'repopulate' regions of the cerebellum that lacked sufficient granule neurons. This observation suggests that cells with the potential for multiple fates 'shifted' their mode of differentiation to compensate for a deficiency in a particular cell type.

When compared with endogenous NSC differentiation in normal cerebella, most of the donor NSCs in regions deficient in granule neurons pursued a granule neuron phenotype in preference to other neuronal phenotypes suggesting that environmental signals may play a role in 'pushing' undifferentiated, multipotent cells towards replacing the missing cell type.

In a pilot study using another mouse mutant model, active communication between the graft and host cells has also been demonstrated. In the *reeler* (*rl*) mouse, the laminar assignment of neurons in the cortex is profoundly abnormal primarily due to a mutation in the gene encoding the secreted extracellular matrix molecule (ECM), Reelin. In this genetic model, NSC transplantation was done at birth via the intracerebroventricular method with the aim of not only replacing developmentally impaired cells, but also help correct certain aspects of the abnormal brain cytoarchitecture [55]. Investigators reported that the grafted cells were able to replace missing neurons, but more importantly these neurons were found to be in correct laminar position suggesting the possibility that the differentiated NSCs were able to provide molecules (perhaps including Reelin) to guide proper histogenesis. Comparison of the brain cytoarchitecture between the mutant and wild-type mice showed that the laminar appearance of neurons between these two groups was similar. These findings suggest that CNS disorders characterized by abnormal brain cytoarchitecture may also benefit from stem cell-based therapy.

Many CNS diseases, particularly those of genetic origin, are characterized by global degeneration or dysfunction, therefore mutants characterized by CNS-wide white matter disease may provide an ideal model for testing the overall effectiveness of neural cell replacement therapy. The *shiverer* (*shi*) is an appropriate model for widespread CNS white matter disease since the oligodendroglia of this dysmyelinated mouse mutant are dysfunctional because they lack the myelin basic protein gene which is essential for effective myelination [56]. In this mutant model, NSCs were transplanted at birth via the intracerebroventricular technique for diffuse engraftment. Investigators found that a vast majority of donor cells differentiated into oligodendroglia and a subgroup of these glial cells were able to myelinate approximately 40% of host axonal processes. Furthermore, some of the mice demonstrated a decrease in the symptomatic tremor caused by dysmyelination. These results suggest that global CNS pathologies may be amenable to cell replacement. More broadly, findings from these studies have implications for the treatment of neurodevelopmental disorders especially with genetic origins.

The graft-induced "regenerative phenomenon" seen in the above studies is possibly mediated by cellular and molecular mechanisms that modified the brain environment such that intrinsic, albeit latent, regenerative responses by the host were either being triggered, uncovered, or amplified (Fig. 1). It is commonly thought that the observed repair or regeneration seen after NSC transplantation may be attributed solely to the capacity of grafted cells to either deliver the missing neuroactive substances or replace dysfunctional cells. On the other hand, the notion that the host tissue itself may be stimulated by donor-derived cells to release growth promoting molecules so that it can participate in its own repair has been reluctantly acknowledged or otherwise completely ignored; however, based on the results reported in the above studies, this is a thought that should be seriously entertained.

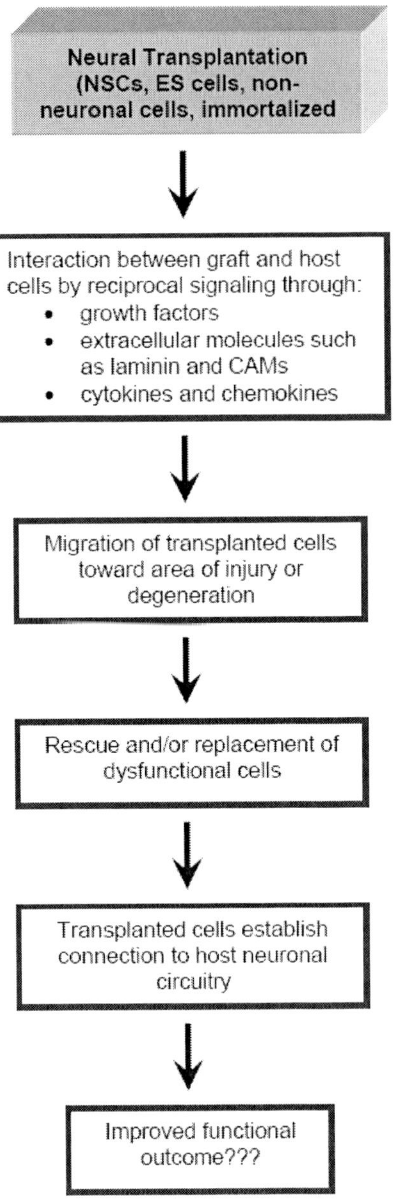

Figure 1. Putative events that occur following neural transplantation. The grafting of NSCs into the damaged CNS initiates a cascade of events starting with the release of signals from donor cells and host tissue to modify their own plasticity-related programs. Depending on the signals released, grafted cells then migrate and repopulate the area of injury where they either: differentiate and replace the dysfunctional neurons or deliver the molecules necessary to enhance the inherent regenerative capacity of the host CNS. The replacement cells then integrate into the cytoarchitecture of the host brain which can lead to functional recovery. The last box have question marks box since the functional significance of graft-induced regeneration and repair is not fully confirmed.

Table 1. Signaling Molecules Involved in Graft/Host Communications. These molecules are generated by either donor or host cells or both to mediate the multifaceted dialogue that occurs between the grafted cells and host tissue. *Abbreviations*: MIP – macrophage inflammatory protein.

Factors Involved in the Dialogue Between Grafted Cells and Host	Functions
Growth factors: • LIF • CNTF • TGF-β • GDNF • BDNF • BMP-2 • FGF • SDNSF	Regulate proliferation and differentiation of transplanted cells
CAMs: • Integrins • L1 glycoprotein • N-cadherins • N-CAM	- Stabilize connections made by transplanted cells into the host neuronal circuitry - Activate various signaling cascade - Support migration of transplanted cells along the extracellular matrix
Cytokines and Chemokines: • IL-6 • TNF-α • MIP-3β • CXCR4 – receptor for stromal cell-derived factor-1	- Supports migration of transplanted cells towards dysfunctional areas - Affects proliferation and differentiation of transplanted cells

A. Possible Factors That Mediate Graft/Host Communication

The long-range effects of grafted tissue seen in the above studies suggest at least a partial role for secreted and diffusible substances mediating the necessary graft/host interaction (Table 1). Graft/host communications contributing to cell differentiation and the 'regenerative phenomenon' seen in the above studies are likely to include processes similar to those regulating plasticity during development [41]. Such processes include, but are not limited to cell - cell interactions through direct contact or mediated by the extracellular matrix (ECM) and the release of diffusible factors such as Sonic hedgehog [57], tissue specific trophic factors [58], bone morphogenic proteins (BMP) [59], neurotrophins [60,61], and cells of the immune system such as cytokines and chemokines [62,63]. Through intricate intracellular signaling pathways, graft/host communication may lead to the modulation of gene transcription defining the fate of both donor and recipient cells.

A group of molecules that has been well-studied in relation to NSCs is the family of neurotrophic factors which are likely to play a key role in graft-induced host plasticity. Various studies have shown that pools of undifferentiated donor progenitor cells spontaneously express growth factors [53,64-68] such as glial cell line-derived neurotrophic factor (GDNF), neurotrophin-3 (NT-3), brain-derived neurotrophic factor (BDNF), LIF, ciliary neurotrophic factor (CNTF), transforming-growth factor-β (TGF-β) or the newly identified stem cell-derived neural stem/progenitor cell supporting factor (SDNSF). For example, undifferentiated donor cells and glia adjacent to rescued dopaminergic neurons in MPTP-treated aged mice were found to express GDNF. The protective effects of GDNF were evident not only on dopaminergic neurons in the mesostriatal system but also in the α-MNs located in the ventral horn of the spinal cord. As well, a two-fold increase in the expression of other growth factors such as LIF, CNTF, and TGF-β has been documented in neuronal progenitor cells. Fibroblast FGF is another neurotrphic factor documented to be involved in regulating neural stem cell proliferation both *in vitro* and *in vivo* [69]. Based on these studies, it is believed that growth factors may be necessary in the proliferation and multi-lineage differentiation of both donor and host NSCs.

Another growth-promoting and guidance molecules involved in the plasticity of the developing and grafted CNS are the ECM molecules such as laminin and cell adhesion molecules (CAMs). Studies have shown that axonal outgrowth and correct targeting of postsynaptic partners depend critically on the binding of growth cone-associated CAMs to their appropriate receptors because cell motility and migration in the ECM substrates are mediated by adhesion receptors called integrins [70-74]. Once the final axonal links were established, CAMs were found to provide stability to the connections suggesting the ability of these molecules to support cell adhesion and to activate various signaling cascades. CAMs that have been identified to support the migration of transplanted cells along ECMs and their contacts with neuronal, glial, immune, and inflammatory cells are: N-CAM, N-cadherin, and the L1 glycoprotein. L1 glycoprotein is the best-characterized molecule in its class and has been shown to be involved in many events involving plasticity in the developing and adult CNS. Evidence suggests that binding between soluble and neuron-bound forms of L1 glycoprotein is important in cell survival, neurite sprouting, and axonal growth [72]. Mice that overexpress L1 glycoprotein showed that an excess of this molecule can accelerate formation of major motor and sensory fiber tracts and promote the development of these tracts [75]. Overexpression of L1 glycoprotein has also led to the enhanced migration of cerebellar granule cells, patterning of nigral dopaminergic neurons and retinal axons, and possibly enhanced neurogenesis. In humans, mutations in the L1 glycoprotein gene result in a complex disorder in the corpus callosum characterized by agenesis, aphasia, spastic paraplegia and hydrocephalus leading to mental retardation [76]. From these reports it seems reasonable to think that the interactions of cell-bound CAMs with each other and with ECM components can possibly mediate the communication between donor and host cells following neural transplant.

Another often-overlooked group of active molecules that may play a role in mediating graft/host communication are the cytokines and chemokines released after CNS injury and during immune response of the host CNS to neural transplantation. Cytokines have been shown to have a profound effect on the differentiation of NSCs into neurons, astrocytes, and oligodendrocytes [3,77-79]. It is presumed that pro-inflammatory cytokines such as tumor necrosis factor-α (TNF-α) and interleukin-1β (IL-1β) may influence the survival of grafted cells by inducing apoptosis and downregulating the expression of the CAM receptors, integrins, thereby interfering with the ability of donor cells to enhance the regenerative capacity of the host CNS. Conversely, the presence of anti-inflammatory cytokines such as interleukin-1 (IL-6) and IL-10 may promote plasticity in the donor and host cells [80,81]. Confounding the complex role of the immune system in mediating graft/host communication after transplantation is the expression of chemokines. Even though both *in vitro* and *in vivo* studies have demonstrated the dependence of transplanted NSCs on chemokines to migrate from the site of implantation to the region of injury [63,82,83], the role of these immune molecules in neural transplantation is far from being understood. Nevertheless, based on our limited understanding of the role of the immune system on the active dialogue that occurs between the donor cells and host brain following neural transplantation, it can be speculated that the migration, and possibly differentiation of transplanted cells may be influenced by the cytokine and chemokine networks.

B. Enhancing Graft/Host Communication

In some instances, implanted NSCs can easily migrate and engraft in the host brain even if the milieu was degenerative or toxic because of intact cytoarchitecture. Nonetheless, in certain circumstances when there is extensive destruction of the CNS cytoarchitecture, even the use of optimal donor cells has minimal chance of surviving, let alone repairing damaged host cells. In these cases, use of 'scaffolds' may be necessary to optimize the communication between donor and host tissue. Indeed, it has been shown that using a three-dimensional highly porous 'scaffolds' composed of polyglycolic acid (PGA) may act as a bridge between donor and host cells in repairing the damaged CNS circuitry [84-86]. PGA is a synthetic, biodegradable, and highly hydrophobic polymer that has been widely used in clinical medicine. Concerns regarding long-term biocompatibility of PGA should be minimal because PGA looses its mechanical strength in approximately 2-4 weeks after implanted in the body [86]. This length of time is enough to provide an initial matrix to guide cellular organization and growth, allow diffusion of nutrients to the transplanted cells, and become vascularized [84,85]. The efficacy of PGA has been reported in NSC transplant studies involving the brain and spinal cord. At the start, NSCs were co-cultured with PGA *in vitro* for 4 days to allow for the donor cells to adhere to the scaffold and migrate throughout the matrix then the NSC-PGA complex was transplanted in the area of infarction in an experimental HI injury model [84,86]. The investigators reported that the NSC-PGA complex 'repopulated' the area of infarction and became vascularized by the host tissue. Furthermore, with the use of DiI and biotinylated dextrose amine (BDA) as tracers, it was documented that neurite outgrowth of host and donor origins enwrapped the polymer fibers often interconnecting with each other and extended as far as the opposite brain hemisphere. These data suggest that the PGA scaffold may be able to act as an artificial ECM to maximize the reciprocal interaction between the NSC and host tissue.

In a parallel study, NSC seeded on a PGA-based scaffold was transplanted in adult rats with experimentally hemisectioned spinal cord injury [84]. Investigators in this study reported a significant improvement in animal movement following transplantation and at the same time a reduction of necrosis in the surrounding parenchyma was seen, and extensive secondary cell loss, inflammation, and formation of a glial scar were also prevented. Again, using DiI and BDA for tract tracing and GAP-43 (marker for axonal growth) for immunohistochemistry, it was documented that the host tissue displayed regenerated neurites that are not only derived from donor NSCs but also from the recipient spinal cord. These results suggest that the graft/host communication can augmented to facilitate the repair of damaged neuronal circuitry in the host CNS.

The studies mentioned above provide encouraging evidence that neural tissues can survive transplantation into the adult mammalian brain and spinal cord, integrate and connect with the host nervous system, and influence the host's behavior. Considerable advances have been made over the past decade in understanding the causes of cell death in transplanted tissues, and in developing strategies to improve cell survival, differentiation and long distance axon growth within the host brain. Nevertheless, there are concerns that although grafted cells were able to establish connections with the host brain, the appropriate integration of these connections into the afferent and efferent pathways of the host brain and their contribution to recovery of function have not been fully studied. That is, the functional improvement seen after grafting has not been delineated as different from the spontaneous recovery that occur after CNS injury. It is possible that circuit reconstruction although necessary, might not be sufficient for full functional recovery. There is some validity to this concern since during ontogeny, the growing animal must not only develop the right anatomical structures and systems, but also acquire and refine appropriate patterns of behavior through learning and experience [87]. The influence of experience and physical activity on CNS plasticity has each been extensively investigated in its own right. Data from animals and humans suggest that appropriate rehabilitation through experience, practice, and retraining is necessary to aid spontaneous recovery and reacquire lost function after CNS injury [88-93]. But the degree to which these rehabilitation strategies can enhance the active communication between graft and host cells is not clear.

Table 2. EC Studies on Rehabilitation Effects on Graft Survival and Function.

Injury Model	Graft Source	Rehabilitation Strategy	Morphological Results	Functional Results	References
Fimbria-fornix aspiration lesion	Fetal septal tissue	Environmental enrichment	Increased neurite outgrowth in the hippocampus	Improved performance in the Hebb-Williams maze	100
Focal ischemia (MCAO)	Fetal neocortical tissue	Environmental enrichment	No effect on size of infarction but decreased thalamic atrophy was seen	Improved posture and performance in traversing the rotating pole	99 and 101
Lesion of the nigrostriatal dopamine pathway	Fetal striatal tissue	Enriched environment	Increased graft survival and formation of dopaminergic neurons	Improved performance in the delayed alternation and rotation tasks	19, 96 and 98
Cortical aspiration	Fetal cortex	Environmental enrichment	No effects on lesion size	Improved performance in the beam walking task	97
Lesion of the striatum	Fetal striatal tissue	Environmental enrichment	Enriched housing condition increased the development of striatal-like neurons	Improved performance in the staircase walking task	102

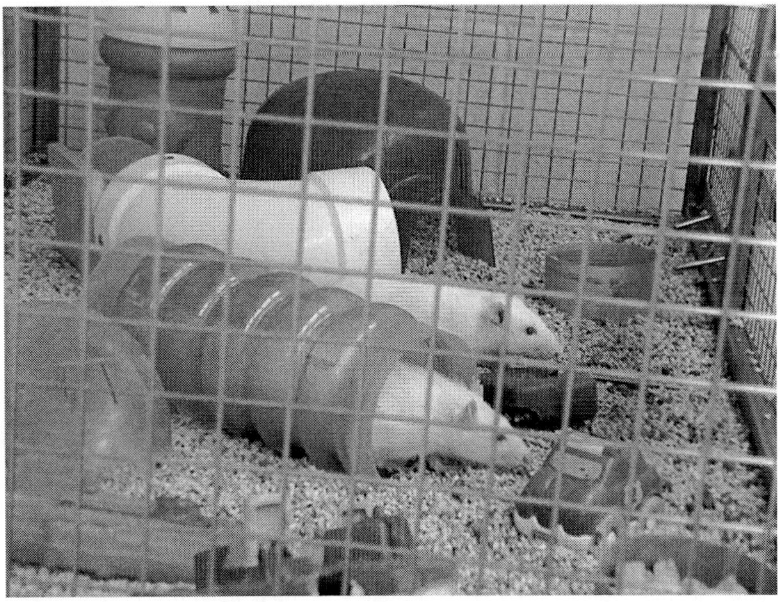

Figure 2. Complex Environment Housing. Rats are usually housed together in a cage filled with a variety of objects. Objects in the home cage are changed at regular intervals to maintain novelty.

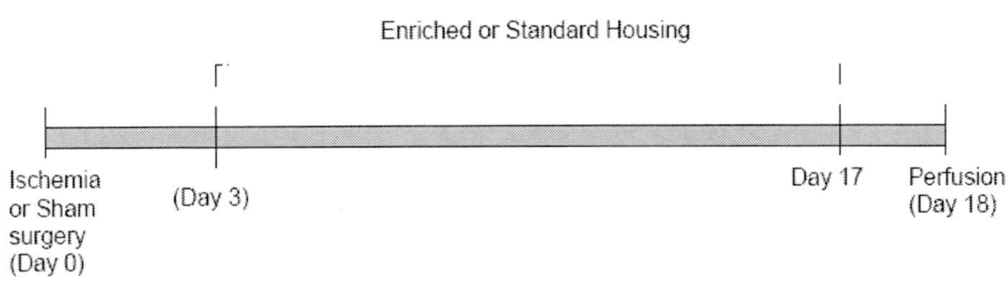

(A)

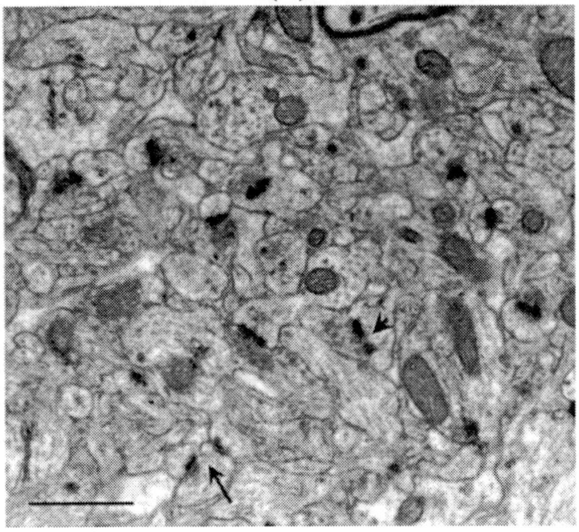

(B)

Figure 3. (Continued on next page)

	Multiple Synaptic Boutons	Perforated PSD
Ischemia EC	3.73 ± 0.39*	2.31 ± 0.38*
Ischemia SC	1.91 ± 0.25	1.38 ± 0.33
Sham EC	4.14 ± 0.42*	2.73 ± 0.42*
Sham SC	1.82 ± 0.44	1.57 ± 0.22

(C)

Figure 3. Enhanced Morphological Plasticity After Cerebral Ischemia May be Mediated by Behavioral Experience (modified from Briones et al., 2004). (A) Study design. (B) Electron micrograph of the stratum radiatum in the hippocampal area printed at a final magnification of 40,000x illustrating multiple synaptic boutons (long arrow) and perforated synapses (short arrow). Multiple synaptic boutons are synapses formed between an individual axonal bouton and more than one dendritic processes (shafts or spines) while perforated synapses are identified by the presence of a completely partitioned and/or interrupted post-synaptic density. These types of synapse are putatively associated with enhanced efficacy in neurotransmission and a major component of behavioral experience-related plasticity. (C) Number of multiple synaptic boutons and synapses with perforated postsynaptic density per neuron based on stereological analysis. Data are 10^6 synapses per neuron (synaptic density/neuronal density) ± standard error of the mean. *$p < 0.05$. *Abbreviations*: EC – enriched housing, SC – control group, PSD – postsynaptic density. Scale bar = 1 μm.

Although limited, experimental evidence suggests that rehabilitation training may be important in enhancing the plasticity of, and functional recovery provided by neural grafts (Table 2). The mechanisms by which behavioral experience can influence brain structure and function first received attention after Hebb's observations and theoretical proposals that learning is represented in the brain by synaptic changes in response to repeated concurrent activation [94]. These fundamental concepts were subsequently confirmed at the cellular and molecular levels in various organisms ranging from simple to complex [95]. The inherent regenerative capacity of the adult brain to respond to injury may also be influenced by behavioral experience [90]. Our group has demonstrated that enriched housing condition (Fig. 2) following global cerebral ischemia enhanced the spontaneous recovery from injury evidenced by the alteration in synaptic morphology at the site of infarction (Fig. 3). Thus, it is possible that the intrinsic plasticity of the adult CNS to recover from injury may be augmented by behavioral experience. Consequently, the possibility exists that rehabilitation strategies following neural transplantation may enhance the functional integration of neural grafts into the host neuronal circuitry leading to complete behavioral recovery.

The literature on the behavioral effects of rehabilitation training following cell-based therapy is very limited. Some studies have been shown that grafts that are rich in cholinergic neurons derived from the embryonic basal forebrain were able to reverse various cognitive impairments associated with cholinergic depletion in the rat cortex and hippocampus caused by ageing or experimental lesions [19,96-102]. In particular, grafted cells in the dorsal neocortex resulted in increased cholinergic fiber outgrowth that was greater in rats that were housed in an enriched or complex environment (EC) as compared to rats kept in standard laboratory cages. The difference in cholinergic fiber outgrowth seen in these studies was particularly marked at 4 weeks after grafting, but seemed to decrease by 10 weeks, suggesting that the greatest effect of complex environment housing might be during the initial interactions between the graft and host cells. Interestingly, the reports on behavioral recovery following EC housing and neural transplantation are conflicting where others demonstrated amelioration in functional deficits while others have shown no improvement in behavior. These conflicting results may be a function of differences in behavioral tests used, length of time in EC, and timing of grafts after injury. The behavioral test used ranged from the simple task of motor asymmetry, such as rotation, postural position and balance on a rotating rod to the more complex test of skilled forelimb reaching task and maze learning. Additionally, the length of EC housing used in these studies ranged from 2 to 10 months while timing of grafts range from immediately after to several days after lesion. Timing of graft after injury may be the most important variable because it is possible that delaying the lesion - graft interval may reduce the opportunities for the grafts to establish the necessary afferent and efferent innervations to become fully functional. From these studies, it is clear that the role of rehabilitation training in mediating the successful communication between the grafted cells and host tissue deserves additional investigation. Since neuronal reorganization that occurs after CNS injury have been compared to the plasticity observed in development, involving sprouting and pruning stages, each under behavioral experience-dependent control [87], it is possible that a similar mechanism may be necessary for the 'appropriate' integration of grafted cell into the host circuitry.

CONCLUSION

In this review, the multifaceted dialogue that occurs between the graft and host tissue, and the graft evoked host plasticity has been highlighted as central in understanding the role of neurotransplantation in restorative medicine. The various mechanisms that may mediate the active communication between the graft and host tissue have also been discussed although the role of some molecules (e.g. cytokines and chemokines) are less understood than others (e.g. growth factors and CAMs). Despite our continuing efforts to gain insight on the interactions between graft and host tissue, NSC transplantation after CNS injury is still fraught with problems such as inconsistent and poor cell survival, and limited differentiation of donor cells to neuronal versus glial phenotypes. To face these challenges, further studies need to be done on the changes that occur in the CNS environment during various types of injury as well as the factors in the environment that might interfere with NSC survival and differentiation. As well, since it is commonly acknowledged that the CNS environment after injury may not be accommodating to neural grafting, more attention is needed on how to shift the balance between permissive and non-permissive milieu to favor successful transplantation. Lastly, consideration must be given to the fact that replacing lost cells and reconstructing damaged circuits of the brain although necessary, may not be sufficient for recovery of function after injury. Thus, the possibility that neural transplantation and rehabilitation training may have complementary roles in promoting full functional recovery deserves further attention.

REFERENCES

[1] Gage FH, Kempermann G, Palmer TD, Peterson DA, Ray J: Multipotent progenitor cells in the adult dentate gyrus. *Journal of Neurobiology* 1998, 36:249-266.
[2] Altman J, Das GD: Autoradiographic examination of the effects of enriched environment on the rate of glial multiplication in the adult rat brain. *Nature* 1964, 204:1161-1163.
[3] Xiao BG, Link H: Immune regulation within the central nervous system. *Journal of Neurological Science* 1998, 157:1-12.
[4] Levison SW, Goldman JE: Multipotential and lineage restricted precursors coexist in the mammalian perinatal subventicular zone. *Journal of Neuroscience Research* 1997, 48:83-94.
[5] Mayer-Proschel M, Kalyani AJ, Mujtaba T, Rao MS: Isolation of lineage-restricted neuronal precursors from multipotent neuroepithelial stem cells. *Neuron* 1997, 19:773-785.
[6] Clarke DL, Johansson CB, Wilbertz J, Veress B, Nilsson E, Karlstrom H, Lendahl U, Frisen J: Generalized Potential of Adult Neural Stem Cells. *Science* 2000, 288:1660-1663.
[7] Meyerrose TE, Herrbrich P, Hess DA, Nolta JA: Immune-deficient mouse models for analysis of human stem cells. *Biotechniques* 2003, 35:1262-1272.
[8] Ourednik V, Ourednik J, Flax JD, Zawada WM, Hutt C, Yang C, Park KI, Kim SU, Sidman RL, Freed CR, et al.: Segregation of human neural stem cells in the developing primate forebrain. *Science* 2001, 293:1820-1824.
[9] Lois C, Alvarez-Buylla A: Proliferating subventricular zone cells in the adult mammalian forebrain can differentiate into neurons and glia. *Proceedings National Academy of Science* 1993, 90:2074-2077.
[10] Johansson CB, Momma S, Clarke DL, Risling M, Lendahl U, Frisen J: Identification of neural stem cell in the adult mammalian central nervous system. *Cell* 1999, 96:25-34.
[11] Carlen M, Cassidy RM, Brismar H, Smith GA, Enquist LW, Frisen J: Functional Integration of Adult-Born Neurons. *Current Biology* 2002, 12:606-608.
[12] Palmer TD, Schwartz PH, Taupin P, Kaspar B, Stein SA, Gage FH: Cell culture: progenitor cells from human brain after death. *Nature* 2001, 411:42-43.
[13] Labat ML: Stem cells and the promise of eternal youth: embryonic versus adult stem cells. *Biomedecine & Pharmacotherapy* 2001, 55:179-185.
[14] Flax JD, Aurora S, Yang C: Engraftable human neural stem cells respond to developmental cues, replace neurons, and express foreign genes. *Nature Biotechnology* 1998, 16:1033-1039.
[15] Bain G, Kitchens D, Yao M, Huettner JE, Gootlieb DI: Embryonic stem cells express neuronal properties in vitro. *Developmental Biology* 1995, 168:342-357.
[16] Liu S, Qu Y, Stewart TJ, Howard MJ, Chakrabortty S, Holekamp TF, McDonald JW: Embryonic stem cells differentiate into oligodendrocytes and myelinate in culture and

after spinal cord transplantation. *Proceedings National Academy of Science* 2000, 97:6126-6131.

[17] Brustle O, Jones KN, Learish RD, Karram K, Choudhary K, Wiestler OD, Duncan ID, McKay RD: Embryonic stem cell-derived glial precursors: a source of myelinating transplants. *Science* 1999, 285:754-756.

[18] Sorensen JC, Grabowski M, Zimmer J, Johansson BB: Fetal neocortical tissue blocks implanted in brain infarction of adult rats interconnect with the host brain. *Experimental Neurology* 1996, 138:227-235.

[19] Döbrössy MD, Dunnett SB: Motor training effects on recovery of function after striatal lesions and striatal grafts. *Experimental Neurology* 2003, 184:274-284.

[20] Chu K, Kim M, Park K-I, Jeong S-W, Park H-K, Jung K-H, Lee S-T, Kang L, Lee K, Park D-K: Human neural stem cells improve sensorimotor deficits in the adult rat brain with experimental focal ischemia. *Brain Research* 2004, 1016:145-153.

[21] Englund U, Bjorklund A, Wictorin K, Lindvall O, Kokaia M: Grafted neural stem cells develop into functional pyramidal neurons and integrate into host cortical circuitry. *Proceedings National Academy of Science* 2002, 99:17089-17094.

[22] Wernig M, Benninger F, Schmandt T, Rade M, Tucker KL, Bussow H, Beck H, Brustle O: Functional Integration of embryonic stem cell-derived neurons in vivo. *Journal of Neuroscience* 2004, 24:5258-5268.

[23] Freed CR, Greene PE, Breeze RE, Tsai W-Y, DuMouchel W, Kao R, Dillon S, Winfield H, Culver S, Trojanowski JQ, et al.: Transplantation of embryonic dopamine neurons for severe Parkinson's disease. *New England Journal of Medicine* 2001, 344:710-719.

[24] Kirik D, Björklund A: Histological analysis of fetal dopamine cell suspension grafts in two patients with Parkinson's disease gives promising results. *Brain* 2005, 128:1478-1479.

[25] Englund U, Fricker-Gates RA, Lundberg C, Björklund A, Wictorin K: Transplantation of human neural progenitor cells into the neonatal rat brain: extensive migration and differentiation with long-distance axonal projections. *Experimental Neurology* 2002, 173:1-21.

[26] Eriksson C, Björklund A, Wictorin K: Neuronal differentiation following transplantation of expanded mouse neurosphere cultures derived from different embryonic forebrain regions. *Experimental Neurology* 2003, 184:615-635.

[27] Jensen JB, Björklund A, Parmar M: Striatal neuron differentiation from neurosphere-expanded progenitors depends on Gsh2 expression. *Journal of Neuroscience* 2004, 24:6958-6967.

[28] Tabar V, Panagiotakos G, Greenberg ED, Chan BK, Sadelain M, Gutin PH, Studer L: Migration and differentiation of neural precursors derived from human embryonic stem cells in the rat brain. *Nature Biotechnology* 2005, 23:601-606.

[29] Studer L, Tabar V, McKay R: Transplantation of expanded mesencephalic precursors leads to recovery in parkinsonian rats. *Nature Neuroscience* 1998, 1:290-295.

[30] Björklund A, Lindvall O: Cell replacment therapies for central nervous system disorders. *Nature Neuroscience* 2000, 3:537-544.

[31] Veizovic T, Beech JS, Stroemer RP, Watson WP, Hodges H: Resolution of stroke deficits following contralateral grafts of conditionally immortal neuroepithelial stem cells. *Stroke* 2001, 32:1012-1019.

[32] Terada N, Hamazaki T, Oka M, Hoki M, Mastalerz DM, Nakano Y, Meyer EM, Morel L, Petersen BE, Scott EW: Bone marrow cells adopt the phenotype of other cells by spontaneous cell fusion. *Nature* 2002, 416:542-545.
[33] Kleppner SR, Robinson KA, Trojanowski JQ, Lee VM: Transplanted human neurons derived from a teratocarcinoma cell line mature, integrate, and survive for over 1 year in the nude mouse brain. *Journal of Comparative Neurology* 1995, 357:618-632.
[34] Borlongan CV, Tajima Y, Trojanowski JQ, Lee VM, Sanberg PR: Transplantation of cryopreserved human embryonal carcinoma-derived neurons (NT2N cells) promotes functional recovery in ischemic rats. *Experimental Neurology* 1998, 149:310-321.
[35] Kondziolka D, Wechsler L, Goldstein S, Meltzer C, Thulbon KR, Gebel J, Jannetta PJ, DeCesare S, Elder EM, McGrogan M, et al.: Transplantation of cultured human neuronal cells for patients with stroke. *Neurology* 2000, 55:565-569.
[36] Saporta S, Makoui AS, Willing AE, Daadi M, Cahill DW, Sanberg PR: Functional recovery after complete contusion injury to the spinal cord and transplantation of human neuroteratocarcinoma neurons in rats. *Journal of Neurosurgery* 2002, 97:63-68.
[37] Snyder EY, Deitcher DL, Walsh CA, Arnold-Aldea S, Hartwieg EA, Cepko CL: Multipotent neural cell lines can engraft and participate in development of mouse cerebellum. *Cell* 1992, 68:33-51.
[38] Park K: Transplantation of neural stem cells: cellular and gene therapy for hypoxic-ischemic brain injury. *Yonsei Medical Journal* 2000, 41:825-835.
[39] Franklin RJM, Bayley SA, Blakemore WF: Transplanted CG4 Cells (an oligodendrocyte progenitor cell line) survive, migrate, and contribute to repair of areas of demyelination in X-Irradiated and damaged spinal cord but not in normal spinal cord. *Experimental Neurology* 1996, 137:263-276.
[40] Tourbah A, Linnington C, Bachelin C, Avellana-Adalid V, Wekerle H, A. Baron-Van Evercooren: Inflammation promotes survival and migration of the CG4 oligodendrocyte progenitors transplanted in the spinal cord of both inflammatory and demyelinated EAE rats. *Journal of Neuroscience Research* 1997, 50:853-861.
[41] Ourednik J, Ourednik W, Loos Vd: Do foetal neural grafts induce repair by the injured juvenile neocortex? *Neuroreport* 1993, 5:133-136.
[42] Andres FL, Van der Loos H: Removal and re-implantation of the parietal cortex of the neonatal mouse: consequences for the barrel field. *Brain Reseach* 1985, 352:115-121.
[43] Ourednik J, Ourednik w, Mitchell DE: Remodeling of lesioned kitten visual cortex after xenotransplantation of fetal mouse neopallidium. *Journal of Comparative Neurology* 1998, 395:91-111.
[44] Ourednik V, Ourednik J: Graft/host relationships in the developing and regenerating CNS of mammals. *Annals New York Academy of Science* 2005, 1049:172-184.
[45] Valoušková V, Gálik J: Unilateral grafting of fetal neocortex into a cortical cavity improves healing of a symmetric lesion in the contralateral cortex of adult rats. *Neuroscience Letters* 1995, 186:103-106.
[46] Ourednik J, Ourednik V, Lynch WP, Schachner M, Snyder EY: Neural stem cells display an inherent mechanism for rescuing dysfunctional neurons. *Nature Biotechnology* 2002, 20:1103-1110.
[47] Fujiwara Y, Tanaka N, Ishida O, Fujimoto Y, Murakami T, Kajihara H, Yasunaga Y, Ochi M: Intravenously injected neural progenitor cells of transgenic rats can migrate to

the injured spinal cord and differentiate into neurons, astrocytes and oligodendrocytes. *Neuroscience Letters* 2004, 366:287-291.

[48] McDonald JW, Becker D, Holekamp TF, Howard M, Liu S, Lu A, Lu J, Platik MM, Qu Y, Stewart T, et al.: Repair of the injured spinal cord and the potential of embryonic stem cell transplantation. *Journal of Neurotrauma* 2004, 21:383-393.

[49] Pfeifer K, Vroemen M, Blesch A, Weidner N: Adult neural progenitor cells provide a permissive guiding substrate for corticospinal axon growth following spinal cord injury. *European Journal of Neuroscience* 2004, 20:1695-1704.

[50] Snyder EY, Yoon C, Flax JD, Macklis JD: Multipotent neural precursors can differentiate toward replacement of neurons undergoing targeted apoptotic degeneration in adult mouse neocortex. *Proceedings National Academy of Science* 1997, 94:663-668.

[51] Park KI, Liu S, Flax JD, Nissim S, Stieg PE, Synder EY: Transplantation of neuronal progenitor and stem-like cells: development insights may suggest new therapies for spinal cord and other CNS dysfunction. *Journal of Neurotrauma* 1999, 16:675-687.

[52] Liu Y, Himes BT, Solowska J, Moul J, Chow SY, Park KI, Tessler A, Murray M, Snyder EY, Fischer I: Intraspinal Delivery of Neurotrophin-3 Using Neural Stem Cells Genetically Modified by Recombinant Retrovirus. *Experimental Neurology* 1999, 158:9-26.

[53] Himes BT, Liu Y, Solowska JM, Snyder EY, Fischer I, Tessler A: Transplants of cells genetically modified to express neurotrophin-3 rescue axotomized Clarke's nucleus neurons after spinal cord hemisection in adult rats. *Journal of Neuroscience Research* 2001, 65:549-564.

[54] Rosario C, Yandava B, Kosaras B, Zurakowski D, Sidman R, Snyder E: Differentiation of engrafted multipotent neural progenitors towards replacement of missing granule neurons in meander tail cerebellum may help determine the locus of mutant gene action. *Development* 1997, 124:4213-4224.

[55] Park KI, Ourednik J, Ourednik V, Taylor RM, Aboody KS, Auguste KI, Lachyankar MB: Global gene and cell replacement strategies via stem cells. *Gene Therapy* 2002, 9:613-624.

[56] Yandava BD, Billinghurst L, Synder EY: "Global"cell replacement is feasible via neural stem cell transplantation: evidence from the dysmyelinated shrverer mouse brain. *Proceedings National Academy of Science* 1999, 96:7029-7034.

[57] Rowitch DH, St.-Jacques B, Lee SMK, Flax JD, Snyder EY, McMahon AP: Sonic hedgehog Regulates Proliferation and Inhibits Differentiation of CNS Precursor Cells. *Journal of Neuroscience* 1999, 19:8954-8965.

[58] Lu P, Jones LL, Snyder EY, Tuszynski MH: Neural stem cells constitutively secrete neurotrophic factors and promote extensive host axonal growth after spinal cord injury. *Experimental Neurology* 2003, 181:115-129.

[59] Kleber M, Lee H-Y, Wurdak H, Buchstaller J, Riccomagno MM, Ittner LM, Suter U, Epstein DJ, Sommer L: Neural crest stem cell maintenance by combinatorial Wnt and BMP signaling. *Journal of Cell Biology* 2005, 169:309-320.

[60] Sommer L, Rao MS: Neural stem cells and regulation of cell number. *Progress in Neurobiology* 2002, 66:1-8.

[61] Philips MF, Mattiasson G, Wieloch T, Björklund A, Johansson BB, Tomasevic G, Matinez-Serrano A, Lenzlinger PM, Sinson G, Grady MS, et al.: Neuroprotective and

behavioral efficacy of nerve growth factor-transfected hippocampal progenitor cell transplants after experimental brain injury. *Journal of Neurosurgery* 2001, 94:765-774.

[62] Wuu YD, Pampfer S, CVanderheyden I, Lee KH, De Hertogh R: Impact of tumor necrosis factor alpha on mouse embryonic stem cells. *Biology of Reproduction* 1998, 58:1416-1424.

[63] Rezaie P, Trillo-Pazos G, Everall IP, Male DK: Expression of beta-chemokines and chemokine receptors in human fetal astrocyte and microglial co-cultures: potential role of chemokines in the developing CNS. *Glia* 2002, 37:64-75.

[64] Ahn Y-H, Bensadoun J-C, Aebischer P, Zurn AD, Seiger A, Bjorklund A, Lindvall O, Wahlberg L, Brundin P, Kaminski Schierle GS: Increased fiber outgrowth from xeno-transplanted human embryonic dopaminergic neurons with co-implants of polymer-encapsulated genetically modified cells releasing glial cell line-derived neurotrophic factor. *Brain Research Bulletin* 2005, 66:135-142.

[65] Rolletschek A, Chang H, Guan K, Czyz J, Meyer M, Wobus AM: Differentiation of embryonic stem cell-derived dopaminergic neurons is enhanced by survival-promoting factors. *Mechanisms of Development* 2001, 105:93-104.

[66] Toda H, Tsuji M, Nakano I, Kobuke K, Hayashi T, Kasahara H, Takahashi J, Mizoguchi A, Houtani T, Sugimoto T, et al.: Stem cell-derived neural stem/progenitor cell supporting factor is an autocrine/paracrine survival factor for adult neural stem/progenitor cells. *Journal of Biological Chemistry* 2003, 278:35491-35500.

[67] Galli R, Pagano SF, Gritti A, Vescovi AL: Regulation of neuronal differentiation in human CNS stem cell progeny by leukemia inhibitory factor. *Developmental Neuroscience* 2000, 22:86-95.

[68] Manabe Y, Nagano I, Gazi MS, Murakami T, Shiote M, Shoji M, Kitagawa H, Abe K: Glial cell line-derived neurotrophic factor protein prevents motor neuron loss of transgenic mice model for amyotrophic lateral sclerosis. *Neurological Research* 2003, 25:195-200.

[69] Kinkl N, Hageman GS, Sahel JA, Hicks D: Fibroblast growth factor receptor (FGFR) and candidate signaling molecule distribution within rat and human retina. *Molecular Vision* 2002, 8:149-160.

[70] Cremer H, Chazal G, Goridis C, Represa A: NCAM is essential for axonal growth and fasciculation in the hippocampus. *Molecular and Cellular Neuroscience* 1997, 8:323-335.

[71] Dihne M, Bernreuther C, Sibbe M, Paulus W, Schachner M: A new role for the cell adhesion molecule L1 in neural precursor cell proliferation, differentiation, and transmitter-specific subtype generation. *Journal of Neuroscience* 2003, 23:6638-6650.

[72] Ourednik J, Ourednik V, Bastmeyer M, Schachner M: Ectopic expression of the neural cell adhesion molecule L1 in astrocytes leads to changes in the development of the corticospinal tract. *European Journal of Neuroscience* 2001, 14:1464-1476.

[73] Brummendorf T, Kenwrick S, Rathjen FG: Neural cell recognition molecule L1: from cell biology to human hereditary brain malformations. *Current Opinion in Neurobiology* 1998, 8:87-97.

[74] Huang EJ, Reichardt LF: Neurotrophins: roles in neuronal development and function. *Annual Review in Neuroscience* 2001, 24:677-736.

[75] Ourednik V, Schachner M, Snyder EY, Lynch WP, Ourednik J: Rescue of impaired host dopaminergic neurons and the role of overexpressed neural cell adhesion molecule

L1 in aged mice grafted with neural stem cells (NSCs). *Experimental Neurology* 2003, 181:101.

[76] Kamiguchi H, Hlavin ML, Yamasaki M, Lemmon V: Adhesion molecules and inherited diseases of the human nervous system. *Annual Review in Neuroscience* 1998, 21:97-125.

[77] Imitola J, Comabella M, Chandraker AK, Dangond F, Sayegh MH, Synder EY, Khoury SJ: Neural stem/progenitor cells express co-stimulatory molecules that are differentially upregulated by inflammatory and apoptotic stimuli. *American Journal of Pathology* 2004, 164:1615-1625.

[78] Cammer W: Effects of TNF-alpha on immature and mature oligodendrocytes and their progenitors in vitro. *Brain Reseach* 2000, 864:213-219.

[79] Shohami E, Ginis I, Hallenbeck JM: Dual role of tumor necrosis factor alpha in brain injury. *Cytokine Growth Factor Reviews* 1999, 10:119-130.

[80] Qin L, Chavin KD, Ding Y, Tahara H, Favaro JP, Woodward JE, Suzuki T, Robbins PD, Lotze MT, Bromberg JS: Retro-virus mediated gene transfer of viral IL-10 gene prolongs murine cardiac allograft survival. *Journal of Immunology* 1996, 156:2316-2323.

[81] Penkowa M, Giralt M, Lago N, Camats J, Carrasco J, Hernandez J, Molinero A, Campbell IL, Hidalgo J: Astrocyte-targeted expression of IL-6 protects the CNSagainst a focal brain injury. *Experimental Neurology* 2003, 181:130-148.

[82] Tran PB, Miller RJ: Chemokine receptors in the brain: a developing story. *Journal of Comparative Neurology* 2003, 457:1-6.

[83] Imitola J, Raddassi K, Park KI, Mueller F-J, Nieto M, Teng YD, Frenkel D, Li J, Sidman RL, Walsh CA, et al.: Directed migration of neural stem cells to sites of CNS injury by the stromal cell-derived factor 1-α/CXC chemokine receptor 4 pathway. *Proceedings National Academy of Science* 2004, 101:18117-18122.

[84] Teng YD, Lavik EB, Qu X, Park KI, Ourednik J, Zurakowski D, Langer R, Snyder EY: Functional recovery following traumatic spinal cord injury mediated by a unique polymer scaffold seeded with neural stem cells. *Proceedings National Academy of Science* 2002, 99:3024-3029.

[85] Bakshi A, Fisher O, Dagci T, Himes BT, Fischer I, Lowman A: Mechanically engineered hydrogel scaffolds for axonal growth and angiogenesis after transplantation in spinal cord injury. *J Neurosurgery of Spine* 2004, 1:322-329.

[86] Park KI, Teng YD, Snyder EY: The injured brain interacts reciprocally with neural stem cells supported by scaffolds to reconstitute lost tissue. *Nature Biotechnology* 2002, 20:1111-1117.

[87] Xerri C, Coq JO, Merzenich MM, Jenkins WM: Experience-induced plasticity of cutaneous maps in the primary somatosensory cortex of adult monkey and rats. *Journal of Physiology (Paris)* 1996, 90:277-287.

[88] Robertson IH, Murre JMJ: Rehabilitation of brain damage: brain plasticity and principles of guided recovery. *Psychological Bulletin* 1999, 125:544-575.

[89] Jones TA, Chu CJ, Grande LA, Gregory AD: Motor skills training enhances lesion-induced structural plasticity in the motor cortex of adult rats. *The Journal of Neuroscience* 1999, 19:10153-10163.

[90] Briones TL, Suh E, Jozsa L, Hattar H, Chai J, Wadowska M: Behaviorally-induced ultrastructural plasticity in the hippocampal region after cerebral ischemia. *Brain Research* 2004, 997:137-146.
[91] Luke LM, Allred RP, Jones TA: Unilateral ischemic sensorimotor cortical damage induces contralesional synaptogenesis and enhances skilled reaching with the ipsilateral forelimb in adult male rats. *Synapse* 2004, 54:187-199.
[92] Briones TL, Therrien B, Metzger B: Effects of environment on enhancing functional plasticity following cerebral ischemia. *Biological Research for Nursing* 2000, 1:299-309.
[93] Young D, Lawlor PA, Leone P, Gragunow M, During MJ: Environmental enrichment inhibits spontaneous apoptosis, prevents seizures and is neuroprotective. *Nature Medicine* 1999, 5:448-453.
[94] Hebb DO: *The Organization of Behavior*. New York: Wiley; 1949.
[95] van Praag H, Kempermann G, Gage FH: Neural consequences of environmental enrichment. *Nature Reviews Neuroscience* 2000, 1:191-198.
[96] Döbrössy MD, Le Moal M, Montaron M-F, Abrous N: Influence of environment on the efficacy of intrastriatal dopaminergic grafts. *Experimental Neurology* 2000, 165:172-183.
[97] Christie MA, Dalrymple-Alford JC: Behavioural consequences of frontal cortex grafts and enriched environments after sensorimotor cortex lesions. *Journal of Neural Transplantation and Plasticity* 1995, 5:199-210.
[98] Döbrössy MD, Dunnett SB: Environmental enrichment affects striatal graft morphology and functional recovery. *European Journal of Neuroscience* 2004, 19:159-168.
[99] Grabowski M, Sorensen JC, Mattsson B, Zimmer J, Johansson BB: Influence of an enriched environment and cortical grafting on functional outcome in brain infarcts of adult rats. *Experimental Neurology* 1995, 133:96-102.
[100] Kelche C, Dalrymple-Alford JC, Will B: Housing condition modulate the effects of intracerebral grafts in rats with brain lesions. *Behavioral Brain Research* 1988, 28:287-295.
[101] Mattsson B, Sorensen JC, Zimmer J, Johansson BB: Neural grafting to experimental neocortical infarcts improves behavioral outcome and reduces thalamic atrophy in rats housed in enriched but not in standard environments. *Stroke* 1997, 28:1225-1231.
[102] Döbrössy MD, Dunnett SB: Training specificity, graft development and graft-mediated functional recovery in a rodent model of Huntington's disease. *Neuroscience* 2005, 132:543-552.

In: Perspectives in Stem Cell Research ISBN: 978-1-61122-985-1
Editors: Brenda M. Davis and Christopher B. Halton © 2011 Nova Science Publishers, Inc.

Chapter IX

RETROVIRUS VECTOR SILENCING IN STEM CELLS

Shuyuan Yao and James Ellis*
Developmental Biology Program
Hospital for Sick Children
555 University Ave. Toronto, Canada
Ontario, Canada M5G 1X8
and Department of Molecular & Medical Genetics
University of Toronto, Canada

ABSTRACT

Retrovirus vectors suffer severe gene silencing in stem cells that hampers their use in stem cell gene therapy. Transduced retrovirus vector can be completely silenced, or dynamically silenced in a subset of cells resulting in variegation. Expressing retrovirus also can be extinguished during stem cell differentiation. Multiple epigenetic modifications including histone modifications and DNA methylation are functionally involved in establishing and maintaining retrovirus silencing via the formation of silent chromatin. A model is proposed that the balance of epigenetic effects at the integration site and retroviral silencer elements on the vectors determines the decision to be silent, variegated or expressing in stem cells. Silencing resistant retrovirus vectors have been developed by removal of these silencer elements, and silencing in stem cells may ultimately be blocked using appropriate insulator elements.

Gene therapy holds the potential to treat cancer, inherited or acquired monogenic disorders and other diseases. A broad arsenal of gene transfer systems is currently available and is still expanding. Among them, the retrovirus vector system has attracted a lot of interest for high efficiency transfer into a wide range of cell types and stable integration into the host genome. Because of their ability to repopulate an entire system, stem cells are often targets

* Corresponding author: James Ellis. Telephone: (416) 813-7295. Fax: (416)813-8883. E-mail: jellis@sickkids.ca

for therapeutic gene delivery. The use of retrovirus vectors has been particularly valuable for introducing and expressing foreign genes in stem cells, for genetic marking of stem cells to trace their differentiation and for mutating and tagging genes associated with specific phenotypes. However, the use of retrovirus vectors has been significantly hampered by gene silencing of retrovirus vector expression in primitive cell types such as embryonic stem (ES) cells, embryonal carcinoma (EC) cells, hematopoietic stem cells (HSC) and early embryos. Understanding retrovirus vector silencing and its mechanisms will benefit the development of retrovirus based stem cell gene transfer vectors and the design of stem cell based gene therapy strategies.

1. Background and Phenomena

1.1. Retrovirus Silencing

Retrovirus silencing was documented as early as 1975 in the study of Moloney Murine Leukemia Virus (Mo-MuLV) infection of 4-8 cell stage mouse preimplantation embryos [Jaenisch et al., 1975]. Although one of the animals raised from infected embryos developed leukemia, no virus was detected from the infected embryos by both co-cultivated viral infection plaque forming assay and electron microscopy. Preimplantation mouse embryos are susceptible to virus integration but cannot express viral functions. In contrast, midgestation stage embryos or newborn mice can be successfully infected by Mo-MuLV and produce viral proteins [Jaenisch, 1980]. Non-virus-producing cell lines derived from a mouse embryo carrying a genetically transmitted Mo-MuLV genome can be reactivated by 5-bromodeoxyuridine (BrdU) to express viral p30 protein in almost all the cells and produce infectious virus in some of the cells [Bacheler et al., 1979]. Clearly, there is a block in preimplantation embryos making them non-permissive to Mo-MuLV gene expression and viral production.

Murine embryonic carcinoma (EC) cells share with preimplantation embryos the potential to differentiate into all three germinal layer cells [Illmensee and Mintz, 1976]. EC cells have been used as an *in vitro* model to study retrovirus silencing in preimplantation embryos. Among the many publications describing retrovirus silencing in EC cells [Gautsch, 1980; Peries et al., 1977; Teich et al., 1977], Speers et al convincingly demonstrated it by picking single cell clones from Mo-MuLV infected EC cells [Speers et al., 1980]. While viral protein and viral production were never observed in undifferentiated EC cells, after differentiation and BrdU drug treatment 2 of 4 clones were reactivated to express viral p30 protein and produce virus particles. The reactivation indicates that retrovirus can be infected into EC cells and that the lack of viral production is due to a block in retrovirus expression. Comparison of the same retrovirus infection in EC cells and differentiated cells is a useful model to study retrovirus silencing.

The features of retrovirus silencing can be summarized as being most prevalent in primitive cells, heritable and transcriptional. Both preimplantation embryo cells and EC cells are primitive cells in their early differentiation stages. Other more differentiated cells are permissive for retrovirus expression indicating that retrovirus silencing is primitive cell type specific. Silent retrovirus is kept silenced during culture, during *in vitro* and *in vivo* differentiation, and even during passage from generation to generation. Therefore, the silenced retrovirus state is heritable. The silent provirus genome is intact and functional [Speers et al., 1980; Stewart et al., 1982]. Retrovirus silencing happens after viral integration and before mRNA translation. In fact, Gautsch and Wilson showed that retrovirus expressing EC cells produce 400-700 fold higher virus based nascent RNA than silent EC cells [Gautsch and Wilson, 1983]. Obviously, transcriptional gene silencing plays an important role in retrovirus silencing, although post-transcriptional silencing of retrovirus has been reported in differentiated cells [Gao et al., 2002].

1.2. Retrovirus Vector Silencing

Retrovirus vectors are derived from isolated retroviruses to transfer and integrate foreign genes into target cells. Retrovirus vectors are created by removing viral genes, leaving only the cis-acting sequences necessary for a single round of replication to avoid vector multiplication and spread to other cells [Buchschacher and Wong-Staal, 2000]. Retrovirus silencing was originally observed with infectious retrovirus. With the development of retrovirus vectors, more and more vectors with easily detectable reporter genes have been used in stem cells gene transfer. The use of retrovirus vectors extends retrovirus silencing studies into other types of primitive cells such as embryonic stem (ES) cells [Cherry et al., 2000; Laker et al., 1998], hematopoietic stem cells (HSC) [Challita and Kohn, 1994; Klug et al., 2000; Lange and Blankenstein, 1997] and hematopoietic progenitor cells [Zentilin et al., 2000]. Retrovirus vector silencing is also found in human SRCs (SCID repopulating cells, a type of HSC), confirming that retroviral silencing occurs in humans and thus will likely pose a significant problem to clinical application of retroviral mediated gene therapy [Guenechea et al., 2001]. The use of retrovirus vectors helped to identify several types of retrovirus vector silencing phenomena. In the literature, retrovirus vector silencing has referred to any phenomena related to non-expression of genes from an integrated retrovirus vector. In the early retrovirus silencing studies, Mo-MuLV was extensively used. Since Mo-MuLV induces severe silencing in EC cells, those studies were focused on silencing established directly after viral infection. Later studies using wildtype or modified retrovirus vectors found the existence of variegated expression and extinction during differentiation or long-term culture.

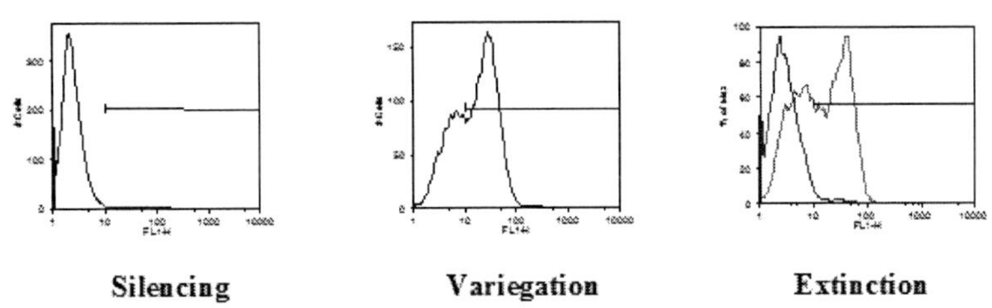

Figure 1. Retrovirus vector silencing, variegation and extinction in embryonic stem cells. Flow cytometry for eGFP expression shows retrovirus vector silencing, variegation and extinction. While silent retrovirus does not espress in any cells, variegated retrovirus expresses in some cells but is silent in others. In extinction, a variegated retrovirus in ES cells (dotted line) is silenced after differentiation (solid line) [Yao, 2004].

1.2.1. Retrovirus vector variegation

Retrovirus vectors can be silenced at different levels. The most extreme example is that the retrovirus vector is totally shut down with no transgene expression. Less well known is that it can be variegated in which retrovirus integrated at the same integration site is either silent or expressing (Figure 1). Single cell derived clones picked from MESV based vector transduced murine ES cells showed a varied percentage of positive cells among different clones and varied expression level among cells in the same clone [Laker et al., 1998]. Variegation of the MSCV retrovirus vector in transduced ES cells was also reported by Christopher Klug's laboratory [Swindle et al., 2004]. In their work about 35% (21 out of 55) of the integrated provirus showed variegated expression. An interesting feature of variegated retrovirus is instability. Sorted expressing and non-expressing cells from the variegated clones revert to the variegated expression pattern after brief expansion [Swindle et al., 2004]. Clones picked from a variegated clone by limit dilution are also variegated (Yao, S. et al., unpublished data). Unstable variegated clones were also isolated from retrovirus transduced de novo methylase null (dnmt3a-/-3b-/-) ES cells [Yao, 2004]. Therefore, variegation represents a dynamic silencing phenomenon occuring on some of the integrated retroviral proviruses in ES cells. Variegated expression was also observed in retrovirus vector transduced hematopoietic progenitor cell clones [Zentilin et al., 2000].

The expressing and non-expressing cells of the variegated clones contain the same retrovirus vector with the same integration site. Reactivation of the non-expressing cells with 5-AzaC in wildtype variegated ES cells further shows that the retrovirus vector in these cells is intact and functional [Yao, 2004]. Therefore, variegated retrovirus expression is due to epigenetic regulation.

1.2.2. Retrovirus vector extinction after long-term culture

Retrovirus silencing can occur at different time points. Retrovirus expression can be shut down immediately post-integration which results in no transgene expression at any time. In silent preimplantation embryos no virus production was observed from both co-culture plaque forming assay and electron microscopy [Jaenisch et al., 1975]. With EC cells, the nascent RNA produced in silent EC cells is the same as uninfected EC cell control [Niwa et al., 1983]. This kind of silencing is also observed in ES cells [Laker et al., 1998] and long-term HSC cells [Klug et al., 2000]. In contrast, retrovirus that initially express may be silenced in a process known as extinction (Figure 1). Extinction is often observed after long term culture. For example, a GFP retrovirus vector is subject to extinction where both the percentage of cells that are GFP positive and the GFP expression level decrease in tranduced murine ES cells after 26 days of passage and culture [Cherry et al., 2000]. Retrovirus vector extinction was also observed in hematopoietic cell lines [McInerney et al., 2000]. Long-term extinction also occurs *in vivo*. Mo-MuLV based retrovirus vector transduced HSC can be assayed as colony forming units-spleen (CFU-S) generated after serial transplantation of infected born marrow cells. While high level gene expression was achieved in all of the primary CFU-S and tissues of the reconstituted marrow transplantation recipients, vector expression is inactive in >90% of the secondary CFU-S and 100% of the third CFU-S [Challita and Kohn, 1994]. Since the primary CFU-S is derived from a committed progenitor cell restricted to the myeloid lineage, this result suggests retrovirus vector in HSC cells is extinguished during serial transplantation. Interestingly, stable transgene expression can be achieved after long-term culture. The factors that control the decision for long-term transgene extinction are not yet clear.

1.2.3. Retrovirus vector extinction after differentiation

In vivo and *in vitro* differentiation of retrovirus vector infected primitive cells can also induce extinction of transgene expression. MESV based retrovirus vector transduced ES cell clones are subject to extinction after *in vitro* differentiation. This was observed with two different reporter genes (LacZ and IL3neoR) and in two different ES cell lines (W9.5 and R1). MESV vector expression was also extinguished after *in vivo* differentiation by making ES cell derived embryos [Laker et al., 1998]. Extinction of retrovirus vectors was also reported after differentiation of HSC. Retrovirus vector expression in transduced long-term HSC was extinguished when differentiated into lymphoid cell populations after transplantation [Klug et al., 2000]. When retrovirus transduced ES cell clones were subjected to 8 days *in vitro* differentiation, extinction occurred primarily on the variegated clones [Yao, 2004], suggesting retrovirus extinction during differentiation may be a consequence of variegation.

1.2.4. Implications of retrovirus vector silencing

Retrovirus vector silencing is a heterogeneous phenomena. The existence of different kinds of silencing on retrovirus vectors implies that a constant monitoring system exists in cells to ensure genomic integrity. The identification of these different retrovirus silencing phenomena are beneficial in terms of evaluating new designs for retrovirus vectors and new gene therapy strategies. Because most of the *ex vivo* transplantation experiments use expressing cells obtained by drug selection or FACS sorting, variegated expressing cells are not excluded. The existence of the unstable variegated expressing cells and their extinction during differentiation may account for some of the unsuccessful gene therapy transplants. Therefore, methods should be developed to distinguish expressing cells and variegated expressing cells before therapeutic transplantation.

1.3. Lentivirus Vector Silencing

1.3.1. Lentivirus vector

The newest and perhaps most promising vectors developed for the infection of non-dividing quiescent stem cells are Lentiviral vectors. Lentivirus vectors gained popularity since Naldini et al [Naldini et al., 1996] demonstrated in 1996 that human immunodeficiency virus type 1 (HIV-1) based vectors were capable of transducing nondividing cells. Conventional retrovirus vectors are limited by their inability to infect terminally differentiated and nondividing cell types. Lentivirus vectors do not rely on the passive mechanism of nuclear envelope breakdown during the cell cycle to gain entry to the nucleus. Instead they utilize active transport mechanisms and achieve entry through the nucleopore [Chicurel, 2000]. This feature is particularly relevant when infecting slowly dividing stem cells, because a greater transduction efficiency is achieved in comparison to Mo-MuLV based retroviruses [Uchida et al., 1998]. Experiments with Lentiviruses have shown that they are able to efficiently transduce human SRCs [Schilz et al., 1998; Woods et al., 2000], which will be necessary for extending findings in mice to clinical trials.

Like Mo-MuLV, HIV-1 was selected for deriving gene transfer vectors for its well understood viral biology and extensively studied molecular biology. Other Lentiviruses also have been used to develop gene transfer vectors [Quinonez and Sutton, 2002]. Three refinements have been achieved to improve HIV-1 based Lentivirus vector usability and especially safety: Lentivirus vector particle pseudotyping, improvement of the packaging constructs and cell lines [Dull et al., 1998; Kim et al., 1998; Naldini et al., 1996; Naldini and Verma, 2000; Zufferey et al., 1997], and self-inactivating deletions in SIN-Lentivirus vector LTRs [Iwakuma et al., 1999; Miyoshi et al., 1998; Zufferey et al., 1998]. Other cis-acting elements such as the central polypurine tract (cppt) [Sirven et al., 2000; Sirven et al., 2001], Rev response element (RRE) [May et al., 2000] and woodchuck posttranscriptional element (WPRE) [Zufferey et al., 1999] were also included into Lentivirus vectors to improve viral titer or viral expression.

1.3.2. Lentivirus vector silencing

Lentivirus is subject to some gene silencing effects in primitive cells. Lentivirus vector silencing was documented in transduced murine hematopoietic progenitor cells. Primitive hematopoietic progenitor cells were transduced with HIV-1 based Lentivirus vector expressing the green fluorescent protein (GFP) gene and then plated for hematopoietic progenitor cell assays. The primary colonies formed are mosaic for GFP expression. When secondary colonies were cultured from the primary colonies 13% of them are GFP negative while PCR analysis showed the existence of Lentivirus provirus [Mikkola et al., 2000]. While this report showed that Lentivirus vector silencing occurs at least at the progenitor stage, we reported Lentivirus silencing in ES cells by identification of silent single copy vector transduced ES cell clone [Yao, 2004]. Lentivirus was also reported to extinguish during ES cell differentiation into CD34+ hematopoietic progenitor cells [Hamaguchi et al., 2000; Ma et al., 2003].

Some reports suggest there is no gene silencing in Lentivirus vector transduced primitive cells and during their differentiation [Lois et al., 2002; Pfeifer et al., 2002]. In Pfeifer's work, a SIN Lentivirus vector with *cppt* and WPRE was used to harbor either PGK or CAG (contains a modified chicken β-actin promoter and enhancer sequence from cytomegalovirus) promoter driven eGFP or LacZ genes. With multiplicity of infection (moi) of 5, about 50% of the cells are GFP positive with an integrated provirus copy of 1 to 3. An moi of 50 was needed to reach 100% positive cells in both murine and human ES cells. Transduced ES cell colonies stayed GFP positive when differentiated into EBs *in vitro* and into teratomas *in vivo*. Transduced ES cells can be readily used to make chimeras by blastocyst injection, and transgene expression was achieved in most of the organs and transmitted through the germ line. Infected eight-cell stage embryos showed transgene expression after 48 hours and expression continued during embryogenesis and after birth. Lois also reported that Lentivirus vectors escaped developmental silencing during embryogenesis [Lois et al., 2002].

Copy number differences may account for the conflicting observations on Lentivirus vector silencing. Multiple provirus copies can exist in one cell and an expressing provirus can mask silent provirus in the same cell. Single cell clones with a single functionally intact provirus are the ideal systems for Lentivirus silencing studies.

1.4. Retrovirus Silencing is Epigenetic

Epigenetics by definition is "the study of mitotically and/or meiotically heritable changes in the function of a gene that cannot be explained by changes in its DNA sequences" [Russo, 1996]. Epigenetic regulation plays a key role in achievement of developmental differentiation and maintenance of cell lineage identities [McNairn and Gilbert, 2003].

Expression of a retrovirus is controlled by cellular epigenetic regulation mechanisms. Indeed, a silent retrovirus stays silent after cell division, embryonic and postnatal development indicating that retrovirus silencing is heritable. The lack of expression of a silent retrovirus is not due to DNA sequence mutations. A silent retrovirus can be reactivated at least partially by drugs such as 5-bromodeoxyuridine (BrdU) [Bacheler et al., 1979] and the methylation inhibitor 5-azacytidine (5-AzaC) [Stewart et al., 1982] demonstrating that the integrated retrovirus is functional. The existence of variegated retrovirus vectors is another excellent demonstration of epigenetic regulation in retrovirus silencing. Cell clones with a variegated vector show intraclonal mosaicness with vector expression. Since the integrated retrovirus vector and its flanking endogenous genes are identical in different cells from the same clone, the variation of vector expression cannot be explained by DNA sequence differences. According to the definition of epigenetics, retrovirus silencing is an epigenetic phenomenon.

2. Epigenetic Gene Silencing Background

It is well accepted that chromatin structure plays an important role in controlling and modulating eukaryotic gene expression [Wolffe and Guschin, 2000]. The basic unit of chromatin is the nucleosome composed of histone components with DNA wrapped around. In each nucleosome there is an octamer of histone H2A, H2B, H3 and H4. The histones forming the basic nucleosomal octamer are called core histones. About 145bp of DNA wraps 1.65 turns around the octamer. Linker DNA, the DNA between adjacent histone octamers, varies in length in different species and in metazoan is bound by linker histones such as histone H1. Arrays of nucleosomes form 30nm diameter chromatin fibers, and linker histone H1 is involved in this process [Graziano et al., 1994]. Chromatin can be bound by non-histone proteins which are referred to as chromatin factors. Like linker histones the binding of chromatin factors induces special chromatin conformations. Heterochromatin, which was originally a term to define cytologically condensed regions of the genome throughout the cell cycle, is now widely used to refer to any silent chromatin domain. Correspondingly, euchromatin refers to active chromatin domains. Chromatin is the platform of gene transcription in eukaryotic cells.

Epigenetic silencing is achieved by establishing and maintaining a relatively inaccessible repressive chromatin domain [Grewal and Moazed, 2003; Wolffe and Matzke, 1999]. DNA methylation and other chromatin modifications induce a silent chromatin conformation by either recruiting repressive chromatin proteins or avoiding positive chromatin protein binding. These epigenetic chromatin modifications serve as heritable silencing marks to pass silent chromatin conformation through cell division [Moazed, 2001]. The inaccessibility of silent chromatin can be studied by its insensitivity to DNase digestion. Chromatin modifications can be studied by chromatin imunoprecipitation (ChIP) assays using modification specific antibodies [Crane-Robinson et al., 1999].

2.1. DNA Methylation Induced Gene Silencing

About 70-80% of the CpG dinucleotides are methylated at cytosine in mammalian cells. Early stage embryos of mammals experience a dramatic demethylation and remethylation [Santos et al., 2002]. These processes are believed to be essential in determining somatic DNA methylation patterns and critical for proper development of the embryo. Treatment with the methylation inhibitor 5-azacytidine or by genetically reducing overall genomic methylation levels through gene targeting of the methyltransferases can reactivate some gene expression. In fact, knockout of the mouse DNA methyltransferase Dnmt1 is embryonic lethal [Li et al., 1992]. These results show that DNA methylation plays a critical role in gene expression and development.

2.1.1. DNA methyltransferases

Three DNA methyltransferases have been identified in mammals (Figure 2A). Dnmt1 is the maintenance methylase with a preference for hemi-methylated DNA. It co-localizes with replication forks [Leonhardt et al., 1992]. The recent finding that Dnmt1 interacts with the clamping protein PCNA in the replication complex is consistent with the maintenance function of Dnmt1 [Iida et al., 2002]. Knocking down dnmt1 expression by antisense oligonucleotides triggers the intra-S-phase arrest of DNA replication [Milutinovic et al., 2003]. Dnmt3a and 3b are the two known de novo methylases [Okano et al., 1999; Xie et al., 1999]. Recent publications also demonstrate that Dnmt3a and 3b function in DNA methylation maintenance by assisting Dnmt1 [Liang et al., 2002].

Knocking out these two de novo methylases does not reduce the overall methylation levels in the genome. However, it does affect methylation on some genes such as endogenous and exogenous retrovirus, imprinting genes and satellite repeats. The dnmt3a knock out mice die 3 to 4 weeks after birth, while the dnmt3b knockout embryos do not develop further than 9.5 days after fertilization [Okano et al., 1999]. Dnmt3a and 3b have different isoforms. The existence of different isoforms in different cell types may determine the different methylation patterns on their genomic DNA. Dnmt2 has a domain homologous with other methylase catalyzing domains. No methylation activity by Dnmt2 has been observed [Okano et al., 1998], but *in vivo* antibody labeling does show Dnmt2 binding to genomic DNA [Liu et al., 2003]. Dnmt3L (dnmt3 like) shares homology with 3a and 3b, but lacks a functional catalytic domain. Dnmt3L assists other methylases in targeting maternal imprinted genes [Hata et al., 2002].

3.1.2. Methylated DNA Binding Proteins And Gene Repression

DNA methylation can result in two modes of repression which are likely biologically relevant. First, methylation of DNA may interfere with trans-acting factors binding to the cognate DNA sequence. The transcriptional activator CpG binding protein (CGBP) serves as an example. This protein exhibits a unique binding specificity for DNA elements that contain unmethylated CpG motifs [Voo et al., 2000]. Knocking out CGBP is embryonic lethal demonstrating that this protein is crucial for early embryogenesis [Carlone and Skalnik,

2001]. The second mode of repression involves recruiting proteins to methyl-CpG (Figure 2B). The first methyl-CpG binding protein identified was MeCP2 [Lewis ct al., 1992]. Dissection of MeCP2 revealed that an 85 amino acid methyl-CpG binding domain (MBD) can bind nonspecifically to one or more symmetrically methylated CpGs [Nan et al., 1993]. By searching expressed sequence tag (EST) databases, four other methyl-CpG binding proteins were identified named MBD1, MBD2, MBD3 and MBD4. MBD4 participates in DNA damage repair [Ballestar and Wolffe, 2001]. The other 4 MBD containing proteins have been implicated in methylation-dependent repression of transcription [Bird and Wolffe, 1999].

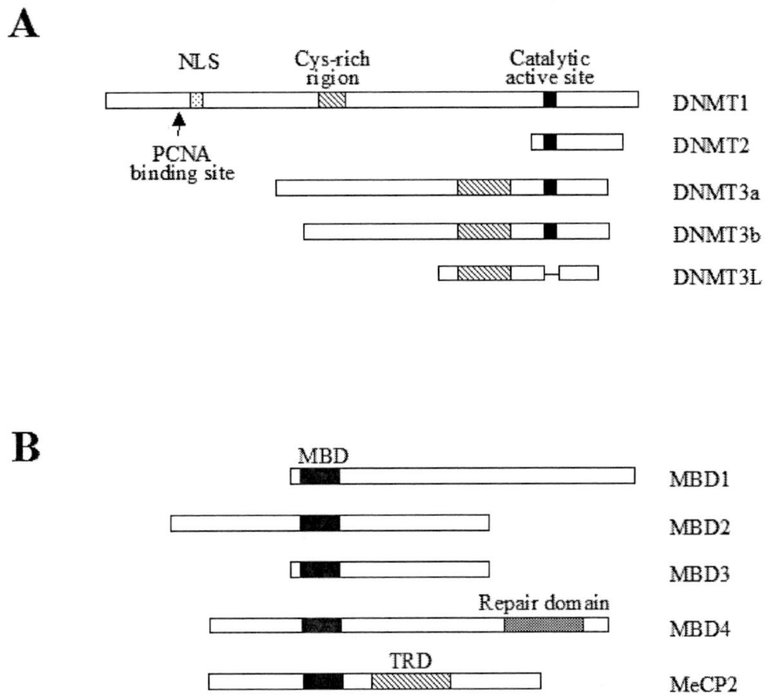

Figure 2. Mammalian DNA methyl-transferases and methylated DNA binding proteins. A). Mammalian DNA methyl-transferases. The methyl-transferase catalytic sites locate at the C-terminal. DNMT3L does not have a catalytic site. HDAC complex binds at the Cys-rich rigion. There is a NLS domain and a replication protein PCNA binding site at DNMT1 N-terminus. B). Mammalian methylated DNA binding proteins. MBD, methyl-CpG binding domain. The DNA repair domain of MBD4 locates at its C-terminus. MeCP2 has a transcription repression domain TRD [Bird and Wolffe, 1999].

Nan et al [Nan et al., 1997] identified the transcriptional repression domain (TRD) in MeCP2 responsible for long-range repression *in vivo*. The TRD domain was later found to be associated with a corepressor complex containing sin3 and a histone deacetylase (HDAC) [Jones et al., 1998; Nan et al., 1998]. HDAC and other repressors were also found to associate with MBD1, MBD2 and MBD3 [Ballestar and Wolffe, 2001]. These findings established a direct causal relationship between DNA methylation and gene repression via chromatin modification. Recent publications further show that MeCP2 complexed with Sin3a is targeted directly to some promoters and represses gene expression [Chen et al., 2003; Martinowich et al., 2003; Stancheva et al., 2003]. However, lines of evidence suggest that other pathways may exist in MeCP2 induced gene repression. First, binding of MeCP2 can form a specific secondary condensed structure *in vitro* [Georgel et al., 2003]. Second, recent publications demonstrate that MeCP2 associates with histone methyltransferase *in vivo* and directs repressive histone Lys9 methylation [Fuks et al., 2003a; Fuks et al., 2003b].

2.2. Chromatin Structure and Gene Silencing

Silent chromatin structure can be induced by histone covalent modification, or by linker histones or other accessory chromatin proteins. All histone proteins share similar structural characteristics. They have a globular domain essential for histone interaction with each other in nucleosomes [Wolffe and Guschin, 2000]. Flanking the globular domain, histones can have one or two non-structured tail domains that can be heavily covalently modified. Modification includes phosphorylation, acetylation, methylation, ADP ribosylation and ubiquitination [Berger, 2002]. Each of these modifications combined with their position on different histones has been reported to relate to different chromatin functions and chromatin structural alterations [Cheung et al., 2000]. In addition, findings of the interplay between these modifications on the same histone tail add another layer of complexity. Notably, histones are not the only proteins whose functions are regulated by post-translational modifications. Enzymes responsible for histone modification such as kinases are also involved in signaling transduction pathways. It was proposed that signaling pathways act directly on chromatin components to regulate different DNA-templated processes [Cheung et al., 2000]. Histone tail modifications and their combinatorial functions have been referred to as a Histone Code [Strahl and Allis, 2000].

2.2.1. Histone Modification And Gene Silencing

Core histone deacetylation and methylation have been found to strongly correlate with gene silencing. Studies of bulk acetylation levels in yeast have shown that up to 13 of the 30 tail lysine residues in a histone octamer are acetylated [Roth et al., 2001]. Histone acetylation levels are maintained by the opposing actions of histone acetyltransferase (HAT) and histone deacetylase (HDAC) complexes [Reid et al., 2000; Vogelauer et al., 2000]. Both HATs and HDACs act as part of large complexes. There are multiple mechanisms by which deacetylation of histone tails might facilitate transcription silencing. Deacetylation may stabilize the interaction between histones and DNA by alteration of the N-terminal charge; or may facilitate the internucleosomal interaction via the histone tail; or may recruit additional chromatin accessory proteins [Narlikar et al., 2002]. Also, deacetylation of histone tails may facilitate other modifications on the same histone tail which may induce further chromatin alteration.

Histone lysine methylation occurs on lysine residues 4, 9, 27 and 36 in H3, position 20 in H4 and also the H1 amino terminus. Suv39 is the first histone methyltransferase (HMTase) to be identified. Identification of the HMTase catalytic domain (Suv39-E(z)-Trithorax domain, SET domain) led to the identification of more than 70 gene sequences containing SET domain in mammals. Suv39h, G9a and Ezh2 are involved in histone H3 Lys9 and Lys27 methylation [Cao et al., 2002; Czermin et al., 2002; Rea et al., 2000; Tachibana et al., 2001]. Suv39h induced histone H3 Lys9 methylation can be bound by HP1 and induce heterochromatin [Peters et al., 2001]. Suv39h is also reported to be involved in repression of euchromatic genes [Nielsen et al., 2001]. Lys27 tri-methylation is observed in X-inactivation and bound by PcG proteins [Cao et al., 2002]. Histone H3 Lys4 methylation is induced by another SET protein MLL and associates with gene expression [Milne et al., 2002]. Interestingly, both Ezh2 and MLL are polycomb/trithrox group (PcG/trxG) proteins. PcG/trxG are involved in epigenetic cellular memory in *Drosophila* [Pirrotta, 1998]. These findings suggest that histone H3 Lys9 and Lys4 tri-methylation may serve as signals for eukaryotic epigenetic regulation memory.

2.2.2. Accessory Chromatin Proteins And Gene Silencing

In addition to nucleosomes, the chromatin fiber contains a diversity of other accessory proteins including linker histone and other non-histone proteins. The binding of linker histone H1 is dynamic [Lever et al., 2000; Misteli et al., 2000]. The displacement of H1 is modulated by cdk2 mediated phosphorylation [Bhattacharjee et al., 2001; Horn et al., 2002]. The binding of linker histone H1 is believed to form a closed chromatin conformation [Karymov et al., 2001] and induce gene silencing on some genes but not all [Shen and Gorovsky, 1996].

Non-histone chromatin accessory proteins are the proteins present in some chromatin structures, which are not essential to form a functional chromatin structure. This includes methylated DNA binding proteins (MBDs), heterochromatin protein 1 (HP1) [Eissenberg and Elgin, 2000], silencing information regulator (Sir) [Shore, 2000], high mobility group (HMG) proteins [Ner and Travers, 1994] and PcG/TrxG proteins etc. The binding of these factors can alter chromatin structure. Some chromatin factors alter chromatin structure via histone tail covalent modification. For example, PcG protein Ezh2 catalyzes histone H3 Lysine27 tri-methylation [Czermin et al., 2002]. Others can form higher order chromatin structures like linker H1, HP1 [Eissenberg and Elgin, 2000] and PcG proteins [Sewalt et al., 2002]. A common character of most chromatin accessory proteins is their ability to form polymers which can spread a specific chromatin conformation into and subsequently silence flanking DNA sequences.

2.3. Gene Silencing Network

Broad interplay among different chromatin alterations has been reported. Interplay can happen between the same levels of chromatin alterations. For example, MeCP2 was reported to replace linker histone H1 *in vitro* [Nan et al., 1997]. Lys9 deacetylation is proposed as a prerequisite for methylation at the same lysine residual [Cheung et al., 2000]. However, often the interplay is between different chromatin alteration levels. Histone tail modification such as H3 Lys9 methylation determines chromatin accessory protein binding. MeCP2 bound on methylated DNA can induce histone H3 deacetylation and methylation [Fuks et al., 2003b]. Also, H3 methylation is reported to direct DNA methylation in yeast [Schramke and Allshire, 2003] and plants [Jackson et al., 2002]. Chromatin modifications such as DNA methylation and histone modifications can be recognized by specific binding proteins. The binding proteins can subsequently recruit other chromatin modification enzymes to the same gene. As a result multiple chromatin modifications and multiple chromatin alterations co-exist on the same gene to enforce chromatin structures, be it condensed or open. It is reasonable to hypothesize that DNA methylation, histone modifications, and chromatin factor binding are all parts of a gene repression network. They function separately and cooperatively to achieve an inaccessible chromatin conformation.

2.4. Variegated Epigenetic Silencing

Variegated epigenetic silencing is observed in *Drosophila*, yeast and transgenic mice and is designated as position effect variegation (PEV). The prototype PEV phenomenon was observed in *Drosophila*. When a normally active euchromatic gene is translocated into the boundary between heterochromatin and euchromatin, its expression is shut down in a portion of the cells due to the spreading of condensed heterochromatin into the translocated gene. PEV of the eye color *white* gene results in the eye color mosaicness in *Drosophilia*. Massive genetic screens led to the identification of a large amount of PEV modifier genes in *Drosophila* [Schotta et al., 2002]. Among them, some can induce chromatin modification and structural alteration [Schotta et al., 2002].

PEV is also observed in transgenic mice. Transgene expression in mouse lines with multicopy transgenes does not correlate with the number of integrated transgene copies indicating an important role for integration sites. Transgene "copy number independent and position dependent" expression can be avoided by inclusion of locus control regions (LCR). LCRs are gene regulatory elements in mammals and birds that can overcome the repressive effects associated with heterochromatic transgene locations to promote position-independent and copy number-dependent transgene expression [Kioussis and Festenstein, 1997]. Transgenes with partially deleted LCRs located at the edge of centromeric heterochromatin regions are subject to PEV [Festenstein et al., 1996; Milot et al., 1996]. Using these PEV mouse lines, Milot and others have shown that PEV is controlled by the balance of positive transcription factors (Sp1 and EKLF) and repressive chromatin modifiers (Suv39H1, HP1, and PcG proteins) [Festenstein et al., 1999; Lundgren et al., 2000; McMorrow et al., 2000]. Interestingly, while most of the PEV in transgenic mice occurs when transgenes are located in heterochromatin, a recent paper demonstrates that PEV also can be established in non-centromeric regions [Ayyanathan et al., 2003].

3. Model Systems Used in Retrovirus Silencing Studies

From the first retrovirus silencing experiment done over 20 years ago, different model systems have been used. In general the model systems used for retrovirus silencing can be categorized into two groups: infection models and transfection models. In infection models, retrovirus or retrovirus vectors are infected into primitive cell types. In transfection models, retrovirus DNA sequences with or without modifications are introduced into different cell types. Both of these models have provided useful information on retrovirus silencing. Understanding the advantages and disadvantages of these systems is crucial to compare the data from different publications. The proper usage of retrovirus silencing systems is also important for the development of silencing-resistant retrovirus vectors.

3.1. Infection Models

In the infection models, retrovirus or retrovirus vectors are infected into preimplantation embryos, EC, ES or HSC. Comparison of retrovirus vector expression in primitive cells and mature cells is commonly used to determine retrovirus silencing effects. The existence of provirus DNA is used to determine successful viral infection. When wildtype retrovirus is used, infectious viral particles and viral protein expression are used to detect retrovirus expression. Expression of retrovirus vectors is detected by the expression of reporter genes. Because retrovirus vector infected cells cannot make infectious retrovirus vectors, it can avoid the virus spread problem associated with wildtype retrovirus infection. The existence of easily detectable reporter genes gives retrovirus vectors another advantage. Retrovirus vector infection models provide a unique opportunity to study different types of retrovirus silencing phenomena and their mechanisms. An infection model is also important to evaluate novel silencing-resistant retrovirus vector design.

Multiple copy provirus integration is a potential problem in infection models. The existence of expressing retrovirus vector can mask silent vectors in the same cell. The silent retrovirus vector transduced cells are also mixed with an excess of untransduced cells. The isolation and identification of single copy vector transduced cell lines are crucial to retrovirus silencing study. The use of *in vitro* cultured primitive cells facilitates the isolation and identification of silent retrovirus. The existence of homologous endogenous retrovirus in the mouse genome is another potential problem. It makes the determination of viral integration difficult. This problem can be avoided by careful design of retrovirus vectors.

Recently, HSC were used as model systems mainly because of their potential use in blood disease gene therapy. Research on HSC is always hampered by the lack of identity of HSC cells [Trevisan and Iscove, 1995]. Because the absolute purification of HSC is not possible, it is difficult to distinguish retrovirus expression in transduced HSC cells from other progenitor cells. One way to avoid this problem is serial transplantation. Since only HSC cells can survive after serial transplantation, the expression of the retrovirus vectors has to derive from HSC cells [Challita and Kohn, 1994].

3.2. Transfection Models

To study the involvement of DNA methylation in retrovirus silencing, two different transfection systems were introduced. M. Lorincz transfected *in vitro* methylated or unmethylated retrovirus sequences into a specific integration site in murine erythroleukemia (MEL) cells [Lorincz et al., 2001; Lorincz et al., 2002]. While this system can clearly determine whether DNA methylation functions in retrovirus silencing, the disadvantage is that the result might heavily depend on the integration site being used. Transgenic *Drosophila* also can be used to investigate the involvement of DNA methylation in retrovirus silencing. *Drosophila* was long believed to be a methylation-free system [Urieli-Shoval et al., 1982]. D. Pannell in our laboratory established that retrovirus sequences function as silencers in transgenic *Drosophila* suggesting that retrovirus silencing can be established independent of DNA methylation [Pannell et al., 2000]. However, a small amount of DNA methylation is detected in *Drosophila* especially in early embryos [Lyko et al., 2000]. The function of this DNA methylation is not yet clear. Nevertheless, the DNA methylation in *Drosophila* is not likely the same as in mammals, because the methylase being used is homologous to Dnmt2 [Hung et al., 1999] while Dnmt2 is not functional as a methylase in mammals [Okano et al., 1998]. The use of these two models has provided great information on whether and how DNA methylation is involved in retrovirus silencing.

Transfection models were also used to identify and modify silencer elements in retrovirus vectors. When a retrovirus sequence was linked to an LCR β-globin reporter gene and microinjected into fertilized mouse eggs, silencing of the reporter gene by the retrovirus sequence was detected in fetal liver [McCune and Townes, 1994; Osborne et al., 1999]. Transgene DNA and its expression were evaluated in each embryo. The silencing effect was evaluated by the percentage of expressing embryos and their expression levels. Since transgene expression suffers from PEV, a strong reporter gene that can promote position independent transgene expression is important to this model, and therefore a human LCR β-globin cassette was used as the reporter gene for retrovirus silencers. The human β-globin LCR is composed of four DNase I-hypersensitive sites all of which are required for full LCR activity [Pasceri et al., 1998]. The reporter cassette we used contains a 3.0-kb LCR(5'HS2 to 5'HS4) linked to the human β-globin transgene and directs 16 to 71% expression at all integration sites [Ellis et al., 1997]. The transgenic mouse model is very useful for evaluation of modifications to retrovirus vector silencer elements and development of silencing resistant retrovirus vectors.

4. Retrovirus Vector Silencing Mechanisms

4.1. Genome Defence Hypothesis

During the course of evolution, cells have been exposed to foreign DNAs. Intragenomic parasites are one of the important pathways for cellular genomes to obtain new genes. But integration of intragenomic parasites can cause endogenous gene damage and misregulation, so is potentially harmful. Genome defence systems may have developed during evolution to ensure genome integrity [Doerfler, 1991]. The genome defense hypothesis contends that cytosine methylation arose in mammals to restrict expression of intragenomic parasites [Walsh and Bestor, 1999]. Evidence supporting the genome defense hypothesis stems from the finding that the LTRs of retrotransposable elements such as L1s, IAPs, and endogenous retroviruses are all heavily methylated at CpG dinucleotides [Yoder et al., 1997a; Yoder et al., 1997b]. Further evidence supporting a role for methylation in genome defense comes from the finding that the IAP class of endogenous retrovirus becomes reactivated in ES cells that are null for the maintenance methyltransferase Dnmt1 [Walsh et al., 1998]. Notably DNA methylation is also involved in the restriction-modification system of bacterial defense function indicating that DNA methylation is an old player in cell defense [Bestor, 1990].

4.2. DNA Methylation and Retrovirus Silencing

4.2.1. Functional Role Of DNA Methylation In Retrovirus Silencing

Silencing of retrovirus is often accompanied by high density cytosine methylation [Jahner et al., 1982; Stewart et al., 1982]. The methylation inhibiting drug 5-azacytidine (5-AzaC) has been used to reactivate silent provirus in EC cells [Stewart et al., 1982]. The Jaenisch laboratory demonstrated that *in vitro* methylated retrovirus DNA is not infectious in cells, but treatment of the recipient cells with 5-AzaC reactivated infectious virus [Simon et al., 1983]. A functional role of DNA methylation in retrovirus silencing and extinction has been demonstrated [Cherry et al., 2000; Lorincz et al., 2000; Lorincz et al., 2001]. Recently Swindle et al [Swindle et al., 2004] also showed a causal role of DNA methylation in establishment and maintenance of retrovirus silencing by mutating the LTR promoter region CpGs.

It is proposed that the binding of MBD proteins on methylated DNA recruits HDACs and subsequently represses gene expression [Ballestar and Wolffe, 2001; Jones et al., 1998; Nan et al., 1998]. MeCP2 is recruited to silent retrovirus sequence [Lorincz et al., 2001; Yao, 2004]. However, no reactivation was observed by the HDAC inhibitor TSA or sodium butyrate alone in silent ES cells [Yao, 2004]. Clearly mechanisms other than histone deacetylation exist in the DNA methylation dependent retrovirus silencing pathway.

4.2.2. DNA Methylation Independent Pathway Of Retrovirus Silencing

While there is data supporting a causal role of DNA methylation in retrovirus silencing, several lines of data suggest other mechanisms may also exist. First, 5-AzaC reactivation of silent retrovirus is only partial. This suggests that other methylation-independent mechanisms are actively silencing some of retroviruses in these cells. Second, retrovirus silencing is established much earlier than DNA methylation. Silencing occurs in EC cells 2 days post-infection whereas methylation is not detectable until 8-16 days [Gautsch and Wilson, 1983; Niwa et al., 1983]. Third, retrovirus silencing can be established in *Drosophila.* Because *Drosophila* is a DNA methylation free environment, this result suggests that DNA methylation is not essential for retrovirus silencing [Pannell et al., 2000]. Fourth, among the identified silencers in retrovirus LTR, the promoter is the only CpG-rich silencer. DNA methylation induced retrovirus silencing cannot account for the other silencers function.

Dnmt3a and 3b are the only de novo methylases known to methylate exogenous transduced retrovirus. Identification of silent retrovirus in dnmt3ab knockout ES cells is the best way to test the existence of DNA methylation independent retrovirus silencing pathway. In deed, silent single copy retrovirus vector transduced dnmt3ab-/- ES cell clones were identified in our lab. DNA methylation sensitive digestion confirmed no DNA methylation on the integrated retrovirus [Yao, 2004], demonstrating the existence of a DNA methylation independent retrovirus silencing pathway.

4.2.3. Relationship Between DNA Methylation Dependent And Independent Pathways

Recently, multiple pathways functioning stepwise in retrovirus silencing have been proposed. MoMLV vector infected MEL cells that initially expressed were sorted and silencing was examined over time. It was found that an initial extinction event is reversible by the HDAC inhibitor trichostatin A (TSA). At later time points, reactivation of expression required 5-AzaC in conjunction with trichostatin A, suggesting that methylation is a secondary step associated with maintenance of silencing [Lorincz et al., 2000; Lorincz et al., 2002]. By studying retrovirus infected ES cell long-term culture extinction, S. Cherry also proposed that there are DNA-methylation independent pathways at early stages and dependent pathways at later stages in retrovirus silencing [Cherry et al., 2000]. However, retrovirus silencing occurs in *do novo* methylase null ES cells [Yao, 2004]. Therefore, both DNA methylation dependent and independent pathways are capable of maintaining retrovirus silencing. We propose that DNA methylation dependent and independent pathways function in parallel in gene repression.

4.3. Chromatin Conformation in Retrovirus Silencing

Retrovirus provirus is integrated into the host genome and inherited with other endogenous genes [Breindl et al., 1979]. Epigenetic mechanisms such as histone modification and chromatin accessory protein binding may therefore also function on integrated provirus DNA. In 1979, Breindl and Jaenisch published that the chromatin conformation of transduced retrovirus is altered in the permissive and non-permissive tissue of the same mouse line by comparing their sensitivity to DNase digestion. In the non-permissive tissue in which the infected retrovirus is silent, the provirus is more resistant to DNase I digestion suggesting a condensed conformation [Breindl and Jaenisch, 1979]. DNase I hypersensitive site alteration was also observed in an endogenous allele mutated by Mo-MuLV insertion [Breindl et al., 1984].

Retrovirus sequence can silence the linked human LCR□-globin transgene in transgenic mice. Using ChIP assay, we have shown that the retrovirus silenced transgene is marked by silent chromatin characterized by histone H3 deacetylation and linker histone H1 [Pannell et al., 2000]. These results demonstrate that histone modifications are involved in retrovirus silencing. A similar silent chromatin is formed on the silent retrovirus vectors in genuine infected ES cells as well as the silenced retrovirus in variegated ES cells [Yao, 2004]. As in wildtype ES cells, silent retrovirus vectors in *dnmt3ab-/-* cells are also marked by histone H3 deacetylation and linker histone H1 binding [Yao, 2004]. The existence of similar chromatin conformation on silent retrovirus regardless of DNA methylation shows that silent chromatin is a universal mark for retrovirus silencing.

No reactivation was observed by TSA treatment on retrovirus silenced transgene in transgenic mice [Pannell et al., 2000] and silenced retrovirus in transduced ES cells [Yao, 2004]. TSA treament can increase the acetylation level of silenced transgene in transgenic mice, however TSA treatment cannot remove the linker histone H1 (unpublished data). These results suggest an important role for histone H1 in maintaining retrovirus silencing. The binding of histone H1 in silent *dnmt3ab-/-* cells is more abundant than in wildtype ES cells [Yao, 2004]. Since MeCP2 can replace histone H1 in binding linker DNA [Nan et al., 1997], we propose there is a compensatory competition between H1 and MeCP2 binding. When

MeCP2 cannot bind, histone H1 will take over to maintain silent chromatin. This dynamic interplay of different pathways directs silent chromatin formation and maintenance.

5. RETROVIRUS SILENCING INSULATION

5.1. Retrovirus Vectors That Resist Silencing

The existence of retrovirus silencing in stem cells indicates the need to develop silencing-resistant retrovirus vectors. Development of such retrovirus vectors started with the isolation of EC cell permissive retrovirus strains and continued with the identification and removal of silencer elements from retrovirus vectors. Self-inactivating (SIN) retrovirus vectors are vectors with a deletion in 3'LTR promoter region so that there are no functional promoters in any of the provirus LTRs after vector transduction. Although SIN retrovirus vectors were originally developed to improve vector safety, the extreme deletion of the retrovirus sequences in SIN vectors also reduces retrovirus silencing. Combining these efforts, many retrovirus vectors have been developed for stem cell gene transfer and gene therapy.

The identification and characterization of multiple silencer elements in retrovirus vectors paved the way for the construction of numerous modified vectors that lack these sequences. Silencer elements are DNA binding sites for trans-acting factors that directly or indirectly reduce transcription at promoters. At least four separate silencer elements located in the LTRs and the adjacent primer binding site (PBS) have been identified in retrovirus vectors. The LTR promoter is CpG rich serving as a potential silencer [Osborne et al., 1999; Swindle et al., 2004]. The Negative Control Region (NCR) was identified in the upstream region of the LTR which reduces virus expression [Flanagan et al., 1989]. Mutations in the direct repeat (DR) of the LTR enhancer were found to increase expression in stem cells [Hilberg et al., 1987]. The groups of Jaenisch and Goff found mutant PBS sites that increased expression from the LTR [Barklis et al., 1986; Colicelli and Goff, 1986]. Several negative trans-acting factors had been found to bind these silencer elements. Specifically, the multi-functional transcriptional regulator YY-1 binds to NCR [Flanagan et al., 1992], six distinct nuclear factors bind to each of the DRs [Speck and Baltimore, 1987], and the PBS is bound by factor A [Petersen et al., 1991]. In addition, the embryonic LTR-binding protein (ELP) [Tsukiyama and Niwa, 1992] was found to bind between the NCR and DR [Tsukiyama et al., 1989]. It has been shown that no single silencer element is sufficient to induce complete silencing [Osborne et al., 1999], suggesting that silencer elements additively increase the probability of silencing via multiple mechanisms.

Mo-MuLV is one of the earliest retrovirus isolated and studied. Given its well understood biology and its ability to efficiently infect a wide range of cells, Mo-MuLV has been widely used to derive retrovirus vectors. One problem for wildtype Mo-MuLV vectors is they are not permissive in ES or EC cells because of the poor functionality of Mo-MuLV LTR enhancer in these cells [Tsukiyama et al., 1989]. PCMV is a mutant form of myeloproliferative sarcoma virus (MPSV) containing a deletion of one of the enhancer DRs, as well as a mutation in the ELP binding site and a point mutation that introduces an Sp1 binding site [Hilberg et al., 1987]. Although the PCMV enhancer is functional in both EC and ES cells,

PCMV derived vectors are still restricted in ES cells [Grez et al., 1990]. Combination of the PCMV LTR with a PBS from an integration-defective Mo-MuLV mutant dl587rev [Colicelli and Goff, 1987] which does not bind factor A, yields the murine embryonic stem cell virus (MESV) [Grez et al., 1990]. Hawley et al further refined the MESV vector to increase titers by including an extended packaging signal from the LN vector and an upstream gag sequence from Moloney murine sarcoma virus, (MoMSV) resulting in MSCV [Hawley, 1994]. MSCV retains silencer elements such as the NCR, one of the DRs, and the CpG rich promoter.

Substitution of the MoMLV enhancer has been another approach to improve retrovirus vector expression in primitive cells. The MPSV (myeloproliferative sarcoma virus) enhancer had been shown to have increased expression in EC cells [Hilberg et al., 1987]. Substitution of the Mo-MuLV LTR with the MPSV LTR in conjunction with the dl587rev PBS yielded the MD (MPSV, dl587rev) vector [Challita et al., 1995]. Unfortunately, the expression from the MD vector did not significantly increase. However, the MND (MPSV, NCR, dl587rev) vector derived from a deletion of the NCR in the MD vector did show substantial improvement with expression in 43% of infected EC cells [Challita et al., 1995]. The MND vector also showed significantly increased expression in murine hematopoietic stem cells (HSCs) [Robbins et al., 1998].

Finally, SIN retrovirus vectors have steadily gained popularity due to the decreased probability that these vectors will undergo recombination leading to the generation of a rescued infectious virus. The first Mo-MuLV-based SIN retrovirus vector used a 299bp deletion in the 3'LTR that removes most of the DR and the promoter, but retains the NCR and wild-type PBS [Yu et al., 1986]. More recently the HSC1 vector was constructed in our laboratory by deletion of the entire NCR, DR, and part of the CpG rich promoter sequence in MSCV which retains the mutant PBS. HSC1 vector directs neo expression in 71% of transduced EC cells, offering a further improvement still [Osborne et al., 1999]. The HSC1 vector is particularly attractive both for its ability to express in non-permissive environments and its SIN properties.

SIN-Lentivirus vectors were created for safety reasons and may express better in primitive cell types due to the deletion of potential silencer sequences from the LTRs [Miyoshi et al., 1998]. Indeed, SIN-Lentivirus vector has been shown to transduce more efficiently into a broad range of cell types with higher expression levels compared with vectors with intact LTRs [Miyoshi et al., 1998]. Notably, the experience and knowledge gained in developing retrovirus vectors are well transferred into Lentivirus vector development.

In summary, progressive deletion or mutation of silencer sequences has lead to the development of retroviral vectors that have an increased probability of expression in primitive cell types. However, none of the current vectors are able to express at all integration sites despite mutations in all known retroviral silencer elements, suggesting that novel silencer elements remain to be discovered and may reside in the essential sequences of retrovirus vectors. In this consideration, insulation of the retrovirus silencer elements should be the next step in development of silencing resistant vectors.

5.2. Insulator Elements

The eukaryotic nucleus is organized into active and inactive domains [Weintraub and Groudine, 1976]. Within each chromosomal domain, each gene is embedded within a chromosomal environment of other DNA sequences that have the potential to affect its expression. Boundary elements such as insulators are needed to keep different domains and genes functioning separately. Insulators are defined as DNA elements located between different functional chromosomal domains that keep each of these domains functioning properly. In practice, insulators are defined by two assays: Enhancer Effect Blocking Assay [Kellum and Schedl, 1991] and Position Effect Protection Assay [Kellum and Schedl, 1992] (Figure 3A). Insulators can block the enhancing effect of an enhancer on a promoter. Transgenes in different integration sites suffer from PEV. Flanking transgenes with insulators can block position effects and promote position-independent transgene expression. Insulator elements themselves should have no enhancer, silencer or promoter activity. In other words, insulator elements should be neutral to make sure the blocking effect observed in these two assays is the result of true insulation. Insulator elements have silencer blocking activity. Otte and collegues showed that insulators block silencing effects of LexA silencing factor fusion proteins recruited to episomal reporter genes in human cells [van der Vlag et al., 2000]. Insulator silencer blocking activity was also tested in transgenic *Drosophila* [Barolo and Levine, 1997; Cai and Levine, 1995]. Insulator elements are found in *Drosophila* (*gypsy*, scs/scs', Fab-7, Fab-8, etc.) yeast (HMR, STAR etc.), sea urchin (sns), birds (cHS4) and mammals (H19/Ig2f, BEAD-1, HS5, etc.) [Bell and Felsenfeld, 1999]. Among them, chicken HS4 (cHS4), *Drosophila gypsy* and Scs are three well studied insulator elements.

Insulator elements were first discovered in *Drosophilia*. Scs/Scs' (special chromatin structures) insulators are located at the boundaries of the heat-shock *hsp70* gene and protect it from stimulation by neighboring genes [Udvardy et al., 1985]. These elements were shown to protect white transgenes against chromosomal position effects to produce uniform eye color [Kellum and Schedl, 1991]. Later the same group also showed that scs/scs' can block enhancer effects [Kellum and Schedl, 1992]. BEAF-32A and BEAF-32B (a boundary-element-associated factor of 32kDa) were found to bind to scs' [Hart et al., 1997; Zhao et al., 1995]. Zest-white-5 (Zw-5) binds to scs insulator [Gaszner et al., 1999]. BEAF was found to locate at hundreds of interbands and many puff boundaries on polytene chromosomes[Zhao et al., 1995].

Gypsy insulator is another *Drosophila* insulator that has been extensively studied. It was originally found in the 5' non-translated region of *Drosophila gypsy* retrotransposon [Geyer and Corces, 1992]. Insertion of the *gypsy* retrotransposon in the yellow gene blocks enhancers located upstream of the insertion site causing abnormal eye pigmentation. A 430-bp fragment of the 5' non-translated region was found to be responsible for this blocking. *Gypsy* insulator was also reported to protect a DNA replication origin from position effects [Lu and Tower, 1997] and to block polycomb group (PcG) protein induced gene repression [Mallin et al., 1998]. Interestingly, when multiple *gypsy* insulators were placed between an enhancer and promoter, or the enhancer was flanked with two *gypsy* insulators no insulation was observed [Cai and Shen, 2001; Melnikova et al., 2002; Muravyova et al., 2001]. Su(Hw) (Suppressor Hairy-wing) protein is required for *gypsy* insulator enhancer-blocking activity in *Drosophila*, and the *mod(mdg4)* gene is also involved [Gause et al., 2001; Gdula et al., 1996; Ghosh et al., 2001]. These two proteins direct *gypsy* insulator DNA to the nuclear periphery

[Gerasimova et al., 2000]. No Su(Hw) homologue has been found in mammalian cells, but *gypsy* insulator was found to be bound by mammalian nuclear matrix proteins and function as a matrix attachment region (MAR) element [Nabirochkin et al., 1998]. Most recently the *gypsy* insulator was also reported to serve as a MAR in *Drosophila* [Byrd and Corces, 2003]. MAR elements are binding sites for nuclear scaffold proteins *in vitro* and are proposed to attach chromatin to the nuclear matrix *in vivo* [Dickinson et al., 1992]. It is proposed that some MAR elements can shield transgenes from the influence of flanking genes [Allen et al., 2000; Bonifer et al., 1994].

The first and the best-characterized vertebrate insulator element is the cHS4 insulator of the chicken β-globin gene (Figure 3B). The β-globin locus in chicken erythrocytes contains a 33-kb domain of open chromatin and a 16-kb stretch of heterochromatin [Litt et al., 2001a; Litt et al., 2001b]. Upstream of this 16-kb heterochromatin domain is the folate receptor gene which is regulated distinctly from that of globin genes [Prioleau et al., 1999]. The 1.2kb cHS4 insulator is located at the boundary between the active globin domain and the heterochromatin domain. cHS4 insulator showed position effect protection activity [Chung et al., 1993] and enhancer blocking activity [Chung et al., 1997]. It blocks the spreading of histone deacetylation from heterochromatin but not DNA methylation [Mutskov et al., 2002]. A 250-bp CpG island that contains the constitutive DNase I hypersensitive site was found to retain most of the insulating activity. This 250-bp core element is used as a dimer to achieve full insulation [Chung et al., 1997]. Further dissection of the 250-bp core element found that only the footprint II bound by CTCF is required for enhancer blocking activity [Bell et al., 1999]. CTCF is a ubiquitous zinc-finger DNA-binding protein which recognizes multiple DNA sequences [Burcin et al., 1997; Klenova et al., 1998].

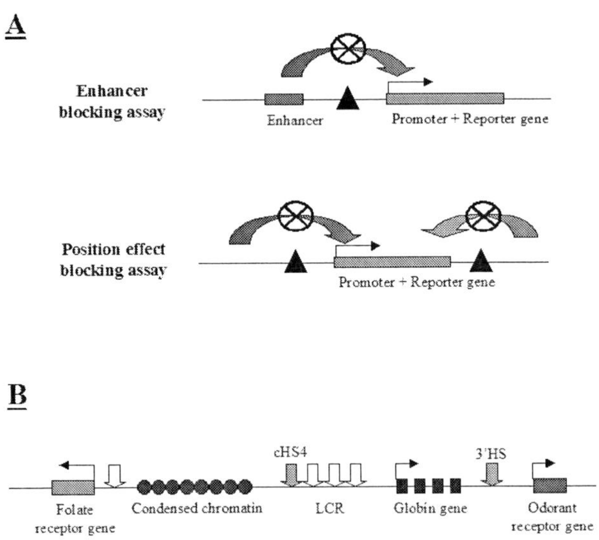

Figure 3. Insulator element. A. Two assays used to define insulator elements. In the enhancer blocking assay, the insulator element (black triangle) located between the enhancer and promoter will block the enhancer effect. In the position effect blocking assay, flanking the transgene with the insulator elements will protect the transgene from position effects from flanking endogenous genes. B, location of chicken HS4 insulator in the globin gene locus. cHS4 and 3'HS are two identified insulator elements functioning as boundary elements between different chromatin domains [Recillas-Targa et al., 2002]. See text for detail.

CTCF is involved in multiple functions such as gene silencing, gene activation, X-inactivation and insulator activity [Lutz et al., 2000]. Position effect protecting activity of the cHS4 core element does not require CTCF binding and resides in the other binding sites in the core element [Recillas-Targa et al., 2002]. The proteins responsible for position effect protection are not known.

5.3. Insulation of Retrovirus and Lentivirus Silencing

Expression of integrated retrovirus may be influenced by the flanking chromosomal environment of the integration site [Verma and Somia, 1997]. On the other hand, insertion of retrovirus also can induce insertional gene activation or repression [Breindl et al., 1984]. All retrovirus vectors contain LTRs and *gag* sequences that harbor known [Challita et al., 1995] and unidentified [Osborne et al., 1999] silencers. These elements can silence the transgene harbored in the retrovirus vector and potentially genomic genes flanking the integration site. Similarly, constant high expression of the retrovirus vector can activate flanking genes. Insulators are *cis*-acting elements and theoretically can be used to block retrovirus silencing spread and protect a transgene harbored inside a retrovirus vector. In addition, insulator elements also can be used to block silencing or activating effects of retrovirus sequences and protect the genes flanking the integration sites.

The monomer 1.2-kb cHS4 insulator has been used in retrovirus and Lentivirus vectors with limited success. Insertion of cHS4 into a Mo-MuLV construct 3'LTR can be faithfully duplicated into two LTRs after retroviral integration. The insulated retrovirus promotes an increased probability of expression at random chromosomal integration sites in MEL cells. Unfortunately, improved reporter gene eGFP expression was not observed when used to infect ES cells [Rivella et al., 2000]. Similar retrovirus vectors based on the MSCV vector were constructed by D. Emery [Emery et al., 2000]. cHS4 in one orientation in MSCV LTRs supports high percentage GFP positive cells and high GFP expression level in both 3T3 and bone marrow derived blood cells. However extinction of retrovirus expression was observed in long-term reconstituted mice. Further experiments showed that cHS4 insulators in the LTRs dramatically decrease gene expression from an internal pgk promoter. In addition, severe differentiation extinction was observed regardless of the existence of cHS4 insulator [Yannaki et al., 2002]. At the same time, the same vector harboring a γ-globin cassette was able to successfully reduce gene silencing [Emery et al., 2002]. Notably, the γ-globin expression cassette used in this vector has its own enhancer. Similarly, cHS4 also failed to protect Lentivirus vector when located in LTRs in transduced CD34+ blood cells [Ramezani et al., 2003]. However, when the insertion of cHS4 in LTRs was combined with insertion of a matrix attachment region (MAR) element, higher and uniform gene expression was achieved [Ramezani and Hawley, 2003]. The same vector was also reported to support better gene expression in human ES cells although long term culture extinction was not avoided [Ma et al., 2003].

Use of insulators in retrovirus or Lentivirus vectors is mostly unsuccessful due to the lack of knowledge of retrovirus silencer blocking. Current insulator assays define the enhancer blocking activity and position effect protection activity of insulator elements. However, retrovirus silencer blocking activity is different from these two activities. Retrovirus silencing is a negative effect on the transgene from retrovirus sequences. Blocking a retrovirus silencer is not the same as blocking enhancer effects. Also, silencer blocking is not necessarily equal to position effect protection. In retrovirus vectors, the transgene is flanked by retrovirus silencers from both the 5' and 3'LTR. Retrovirus silencers may affect the transgene more than the flanking genomic DNA sequences simply because they are closer to the transgene. Our and other reports all show that blocking position effects by flanking retrovirus vectors with insulators is not sufficient to avoid silencing [Emery et al., 2000; Rivella et al., 2000; Yao et al., 2003]. An assay specific for retrovirus silencer blocking is needed to identify insulator elements suitable to be used in retrovirus vectors. In our work, an LCR □-globin expression cassette is used as a reporter transgene to evaluate the blocking of retrovirus silencer effects in transgenic mouse fetal liver cells [Yao et al., 2003]. Retrovirus sequences can silence this LCR β-globin transgene when linked directly [Osborne et al., 1999; Pannell et al., 2000]. Insulators with retrovirus silencer blocking activity will be able to protect transgene expression when inserted between the transgene and retrovirus sequence. Using this assay we screened different insulator elements and found that cHS4 has the ability to block retrovirus silencers [Yao et al., 2003]. The identification of retrovirus silencer blocking insulator elements is important to the design of insulated retrovirus vectors to avoid retrovirus silencing.

Using our retrovirus silencer blocking assay, we also showed retrovirus silencer blocking activity is independent of CTCF binding [Yao et al., 2003]. CTCF binding is the common feature for vertebrate insulator element enhancer blocking activities [Bell et al., 1999]. Therefore, this result further supports retrovirus silencer blocking activity is different from enhancer blocking activity. When the cHS4 dimer core insulator is used to flank the LCR □-globin reporter gene, full levels of expression were observed in the transgenic mice [Yao et al., 2003]. This result suggests the transgene in a retrovirus vector needs to be flanked by insulators to achieve full protection. However, flanking the reporter gene in retrovirus vectors with the cHS4 dimer core insulator failed to produce high titer virus suggesting another non-homologous insulator is needed to combine with cHS4 [Yao et al., 2003].

No silencer blocking activity was observed with *gypsy* and Scs insulator. However the *gypsy* insulator was observed to increase transgene expression when located in the retrovirus LTRs. cHS4, on the other hand, does not increase transgene expression in the same configuration. This result indicates that the *gypsy* insulator does not increase transgene expression by blocking retrovirus silencers [Yao et al., 2003]. *Gypsy* was reported to function as a MAR element in both *Drosophila* [Byrd and Corces, 2003] and mammalian cells [Nabirochkin et al., 1998]. The increase of transgene expression by *gypsy* in retrovirus vectors may be due to its ability to tether the transgene to the nuclear matrix. Regardless of the mechanism, the increase of transgene expression by *gypsy* insulator can be used to design high expressing retrovirus vectors.

An ideal insulated retrovirus vector would be able to protect both the internal transgene and the integration site flanking endogenous genes. Currently all the insulated retrovirus vectors use insulators located in LTRs and aim to block position effects from the flanking sequences and to prevent induction of insertional activation. However, some of the retrovirus silencers especially those located in 5'LTR and *gag* sequences are left between the two insulators and adjacent to the transgene. To completely protect the transgene, two different insulators should be used, one located in the U3 region of LTRs, the other between 5'LTR-PBS and the internal transgene. In this configuration, the transgene will be flanked by two insulators to achieve high expression and the flanking genomic genes will also be partially insulated from the integrated retrovirus vector.

6. Retrovirus Silencing Model

Although retrovirus vector silencing has long been documented, there is still argument about whether retrovirus silencing is solely due to position effects. Although the integration site flanking chromatin may be involved in the decision, the silencing of retrovirus vectors is mainly due to effects induced by the silencer elements in retrovirus vector sequences. Multiple silencer elements have been identified in retrovirus LTR and *gag* sequences [Challita et al., 1995; Osborne et al., 1999]. Osborne et al also demonstrate that deletions in the SIN retrovirus vectors are not enough to remove all the silencer elements [Osborne et al., 1999]. Transgene experiments show that both retrovirus and Lentivirus sequences are dominant silencers in both transgenic mice and *Drosophilia* [Pannell et al., 2000]. Direct evidence comes from blocking of retrovirus silencers by insulators. After the genomic position effect is blocked, retrovirus sequences are still silenced in transgenic mice [Yao et al., 2003]. Our and other results also show that flanking the retrovirus vector with insulators failed to avoid silencing on both retrovirus and Lentivirus vectors [Emery et al., 2000; Ramezani et al., 2003; Yannaki et al., 2002; Yao et al., 2003].

Present models account for transgene expression variegation by proposing that the cell equates the balance between positive and negative factors located in both the transgene and the flanking sequences [Dillon and Festenstein, 2002]. We propose that this can be readily applied to retrovirus silencing. The silencer elements in retrovirus vectors are dominant elements that recruit negative factors in stem cells. The transgenes harbored in the vectors bear positive elements such as enhancer, promoter or LCR sequences. The integration site flanking sequences can be either positive or negative. The final expressing state of the transgene is the sum of all the negative and positive effects of all of the recruited factors. We proposed that a negative integration environment permits the establishment of silent chromatin on the integrated retrovirus vectors. On the other hand, when a provirus locates in a constantly active domain the chromatin environment will not permit the silencing machinery to establish silent chromatin on the retrovirus vector. As a result, the integrated retrovirus will continue to express even after differentiation, but only to low levels because of continued binding by the stem cell silencing factors. The variegated retrovirus vector may reflect the recruitment of silencing proteins by retrovirus silencers into an otherwise active chromatin environment that is near heterochromatin. During differentiation of ES cells, some genomic domains are progressively silenced [Rasmussen, 2003]. Correspondingly, provirus located in these regions may also be shut down resulting in extinction (Figure 4.).

Since the Mo-MuLV enhancer is almost non-functional in ES cells [Tsukiyama et al., 1989], the balance of the positive and negative factors lean to the negative side. This explains why Mo-MuLV can induce stronger silencing compared to MSCV [Hawley, 1994]. This balance model also can explain why the inclusion of LCR or MARs elements in retrovirus vectors can limit silencing effects [Emery et al., 2002; Ma et al., 2003; Ramezani et al., 2003]. This model emphasizes the silencers as the main determinant of the retrovirus silencing, but does not underestimate the importance of the integration site flanking sequences.

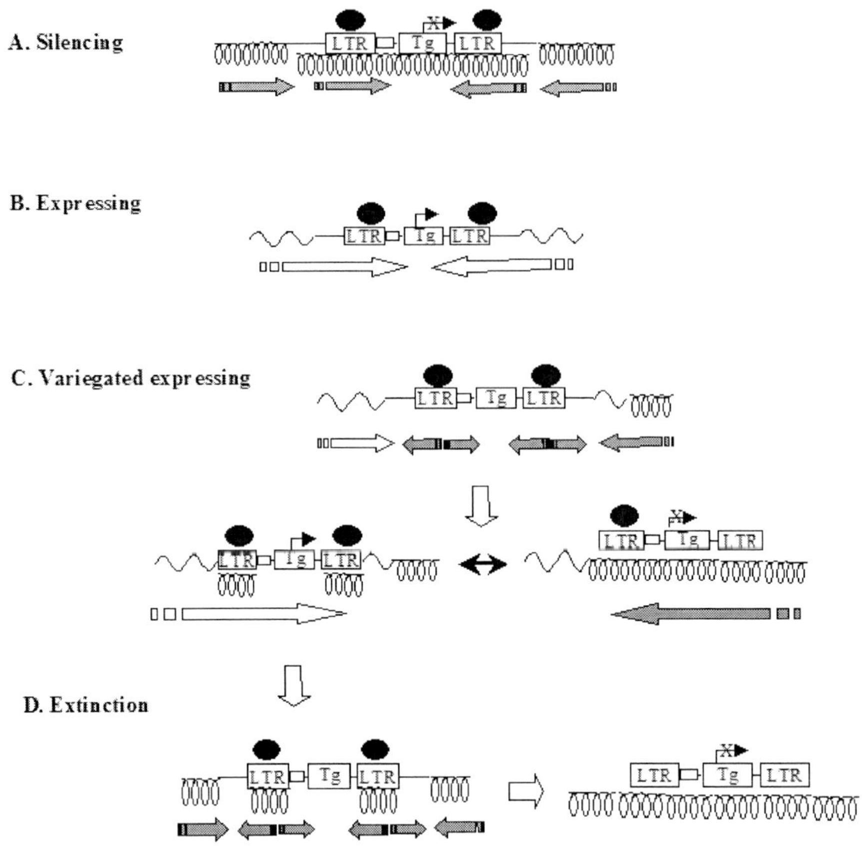

Figure 4. Retrovirus silencing hypothetical model. A). When the retrovirus vector is integrated into heterochromatin, the formation of silent chromatin on the LTRs and the spread of flanking heterochromatin establish silencing. B). When the retrovirus vector is integrated into extremely active euchromatin, the spread of active effects from the flanking gene inhibits the establishment of silent chromatin on LTRs. C). When the retrovirus vector integrates into euchromatin, variegated expression will be established by the balance of the spreading of silent effects from LTRs and the spread of active effects from euchromatin. D). During differentiation, the flanking euchromatin turns into heterochromatin and the transgene will be extinguished by the spreading of silencing effects from both LTRs and flanking heterochromatin. The black circle represents silencing factors.

7. Future Directions

7.1. Role of Integration Site in Determining Retrovirus Silencing

Our model proposes that the integration site is involved to some degree in the decision to silence retrovirus in stem cells. To test this model, the relationship between retrovirus vector expression status and its integration site needs to be investigated. The effect of the integrated retrovirus vector on the flanking genomic genes also needs to be studied. The inverse PCR technique has been combined with bioinformatics research to successfully identify large number of integration sites in retrovirus and Lentivirus infected bulk cell populations [Schroder et al., 2002; Wu et al., 2003]. After identification of the integration sites and their chromatin features, the relationship between retrovirus silencing and the integration environment can be studied.

7.2. Retrovirus Silencing in Somatic Stem Cells

Because of the ethical problems associated with using human ES cells, somatic stem cells have been the center of attention for gene therapy. The finding of somatic stem cell plasticity [Bjornson et al., 1999; Martin-Rendon and Watt, 2003] further emphasizes the importance of somatic stem cell studies. Although retrovirus and Lentivirus silencing have been documented in HSC, the understanding of this silencing and its mechanisms are limited. The lack of identity of HSC makes it difficult to monitor single HSC clones and their differentiation. As a result, the identification of different silencing phenomena and investigation of their mechanisms are restricted. In addition, whether other somatic stem cells retain retrovirus silencing pathways that may interfere with gene therapy needs to be addressed. The neural stem cell (NSC) has the potential to be used to study retrovirus silencing. Theoretically, a single neurosphere can be derived from a single NSC. Therefore, isolation of single NSC derived neurospheres can be used to identify retrovirus silencing or variegation. NSC have the potential to differentiate into three types of neural cells: astrocytes, oligodendrocytes and neurons [McKay, 1997]. Differentiation of single NSC derived neurospheres can be used to study retrovirus extinction.

CONCLUSION

In conclusion, retrovirus and Lentivirus silencing are heterogeneous epigenetic phenomena that involve induction of inheritable silent chromatin on integrated retroviruses. While every integrated retrovirus has the potential to be silenced, silent chromatin only can be established in a permissive genomic environment. Retrovirus silencing is achieved by cooperation of multiple cellular gene repression mechanisms to induce either static or dynamic silent chromatin conformations resulting in retrovirus silencing and variegated expression. Silent chromatin serves as the inheritable epigenetic mark that can be passed through DNA replication during cell division. The silent chromatin formed on the retrovirus vector sequences can spread into the flanking genes. Spread of retrovirus silencing can be blocked by insulator elements. Finally, insulator elements with retrovirus silencer blocking activity can be used to design silencing resistant retrovirus and Lentivirus vectors.

References

Allen, G. C., Spiker, S., and Thompson, W. F. (2000). Use of matrix attachment regions (MARs) to minimize transgene silencing. *Plant Mol Biol 43*, 361-376.

Ayyanathan, K., Lechner, M. S., Bell, P., Maul, G. G., Schultz, D. C., Yamada, Y., Tanaka, K., Torigoe, K., and Rauscher, F. J., 3rd (2003). Regulated recruitment of HP1 to a euchromatic gene induces mitotically heritable, epigenetic gene silencing: a mammalian cell culture model of gene variegation. *Genes Dev 17*, 1855-1869.

Bacheler, L., Jaenisch, R., and Fan, H. (1979). Highly inducible cell lines derived from mice genetically transmitting the Moloney murine leukemia virus genome. *J Virol 29*, 896-906.

Ballestar, E., and Wolffe, A. P. (2001). Methyl-CpG-binding proteins. Targeting specific gene repression. *Eur J Biochem 268*, 1-6.

Barklis, E., Mulligan, R. C., and Jaenisch, R. (1986). Chromosomal position or virus mutation permits retrovirus expression in embryonal carcinoma cells. *Cell 47*, 391-399.

Barolo, S., and Levine, M. (1997). hairy mediates dominant repression in the Drosophila embryo. *Embo J 16*, 2883-2891.

Bell, A. C., and Felsenfeld, G. (1999). Stopped at the border: boundaries and insulators. *Curr Opin Genet Dev 9*, 191-198.

Bell, A. C., West, A. G., and Felsenfeld, G. (1999). The protein CTCF is required for the enhancer blocking activity of vertebrate insulators. *Cell 98*, 387-396.

Berger, S. L. (2002). Histone modifications in transcriptional regulation. *Curr Opin Genet Dev 12*, 142-148.

Bestor, T. H. (1990). DNA methylation: evolution of a bacterial immune function into a regulator of gene expression and genome structure in higher eukaryotes. *Philos Trans R Soc Lond B Biol Sci 326*, 179-187.

Bhattacharjee, R. N., Banks, G. C., Trotter, K. W., Lee, H. L., and Archer, T. K. (2001). Histone H1 phosphorylation by Cdk2 selectively modulates mouse mammary tumor virus transcription through chromatin remodeling. *Mol Cell Biol 21*, 5417-5425.

Bird, A. P., and Wolffe, A. P. (1999). Methylation-induced repression--belts, braces, and chromatin. *Cell 99*, 451-454.

Bjornson, C. R., Rietze, R. L., Reynolds, B. A., Magli, M. C., and Vescovi, A. L. (1999). Turning brain into blood: a hematopoietic fate adopted by adult neural stem cells in vivo. *Science 283*, 534-537.

Bonifer, C., Yannoutsos, N., Kruger, G., Grosveld, F., and Sippel, A. E. (1994). Dissection of the locus control function located on the chicken lysozyme gene domain in transgenic mice. *Nucleic Acids Res 22*, 4202-4210.

Breindl, M., Doehmer, J., Willecke, K., Dausman, J., and Jaenisch, R. (1979). Germ line integration of Moloney leukemia virus: identification of the chromosomal integration site. *Proc Natl Acad Sci U S A 76*, 1938-1942.

Breindl, M., Harbers, K., and Jaenisch, R. (1984). Retrovirus-induced lethal mutation in collagen I gene of mice is associated with an altered chromatin structure. *Cell 38*, 9-16.

Breindl, M., and Jaenisch, R. (1979). Conformation of Moloney murine leukaemia proviral sequences in chromatin from leukaemic and nonleukaemic cells. *Nature 277*, 320-322.

Buchschacher, G. L., Jr., and Wong-Staal, F. (2000). Development of lentiviral vectors for gene therapy for human diseases. *Blood 95*, 2499-2504.

Burcin, M., Arnold, R., Lutz, M., Kaiser, B., Runge, D., Lottspeich, F., Filippova, G. N., Lobanenkov, V. V., and Renkawitz, R. (1997). Negative protein 1, which is required for function of the chicken lysozyme gene silencer in conjunction with hormone receptors, is identical to the multivalent zinc finger repressor CTCF. *Mol Cell Biol 17*, 1281-1288.

Byrd, K., and Corces, V. G. (2003). Visualization of chromatin domains created by the gypsy insulator of Drosophila. *J Cell Biol 162*, 565-574.

Cai, H., and Levine, M. (1995). Modulation of enhancer-promoter interactions by insulators in the Drosophila embryo. *Nature 376*, 533-536.

Cai, H. N., and Shen, P. (2001). Effects of cis arrangement of chromatin insulators on enhancer-blocking activity. *Science 291*, 493-495.

Cao, R., Wang, L., Wang, H., Xia, L., Erdjument-Bromage, H., Tempst, P., Jones, R. S., and Zhang, Y. (2002). Role of histone H3 lysine 27 methylation in Polycomb-group silencing. *Science 298*, 1039-1043.

Carlone, D. L., and Skalnik, D. G. (2001). CpG binding protein is crucial for early embryonic development. *Mol Cell Biol 21*, 7601-7606.

Challita, P. M., and Kohn, D. B. (1994). Lack of expression from a retroviral vector after transduction of murine hematopoietic stem cells is associated with methylation in vivo. *Proc Natl Acad Sci U S A 91*, 2567-2571.

Challita, P. M., Skelton, D., el-Khoueiry, A., Yu, X. J., Weinberg, K., and Kohn, D. B. (1995). Multiple modifications in cis elements of the long terminal repeat of retroviral vectors lead to increased expression and decreased DNA methylation in embryonic carcinoma cells. *J Virol 69*, 748-755.

Chen, W. G., Chang, Q., Lin, Y., Meissner, A., West, A. E., Griffith, E. C., Jaenisch, R., and Greenberg, M. E. (2003). Derepression of BDNF transcription involves calcium-dependent phosphorylation of MeCP2. *Science 302*, 885-889.

Cherry, S. R., Biniszkiewicz, D., van Parijs, L., Baltimore, D., and Jaenisch, R. (2000). Retroviral expression in embryonic stem cells and hematopoietic stem cells. *Mol Cell Biol 20*, 7419-7426.

Cheung, P., Allis, C. D., and Sassone-Corsi, P. (2000). Signaling to chromatin through histone modifications. *Cell 103*, 263-271.

Chicurel, M. (2000). Virology. Probing HIV's elusive activities within the host cell. *Science 290*, 1876-1879.

Chung, J. H., Bell, A. C., and Felsenfeld, G. (1997). Characterization of the chicken beta-globin insulator. *Proc Natl Acad Sci U S A 94*, 575-580.

Chung, J. H., Whiteley, M., and Felsenfeld, G. (1993). A 5' element of the chicken beta-globin domain serves as an insulator in human erythroid cells and protects against position effect in Drosophila. *Cell 74*, 505-514.

Colicelli, J., and Goff, S. P. (1986). Isolation of a recombinant murine leukemia virus utilizing a new primer tRNA. *J Virol 57*, 37-45.

Colicelli, J., and Goff, S. P. (1987). Identification of endogenous retroviral sequences as potential donors for recombinational repair of mutant retroviruses: positions of crossover points. *Virology 160*, 518-522.

Crane-Robinson, C., Myers, F. A., Hebbes, T. R., Clayton, A. L., and Thorne, A. W. (1999). Chromatin immunoprecipitation assays in acetylation mapping of higher eukaryotes. *Methods Enzymol 304*, 533-547.

Czermin, B., Melfi, R., McCabe, D., Seitz, V., Imhof, A., and Pirrotta, V. (2002). Drosophila enhancer of Zeste/ESC complexes have a histone H3 methyltransferase activity that marks chromosomal Polycomb sites. *Cell 111*, 185-196.

Dickinson, L. A., Joh, T., Kohwi, Y., and Kohwi-Shigematsu, T. (1992). A tissue-specific MAR/SAR DNA-binding protein with unusual binding site recognition. *Cell 70*, 631-645.

Dillon, N., and Festenstein, R. (2002). Unravelling heterochromatin: competition between positive and negative factors regulates accessibility. *Trends Genet 18*, 252-258.

Doerfler, W. (1991). Patterns of DNA methylation--evolutionary vestiges of foreign DNA inactivation as a host defense mechanism. A proposal. *Biol Chem Hoppe Seyler 372*, 557-564.

Dull, T., Zufferey, R., Kelly, M., Mandel, R. J., Nguyen, M., Trono, D., and Naldini, L. (1998). A third-generation lentivirus vector with a conditional packaging system *J Virol 72*, 8463-8471.

Eissenberg, J. C., and Elgin, S. C. (2000). The HP1 protein family: getting a grip on chromatin. *Curr Opin Genet Dev 10*, 204-210.

Ellis, J., Pasceri, P., Tan-Un, K. C., Wu, X., Harper, A., Fraser, P., and Grosveld, F. (1997). Evaluation of beta-globin gene therapy constructs in single copy transgenic mice. *Nucleic Acids Res 25*, 1296-1302.

Emery, D. W., Yannaki, E., Tubb, J., Nishino, T., Li, Q., and Stamatoyannopoulos, G. (2002). Development of virus vectors for gene therapy of beta chain hemoglobinopathies: flanking with a chromatin insulator reduces gamma-globin gene silencing in vivo. *Blood 100*, 2012-2019.

Emery, D. W., Yannaki, E., Tubb, J., and Stamatoyannopoulos, G. (2000). A chromatin insulator protects retrovirus vectors from chromosomal position effects. *Proc Natl Acad Sci U S A 97*, 9150-9155.

Festenstein, R., Sharghi-Namini, S., Fox, M., Roderick, K., Tolaini, M., Norton, T., Saveliev, A., Kioussis, D., and Singh, P. (1999). Heterochromatin protein 1 modifies mammalian PEV in a dose- and chromosomal-context-dependent manner. *Nat Genet 23*, 457-461.

Festenstein, R., Tolaini, M., Corbella, P., Mamalaki, C., Parrington, J., Fox, M., Miliou, A., Jones, M., and Kioussis, D. (1996). Locus control region function and heterochromatin-induced position effect variegation. *Science 271*, 1123-1125.

Flanagan, J. R., Becker, K. G., Ennist, D. L., Gleason, S. L., Driggers, P. H., Levi, B. Z., Appella, E., and Ozato, K. (1992). Cloning of a negative transcription factor that binds to the upstream conserved region of Moloney murine leukemia virus. *Mol Cell Biol 12*, 38-44.

Flanagan, J. R., Krieg, A. M., Max, E. E., and Khan, A. S. (1989). Negative control region at the 5' end of murine leukemia virus long terminal repeats. *Mol Cell Biol 9*, 739-746.

Fuks, F., Hurd, P. J., Deplus, R., and Kouzarides, T. (2003a). The DNA methyltransferases associate with HP1 and the SUV39H1 histone methyltransferase. *Nucleic Acids Res 31*, 2305-2312.

Fuks, F., Hurd, P. J., Wolf, D., Nan, X., Bird, A. P., and Kouzarides, T. (2003b). The methyl-CpG-binding protein MeCP2 links DNA methylation to histone methylation. *J Biol Chem 278*, 4035-4040.

Gao, G., Guo, X., and Goff, S. P. (2002). Inhibition of retroviral RNA production by ZAP, a CCCH-type zinc finger protein. *Science 297*, 1703-1706.

Gaszner, M., Vazquez, J., and Schedl, P. (1999). The Zw5 protein, a component of the scs chromatin domain boundary, is able to block enhancer-promoter interaction. *Genes Dev 13*, 2098-2107.

Gause, M., Morcillo, P., and Dorsett, D. (2001). Insulation of enhancer-promoter communication by a gypsy transposon insert in the Drosophila cut gene: cooperation between suppressor of hairy-wing and modifier of mdg4 proteins. *Mol Cell Biol 21*, 4807-4817.

Gautsch, J. W. (1980). Embryonal carcinoma stem cells lack a function required for virus replication. *Nature 285*, 110-112.

Gautsch, J. W., and Wilson, M. C. (1983). Delayed de novo methylation in teratocarcinoma suggests additional tissue-specific mechanisms for controlling gene expression. *Nature 301*, 32-37.

Gdula, D. A., Gerasimova, T. I., and Corces, V. G. (1996). Genetic and molecular analysis of the gypsy chromatin insulator of Drosophila. *Proc Natl Acad Sci U S A 93*, 9378-9383.

Georgel, P. T., Horowitz-Scherer, R. A., Adkins, N., Woodcock, C. L., Wade, P. A., and Hansen, J. C. (2003). Chromatin compaction by human MeCP2. Assembly of novel secondary chromatin structures in the absence of DNA methylation. *J Biol Chem 278*, 32181-32188.

Gerasimova, T. I., Byrd, K., and Corces, V. G. (2000). A chromatin insulator determines the nuclear localization of DNA. *Mol Cell 6*, 1025-1035.

Geyer, P. K., and Corces, V. G. (1992). DNA position-specific repression of transcription by a Drosophila zinc finger protein. *Genes Dev 6*, 1865-1873.

Ghosh, D., Gerasimova, T. I., and Corces, V. G. (2001). Interactions between the Su(Hw) and Mod(mdg4) proteins required for gypsy insulator function. *Embo J 20*, 2518-2527.

Graziano, V., Gerchman, S. E., Schneider, D. K., and Ramakrishnan, V. (1994). Histone H1 is located in the interior of the chromatin 30-nm filament. *Nature 368*, 351-354.

Grewal, S. I., and Moazed, D. (2003). Heterochromatin and epigenetic control of gene expression. *Science 301*, 798-802.

Grez, M., Akgun, E., Hilberg, F., and Ostertag, W. (1990). Embryonic stem cell virus, a recombinant murine retrovirus with expression in embryonic stem cells. Proc Natl Acad Sci U S A *87*, 9202-9206.

Guenechea, G., Gan, O. I., Dorrell, C., and Dick, J. E. (2001). Distinct classes of human stem cells that differ in proliferative and self-renewal potential. *Nat Immunol 2*, 75-82.

Hamaguchi, I., Woods, N. B., Panagopoulos, I., Andersson, E., Mikkola, H., Fahlman, C., Zufferey, R., Carlsson, L., Trono, D., and Karlsson, S. (2000). Lentivirus vector gene expression during ES cell-derived hematopoietic development in vitro. *J Virol 74*, 10778-10784.

Hart, C. M., Zhao, K., and Laemmli, U. K. (1997). The scs' boundary element: characterization of boundary element-associated factors. *Mol Cell Biol 17*, 999-1009.

Hata, K., Okano, M., Lei, H., and Li, E. (2002). Dnmt3L cooperates with the Dnmt3 family of de novo DNA methyltransferases to establish maternal imprints in mice. *Development 129*, 1983-1993.

Hawley, R. G. (1994). High-titer retroviral vectors for efficient transduction of functional genes into murine hematopoietic stem cells. *Ann N Y Acad Sci 716*, 327-330.

Hilberg, F., Stocking, C., Ostertag, W., and Grez, M. (1987). Functional analysis of a retroviral host-range mutant: altered long terminal repeat sequences allow expression in embryonal carcinoma cells. *Proc Natl Acad Sci U S A 84*, 5232-5236.

Horn, P. J., Carruthers, L. M., Logie, C., Hill, D. A., Solomon, M. J., Wade, P. A., Imbalzano, A. N., Hansen, J. C., and Peterson, C. L. (2002). Phosphorylation of linker histones regulates ATP-dependent chromatin remodeling enzymes. *Nat Struct Biol 9*, 263-267.

Hung, M. S., Karthikeyan, N., Huang, B., Koo, H. C., Kiger, J., and Shen, C. J. (1999). Drosophila proteins related to vertebrate DNA (5-cytosine) methyltransferases. *Proc Natl Acad Sci U S A 96*, 11940-11945.

Iida, T., Suetake, I., Tajima, S., Morioka, H., Ohta, S., Obuse, C., and Tsurimoto, T. (2002). PCNA clamp facilitates action of DNA cytosine methyltransferase 1 on hemimethylated DNA. *Genes Cells 7*, 997-1007.

Illmensee, K., and Mintz, B. (1976). Totipotency and normal differentiation of single teratocarcinoma cells cloned by injection into blastocysts. *Proc Natl Acad Sci U S A 73*, 549-553.

Iwakuma, T., Cui, Y., and Chang, L. J. (1999). Self-inactivating lentiviral vectors with U3 and U5 modifications. *Virology 261*, 120-132.

Jackson, J. P., Lindroth, A. M., Cao, X., and Jacobsen, S. E. (2002). Control of CpNpG DNA methylation by the KRYPTONITE histone H3 methyltransferase. *Nature 416*, 556-560.

Jaenisch, R. (1980). Retroviruses and embryogenesis: microinjection of Moloney leukemia virus into midgestation mouse embryos. *Cell 19*, 181-188.

Jaenisch, R., Fan, H., and Croker, B. (1975). Infection of preimplantation mouse embryos and of newborn mice with leukemia virus: tissue distribution of viral DNA and RNA and leukemogenesis in the adult animal. *Proc Natl Acad Sci U S A 72*, 4008-4012.

Jahner, D., Stuhlmann, H., Stewart, C. L., Harbers, K., Lohler, J., Simon, I., and Jaenisch, R. (1982). De novo methylation and expression of retroviral genomes during mouse embryogenesis. *Nature 298*, 623-628.

Jones, P. L., Veenstra, G. J., Wade, P. A., Vermaak, D., Kass, S. U., Landsberger, N., Strouboulis, J., and Wolffe, A. P. (1998). Methylated DNA and MeCP2 recruit histone deacetylase to repress transcription. *Nat Genet 19*, 187-191.

Karymov, M. A., Tomschik, M., Leuba, S. H., Caiafa, P., and Zlatanova, J. (2001). DNA methylation-dependent chromatin fiber compaction in vivo and in vitro: requirement for linker histone. *Faseb J 15*, 2631-2641.

Kellum, R., and Schedl, P. (1991). A position-effect assay for boundaries of higher order chromosomal domains. *Cell 64*, 941-950.

Kellum, R., and Schedl, P. (1992). A group of scs elements function as domain boundaries in an enhancer-blocking assay. *Mol Cell Biol 12*, 2424-2431.

Kim, V. N., Mitrophanous, K., Kingsman, S. M., and Kingsman, A. J. (1998). Minimal requirement for a lentivirus vector based on human immunodeficiency virus type 1. *J Virol 72*, 811-816.

Kioussis, D., and Festenstein, R. (1997). Locus control regions: overcoming heterochromatin-induced gene inactivation in mammals. *Curr Opin Genet Dev 7*, 614-619.

Klenova, E. M., Fagerlie, S., Filippova, G. N., Kretzner, L., Goodwin, G. H., Loring, G., Neiman, P. E., and Lobanenkov, V. V. (1998). Characterization of the chicken CTCF genomic locus, and initial study of the cell cycle-regulated promoter of the gene. *J Biol Chem 273*, 26571-26579.

Klug, C. A., Cheshier, S., and Weissman, I. L. (2000). Inactivation of a GFP retrovirus occurs at multiple levels in long-term repopulating stem cells and their differentiated progeny. *Blood 96*, 894-901.

Laker, C., Meyer, J., Schopen, A., Friel, J., Heberlein, C., Ostertag, W., and Stocking, C. (1998). Host cis-mediated extinction of a retrovirus permissive for expression in embryonal stem cells during differentiation. *J Virol 72*, 339-348.

Lange, C., and Blankenstein, T. (1997). Loss of retroviral gene expression in bone marrow reconstituted mice correlates with down-regulation of gene expression in long-term culture initiating cells. *Gene Ther 4*, 303-308.

Leonhardt, H., Page, A. W., Weier, H. U., and Bestor, T. H. (1992). A targeting sequence directs DNA methyltransferase to sites of DNA replication in mammalian nuclei. *Cell 71*, 865-873.

Lever, M. A., Th'ng, J. P., Sun, X., and Hendzel, M. J. (2000). Rapid exchange of histone H1.1 on chromatin in living human cells. *Nature 408*, 873-876.

Lewis, J. D., Meehan, R. R., Henzel, W. J., Maurer-Fogy, I., Jeppesen, P., Klein, F., and Bird, A. (1992). Purification, sequence, and cellular localization of a novel chromosomal protein that binds to methylated DNA. *Cell 69*, 905-914.

Li, E., Bestor, T. H., and Jaenisch, R. (1992). Targeted mutation of the DNA methyltransferase gene results in embryonic lethality. *Cell 69*, 915-926.

Liang, G., Chan, M. F., Tomigahara, Y., Tsai, Y. C., Gonzales, F. A., Li, E., Laird, P. W., and Jones, P. A. (2002). Cooperativity between DNA methyltransferases in the maintenance methylation of repetitive elements. *Mol Cell Biol 22*, 480-491.

Litt, M. D., Simpson, M., Gaszner, M., Allis, C. D., and Felsenfeld, G. (2001a). Correlation between histone lysine methylation and developmental changes at the chicken beta-globin locus. *Science 293*, 2453-2455.

Litt, M. D., Simpson, M., Recillas-Targa, F., Prioleau, M. N., and Felsenfeld, G. (2001b). Transitions in histone acetylation reveal boundaries of three separately regulated neighboring loci. *Embo J 20*, 2224-2235.

Liu, K., Wang, Y. F., Cantemir, C., and Muller, M. T. (2003). Endogenous assays of DNA methyltransferases: Evidence for differential activities of DNMT1, DNMT2, and DNMT3 in mammalian cells in vivo. *Mol Cell Biol 23*, 2709-2719.

Lois, C., Hong, E. J., Pease, S., Brown, E. J., and Baltimore, D. (2002). Germline transmission and tissue-specific expression of transgenes delivered by lentiviral vectors. *Science 295*, 868-872.

Lorincz, M. C., Schubeler, D., Goeke, S. C., Walters, M., Groudine, M., and Martin, D. I. (2000). Dynamic analysis of proviral induction and De Novo methylation: implications for a histone deacetylase-independent, methylation density-dependent mechanism of transcriptional repression. *Mol Cell Biol 20*, 842-850.

Lorincz, M. C., Schubeler, D., and Groudine, M. (2001). Methylation-mediated proviral silencing is associated with MeCP2 recruitment and localized histone H3 deacetylation. *Mol Cell Biol 21*, 7913-7922.

Lorincz, M. C., Schubeler, D., Hutchinson, S. R., Dickerson, D. R., and Groudine, M. (2002). DNA methylation density influences the stability of an epigenetic imprint and Dnmt3a/b-independent de novo methylation. *Mol Cell Biol 22*, 7572-7580.

Lu, L., and Tower, J. (1997). A transcriptional insulator element, the su(Hw) binding site, protects a chromosomal DNA replication origin from position effects. *Mol Cell Biol 17*, 2202-2206.

Lundgren, M., Chow, C. M., Sabbattini, P., Georgiou, A., Minaee, S., and Dillon, N. (2000). Transcription factor dosage affects changes in higher order chromatin structure associated with activation of a heterochromatic gene. *Cell 103*, 733-743.

Lutz, M., Burke, L. J., Barreto, G., Goeman, F., Greb, H., Arnold, R., Schultheiss, H., Brehm, A., Kouzarides, T., Lobanenkov, V., and Renkawitz, R. (2000). Transcriptional repression by the insulator protein CTCF involves histone deacetylases. *Nucleic Acids Res 28*, 1707-1713.

Lyko, F., Ramsahoye, B. H., and Jaenisch, R. (2000). DNA methylation in Drosophila melanogaster. *Nature 408*, 538-540.

Ma, Y., Ramezani, A., Lewis, R., Hawley, R. G., and Thomson, J. A. (2003). High-level sustained transgene expression in human embryonic stem cells using lentiviral vectors. *Stem Cells 21*, 111-117.

Mallin, D. R., Myung, J. S., Patton, J. S., and Geyer, P. K. (1998). Polycomb group repression is blocked by the Drosophila suppressor of Hairy-wing [su(Hw)] insulator. *Genetics 148*, 331-339.

Martinowich, K., Hattori, D., Wu, H., Fouse, S., He, F., Hu, Y., Fan, G., and Sun, Y. E. (2003). DNA methylation-related chromatin remodeling in activity-dependent BDNF gene regulation. *Science 302*, 890-893.

Martin-Rendon, E., and Watt, S. M. (2003). Exploitation of stem cell plasticity. *Transfus Med 13*, 325-349.

May, C., Rivella, S., Callegari, J., Heller, G., Gaensler, K. M., Luzzatto, L., and Sadelain, M. (2000). Therapeutic haemoglobin synthesis in beta-thalassaemic mice expressing lentivirus-encoded human beta-globin. *Nature 406*, 82-86.

McCune, S. L., and Townes, T. M. (1994). Retroviral vector sequences inhibit human beta-globin gene expression in transgenic mice. *Nucleic Acids Res 22*, 4477-4481.

McInerney, J. M., Nawrocki, J. R., and Lowrey, C. H. (2000). Long-term silencing of retroviral vectors is resistant to reversal by trichostatin A and 5-azacytidine. *Gene Ther 7*, 653-663.

McKay, R. (1997). Stem cells in the central nervous system. *Science 276*, 66-71.

McMorrow, T., van den Wijngaard, A., Wollenschlaeger, A., van de Corput, M., Monkhorst, K., Trimborn, T., Fraser, P., van Lohuizen, M., Jenuwein, T., Djabali, M., *et al.* (2000). Activation of the beta globin locus by transcription factors and chromatin modifiers. *Embo J 19*, 4986-4996.

McNairn, A. J., and Gilbert, D. M. (2003). Epigenomic replication: linking epigenetics to DNA replication. *Bioessays 25*, 647-656.

Melnikova, L., Gause, M., and Georgiev, P. (2002). The gypsy insulators flanking yellow enhancers do not form a separate transcriptional domain in Drosophila melanogaster: the enhancers can activate an isolated yellow promoter. *Genetics 160*, 1549-1560.

Mikkola, H., Woods, N. B., Sjogren, M., Helgadottir, H., Hamaguchi, I., Jacobsen, S. E., Trono, D., and Karlsson, S. (2000). Lentivirus gene transfer in murine hematopoietic progenitor cells is compromised by a delay in proviral integration and results in transduction mosaicism and heterogeneous gene expression in progeny cells. *J Virol 74*, 11911-11918.

Milne, T. A., Briggs, S. D., Brock, H. W., Martin, M. E., Gibbs, D., Allis, C. D., and Hess, J. L. (2002). MLL targets SET domain methyltransferase activity to Hox gene promoters. *Mol Cell 10*, 1107-1117.

Milot, E., Strouboulis, J., Trimborn, T., Wijgerde, M., de Boer, E., Langeveld, A., Tan-Un, K., Vergeer, W., Yannoutsos, N., Grosveld, F., and Fraser, P. (1996). Heterochromatin effects on the frequency and duration of LCR-mediated gene transcription. *Cell 87*, 105-114.

Milutinovic, S., Zhuang, Q., Niveleau, A., and Szyf, M. (2003). Epigenomic stress response. Knockdown of DNA methyltransferase 1 triggers an intra-S-phase arrest of DNA replication and induction of stress response genes. *J Biol Chem 278*, 14985-14995.

Misteli, T., Gunjan, A., Hock, R., Bustin, M., and Brown, D. T. (2000). Dynamic binding of histone H1 to chromatin in living cells. *Nature 408*, 877-881.

Miyoshi, H., Blomer, U., Takahashi, M., Gage, F. H., and Verma, I. M. (1998). Development of a self-inactivating lentivirus vector. *J Virol 72*, 8150-8157.

Moazed, D. (2001). Common themes in mechanisms of gene silencing. *Mol Cell 8*, 489-498.

Muravyova, E., Golovnin, A., Gracheva, E., Parshikov, A., Belenkaya, T., Pirrotta, V., and Georgiev, P. (2001). Loss of insulator activity by paired Su(Hw) chromatin insulators. *Science 291*, 495-498.

Mutskov, V. J., Farrell, C. M., Wade, P. A., Wolffe, A. P., and Felsenfeld, G. (2002). The barrier function of an insulator couples high histone acetylation levels with specific protection of promoter DNA from methylation. *Genes Dev 16*, 1540-1554.

Nabirochkin, S., Ossokina, M., and Heidmann, T. (1998). A nuclear matrix/scaffold attachment region co-localizes with the gypsy retrotransposon insulator sequence. J *Biol Chem 273*, 2473-2479.

Naldini, L., Blomer, U., Gallay, P., Ory, D., Mulligan, R., Gage, F. H., Verma, I. M., and Trono, D. (1996). In vivo gene delivery and stable transduction of nondividing cells by a lentiviral vector. *Science 272*, 263-267.

Naldini, L., and Verma, I. M. (2000). Lentiviral vectors. *Adv Virus Res 55*, 599-609.

Nan, X., Campoy, F. J., and Bird, A. (1997). MeCP2 is a transcriptional repressor with abundant binding sites in genomic chromatin. *Cell 88*, 471-481.

Nan, X., Meehan, R. R., and Bird, A. (1993). Dissection of the methyl-CpG binding domain from the chromosomal protein MeCP2. *Nucleic Acids Res 21*, 4886-4892.

Nan, X., Ng, H. H., Johnson, C. A., Laherty, C. D., Turner, B. M., Eisenman, R. N., and Bird, A. (1998). Transcriptional repression by the methyl-CpG-binding protein MeCP2 involves a histone deacetylase complex. *Nature 393*, 386-389.

Narlikar, G. J., Fan, H. Y., and Kingston, R. E. (2002). Cooperation between complexes that regulate chromatin structure and transcription. *Cell 108*, 475-487.

Ner, S. S., and Travers, A. A. (1994). HMG-D, the Drosophila melanogaster homologue of HMG 1 protein, is associated with early embryonic chromatin in the absence of histone H1. *Embo J 13*, 1817-1822.

Nielsen, S. J., Schneider, R., Bauer, U. M., Bannister, A. J., Morrison, A., O'Carroll, D., Firestein, R., Cleary, M., Jenuwein, T., Herrera, R. E., and Kouzarides, T. (2001). Rb targets histone H3 methylation and HP1 to promoters. *Nature 412*, 561-565.

Niwa, O., Yokota, Y., Ishida, H., and Sugahara, T. (1983). Independent mechanisms involved in suppression of the Moloney leukemia virus genome during differentiation of murine teratocarcinoma cells. *Cell 32*, 1105-1113.

Okano, M., Bell, D. W., Haber, D. A., and Li, E. (1999). DNA methyltransferases Dnmt3a and Dnmt3b are essential for de novo methylation and mammalian development. *Cell 99*, 247-257.

Okano, M., Xie, S., and Li, E. (1998). Dnmt2 is not required for de novo and maintenance methylation of viral DNA in embryonic stem cells. *Nucleic Acids Res 26*, 2536-2540.

Osborne, C. S., Pasceri, P., Singal, R., Sukonnik, T., Ginder, G. D., and Ellis, J. (1999). Amelioration of retroviral vector silencing in locus control region beta-globin-transgenic mice and transduced F9 embryonic cells. *J Virol 73*, 5490-54196.

Pannell, D., Osborne, C. S., Yao, S., Sukonnik, T., Pasceri, P., Karaiskakis, A., Okano, M., Li, E., Lipshitz, H. D., and Ellis, J. (2000). Retrovirus vector silencing is de novo methylase independent and marked by a repressive histone code. *Embo J 19*, 5884-5894.

Pasceri, P., Pannell, D., Wu, X., and Ellis, J. (1998). Full activity from human beta-globin locus control region transgenes requires 5'HS1, distal beta-globin promoter, and 3' beta-globin sequences. *Blood 92*, 653-663.

Peries, J., Debons-Guillemin, M. C., Canivet, M., Emanoil-Ravicovitch, R., Tavitian, A., and Boiron, M. (1977). [Multiplication of murine C-type viruses in mouse teratocarcinoma cell lines]. *Nouv Rev Fr Hematol Blood Cells 18*, 383-390.

Peters, A. H., O'Carroll, D., Scherthan, H., Mechtler, K., Sauer, S., Schofer, C., Weipoltshammer, K., Pagani, M., Lachner, M., Kohlmaier, A., *et al.* (2001). Loss of the Suv39h histone methyltransferases impairs mammalian heterochromatin and genome stability. *Cell 107*, 323-337.

Petersen, R., Kempler, G., and Barklis, E. (1991). A stem cell-specific silencer in the primer-binding site of a retrovirus. *Mol Cell Biol 11*, 1214-1221.

Pfeifer, A., Ikawa, M., Dayn, Y., and Verma, I. M. (2002). Transgenesis by lentiviral vectors: lack of gene silencing in mammalian embryonic stem cells and preimplantation embryos. *Proc Natl Acad Sci U S A 99*, 2140-2145.

Pirrotta, V. (1998). Polycombing the genome: PcG, trxG, and chromatin silencing. *Cell 93*, 333-336.

Prioleau, M. N., Nony, P., Simpson, M., and Felsenfeld, G. (1999). An insulator element and condensed chromatin region separate the chicken beta-globin locus from an independently regulated erythroid-specific folate receptor gene. *Embo J 18*, 4035-4048.

Quinonez, R., and Sutton, R. E. (2002). Lentiviral vectors for gene delivery into cells. DNA *Cell Biol 21*, 937-951.

Ramezani, A., and Hawley, R. G. (2003). Human immunodeficiency virus type 1-based vectors for gene delivery to human hematopoietic stem cells. *Methods Mol Med 76*, 467-492.

Ramezani, A., Hawley, T. S., and Hawley, R. G. (2003). Performance- and safety-enhanced lentiviral vectors containing the human interferon-beta scaffold attachment region and the chicken beta-globin insulator. *Blood 101*, 4717-4724.

Rasmussen, T. P. (2003). Embryonic stem cell differentiation: A chromatin perspective. *Reprod Biol Endocrinol 1*, 100.

Rea, S., Eisenhaber, F., O'Carroll, D., Strahl, B. D., Sun, Z. W., Schmid, M., Opravil, S., Mechtler, K., Ponting, C. P., Allis, C. D., and Jenuwein, T. (2000). Regulation of chromatin structure by site-specific histone H3 methyltransferases. *Nature 406*, 593-599.

Recillas-Targa, F., Pikaart, M. J., Burgess-Beusse, B., Bell, A. C., Litt, M. D., West, A. G., Gaszner, M., and Felsenfeld, G. (2002). Position-effect protection and enhancer blocking by the chicken beta-globin insulator are separable activities. *Proc Natl Acad Sci U S A 99*, 6883-6888.

Reid, J. L., Iyer, V. R., Brown, P. O., and Struhl, K. (2000). Coordinate regulation of yeast ribosomal protein genes is associated with targeted recruitment of Esa1 histone acetylase. *Mol Cell 6*, 1297-1307.

Rivella, S., Callegari, J. A., May, C., Tan, C. W., and Sadelain, M. (2000). The cHS4 insulator increases the probability of retroviral expression at random chromosomal integration sites. *J Virol 74*, 4679-4687.

Robbins, P. B., Skelton, D. C., Yu, X. J., Halene, S., Leonard, E. H., and Kohn, D. B. (1998). Consistent, persistent expression from modified retroviral vectors in murine hematopoietic stem cells. *Proc Natl Acad Sci U S A 95*, 10182-10187.

Roth, S. Y., Denu, J. M., and Allis, C. D. (2001). Histone acetyltransferases. *Annu Rev Biochem 70*, 81-120.

Russo, V. E. A., Martienssen, R.A. and Riggs, A.D. (1996). *Epigenetic Mechanisms of Gene Regulation.* In Cold Spring Harbor Laboratory Press, pp. 1-5.

Santos, F., Hendrich, B., Reik, W., and Dean, W. (2002). Dynamic reprogramming of DNA methylation in the early mouse embryo. *Dev Biol 241*, 172-182.

Schilz, A. J., Brouns, G., Knoss, H., Ottmann, O. G., Hoelzer, D., Fauser, A. A., Thrasher, A. J., and Grez, M. (1998). High efficiency gene transfer to human hematopoietic SCID-repopulating cells under serum-free conditions. *Blood 92*, 3163-3171.

Schotta, G., Ebert, A., Krauss, V., Fischer, A., Hoffmann, J., Rea, S., Jenuwein, T., Dorn, R., and Reuter, G. (2002). Central role of Drosophila SU(VAR)3-9 in histone H3-K9 methylation and heterochromatic gene silencing. *Embo J 21*, 1121-1131.

Schramke, V., and Allshire, R. (2003). Hairpin RNAs and retrotransposon LTRs effect RNAi and chromatin-based gene silencing. *Science 301*, 1069-1074.

Schroder, A. R., Shinn, P., Chen, H., Berry, C., Ecker, J. R., and Bushman, F. (2002). HIV-1 integration in the human genome favors active genes and local hotspots. *Cell 110*, 521-529.

Sewalt, R. G., Lachner, M., Vargas, M., Hamer, K. M., den Blaauwen, J. L., Hendrix, T., Melcher, M., Schweizer, D., Jenuwein, T., and Otte, A. P. (2002). Selective interactions between vertebrate polycomb homologs and the SUV39H1 histone lysine methyltransferase suggest that histone H3-K9 methylation contributes to chromosomal targeting of Polycomb group proteins. *Mol Cell Biol 22*, 5539-5553.

Shen, X., and Gorovsky, M. A. (1996). Linker histone H1 regulates specific gene expression but not global transcription in vivo. *Cell 86*, 475-483.

Shore, D. (2000). The Sir2 protein family: A novel deacetylase for gene silencing and more. *Proc Natl Acad Sci U S A 97*, 14030-14032.

Simon, D., Stuhlmann, H., Jahner, D., Wagner, H., Werner, E., and Jaenisch, R. (1983). Retrovirus genomes methylated by mammalian but not bacterial methylase are non-infectious. *Nature 304*, 275-277.

Sirven, A., Pflumio, F., Zennou, V., Titeux, M., Vainchenker, W., Coulombel, L., Dubart-Kupperschmitt, A., and Charneau, P. (2000). The human immunodeficiency virus type-1 central DNA flap is a crucial determinant for lentiviral vector nuclear import and gene transduction of human hematopoietic stem cells. *Blood 96*, 4103-4110.

Sirven, A., Ravet, E., Charneau, P., Zennou, V., Coulombel, L., Guetard, D., Pflumio, F., and Dubart-Kupperschmitt, A. (2001). Enhanced transgene expression in cord blood CD34(+)-derived hematopoietic cells, including developing T cells and NOD/SCID mouse repopulating cells, following transduction with modified trip lentiviral vectors. *Mol Ther 3*, 438-448.

Speck, N. A., and Baltimore, D. (1987). Six distinct nuclear factors interact with the 75-base-pair repeat of the Moloney murine leukemia virus enhancer. *Mol Cell Biol 7*, 1101-1110.

Speers, W. C., Gautsch, J. W., and Dixon, F. J. (1980). Silent infection of murine embryonal carcinoma cells by Moloney murine leukemia virus. *Virology 105*, 241-244.

Stancheva, I., Collins, A. L., Van den Veyver, I. B., Zoghbi, H., and Meehan, R. R. (2003). A mutant form of MeCP2 protein associated with human Rett syndrome cannot be displaced from methylated DNA by notch in Xenopus embryos. *Mol Cell 12*, 425-435.

Stewart, C. L., Stuhlmann, H., Jahner, D., and Jaenisch, R. (1982). De novo methylation, expression, and infectivity of retroviral genomes introduced into embryonal carcinoma cells. *Proc Natl Acad Sci U S A 79*, 4098-4102.

Strahl, B. D., and Allis, C. D. (2000). The language of covalent histone modifications. *Nature 403*, 41-45.

Swindle, C. S., Kim, H. G., and Klug, C. A. (2004). Mutation of CpGs in the Murine Stem Cell Virus Retroviral Vector Long Terminal Repeat Represses Silencing in Embryonic Stem Cells. *J Biol Chem 279*, 34-41.

Tachibana, M., Sugimoto, K., Fukushima, T., and Shinkai, Y. (2001). Set domain-containing protein, G9a, is a novel lysine-preferring mammalian histone methyltransferase with hyperactivity and specific selectivity to lysines 9 and 27 of histone H3. *J Biol Chem 276*, 25309-25317.

Teich, N. M., Weiss, R. A., Martin, G. R., and Lowy, D. R. (1977). Virus infection of murine teratocarcinoma stem cell lines. *Cell 12*, 973-982.

Trevisan, M., and Iscove, N. N. (1995). Phenotypic analysis of murine long-term hemopoietic reconstituting cells quantitated competitively in vivo and comparison with more advanced colony-forming progeny. *J Exp Med 181*, 93-103.

Tsukiyama, T., and Niwa, O. (1992). Isolation of high affinity cellular targets of the embryonal LTR binding protein, an undifferentiated embryonal carcinoma cell-specific repressor of Moloney leukemia virus. *Nucleic Acids Res 20*, 1477-1482.

Tsukiyama, T., Niwa, O., and Yokoro, K. (1989). Mechanism of suppression of the long terminal repeat of Moloney leukemia virus in mouse embryonal carcinoma cells. *Mol Cell Biol 9*, 4670-4676.

Uchida, N., Sutton, R. E., Friera, A. M., He, D., Reitsma, M. J., Chang, W. C., Veres, G., Scollay, R., and Weissman, I. L. (1998). HIV, but not murine leukemia virus, vectors mediate high efficiency gene transfer into freshly isolated G0/G1 human hematopoietic stem cells. *Proc Natl Acad Sci U S A 95*, 11939-11944.

Udvardy, A., Maine, E., and Schedl, P. (1985). The 87A7 chromomere. Identification of novel chromatin structures flanking the heat shock locus that may define the boundaries of higher order domains. *J Mol Biol 185*, 341-358.

Urieli-Shoval, S., Gruenbaum, Y., Sedat, J., and Razin, A. (1982). The absence of detectable methylated bases in Drosophila melanogaster DNA. *FEBS Lett 146*, 148-152.

van der Vlag, J., den Blaauwen, J. L., Sewalt, R. G., van Driel, R., and Otte, A. P. (2000). Transcriptional repression mediated by polycomb group proteins and other chromatin-associated repressors is selectively blocked by insulators. *J Biol Chem 275*, 697-704.

Verma, I. M., and Somia, N. (1997). Gene therapy -- promises, problems and prospects. *Nature 389*, 239-242.

Vogelauer, M., Wu, J., Suka, N., and Grunstein, M. (2000). Global histone acetylation and deacetylation in yeast. *Nature 408*, 495-498.

Voo, K. S., Carlone, D. L., Jacobsen, B. M., Flodin, A., and Skalnik, D. G. (2000). Cloning of a mammalian transcriptional activator that binds unmethylated CpG motifs and shares a CXXC domain with DNA methyltransferase, human trithorax, and methyl-CpG binding domain protein 1. *Mol Cell Biol 20*, 2108-2121.

Walsh, C. P., and Bestor, T. H. (1999). Cytosine methylation and mammalian development. *Genes Dev 13*, 26-34.

Walsh, C. P., Chaillet, J. R., and Bestor, T. H. (1998). Transcription of IAP endogenous retroviruses is constrained by cytosine methylation. *Nat Genet 20*, 116-117.

Weintraub, H., and Groudine, M. (1976). Chromosomal subunits in active genes have an altered conformation. *Science 193*, 848-856.

Wolffe, A. P., and Guschin, D. (2000). Review: chromatin structural features and targets that regulate transcription. *J Struct Biol 129*, 102-122.

Wolffe, A. P., and Matzke, M. A. (1999). Epigenetics: regulation through repression. *Science 286*, 481-486.

Woods, N. B., Fahlman, C., Mikkola, H., Hamaguchi, I., Olsson, K., Zufferey, R., Jacobsen, S. E., Trono, D., and Karlsson, S. (2000). Lentiviral gene transfer into primary and secondary NOD/SCID repopulating cells. *Blood 96*, 3725-3733.

Wu, X., Li, Y., Crise, B., and Burgess, S. M. (2003). Transcription start regions in the human genome are favored targets for MLV integration. *Science 300*, 1749-1751.

Xie, S., Wang, Z., Okano, M., Nogami, M., Li, Y., He, W. W., Okumura, K., and Li, E. (1999). Cloning, expression and chromosome locations of the human DNMT3 gene family. *Gene 236*, 87-95.

Yannaki, E., Tubb, J., Aker, M., Stamatoyannopoulos, G., and Emery, D. W. (2002). Topological constraints governing the use of the chicken HS4 chromatin insulator in oncoretrovirus vectors. *Mol Ther 5*, 589-598.

Yao, S., Osborne, C. S., Bharadwaj, R. R., Pasceri, P., Sukonnik, T., Pannell, D., Recillas-Targa, F., West, A. G., and Ellis, J. (2003). Retrovirus silencer blocking by the cHS4 insulator is CTCF independent. *Nucleic Acids Res 31*, 5317-5323.

Yao, S., Sukonnik, T., Kean, T., Bharadwaj R.R., Pasceri P. and Ellis J. (2004). Retrovirus silencing, variegation, extinction and memory are controlled by dynamic interplay of multiple epigenetic modifications. *Mol Ther* (*In Press).*

Yoder, J. A., Soman, N. S., Verdine, G. L., and Bestor, T. H. (1997a). DNA (cytosine-5)-methyltransferases in mouse cells and tissues. Studies with a mechanism-based probe. *J Mol Biol 270*, 385-395.

Yoder, J. A., Walsh, C. P., and Bestor, T. H. (1997b). Cytosine methylation and the ecology of intragenomic parasites. *Trends Genet 13*, 335-340.

Yu, S. F., von Ruden, T., Kantoff, P. W., Garber, C., Seiberg, M., Ruther, U., Anderson, W. F., Wagner, E. F., and Gilboa, E. (1986). Self-inactivating retroviral vectors designed for transfer of whole genes into mammalian cells. *Proc Natl Acad Sci U S A 83*, 3194-3198.

Zentilin, L., Qin, G., Tafuro, S., Dinauer, M. C., Baum, C., and Giacca, M. (2000). Variegation of retroviral vector gene expression in myeloid cells. *Gene Ther 7*, 153-166.

Zhao, K., Hart, C. M., and Laemmli, U. K. (1995). Visualization of chromosomal domains with boundary element-associated factor BEAF-32. *Cell 81*, 879-889.

Zufferey, R., Donello, J. E., Trono, D., and Hope, T. J. (1999). Woodchuck hepatitis virus posttranscriptional regulatory element enhances expression of transgenes delivered by retroviral vectors. *J Virol 73*, 2886-2892.

Zufferey, R., Dull, T., Mandel, R. J., Bukovsky, A., Quiroz, D., Naldini, L., and Trono, D. (1998). Self-inactivating lentivirus vector for safe and efficient in vivo gene delivery. *J Virol 72*, 9873-9880.

Zufferey, R., Nagy, D., Mandel, R. J., Naldini, L., and Trono, D. (1997). Multiply attenuated lentiviral vector achieves efficient gene delivery in vivo. *Nat Biotechnol 15*, 871-875.

In: Perspectives in Stem Cell Research ISBN: 978-1-61122-985-1
Editors: Brenda M. Davis and Christopher B. Halton © 2011 Nova Science Publishers, Inc.

Chapter X

Migration of Hematopoietic Stem/Progenitor Cells in Health and Disease

Susannah H. Kassmer, Jeanette Seidel, Bernd Niggemann, Kurt S. Zänker and Thomas Dittmar*

Institute of Immunology, Witten/ Herdecke University,
Stockumer Str. 10, 58448 Witten, Germany

Abstract

Hematopoietic stem/ progenitor cells (HSPC) are a rare population of cells within the bone marrow, which are capable to self-renew and which constantly reproduce all hematopoietic lineages. Transplantation of HSPC collected from peripheral mobilized blood or bone marrow has become more and more significant, e.g., for treatment of hematological diseases. Thereby, the homing and migration capacities of HSPC are of fundamental importance for successful transplantation since HSPC are usually administered intravenously. The multi-step process of HSPC homing, involving adhesion, transendothelial migration and migration across the bone marrow stroma, depends on active migration along a gradient of the chemokine SDF-1α. The potential of HSPC to undergo self-renewing cell divisions has stimulated investigations of *ex vivo* stem cell expansion, which would be valuable to improve the quality of stem cell transplants by increasing the number of stem cells. HSPC can be expanded *in vitro* by supplementation with hematopoietic cytokines, for instance, Flt3-Ligand and stem cell factor (SCF). However, analyses of migratory activity using a collagen matrix migration assay recently revealed a dramatic impact of various hematopoietic cytokines on the SDF-1α-directed migration of these *ex vivo* expanded HSPC.

Most hematopoietic progenitors reside in the bone marrow, however, a small fraction of these motile cells constantly circulate via the blood vessel system during steady state

* Correspondence to: Dr. Thomas Dittmar, Institute of Immunology, Witten/ Herdecke University, Stockumer Str. 10, 58448 Witten, Germany; Phone: +49 2302 926 165; FAX: +49 2302 926 158; E-mail: thomasd@uni-wh.de

homeostasis. During inflammatory conditions, e.g., after (organ) tissue injury, the number of circulating HSPC increases dramatically. Inflammatory chemokines such as IL-8 and GROβ causes a rapid mobilization of HSPC from bone marrow. Conjointly, SDF-1α, released by endothelial cells, attracts HSPC to sites of injury, which thereupon participate in tissue repair. Due to their plasticity and pluripotency as well as their capacity to fuse with other cells, HSPC can transdifferentiate in various cell types such as liver, heart and skeletal muscle, or neurons. However, the directed migration and homing of HSPC to their target tissues underlies the influence of both *start* and *stop* signals. Recent observations indicate a modulating effect of the chemokine IL-8 and even the neurotransmitter GABA on the SDF-1α mediated migratory activity of HSPC. Further elucidation of these mechanisms may facilitate the selective manipulation of HSPC homing to their target tissues.

Thus, it appears that understanding the mechanisms influencing and regulating the migratory processes of HSPC, comprising homing, retention, release and mobilization, may allow the improvement of their clinical applications.

INTRODUCTION

Hematopoietic stem cells (HSC) are a rare population of immature cells within the bone marrow, possessing the ability to self-renew and continuously give rise to all hematopoietic lineages [1]. The application of HSC for the treatment of hematologic malignancies and myeloproliferative disorders requires their inherent migratory capacity, which is fundamental during homing and mobilization. In the 1950s, Dr. E. Donnall Thomas discovered that bone marrow cells infused intravenously repopulated the bone marrow and produced new blood cells. Besides transplantation of HSC from bone marrow, transplantation of HSC collected from peripheral blood after mobilization with granulocyte-colony stimulating factor (G-CSF) or granulocyte macrophage-colony stimulating factor (GM-CSF) has become more and more significant since the early 1990s. After intravenous infusion, successful engraftment depends on directed homing of the transplanted HSC to the bone marrow niche. During the homing process, HSC have to actively migrate along a chemotactic gradient secreted by the bone marrow stroma and endothelium. The engrafted HSC repopulate the bone marrow, leading to generation of maturing blood cells of all lineages as well as maintenance of a small stem cell pool within the host bone marrow. Under healthy conditions, very low levels of these motile cells constantly migrate throughout the bloodstream. The migratory capacity of HSC becomes significant during inflammation and tissue injury, when migrating HSC are attracted to injured or inflamed tissues, and participate in their repair. Under several circumstances, trans-differentiation or fusion of HSC with other cells was observed in injured or inflamed tissues. Within this chapter, we will describe the conditions and factors influencing HSC migration, and briefly discuss the question as to the outcome of trans-differentiation or fusion events when a hematopoietic stem cell is recruited to malignant tissue.

MIGRATION OF HSC DURING MOBILIZATION AND HOMING TO BONE MARROW

Under steady state conditions, HSC reside within their specialized bone marrow niches (Figure 1). They give rise to more committed progenies, which successively differentiate in mature blood cells that migrate into the circulation. However, a very small proportion of primitive hematopoietic stem/ progenitor cells (HSPC) constantly leaves the bone marrow and circulates through the bloodstream (Figure 1). HSPC numbers in the peripheral blood are extremely low, ranging from 0.05-0.1% within the peripheral blood mononuclear cell fraction [2]. The pool of circulating HSPC can be significantly increased by their enforced migration from the bone marrow via administration of cytokines or chemokines, so-called "mobilization". In general, HSPC mobilization from the bone marrow into the bloodstream is induced by frequent injection of the cytokine G-CSF, which activates neutrophil granulocytes to secrete various serin proteases, including elastin and cathepsin G. These proteases then cleave multiple target molecules, such as adhesion molecules, chemokines, and their receptors, on both HSPC and bone marrow stromal cells [3]. For instance, neutrophil elastase, accumulate within the bone marrow, cleaving substrates comprising VCAM-1, vascular endothelial cadherin, CXCR4 and SDF-1α [4, 5]. G-CSF mediated mobilization likely involves CD26, a membrane bound extracellular peptidase expressed by HSPC, which cleaves some of the same target molecules as serine proteases, including SDF-1α, yielding its truncated from. This results in a reduced migratory response to normal SDF-1α, thereby reducing retention of HSPC within the bone marrow and facilitating mobilization into the periphery [6]. Inhibition of CD26 on HSPC increases their SDF-1α directed homing and chemotactic migration [7]. Another substrate of proteases is membrane bound urokinase receptor (uPAR), which plays an important role in short term homing and engraftment, and constitutes a cell-autonomous retention signal for HSPC. In response to G-CSF stimulation, uPAR is proteolytically cleaved by the protease plasmin, leading to formation of soluble uPAR. Soluble uPAR further amplifies mobilization and also promotes HSPC migration [8]. In general, disruption of the SDF-1α/ CXCR4 axis is one of the most important mechanisms causing HSPC mobilization [9], whereas its activation is essential for homing, as will be described below. For instance, the CXCR4 antagonist AMD3100 induced rapid mobilization of HSPC, alone or in addition to G-CSF [10, 11]. Mobilized cells exhibit decreased expression of very late antigen-4 (VLA-4). More important, however, is the reduced functional state of VLA receptors. As migratory responses require the participation of integrins, functional down-regulation of integrins is an important step during the final stages of transmigration through the endothelial sinuses [9].

Homing is defined as the active migration of circulating HSPC across the blood/bone endothelial barrier into the bone marrow compartment (Figure 1) within a fairly short time span. The multi-step process of HSPC homing involving recruitment of circulating HSPC by the bone marrow microvasculature, adhesion, transendothelial migration and migration across the bone marrow stroma, depends on active migration along a gradient of the chemokine SDF-1α [12-15]. SDF-1α plays a major role in migration, proliferation, differentiation and survival of various cell types including HSPC. The CXC chemokine SDF-1α is constitutively expressed in many organs, including bone marrow endothelium and the stem cell rich endosteum region, as well as multiple stromal cell types. SDF forms a decreasing gradient from the marrow extravascular compartment toward the lumen of infiltrating vessels [12, 16, 17], thus promoting homing of transplanted HSPC to bone marrow. The G-protein-coupled chemokine receptor CXCR4, which is expressed by HSPC, binds SDF-1α and thus mediates chemotaxis and Integrin-mediated firm adhesion and transendothelial migration [15]. Integrin activation is mediated by chemokine and cytokine receptors via 'inside out' signaling [18]. Cytokines and chemokines, like, for instance, GM-CSF, IL-3, SCF and SDF-1α, activate integrin function, thereby increasing adhesiveness of human $CD34^+$ bone marrow cells to fibronectin and collagen [19, 20]. Thus, SDF-1α stimulates firm adhesion of HSPC to endothelium and transendothelial migration, which depends on lymphocyte function associated antigen-1 (LFA-1) / ICAM-1 (intracellular adhesion molecule-1) and VLA-4 / VCAM-1 (vascular adhesion molecule-1) interactions [9]. For instance, SDF-1α induced polarization and extravasation of HSPC has been shown to depend on VLA-4 and VLA-5 [13, 14, 21]. P-selectin glycoprotein ligand, the sialomucin receptor for P-selectin, likewise seems to play a key role in homing of HSPC [22, 23]. Polarization is also induced when SDF stimulated cells bind to immobilized hyaloronic acid (HA), and the HA-receptor CD44 is involved in adhesion and immobilization of cells [24]. Transendothelial migration requires the degradation of the basement membrane and thus the production of matrix degrading enzymes, like matrix-metalloproteinases (MMP) [25]. Their expression and secretion by cells crossing the endothelial layer are stimulated by various cytokines and chemokines. Additionally, MMP-9 expressed by bone marrow stromal cells cleaves membrane bound SCF, which then enhances Integrin-mediated binding of HSPC to extracellular matrix components. Exposure of HSPC to SCF upregulates the levels of the homing related molecules CD49e, CD49f, CD54, CXCR4, MMP-4 and MMP-2, leading to increased transmigration and homing potential [26]. After firm adhesion to the bone marrow endostelium, HSPC transmigrate within the marrow to specific sites know as stem cell niches, where their lodgment, proliferation and self-renewal is regulated by a complex interplay of cells, growth factors and adhesion molecules. HSPC predominantly transmigrate to the endosteal region, whereas lineage committed or differentiated cells move away from the endosteal region and into the central marrow region [27, 28]. Our current understanding about the molecules involved in this process is still fragmentary, however, hyaluronic acid, the transmembrane isoform of SCF and osteopontin seem to play a role in transendothelial migration and lodgment of transplanted HSPC within their niche [29]. On human $CD34^+$ HSPC, RHAMM, a receptor for hyaluronic acid, leads to an increase in cell motility, whereby CD44 leads to an increase in adhesion.

THE SDF-1α/ CXCR4 SIGNAL TRANSDUCTION CASCADE

The SDF-1α receptor CXCR4 belongs to the group of 7-transmembrane helix receptors, as SDF-1α signaling via CXCR4 involves a pertussis toxin sensitive $G_{\alpha i}$ protein [30]. Upon SDF binding, PI3-kinase (PI3K), phospholipase C-γ (PLC-γ), protein kinase C (PKC) and $MAPK^{p42/44}$ are activated, finally leading to tyrosine phosphorylation of focal adhesion components such as paxillin, related adhesion focal tyrosine kinase (RAFTK/ pyk2), $p130^{CAS}$, Crk-II, and Crk-L [31, 32]. Furthermore, cell polarization, adhesion to bone marrow stromal cells, chemotaxis and homing of human $CD34^+$ HSPC were shown to depend upon PKC-ζ, representing an atypical PKC subtype independent of calcium or diacylglycerolc [33].

SDF also induces transient activation of molecules implicated in cell survival, like ribosomal S6 kinase and Akt [34], and nuclear factor-κB (NF-κB) [31, 35]. SDF binding to CXCR4 triggers receptor dimerization and activates the JAK/STAT pathway, and thus seems to influence gene regulation [35]. Association of CXCR4 with lipid rafts and colocalization with Rac-1 primes the SDF-directed homing response of HSPC and facilitates activation of Rac-1 [36]. Rac-1 expression is crucial during the engraftment phase of HSPC homing, while lack of Rac-1 and Rac-2 expression leads to massive mobilization of HSPC and impaired hematopoiesis. Thus, Rac proteins seem to regulate homing as well as mobilization processes [37].

Activation of PLC-γ by SDF binding to CXCR4 leads to release of calcium from IP_3 sensitive endoplasmatic reticulum stores. Intracellular calcium ions regulate the structure and function of cytoskeletal proteins like actin. Thus, CXCR4 signaling finally culminates in the highly synchronized processes of actin polymerization, and cytoskeleton reorganization.

Migration of HSPC in Steady State Homeostasis and Tissue Repair

Although most hematopoietic progenitors reside in the bone marrow, a small fraction of these motile cells constantly circulates via the blood system during steady state homeostasis. Continuous remodeling within the bone marrow results in their constant and random release into the circulation. These constitutively migrating cells play a physiological role in the functional reengraftment of unconditioned bone marrow by filling open HSC niches [38]. The fact that HSPC have been isolated from many other tissues besides bone marrow would indicate that circulating cells are in dynamic equilibrium with these other tissues [9]. For instance, HSPC present in substantial numbers in muscle tissue are of bone marrow origin [39, 40]. Krause et al. showed that after transplantation of single cells into irradiated mice, long term repopulating HSPC initiated differentiation of bone marrow derived cells into epithelial cells of the liver, lung, gastrointestinal tract and skin in the absence of tissue injury [41]. An important player in this scenario is SDF-1α as it is the product of resting cells in multiple organs, like bone, lymph node, muscle, lung, skin and liver [42-45]. Thus, transplanted HSPC have been found to home, besides bone marrow, to spleen, liver and lung [46], which likely applies also to circulating HSPC during homeostasis. For instance, human liver bile duct epithelium expresses SDF-1α under steady state conditions, attracting $CD34^+$ hematopoietic progenitors [47]. SDF-1α expressed in human heart and skeletal muscle constantly attracts CXCR4 positive $CD34^+$ HSPC to niches within the muscle tissue [42, 48].

In stress situations, like bleeding, organ injury and inflammation, the number of circulating HSPC increases dramatically. In response to tissue injury, multiple chemical signals in concert with cytokines, growth factors and chemokines like SDF-1α initiate the host response, involving activation and directed migration of leukocytes from the venous system to sites of tissue damage. Activated endothelial cells facilitate rolling of leukocytes on activated members of the selectin family of adhesion molecules (L-P-E-selectin). Cytokine-mediated activation of leukocyte-integrins leads to immobilization and firm adhesion by means of $\alpha_4\beta_1$- and $\alpha_4\beta_7$-integrins binding to VCAM-1, followed by transmigration through the endothelium to sites of injury, facilitated by matrix metalloproteinases.

During inflammation and tissue damage, SDF-1α as well as other chemokines are released from cells within the lesioned areas, attracting migrating HSPC to sites of injury, which thereupon participate in tissue repair. For HSPC, it has been observed that cytokine exposure, which is likely to occur during an inflammatory process, seems to be able to change the homing behavior of circulating HSPC, and to increase homing to tissues other than bone marrow, as murine HSPC exposed to a combination of cytokines showed an increased homing to lung tissue and decreased homing to marrow [46]. The complement anaphylatoxin C3a, which is generated during inflammatory responses, sensitizes the response of human $CD34^+$ HSPC to SDF-1α by potentiating SDF-1α dependent chemotaxis and stimulates MMP-9 secretion and VLA-4 mediated adhesion to VCAM-1 [49].

Various animal models for tissue damage have been used to detect migration and homing of bone marrow derived hematopoietic stem cells to sites of tissue injury. For instance, systemically injected HSPC are attracted to the subretinal space in a murine model of retinal pigment epithelium damage by SDF-1α, C3a, hepatic growth factor (HGF), and leukemia inhibitory factor (LIF) which are released from the injured tissue. HSPC were found to express the tissue specific marker RPE-65 after homing to the subretinal space [50, 51]. In the liver, irradiation or inflammation increases SDF-1α and HGF expression, promoting recruitment and directional migration of $CD34^+$ hematopoietic progenitors, which differentiate into albumin producing cells [47]. In a murine model for hepatic tissue damage, only transplantation of purified HSPC gave rise to donor derived hepatic regeneration [52]. Another important mediator of stem cell homing is hyaluronic acid, which is increasingly expressed in injured tissue, as was recently demonstrated by Herrera et al. in a murine model of tubular injury in the kidney [53]. Expression of hyaluronic acid was crucial in the homing of transplanted stem cells, which subsequently increased renal healing. This finding is interesting in the light of a previous study, in which homing of human $CD34^+$ HSPC to bone marrow was found to depend on binding of hyaluronic acid to its receptor CD44 on the cell surface, whereby a crosstalk between CXCR4 and CD44 seems to be present [24]. Another stress situation leading to increased expression of chemokines is ischemic injury. In ischemic tissues, hypoxic stimuli lead to hypoxia inducible factor-1α (HIF-1α) dependent expression of SDF-1α by endothelial cells, mediating ischemia specific recruitment of circulating progenitor cells [54, 55]. After ischemic injury, SDF-1α expression increases in the kidney and decreases in the bone marrow, causing mobilization of $CD34^+$ HSPC and their subsequent homing to damaged kidney tissue [56]. Bone marrow derived stem cells (BMDC) comprise HSPC and mesenchymal stem cells, which both exhibit high plasticity and a high migratory potential. After ischemia induced by coronary heart occlusion, highly purified BMDC transplanted into mice differentiate into cardiomyocytes and contribute to the formation of functional tissue [57]. Myocardial infarction leads to increased expression of SDF-1α, vascular endothelial growth factor (VEGF), MMP-9, ICAM-1 and VCAM-1 [58], all of which may be involved in promoting recruitment of bone marrow derived cells including HSPC to the injured heart. In the brains of mice recieving focal cerebral ischemia, SDF-1α expression by endothelial cells within the lesioned areas is profoundly increased and leads to the attraction of CXCR4 expressing leukocytes [59], including HSPC. Mobilization of BMDC in mice by treatment with G-CSF and SCF significantly increased the number of bone marrow derived cells expressing neuronal markers within several brain areas, which may become a new strategy for neuronal repair in neurodegenerative diseases [60]. In micc within the subacute phase of cerebral infarction, the same treatment induced attraction of BMDC to the infracted area, associated with improved motor performance and brain function [61]. Thus, it appears that stimulated migration and homing of hematopoietic and other bone marrow derived stem cells may be a valuable process during healing and treatment of tissue injury.

In all the situations described so far, HSPC entering the damaged or inflamed tissue seem to contribute to tissue repair, either by trans-differentiation, or via indirect mechanisms, like secretion of cytokines and attraction of other cells. Trans-differentiation may be due either to the local tissue milieu, which serves as a blueprint for the differentiation of the invading BMDC [62], to cell-fusion events [63], or to a combination of both. HSPC show a high plasticity, as they differentiate into tissue cells even when derived from other embryonic origin, like ectoderm and endoderm, for instance, hepatocytes and neuronal cell types. For instance, bone marrow derived cells were demonstrated to fuse *in vivo* with hepatocytes, purkinje neurons, and cardiomyocytes [64]. However, in these cells, polyploidy and multiple nuclei are well tolerated, as hepatocytes and purkinje neurons tend to be polyploid, and muscle fibers form multinucleated syncytia. Interestingly, a recent study has shown that transplanted BMDC fuse with normal intestinal stem cells in gamma-irradiated mice.

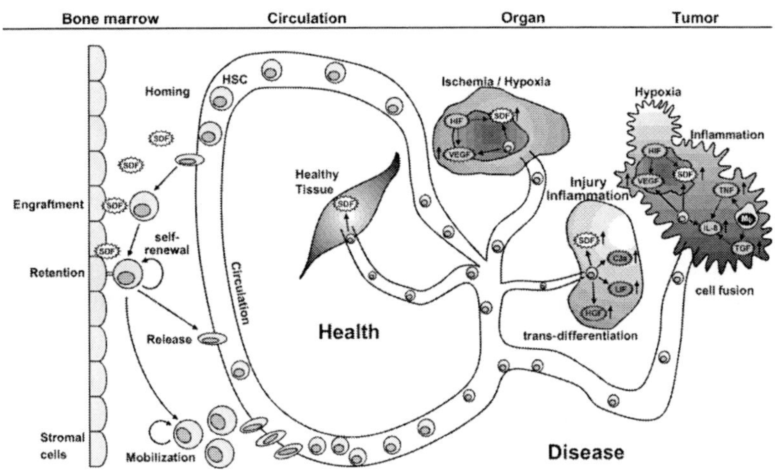

Figure 1. Hematopoietic stem cell migration. Under steady state conditions, HSPC are retained within specialized bone marrow niches supported by stromal cells. HSPC homing to the bone marrow depends on active migration along a gradient of the chemokine SDF-1α, which is secreted by the bone marrow stroma. A very small proportion of primitive HSPC constantly leaves the bone marrow and circulates through the bloodstream. These circulating HSPC enter other tissues, forming a dynamic equilibrium. Mobilization results in proliferation of HSPC and their enforced migration from the bone marrow. During inflammation and tissue damage, SDF-1α as well as other chemokines are released from cells within the lesioned areas, attracting migrating HSPC to sites of injury. These include HGF, C3a and LIF. In ischemic tissues, including tumor tissue, hypoxic stimuli lead to HIF dependent expression of SDF-1α and VEGF. HSPC recruited to injured, inflamed or hypoxic tissue thereupon participate in tissue repair by trans-differentiation. The inflammatory reaction within tumor tissue is mediated by tumor-associated macrophages (Mϕ) secreting TNF-α, IL-8 and TGF-β. Recruitment of HSPC to tumor tissue may result in faulty trans-differentiation, or cell-fusion with transformed cells.

Additionally, they report fusion of BMDC with transformed intestinal stem cells, providing *in vivo* evidence that strongly supports the hypothesis that fusion between circulating hematopoietic cells and transformed intestinal epithelium is involved in intestinal tumorigenesis [65].

The concept that regeneration of liver after bone-marrow transplantation in mice occurs through cell fusion of hepatocytes with HSC progeny has received substantial support by two studies, in which male donor cells derived from bone marrow were injected into female recipients, and fusion of HSPC with liver cells was proven by sex-mismatch of repopulated liver cells [66, 67]. Other groups favor the theory that HSPC trans-differentiate into liver cells. Jang et al. could show via RT-PCR that HSPC exposed to supernatant of damaged or injured liver tissue, up-regulated liver marker expression [68]. Another study by Oh et al. also provides evidence that BMDC plasticity involves trans-differentiation in the absence of fusion.

BMDC were induced *in vitro* to trans-differentiate into insulin producing cells, which showed an architecture and protein expression pattern characteristic of the pancreatic lineage after transplantation into mice [69].

Recruitment of HSPC to Malignant Tissue – Contribution to Carcinogenesis?

Thus, the question arises what will be the outcome of these events of trans-differentiation and fusion, if HSPC enters chronically inflamed or even tumor tissue. Tumor cells produce various cytokines and chemokines, which act in concert to attract leukocytes comprising neutrophils, dendritic cells, macrophages, eosinophils and mast cells, as well as lymphocytes, which in turn secrete an array of cytokines, inflammatory mediators and chemokines. The enhanced proliferation within a tumor tissue results in hypoxic areas and the release of reactive oxygen species, promoting the loss of self-limitation of the mechanisms involved in normal inflammation. The inflammatory reaction is mediated by tumor associated macrophages, which are attracted to tumor tissue via hypoxia, and in turn secrete proinflammatory cytokines, such as TNF-α and chemokines such as monocyte chemo-attractant protein 1, -2, -3 (MCP-1, -2, -3) [70, 71]. But not only cells of the immune system have been shown to enter sites of inflammation. More recently, also hematopoietic stem cells were found at inflammatory sites, in all likelihood recruited by a hypoxia induced SDF-1α-release of the inflamed or tumor tissue [54]. TGF-β and SDF-1α dependent migration of HSPC and homing towards gliomas *in vivo* are induced by hypoxia and irradiation, and, like in ischemic tissue, depend on HIF-1α [72]. However, the fate of HSPC recruited to neoplastic tissue still remains unclear.

Bone marrow-derived stem cells, including HSPC, which are recruited to tumor tissue, encounter this malignant environment as instructing milieu. Thus, stem cells may adopt cancer cells characteristics by trans-differentiation, as the blueprint for this process is given by the local tissue environment, which is defined by a specific pattern of cytokines, chemokines and adhesion molecules, etc. [62]. The second possible mechanism leading to (trans-)differentiation is fusion of a BMDC with a tissue or even a tumor cell. As stated above, HSPC possess the ability to fuse with tissue cells during processes of tissue repair.

Fusion of a BMDC with a tumor cell might increase tumor cell diversity due to chromosomal aberrations and unbalanced chromosome distribution during mitosis [67, 73-75]. Cancer stem cells are certain cells within a tumor tissue sharing similarities to stem cells such as immortality, drug resistance, and responsiveness to chemokines, an undifferentiated phenotype and migratory activity leading to metastasis. It would be conceivable that cancer stem cells result from fusion events of BMDC or tissue stem cells and transformed tissue cells [76-79].

Several studies indicate that a chronically inflamed microenvironment may lead to a faulty set of instructions received by a tissue stem cell, which may then adopt a neoplastic phenotype [62]. For instance, Houghton et al. showed that chronic infection of mice with *helicobacter felis* induced the attraction of BMDC to the stomach, which progress to form intraepithelial cancer [80]. The chronically inflamed tissue within a tumor is characterized by the presence of chemokines, cytokines, reactive oxygen and nitrogen species and proteases, which have an impact on cell-cell communication via gap-junctions and adhesion molecules. Furthermore, reactive oxygen and nitrogen species can cause DNA damage, leading to multiple genetic aberrations. Thus, HSPC and other BMDC entering a chronically inflamed tissue may encounter an altered set of instructions, which then results in a faulty (trans-) differentiation process.

Migration Capacity and Engraftment of *Ex Vivo* Expanded HSPC

The ability of HSPC to self-renew allows them to undergo symmetric cell divisions, yielding two daughter cells retaining the characteristics of the originating cell. This has stimulated investigations of *ex vivo* stem cell expansion, which would be valuable to increase the number of stem cells and thus improve the quality of stem cell transplants. For instance, umbilical cord blood transplants, which are suitable for transplantations of small children, contain only a very limited number of stem cells, and thus, *ex vivo* expansion may allow cord blood transplants to be used in adults [81]. To investigate *ex vivo* expansion and engraftment of HSPC, murine models are frequently used. HSPC can be isolated from murine bone marrow and expanded *in vitro* by supplementation with a variety of hematopoietic cytokines. Recent studies have identified thrombopoietin (TPO), Flt3-ligand (FL), stem cell factor (SCF) and interleukin (IL)-11 as cytokines able to stimulate amplification of primitive murine hematopoietic stem cells *in vitro* [82-87]. Human HSC and HSPC have been successfully expanded *in vitro* by supplementation with combinations of FL, SCF, IL-1β, IL-6, IL-3, G-CSF, GM-CSF and SCF [88, 89]. Megakaryocyte growth and differentiation factor (MGDF) has also been used [81].

HSPC expansion *in vitro* needs to induce self renewing cell divisions, however, proliferation itself may silence the ability of HSPC to home [90]. As stated above, the homing and migration capacities of HSPC cells are of fundamental importance for successful transplantation during treatment of hematological diseases. A number of recent observations suggest a specific influence of cytokines and cytokine combinations on the engraftment potential as well as on the homing ability of HSPC. Initially, Cerny et al. reported a cytokine induced defect in homing to the bone marrow and engraftment potential of murine Lin^- $Sca\text{-}1^+$

HSPC after cultivation in IL-3, IL-6, IL-11 and SCF for 48 hours [91]. Likewise, Ahmed et al. showed an irreversibly impaired homing of human $CD34^+$ HSPC to the bone marrow following 48 hour exposure to FL, SCF, IL-6 and IL-3 [92]. Von Drygalski and colleagues performed transplantation studies using murine bone marrow cells cultivated with three different cytokine combinations (FL, SCF, TPO; FL, SCF, TPO + IL-11 and FL, SCF, TPO, IL-11 + IL-3), and observed decreased 7 months survival rates and poorer donor engraftment of cultured compared to freshly isolated cells [93]. In line with these observations, one recent study analyzing the migratory activity of *ex vivo* expanded HSPC revealed a dramatic impact of various hematopoietic cytokines on SDF-1α-directed migration [94]. Murine $Lin^-c\text{-}kit^+$ (HSPC) were cultivated in the presence of twelve combinations of the hematopoietic cytokines TPO, FL, SCF and IL-11. As SDF-1α is the most potent migratory stimulant for HSPC [95], spontaneous as well as SDF-1α stimulated locomotory activity were measured in a 3D collagen matrix using time lapse video microscopy. Each cytokine combination had a distinct effect on the expansion as well as the SDF-1α-stimulated migratory activity of murine Lin^- $c\text{-}kit^+$ HSPC. For instance, FL and SCF cultivated cells showed a high SDF-response, but only a moderate fold expansion of long term repopulating HSPC. By contrast, cultivation with SCF, TPO and IL-11 resulted in a relatively high fold expansion of HSPC, but absence of an elevated migratory activity in response to SDF stimulation. The differences in the migratory SDF-response were not related to different CXCR4 expression levels, but rather to the differential engagement of the CXCR4 dependent $MAPK^{p42/44}$ and PI3K signal transduction pathways, demonstrating a strong influence of different cytokines and cytokine combinations on signal processing downstream of CXCR4. In cells exhibiting an intermediate to low increase of migratory activity in response to SDF-1α, PI3K and $MAPK^{p42/44}$ pathways are not involved in migration in the presence of SDF-1α, while in cells exhibiting a high response to SDF-stimulation, PI3K and $MAPK^{p42/44}$ are crucial in SDF-1α directed migration [94]. This is in accordance with a study by Fukuda and colleagues, who previously demonstrated differential phosphorylation of key signal transduction proteins induced by FL treatment in human $CD34^+$ HSPC. Flt3-ligand and SDF-1α were observed to synergistically enhance the phosphorylation of $MAPK^{p42/44}$, PI3K and Akt, as well as migratory activity. In cells pretreated with FL for two days, weaker and delayed phosphorylation of $MAPK^{p42/44}$ was observed after SDF-1α stimulation [96]. In another study on *ex vivo* expanded human $CD133^+$ HSPC, analyses of the migratory activity revealed an enhancing effect of IL-6 on the SDF-1α-stimulated migratory activity of these cells [97]. This was due to recruitment of nonmoving cells, and an increase in the speed of actively migrating cells. One of the possible mechanisms underlying the altered migratory and homing capacity of *ex vivo* cultivated HSPC is a dramatically altered adhesion receptor expression and reduced functional binding to the extracellular matrix [98], or delayed deactivation of integrins and sustained attachment. This may result in either impaired engraftment within the bone marrow niche or decreased migratory activity, respectively. The involved mechanisms were further elucidated by Glimm et al. who observed a cell cycle dependent change in *in vivo* stem cell transplantability of $CD34^+$ human cord blood HSPC after 5 days of *ex vivo* expansion. [88]. After cultivation in FL, SCF, IL-3, IL-6 and G-CSF, cells in the G_1 phase of the cell cycle contained at least 85% of the transplantable stem cell activity, suggesting a cell cycle associated change in *in vivo* stem cell homing. A recent study by Yang et al. provides insight into the cell cycle associated processes resulting in homing and engraftment deficiencies of HSPC [99]. In Cdc42 deficient mice, HSPC within the bone marrow enter the active cell cycle, resulting in impaired adhesion, homing, lodging and retention of HSPC within the bone marrow, which also causes a massive egress of HSPC to distal organs and peripheral blood and an engraftment failure. These effects are associated with deregulated β_1-integrin and N-cadherin expression and defective actin organization.

In summary, cytokines commonly used in *ex vivo* expansion protocols seem to influence homing and migration of hematopoietic cells in many different ways, depending on combination with other cytokines, cell type, incubation time, etc. Furthermore, hematopoietic cytokines strongly affect the intracellular signaling machinery of *ex vivo* expanded HSPC and their aptitude to react to SDF-1α stimulation with increased locomotory activity. As therapeutic success is fundamentally dependent on the migration capacity and homing of transplanted HSPC to bone marrow, analysis of SDF-1α-stimulated migratory activity and migration parameters may prove valuable to investigate the effects of *ex vivo* expansion supplements, as these may enhance or even compromise the efficacy of therapy involving HSPC migration.

Identification of Factors Terminating HSPC Migration

The directed migration and homing of HSPC to their target tissues, including inflamed and malignant tissue, underlies the influence of start and stop signals, exerted, apart from CXCR4/SDF-1α interaction, by various factors. In inflammatory responses, the chemokine IL-8 is released by macrophages encountering an antigen, and is therefore present at sites of inflammation. Recent observations indicate a modulating effect of the chemokine IL-8 and even neurotransmitters on the migratory activity of human mobilized $CD133^+$ HSPC (Figure 2A). Human HSPC express the receptors for IL-8, CXCR1 and CXCR2. Co-stimulation of HSPC with IL-8 revealed an inhibitory effect of IL-8 on their SDF-1α induced migratory activity. Thus, IL-8 might be one of the factors responsible for the retention of HSPC at inflammatory sites within a tissue or a tumor. For instance, during development of melanoma, melanoma cells have been found to express IL-8 in response to TGF-β, TNF-α and IL-1α secretion by activated macrophages [100].

Remarkably, the neurotransmitter γ-aminobutyric acid (GABA), which has formerly been mainly associated with neuronal tissues, was recently shown to exert an inhibitory influence on human HSPC-migration (Figure 2B). Therefore, functional characterization of distinct migration parameters revealed the inhibitory effect of GABA on spontaneous and SDF-1α-stimulated migration of HSPC to be primarily attributed to an increase in the average pause length and a decrease in speed and velocity.

GABA-signaling on HSPC was mediated by the $GABA_B$-receptor. Time dependent calcium measurements revealed a decrease in intracellular calcium level after GABA application. Inhibition of calcium release activated calcium (CRAC) channels with BTP-2 indicates that GABA-mediated reduction of HSPC-migration is exerted by inhibitions of CRAC channels, resulting in a decrease of intracellular calcium, which is crucial for cell migration [101].

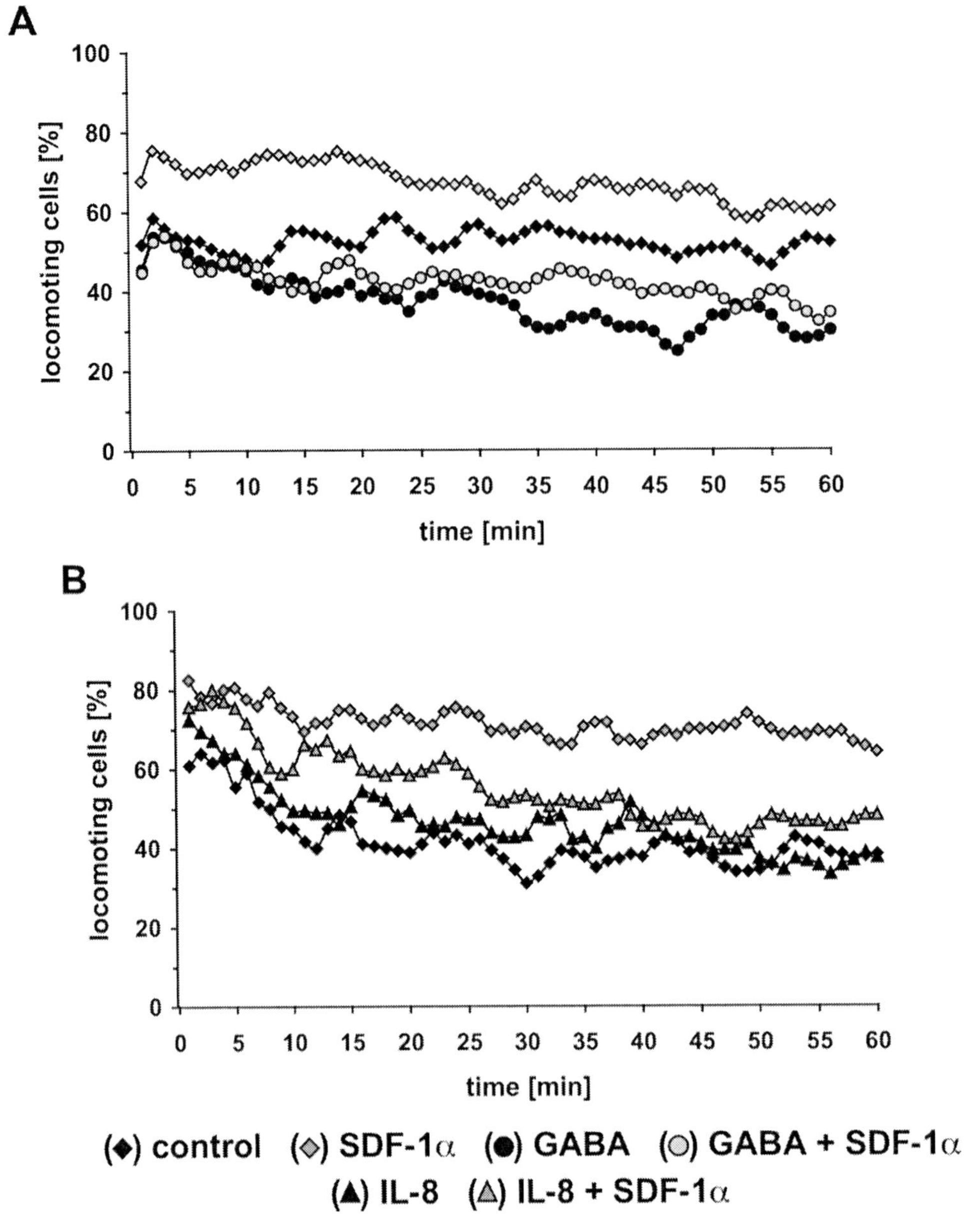

Figure 2. Termination of SDF-1α induced HSPC migration by IL-8 and GABA. Cell migration studies were performed using the 3-dimensional collagen matrix migration assay combined with computer-assisted cell-tracking. Addition of SDF-1α to human $CD133^+$ HSPC from mobilized peripheral blood resulted in an increased locomotory activity (black diamonds) as compared to untreated $CD133^+$ HSPC (grey diamonds). A) The neurotransmitter γ-aminobutyric acid (GABA) efficiently blocks both the spontaneous and SDF-1α induced migration of human $CD133^+$ HSPC. Thereby, GABA signals via the $GABA_B$-receptor, which causes the blockade of calcium release activated calcium (CRAC) channels, thereby inhibiting cell migration. B) The chemokine IL-8 potently inhibits the SDF-1α induced migration of human $CD133^+$ HSPC. Analyses of the appropriate SDF-1α and IL-8 signal transduction cascades indicate that IL-8 likely interrupts the intracellular calcium cycling. Shown are the mean of at least three independent experiments.

CONCLUSIONS

As cytokines used for *ex vivo* expansion extensively influence the engraftment and homing properties of HSPC, the application of in vitro assays allowing the close analysis of the migratory capacity of *ex vivo* cultivated HSPC may prove useful to predict their homing abilities during transplantation procedures. So far, *in vivo* mechanisms of recruitment and mobilization of *in vitro* propagated HSPCs have been extensively investigated, but very little is known about mechanisms terminating HSPC-migration. Further elucidation of these mechanisms may therefore allow the selective manipulation of HSPC homing to their target tissues. This may improve the future use of HSPC in regenerative medicine and may also prove valuable to prevent HSPC from entering malignant tissue. Thus it appears that understanding the mechanisms influencing and regulating the migratory processes of HSPC, comprising homing, retention, release and mobilization, may allow the improvement of their clinical applications.

ACKNOWLEDGMENTS

This work was supported by the Fritz Bender Foundation, Munich, Germany.

REFERENCES

[1] Morrison SJ; Uchida N; Weissman IL. The biology of hematopoietic stem cells. *Annu Rev. Cell Dev. Biol.*, 1995 11, 35-71.

[2] de Wynter EA; Buck D; Hart C; Heywood R; Coutinho LH; Clayton A; Rafferty JA; Burt D; Guenechea G; Bueren JA; Gagen D; Fairbairn LJ; Lord BI; Testa NG. CD34+AC133+ cells isolated from cord blood are highly enriched in long-term culture-initiating cells, NOD/SCID-repopulating cells and dendritic cell progenitors. *Stem Cells*, 1998 16, 387-396.

[3] Weidt C; Niggemann B; Kasenda B; Drell TL; Zänker KS; Dittmar T. Stem cell migration: a quintessential stepping stone to successful therapy. *Curr. Stem Cell Res. Treat*, 2007 2, 89-103.

[4] Levesque JP; Takamatsu Y; Nilsson SK; Haylock DN; Simmons PJ. Vascular cell adhesion molecule-1 (CD106) is cleaved by neutrophil proteases in the bone marrow following hematopoietic progenitor cell mobilization by granulocyte colony-stimulating factor. *Blood*, 2001 98, 1289-1297.

[5] Hermant B; Bibert S; Concord E; Dublet B; Weidenhaupt M; Vernet T; Gulino-Debrac D. Identification of proteases involved in the proteolysis of vascular endothelium cadherin during neutrophil transmigration. *J. Biol. Chem.*, 2003 278, 14002-14012.

[6] Christopherson KW, 2nd; Cooper S; Broxmeyer HE. Cell surface peptidase CD26/DPPIV mediates G-CSF mobilization of mouse progenitor cells. *Blood*, 2003 101, 4680-4686.

[7] Christopherson KW, 2nd; Hangoc G; Mantel CR; Broxmeyer HE. Modulation of hematopoietic stem cell homing and engraftment by CD26. *Science*, 2004 305, 1000-1003.

[8] Tjwa M, Sidenius N, Theunissen K, Moura R, Moons L, Janssens S, Blasi F, Collen D, Carmeliet P. Novel role of plasmin in mobilization and of uPAR in retention of hematopoietic stem/progenitor cells in the bone marrow niche: therapeutic implications. *Blood*, 2004 11, 37a.

[9] Papayannopoulou T. Current mechanistic scenarios in hematopoietic stem/progenitor cell mobilization. *Blood*, 2004 103, 1580-1585.

[10] Larochelle A; Krouse A; Metzger M; Orlic D; Donahue RE; Fricker S; Bridger G; Dunbar CE; Hematti P. AMD3100 mobilizes hematopoietic stem cells with long-term repopulating capacity in nonhuman primates. *Blood*, 2006 107, 3772-3778.

[11] Flomenberg N; DiPersio J; Calandra G. Role of CXCR4 chemokine receptor blockade using AMD3100 for mobilization of autologous hematopoietic progenitor cells. *Acta Haematol*, 2005 114, 198-205.

[12] Lapidot T; Kollet O. The essential roles of the chemokine SDF-1 and its receptor CXCR4 in human stem cell homing and repopulation of transplanted immune-deficient NOD/SCID and NOD/SCID/B2m(null) mice. *Leukemia*, 2002 16, 1992-2003.

[13] Peled A; Petit I; Kollet O; Magid M; Ponomaryov T; Byk T; Nagler A; Ben-Hur H; Many A; Shultz L; Lider O; Alon R; Zipori D; Lapidot T. Dependence of human stem cell engraftment and repopulation of NOD/SCID mice on CXCR4. *Science*, 1999 283, 845-848.

[14] Peled A; Kollet O; Ponomaryov T; Petit I; Franitza S; Grabovsky V; Slav MM; Nagler A; Lider O; Alon R; Zipori D; Lapidot T. The chemokine SDF-1 activates the integrins LFA-1, VLA-4, and VLA-5 on immature human CD34(+) cells: role in transendothelial/stromal migration and engraftment of NOD/SCID mice. *Blood*, 2000 95, 3289-3296.

[15] Aiuti A; Webb IJ; Bleul C; Springer T; Gutierrez-Ramos JC. The chemokine SDF-1 is a chemoattractant for human CD34+ hematopoietic progenitor cells and provides a new mechanism to explain the mobilization of CD34+ progenitors to peripheral blood. *J. Exp. Med.*, 1997 185, 111-120.

[16] Ponomaryov T; Peled A; Petit I; Taichman RS; Habler L; Sandbank J; Arenzana-Seisdedos F; Magerus A; Caruz A; Fujii N; Nagler A; Lahav M; Szyper-Kravitz M; Zipori D; Lapidot T. Induction of the chemokine stromal-derived factor-1 following DNA damage improves human stem cell function. *J. Clin. Invest*, 2000 106, 1331-1339.

[17] Imai K; Kobayashi M; Wang J; Shinobu N; Yoshida H; Hamada J; Shindo M; Higashino F; Tanaka J; Asaka M; Hosokawa M. Selective secretion of chemoattractants for haemopoietic progenitor cells by bone marrow endothelial cells: a possible role in homing of haemopoietic progenitor cells to bone marrow. *Br. J. Haematol.*, 1999 106, 905-911.

[18] Clark EA; Brugge JS. Integrins and signal transduction pathways: the road taken. *Science*, 1995 268, 233-239.

[19] Levesque JP; Leavesley DI; Niutta S; Vadas M; Simmons PJ. Cytokines increase human hemopoietic cell adhesiveness by activation of very late antigen (VLA)-4 and VLA-5 integrins. *J. Exp. Med.*, 1995 181, 1805-1815.

[20] Hidalgo A; Sanz-Rodriguez F; Rodriguez-Fernandez JL; Albella B; Blaya C; Wright N; Cabanas C; Prosper F; Gutierrez-Ramos JC; Teixido J. Chemokine stromal cell-derived factor-1alpha modulates VLA-4 integrin-dependent adhesion to fibronectin and VCAM-1 on bone marrow hematopoietic progenitor cells. *Exp. Hematol.*, 2001 29, 345-355.

[21] Kollet O; Spiegel A; Peled A; Petit I; Byk T; Hershkoviz R; Guetta E; Barkai G; Nagler A; Lapidot T. Rapid and efficient homing of human CD34(+)CD38(-/low)CXCR4(+) stem and progenitor cells to the bone marrow and spleen of NOD/SCID and NOD/SCID/B2m(null) mice. *Blood*, 2001 97, 3283-3291.

[22] Frenette PS; Subbarao S; Mazo IB; von Andrian UH; Wagner DD. Endothelial selectins and vascular cell adhesion molecule-1 promote hematopoietic progenitor homing to bone marrow. *Proc. Natl. Acad. Sci. USA*, 1998 95, 14423-14428.

[23] Ma Q; Jones D; Borghesani PR; Segal RA; Nagasawa T; Kishimoto T; Bronson RT; Springer TA. Impaired B-lymphopoiesis, myelopoiesis, and derailed cerebellar neuron migration in CXCR4- and SDF-1-deficient mice. *Proc. Natl. Acad. Sci. USA*, 1998 95, 9448-9453.

[24] Avigdor A; Goichberg P; Shivtiel S; Dar A; Peled A; Samira S; Kollet O; Hershkoviz R; Alon R; Hardan I; Ben-Hur H; Naor D; Nagler A; Lapidot T. CD44 and hyaluronic acid cooperate with SDF-1 in the trafficking of human CD34+ stem/progenitor cells to bone marrow. *Blood*, 2004 103, 2981-2989.

[25] Chang C; Werb Z. The many faces of metalloproteases: cell growth, invasion, angiogenesis and metastasis. *Trends Cell Biol*, 2001 11, S37-43.

[26] Zheng Y; Watanabe N; Nagamura-Inoue T; Igura K; Nagayama H; Tojo A; Tanosaki R; Takaue Y; Okamoto S; Takahashi TA. Ex vivo manipulation of umbilical cord blood-derived hematopoietic stem/progenitor cells with recombinant human stem cell factor can up-regulate levels of homing-essential molecules to increase their transmigratory potential. *Exp. Hematol*, 2003 31, 1237-1246.

[27] Nilsson SK; Dooner MS; Tiarks CY; Weier HU; Quesenberry PJ. Potential and distribution of transplanted hematopoietic stem cells in a nonablated mouse model. *Blood*, 1997 89, 4013-4020.

[28] Nilsson SK; Johnston HM; Coverdale JA. Spatial localization of transplanted hemopoietic stem cells: inferences for the localization of stem cell niches. *Blood*, 2001 97, 2293-2299.

[29] Nilsson SK; Simmons PJ; Bertoncello I. Hemopoietic stem cell engraftment. *Exp. Hematol*, 2006 34, 123-129.

[30] Dutt P; Wang JF; Groopman JE. Stromal cell-derived factor-1 alpha and stem cell factor/kit ligand share signaling pathways in hemopoietic progenitors: a potential mechanism for cooperative induction of chemotaxis. *J. Immunol.*, 1998 161, 3652-3658.

[31] Ganju RK; Brubaker SA; Meyer J; Dutt P; Yang Y; Qin S; Newman W; Groopman JE. The alpha-chemokine, stromal cell-derived factor-1alpha, binds to the transmembrane G-protein-coupled CXCR-4 receptor and activates multiple signal transduction pathways. *J. Biol. Chem.*, 1998 273, 23169-23175.

[32] Wang JF; Park IW; Groopman JE. Stromal cell-derived factor-1alpha stimulates tyrosine phosphorylation of multiple focal adhesion proteins and induces migration of

hematopoietic progenitor cells: roles of phosphoinositide-3 kinase and protein kinase C. *Blood*, 2000 95, 2505-2513.

[33] Petit I; Goichberg P; Spiegel A; Peled A; Brodie C; Seger R; Nagler A; Alon R; Lapidot T. Atypical PKC-zeta regulates SDF-1-mediated migration and development of human CD34+ progenitor cells. *J. Clin. Invest*, 2005 115, 168-176.

[34] Lee Y; Gotoh A; Kwon HJ; You M; Kohli L; Mantel C; Cooper S; Hangoc G; Miyazawa K; Ohyashiki K; Broxmeyer HE. Enhancement of intracellular signaling associated with hematopoietic progenitor cell survival in response to SDF-1/CXCL12 in synergy with other cytokines. *Blood*, 2002 99, 4307-4317.

[35] Vila-Coro AJ; Rodriguez-Frade JM; Martin De Ana A; Moreno-Ortiz MC; Martinez AC; Mellado M. The chemokine SDF-1alpha triggers CXCR4 receptor dimerization and activates the JAK/STAT pathway. *Faseb J.*, 1999 13, 1699-1710.

[36] Wysoczynski M; Reca R; Ratajczak J; Kucia M; Shirvaikar N; Honczarenko M; Mills M; Wanzeck J; Janowska-Wieczorek A; Ratajczak MZ. Incorporation of CXCR4 into membrane lipid rafts primes homing-related responses of hematopoietic stem/progenitor cells to an SDF-1 gradient. *Blood*, 2005 105, 40-48.

[37] Cancelas JA; Lee AW; Prabhakar R; Stringer KF; Zheng Y; Williams DA. Rac GTPases differentially integrate signals regulating hematopoietic stem cell localization. *Nat. Med.*, 2005 11, 886 891.

[38] Wright DE; Wagers AJ; Gulati AP; Johnson FL; Weissman IL. Physiological migration of hematopoietic stem and progenitor cells. *Science*, 2001 294, 1933-1936.

[39] McKinney-Freeman SL; Jackson KA; Camargo FD; Ferrari G; Mavilio F; Goodell MA. Muscle-derived hematopoietic stem cells are hematopoietic in origin. *Proc. Natl. Acad. Sci. USA*, 2002 99, 1341-1346.

[40] Kawada H; Ogawa M. Bone marrow origin of hematopoietic progenitors and stem cells in murine muscle. *Blood*, 2001 98, 2008-2013.

[41] Krause DS; Theise ND; Collector MI; Henegariu O; Hwang S; Gardner R; Neutzel S; Sharkis SJ. Multi-organ, multi-lineage engraftment by a single bone marrow-derived stem cell. *Cell*, 2001 105, 369-377.

[42] Ratajczak MZ; Majka M; Kucia M; Drukala J; Pietrzkowski Z; Peiper S; Janowska-Wieczorek A. Expression of functional CXCR4 by muscle satellite cells and secretion of SDF-1 by muscle-derived fibroblasts is associated with the presence of both muscle progenitors in bone marrow and hematopoietic stem/progenitor cells in muscles. *Stem Cells*, 2003 21, 363-371.

[43] Kucia M; Jankowski K; Reca R; Wysoczynski M; Bandura L; Allendorf DJ; Zhang J; Ratajczak J; Ratajczak MZ. CXCR4-SDF-1 signalling, locomotion, chemotaxis and adhesion. *J. Mol. Histol.*, 2004 35, 233-245.

[44] Pablos JL; Amara A; Bouloc A; Santiago B; Caruz A; Galindo M; Delaunay T; Virelizier JL; Arenzana-Seisdedos F. Stromal-cell derived factor is expressed by dendritic cells and endothelium in human skin. *Am. J. Pathol.*, 1999 155, 1577-1586.

[45] Rossi D; Zlotnik A. The biology of chemokines and their receptors. *Annu. Rev. Immunol.*, 2000 18, 217-242.

[46] Dooner M; Cerny J; Colvin G; Demers D; Pimentel J; Greer D; Abedi M; McAuliffe C; Quesenberry P. Homing and conversion of murine hematopoietic stem cells to lung. *Blood Cells Mol. Dis.*, 2004 32, 47-51.

[47] Kollet O; Shivtiel S; Chen YQ; Suriawinata J; Thung SN; Dabeva MD; Kahn J; Spiegel A; Dar A; Samira S; Goichberg P; Kalinkovich A; Arenzana-Seisdedos F; Nagler A; Hardan I; Revel M; Shafritz DA; Lapidot T. HGF, SDF-1, and MMP-9 are involved in stress-induced human CD34+ stem cell recruitment to the liver. *J. Clin. Invest.*, 2003 112, 160-169.

[48] Pituch-Noworolska A; Majka M; Janowska-Wieczorek A; Baj-Krzyworzeka M; Urbanowicz B; Malec E; Ratajczak MZ. Circulating CXCR4-positive stem/progenitor cells compete for SDF-1-positive niches in bone marrow, muscle and neural tissues: an alternative hypothesis to stem cell plasticity. *Folia Histochem. Cytobiol.*, 2003 41, 13-21.

[49] Reca R; Mastellos D; Majka M; Marquez L; Ratajczak J; Franchini S; Glodek A; Honczarenko M; Spruce LA; Janowska-Wieczorek A; Lambris JD; Ratajczak MZ. Functional receptor for C3a anaphylatoxin is expressed by normal hematopoietic stem/progenitor cells, and C3a enhances their homing-related responses to SDF-1. *Blood*, 2003 101, 3784-3793.

[50] Li Y; Reca RG; Atmaca-Sonmez P; Ratajczak MZ; Ildstad ST; Kaplan HJ; Enzmann V. Retinal pigment epithelium damage enhances expression of chemoattractants and migration of bone marrow-derived stem cells. *Invest Ophthalmol Vis. Sci.*, 2006 47, 1646-1652.

[51] Atmaca-Sonmez P; Li Y; Yamauchi Y; Schanie CL; Ildstad ST; Kaplan HJ; Enzmann V. Systemically transferred hematopoietic stem cells home to the subretinal space and express RPE-65 in a mouse model of retinal pigment epithelium damage. *Exp. Eye Res.*, 2006 83, 1295-1302.

[52] Lagasse E; Connors H; Al-Dhalimy M; Reitsma M; Dohse M; Osborne L; Wang X; Finegold M; Weissman IL; Grompe M. Purified hematopoietic stem cells can differentiate into hepatocytes in vivo. *Nat. Med.*, 2000 6, 1229-1234.

[53] Herrera MB; Bussolati B; Bruno S; Morando L; Mauriello-Romanazzi G; Sanavio F; Stamenkovic I; Biancone L; Camussi G. Exogenous mesenchymal stem cells localize to the kidney by means of CD44 following acute tubular injury. *Kidney Int.*, 2007 72, 430-441.

[54] Ceradini DJ; Kulkarni AR; Callaghan MJ; Tepper OM; Bastidas N; Kleinman ME; Capla JM; Galiano RD; Levine JP; Gurtner GC. Progenitor cell trafficking is regulated by hypoxic gradients through HIF-1 induction of SDF-1. *Nat. Med.*, 2004 10, 858-864.

[55] Ceradini DJ; Gurtner GC. Homing to hypoxia: HIF-1 as a mediator of progenitor cell recruitment to injured tissue. *Trends Cardiovasc Med.*, 2005 15, 57-63.

[56] Togel F; Isaac J; Hu Z; Weiss K; Westenfelder C. Renal SDF-1 signals mobilization and homing of CXCR4-positive cells to the kidney after ischemic injury. *Kidney Int*, 2005 67, 1772-1784.

[57] Goodell MA; Jackson KA; Majka SM; Mi T; Wang H; Pocius J; Hartley CJ; Majesky MW; Entman ML; Michael LH; Hirschi KK. Stem cell plasticity in muscle and bone marrow. *Ann. N Y Acad. Sci.*, 2001 938, 208-218; discussion 218-220.

[58] Abbott JD; Huang Y; Liu D; Hickey R; Krause DS; Giordano FJ. Stromal cell-derived factor-1alpha plays a critical role in stem cell recruitment to the heart after myocardial infarction but is not sufficient to induce homing in the absence of injury. *Circulation*, 2004 110, 3300-3305.

[59] Stumm RK; Rummel J; Junker V; Culmsee C; Pfeiffer M; Krieglstein J; Hollt V; Schulz S. A dual role for the SDF-1/CXCR4 chemokine receptor system in adult brain: isoform-selective regulation of SDF-1 expression modulates CXCR4-dependent neuronal plasticity and cerebral leukocyte recruitment after focal ischemia. *J. Neurosci.*, 2002 22, 5865-5878.

[60] Corti S; Locatelli F; Strazzer S; Salani S; Del Bo R; Soligo D; Bossolasco P; Bresolin N; Scarlato G; Comi GP. Modulated generation of neuronal cells from bone marrow by expansion and mobilization of circulating stem cells with in vivo cytokine treatment. *Exp. Neurol.*, 2002 177, 443-452.

[61] Kawada H; Takizawa S; Takanashi T; Morita Y; Fujita J; Fukuda K; Takagi S; Okano H; Ando K; Hotta T. Administration of hematopoietic cytokines in the subacute phase after cerebral infarction is effective for functional recovery facilitating proliferation of intrinsic neural stem/progenitor cells and transition of bone marrow-derived neuronal cells. *Circulation*, 2006 113, 701-710.

[62] Dittmar T; Seidel J; Zaenker KS; Niggemann B. Carcinogenesis driven by bone marrow-derived stem cells. *Contrib Microbiol.*, 2006 13, 156-169.

[63] Terada N; Hamazaki T; Oka M; Hoki M; Mastalerz DM; Nakano Y; Meyer EM; Morel L; Petersen BE; Scott EW. Bone marrow cells adopt the phenotype of other cells by spontaneous cell fusion. *Nature*, 2002 416, 542-545.

[64] Alvarez-Dolado M; Pardal R; Garcia-Verdugo JM; Fike JR; Lee HO; Pfeffer K; Lois C; Morrison SJ; Alvarez-Buylla A. Fusion of bone-marrow-derived cells with Purkinje neurons, cardiomyocytes and hepatocytes. *Nature*, 2003 425, 968-973.

[65] Rizvi AZ; Swain JR; Davies PS; Bailey AS; Decker AD; Willenbring H; Grompe M; Fleming WH; Wong MH. Bone marrow-derived cells fuse with normal and transformed intestinal stem cells. *Proc. Natl. Acad. Sci. USA*, 2006 103, 6321-6325.

[66] Quintana-Bustamante O; Alvarez-Barrientos A; Kofman AV; Fabregat I; Bueren JA; Theise ND; Segovia JC. Hematopoietic mobilization in mice increases the presence of bone marrow-derived hepatocytes via in vivo cell fusion. *Hepatology*, 2006 43, 108-116.

[67] Wang X; Willenbring H; Akkari Y; Torimaru Y; Foster M; Al-Dhalimy M; Lagasse E; Finegold M; Olson S; Grompe M. Cell fusion is the principal source of bone-marrow-derived hepatocytes. *Nature*, 2003 422, 897-901.

[68] Jang YY; Collector MI; Baylin SB; Diehl AM; Sharkis SJ. Hematopoietic stem cells convert into liver cells within days without fusion. *Nat. Cell Biol.*, 2004 6, 532-539.

[69] Oh SH; Muzzonigro TM; Bae SH; LaPlante JM; Hatch HM; Petersen BE. Adult bone marrow-derived cells trans-differentiating into insulin-producing cells for the treatment of type I diabetes. *Lab Invest*, 2004 84, 607-617.

[70] Coussens LM; Werb Z. Inflammation and cancer. *Nature*, 2002 420, 860-867.

[71] Balkwill F; Mantovani A. Inflammation and cancer: back to Virchow? *Lancet*, 2001 357, 539-545.

[72] Tabatabai G; Frank B; Mohle R; Weller M; Wick W. Irradiation and hypoxia promote homing of haematopoietic progenitor cells towards gliomas by TGF-beta-dependent HIF-1alpha-mediated induction of CXCL12. *Brain*, 2006 129, 2426-2435.

[73] Sotillo R; Hernando E; Diaz-Rodriguez E; Teruya-Feldstein J; Cordon-Cardo C; Lowe SW; Benezra R. Mad2 overexpression promotes aneuploidy and tumorigenesis in mice. *Cancer Cell*, 2007 11, 9-23.

[74] Weaver BA; Silk AD; Montagna C; Verdier-Pinard P; Cleveland DW. Aneuploidy acts both oncogenically and as a tumor suppressor. *Cancer Cell*, 2007 11, 25-36.

[75] Vassilopoulos G; Wang PR; Russell DW. Transplanted bone marrow regenerates liver by cell fusion. *Nature*, 2003 422, 901-904.

[76] Jamieson CH; Ailles LE; Dylla SJ; Muijtjens M; Jones C; Zehnder JL; Gotlib J; Li K; Manz MG; Keating A; Sawyers CL; Weissman IL. Granulocyte-macrophage progenitors as candidate leukemic stem cells in blast-crisis CML. *N. Engl. J. Med.*, 2004 351, 657-667.

[77] Seidel J; Batistin E; Schwitalla S; Niggemann B; Zänker KS; Dittmar T. Cancer Cell + Stem Cell = Cancer Stem Cell? In: Saitama H. *New Cell Differentiation Research Topics*. Hauppauge, NY: Nova Science Publishers; 2007; 117-151.

[78] Eisenberg LM; Eisenberg CA. Stem cell plasticity, cell fusion, and transdifferentiation. *Birth Defects Res. C Embryo Today*, 2003 69, 209-218.

[79] Ying QL; Nichols J; Evans EP; Smith AG. Changing potency by spontaneous fusion. *Nature*, 2002 416, 545-548.

[80] Houghton J; Stoicov C; Nomura S; Rogers AB; Carlson J; Li H; Cai X; Fox JG; Goldenring JR; Wang TC. Gastric cancer originating from bone marrow-derived cells. *Science*, 2004 306, 1568-1571.

[81] Hofmeister CC; Zhang J; Knight KL; Le P; Stiff PJ. Ex vivo expansion of umbilical cord blood stem cells for transplantation: growing knowledge from the hematopoietic niche. *Bone Marrow Transplant*, 2007 39, 11-23.

[82] Audet J; Miller CL; Eaves CJ; Piret JM. Common and distinct features of cytokine effects on hematopoietic stem and progenitor cells revealed by dose-response surface analysis. *Biotechnol Bioeng*, 2002 80, 393-404.

[83] Ema H; Takano H; Sudo K; Nakauchi H. In vitro self-renewal division of hematopoietic stem cells. *J. Exp. Med.*, 2000 192, 1281-1288.

[84] Miller CL; Eaves CJ. Expansion in vitro of adult murine hematopoietic stem cells with transplantable lympho-myeloid reconstituting ability. *Proc. Natl. Acad. Sci. USA*, 1997 94, 13648-13653.

[85] Ramsfjell V; Bryder D; Bjorgvinsdottir H; Kornfalt S; Nilsson L; Borge OJ; Jacobsen SE. Distinct requirements for optimal growth and In vitro expansion of human CD34(+)CD38(-) bone marrow long-term culture-initiating cells (LTC-IC), extended LTC-IC, and murine in vivo long-term reconstituting stem cells. *Blood*, 1999 94, 4093-4102.

[86] Piacibello W; Sanavio F; Severino A; Dane A; Gammaitoni L; Fagioli F; Perissinotto E; Cavalloni G; Kollet O; Lapidot T; Aglietta M. Engraftment in nonobese diabetic severe combined immunodeficient mice of human CD34(+) cord blood cells after ex vivo expansion: evidence for the amplification and self-renewal of repopulating stem cells. *Blood*, 1999 93, 3736-3749.

[87] Albella B; Segovia JC; Guenechea G; Pragnell IB; Bueren JA. Preserved long-term repopulation and differentiation properties of hematopoietic grafts subjected to ex vivo expansion with stem cell factor and interleukin 11. *Transplantation*, 1999 67, 1348-1357.

[88] Glimm H; Oh IH; Eaves CJ. Human hematopoietic stem cells stimulated to proliferate in vitro lose engraftment potential during their S/G(2)/M transit and do not reenter G(0). *Blood*, 2000 96, 4185-4193.

[89] Haylock DN; To LB; Dowse TL; Juttner CA; Simmons PJ. Ex vivo expansion and maturation of peripheral blood CD34+ cells into the myeloid lineage. *Blood*, 1992 80, 1405-1412.

[90] Verfaillie CM. Hematopoietic stem cells for transplantation. *Nat. Immunol.*, 2002 3, 314-317.

[91] Cerny J; Dooner M; McAuliffe C; Habibian H; Stencil K; Berrios V; Reilly J; Carlson J; Cerny AM; d'Hondt L; Benoit B; Lambert JF; Colvin G; Nilsson S; Becker P; Quesenberry P. Homing of purified murine lymphohematopoietic stem cells: a cytokine-induced defect. *J. Hematother Stem Cell Res.*, 2002 11, 913-922.

[92] Ahmed F; Ings SJ; Pizzey AR; Blundell MP; Thrasher AJ; Ye HT; Fahey A; Linch DC; Yong KL. Impaired bone marrow homing of cytokine-activated CD34+ cells in the NOD/SCID model. *Blood*, 2004 103, 2079-2087.

[93] Von Drygalski A; Alespeiti G; Ren L; Adamson JW. Murine bone marrow cells cultured ex vivo in the presence of multiple cytokine combinations lose radioprotective and long-term engraftment potential. *Stem Cells Dev.*, 2004 13, 101-111.

[94] Kassmer SH; Niggemann B; Zaenker KS; Dittmar T. Cytokine Combinations differentially influence the SDF-1α dependent migratory activity of cultured murine hematopoietic stem and progenitor cells *Biological Chemistry*, 2008 389, 863-872.

[95] Wright DE; Bowman EP; Wagers AJ; Butcher EC; Weissman IL. Hematopoietic stem cells are uniquely selective in their migratory response to chemokines. *J Exp Med*, 2002 195, 1145-1154.

[96] Fukuda S; Broxmeyer HE; Pelus LM. Flt3 ligand and the Flt3 receptor regulate hematopoietic cell migration by modulating the SDF-1alpha(CXCL12)/CXCR4 axis. *Blood*, 2005 105, 3117-3126.

[97] Weidt C; Niggemann B; Hatzmann W; Zanker KS; Dittmar T. Differential effects of culture conditions on the migration pattern of stromal cell-derived factor-stimulated hematopoietic stem cells. *Stem Cells*, 2004 22, 890-896.

[98] Berrios VM; Dooner GJ; Nowakowski G; Frimberger A; Valinski H; Quesenberry PJ; Becker PS. The molecular basis for the cytokine-induced defect in homing and engraftment of hematopoietic stem cells. *Exp Hematol.*, 2001 29, 1326-1335.

[99] Yang L; Wang L; Geiger H; Cancelas JA; Mo J; Zheng Y. Rho GTPase Cdc42 coordinates hematopoietic stem cell quiescence and niche interaction in the bone marrow. *Proc. Natl. Acad. Sci. USA*, 2007 104, 5091-5096.

[100]

[101] Torisu H; Ono M; Kiryu H; Furue M; Ohmoto Y; Nakayama J; Nishioka Y; Sone S; Kuwano M. Macrophage infiltration correlates with tumor stage and angiogenesis in human malignant melanoma: possible involvement of TNFalpha and IL-1alpha. *Int. J. Cancer*, 2000 85, 182-188.

[102] Seidel J; Niggemann B; Punzel M; Fischer J; Zänker KS; Dittmar T. The neurotransmitter gamma-aminobutyric-acid (GABA) is a potent inhibitor of the stromal cell-derived factor-1. *Stem Cells Dev.*, 2007 16, 827-836.

In: Perspectives in Stem Cell Research ISBN: 978-1-61122-985-1
Editors: Brenda M. Davis and Christopher B. Halton

Chapter XI

MORAL AND SCIENTIFIC CONSIDERATIONS IN EMBRYONIC STEM CELL RESEARCH

Zubin Master[1], Daisy Laforce[*2], Marcus McLeod[*3] and Bryn Williams-Jones[*4]

[1]Ottawa Health Research Institute, University of Ottawa
501 Smyth Road, Ottawa, Ontario, Canada K1H 8L6
[2]Department of Philosophy, Simon Fraser University,
8888 University Drive, Burnaby, British Columbia, Canada V5A 1S6
[3]The University of Melbourne, Melbourne, Victoria, Australia 3010
[4]Groupe de recherche en bioéthique and
Département de médecine sociale et préventive, Université de Montréal
C.P. 6128, succ. Centre-ville, Montréal, Québec, Canada H3C 3J7

*Authors have contributed equally to this work.

ABSTRACT

The science of human embryonic stem (hES) cells holds tremendous promise for the discovery of revolutionary cellular therapeutic options for the restoration and regeneration of damaged or destroyed cells and tissues. Yet the fact that the derivation of hES cells from embryos normally results in the destruction of the embryo poses ethical challenges, which for some, amounts to a veritable impasse to the further development of stem cell science. In this article, we review the scientific and ethics literature on hES cells including the use of somatic cell nuclear transfer to generate cloned hES cells for biomedical research and potential clinical applications. The article reviews the various normative theories on the moral status of the human embryo that capture issues ranging from the continuity of embryonic development to cognitive prerequisites for personhood such as sentience, rationality and self-awareness. We also discuss arguments for the symbolic value of human embryos and the need to respect human embryos as potential persons. Beyond issues related to the destruction of human embryos, a number of other ethical issues germane to embryonic stem cell science are also considered, such as the instrumentalization and commercialization of human materials for stem cell research, and the potential social and health risks to women in obtaining and donating oocytes or embryos for hES cell research. Finally, ethical questions arising from the relatively recent development of scientific methods to create new types of embryos for harvesting hES cells are also discussed.

Introduction

Current discourse on the ethics of human embryonic stem (hES) cell research involves a range of stakeholders, which include scientists, ethicists, lawyers, social scientists, religious leaders, politicians, various lobbying organizations, the media and the general public. The diversity of perspectives, values, and agendas involved in this debate make for a very complex space in which to explore and address the ethics of hES cell and embryo research. As with ongoing debates about the legitimacy of and access to abortion, the most widely discussed ethical issue in hES research is the moral status of the human embryo. This focus has clouded other ethical issues related to the ethics of embryo and hES cell research. For example, one must not forget that hES cell research involves the women whose oocytes are obtained in order to create embryos. The possible social, physical and psychological harms to women are also of significant ethical concern.

Despite the multitude of different voices present in the debate over the moral status of the human embryo, certain fact-value distinctions (e.g., is the embryo a person, and does it become so at conception?) create moral impasses that are not easily resolved through ethical debate and public dialogue – these questions invariably require political compromises, decisions that are influenced by factors including economic benefit, global competitiveness, social outrage/acceptance and political expediency. Given the lack of consensus on the moral status of human embryos at the stage of the derivation of hES cells, some commentators understandably question whether embryos should actually be used for hES cell research as it ultimately leads to their destruction. If one grants embryos significant moral status, then conducting research on embryos that results in their destruction is problematic, if not unacceptable, because it treats embryos as only a means for research, rather than as ends in themselves worthy of respectful treatment. The debated moral status of the embryo has had a significant influence on scientific research in North America and Europe, and has led to the development of novel technologies that could potentially eliminate the need to destroy human embryos in the course of hES cell research. Different types of embryonic life have also been created that by virtue of their inability to undergo normal embryonic development could be considered devoid or limited in their moral worth, and thus more permissible to standard forms of hES cell research that would lead to their destruction. However, these approaches are still in the earliest phases of development and contemporary hES cell research still relies primarily on human embryos originally created for reproductive purposes as source material.

In this article, we review the social value of hES cell research through a discussion of the state of hES cell science. We state the potential applications of hES cells in both basic and applied biology, since hES cells may be used to study developmental biology and cancer, and may in the future be used in transplantation medicine for the regeneration of destroyed or diseased cells and tissues. In doing so, we review the various normative theories on the moral status of the human embryo that collectively address issues ranging from the continuity of embryonic development to cognitive prerequisites for personhood such as sentience, rationality, and self-awareness. We also explain arguments for respecting the dignity and the symbolic value of human embryos as potential persons. Other controversial issues examined include the potential harms to women donors, and the instrumentalization and commercialization of human materials for hES cell research. Although this article provides a general overview of the classical themes in the ethics of embryo and hES cell research, we also discuss the ethics of recent scientific methods for deriving hES cells to demonstrate how ethical discourse on the moral status of the human embryo has influenced scientific practices.

The Value of hES Cell Research

Although the majority of ethical challenges associated with hES cell research relate to the treatment of and harms towards the human embryo or to women donors, there are also immediate and potential social and scientific benefits that might arise from this research. The immediate benefits for hES cell research include further understanding of developmental biology and disease as well as the development of embryonic stem (ES) cell-based bioassays for drug testing. Arguably, the most significant long term potential benefit lies in the use of hES cell research to provide a limitless source of biological material for clinical applications in cell replacement therapies. Looking ahead further still, genetic modification could enable the use of hES cells as vectors for gene replacement strategies (not covered in this article) while nuclear transfer (cloning) technology could provide the means to tailor hES cell therapies to individual patients in order to avoid immune recognition and rejection following transplantation.

The Derivation and Biology of hES Cells

Fertilization of an egg by sperm results in the creation of a single cell zygote, which is the first stage of human embryonic development. Mitotic division and cleavage of the zygote continues through to the two, four, and eight cell stages, eventually undergoing compaction to form a morula (approximately sixteen cells). During early cleavage stages, the embryo is considered totipotent, i.e., the cells in the embryo can form any other cell type including extraembryonic tissue. Between days three and five, the human embryo develops into a 100-500 cell blastocyst, consisting of an inner cell mass (ICM) that develops into the embryo proper and a fluid filled cavity known as the blastocoel. The ICM and the blastocoel of the blastocyst are surrounded by an outer trophectoderm layer that forms the placenta. The ICM has the potential to differentiate into primitive ectoderm which ultimately differentiates during gastrulation into the three embryonic germ layers: the ectoderm, mesoderm and endoderm.

Cells from the ICM can be extracted from the blastocyst and cultured under appropriate conditions to form immortalized ES cell lines that are capable of unlimited and undifferentiated proliferation in the presence of leukemia inhibitory factor (LIF), embryonic fibroblasts, human fetal muscle, skin or fibroblasts [1-9] and retain their capacity to form any and all cell types [10;11]. To date, ES cells have been isolated from species including mice [1;2;12-14], chicken [15] hamster [16], pig [17], non-human primates [18;19] and humans [4;6;7;20-26].

The proliferative capacity of ES cell lines is linked to high levels of activity of the enzyme telomerase which adds specific DNA sequence repeats to the ends of eukaryotic chromosomes (known as telomeres). A high telomerase activity is associated with a greater replicative life-span of a cell [27-29]. Human ES cells have been shown to have high telomerase activity after 1 year and 300 population doublings [4;30]. In contrast, diploid human somatic cells do not express high levels of telomerase, have shortened telomeres with age, and enter senescence after a finite proliferative life-span in tissue culture of approximately 50-80 population doublings [31-33]. Human ES cell lines express the specific markers for pluripotent cells such as SSEA-3 and SSEA-4, TRA-2-39, the high molecular weight proteins TRA-1-60 and TRA-1-81, the transcription factors Oct-4 and Nanog, have high alkaline phosphatase enzyme activity and are karyotypically normal [4;30;34]. Genes such as Oct-4 and Nanog maintain pluripotency in ES cells [35;36]. Through the manipulation of the culture conditions, ES cells can undergo restricted differentiation and generate lineage-specific precursors. Studies have shown that mouse ES cells can differentiate into various cell types including hematopoietic precursors [37], neural cells [38], adipocytes [39], muscle cells [40], cardiomyocytes [41], chondrocytes [42] and pancreatic islet cells [43]. Similarly, *in vitro* differentiation and transplantation studies using hES cells indicate the potential to form derivatives of all embryonic germ layers that include gut and secretory epithelium (endoderm) [4;26]; cartilage, bone, cardiomyocytes, smooth muscle, and striated muscle (mesoderm) [4;7;22;23;26]; as well as embryonic ganglia, stratified squamous epithelium, neural epithelium and progenitors (ectodermal in origin) [4;7;22;23;26].

Human ES Cells and Cloning by Somatic Cell Nuclear Transfer

Since ES cells are derived from preimplantation embryos, they exhibit the fundamental properties of high proliferative capacity and potentiality. Preimplantation embryos are created *in vitro* using donated sperm and ova generally produced for reproductive purposes, but they can also be created specifically for research purposes (discussed later in the article). Human ES cells can also be derived from embryos created through parthenogenic means either with or without cloning by somatic cell nuclear transfer (SCNT).

Parthenogenesis is the process (which occurs naturally in some species e.g., reptiles, but not in humans) whereby an oocyte is induced to develop into an embryo without fertilization by a male gamete; as such, parthenogenic embryos only have the genetic material of the female. Mammalian embryonic development can be initiated through parthenogenesis using mechanical, electrical or chemical techniques. Studies have shown that parthenogenic embryos without SCNT cannot reach term in mice, sheep, pigs and rabbits [44-46], suggesting that the lack of paternal gene expression necessary for the development of the trophectoderm and primitive endoderm-extraembryonic tissues prevents any further development of the embryo [44].

Parthenogenesis has been previously described to some extent in non-human primates [47;48], with parthenogenic ES cells isolated in these animals and propagated to the blastocyst stage to create a pluripotent stem cell line that is stable *in vitro* for up to 2 years

[49;50]. These ES cells can differentiate into astrocytes, dopaminergic and serotonergic neurons, spontaneous beating cardiomyocyte-like cells, smooth muscle cells, adipocytes and beating ciliary epithelium cells [50]. Human ES cells have also been derived from parthenogenically activated human oocytes and have developed to the blastocyst stage [51]. Although parthenogenically derived ES cells appear to have many of the characteristics of ES cells derived from blastocysts created through normal fertilization, it remains uncertain whether they are viable and can be used in regenerative medicine since they exclusively contain maternal genes.

ES cells can also be derived from blastocysts created after cloning by SCNT. SCNT involves the transfer of a diploid nucleus from a somatic cell into an enucleated oocyte to make an embryo [52;53]. Embryonic development after SCNT is initiated by parthenogenesis. The use of SCNT to generate embryos which are subsequently implanted and allowed to develop to term as a full organism is commonly referred to as reproductive cloning whereas the same technique used to generate hES cells for potential therapeutic purposes is referred to as therapeutic cloning [52;54;55]. ES cells generated by SCNT are a genetic match to the somatic cell donor and as such, theoretically, would not undergo immune rejection upon transplantation into that donor. Proof of this principle has been shown in the correction of immunodeficient mice using embryonic cells created by nuclear transfer [56].

However, at the cellular level, cloned cells display differences to normal cells in telomere length [57-61], spindle formation [62], as well as chromosomal aberrations [63] and epigenetic expression [64-68] most likely due to the use of an aged nucleus from an adult somatic cell. These cellular defects may also be translated into physical problems in cloned animals. Although the transfer of nuclei from embryonic cells has been previously demonstrated to create live animals visibly free of any pathologies or congenital defects [69-73], similar success has not been seen with animals created by the transfer of nuclei from somatic cells. The cloning of Dolly was the first experimental demonstration that nuclear transfer of a somatic cell nucleus from a large mammal could enable nuclear reprogramming and thus the creation of a new organism [74]. This study was pivotal in demonstrating that normal epigenetic modification that occurs during development is a reversible process [75;76]. However, despite this breakthrough, many of the resulting cloned animals display significant pathologies in organs such as the heart [77;78], kidneys [77;79], lungs [77;78;80;81] and liver [77;79;81]. Moreover, the efficiency of cloning animals is low [76]. A detailed discussion on reproductive cloning is beyond the scope of this paper.

Scientific and Clinical Value in the Applications for hES Cells

The objective of generating clinical grade hES cells in unlimited quantities is for use in cell replacement therapies. Human ES cells exhibit chromosomal and epigenetic stability and have many characteristics that could provide an unlimited and optimal cell source capable of differentiating into a multitude of cell types for the treatment of disorders such as diabetes, Parkinson's disease, Huntington's disease and spinal cord injury [82-84], as well for the regeneration of cells of the heart and immune system.

Risks in Transplantation Therapies Using hES Cells

At present, the use of hES cells poses risks for patients and thus has not yet gone beyond preclinical stages. As is the case with whole organ donations, immunosuppressive drugs may be used to facilitate survival of the allografted hES cells, however these drugs are not without their own side effects including nephrotoxicity, hypertension and immune suppression [85]. The immune rejection problem may theoretically be bypassed through the use of SCNT to create patient-matched hES cells; however, the behavior of hES cells generated by SCNT remains unknown and could have long-term unintended negative consequences. Autologous transplantation, which should ideally avoid the risk of immune rejection common with other tissue transplants, may still be problematic because of the difficulty of ensuring contaminant-free hES cells. The risk of microbiological or viral contamination is common to all types of tissue and organ transplantation [86]. Appropriate screening for potential contamination of hES cells prior to transplantation based on pre-existing organ donation programs can minimize the risk of passing on infectious agents to transplant recipients.

Currently, both mouse fetal fibroblast feeder layers as well as fetal bovine serum within the cell culture media are used to expand hES cells [4;20]; hence cross species contamination of hES cells may also occur from the use of animal feeder cell layers or the use of growth serum [87]. Therefore, hES cells for therapeutic purposes must undergo controlled isolation and expansion to minimize the risk of transmission of retroviruses and other animal pathogens [88]. The expansion of hES cells for therapeutic purposes in the future will require animal-free growth conditions [86;89;90]. As a result, the use of human derived feeder layers based on human derived foreskin fibroblasts [7], human placental fibroblasts [89;91], endometrial cells [92] or adult marrow stromal cells [93] might be a productive means of safely culturing hES cells. Animal-free culture plate substrates such as laminin [94] and fibronectin [95] may also be used to facilitate the growth of hES cells without resorting to the use of animal feeder layers. Avoiding the use of feeder layers altogether to generate unlimited quantities of hES cells may also be achieved with the use of suspension bioreactors. Studies have shown that human and murine neural stem cells can be expanded in a standardized manner in suspension bioreactors for extended periods without the loss of defining stem cell characteristics [96-98]. However, extensive passaging of ES cells may result in chromosomal abnormalities [99;100] and the non-retention of the diploid karyotype [4].

The biological properties of hES cells make them ideal candidates for transplantation therapies due to their proliferative capacity and lineage potentiality. However, these same properties may also pose theoretical or actual risks to transplant recipients. A major risk observed in the transplantation of ES cells is tumor formation [86;87]. More specifically, studies transplanting either human or rodent ES cells have revealed the formation of tumors [84;101]. Although undifferentiated ES cells have been observed to undergo spontaneous differentiation into neuronal phenotypes upon transplantation in rodent models of Parkinson's disease, the formation of teratomas containing cell types from all three germ cell lineages have been observed [84]. As a consequence, and as a means of avoiding teratoma formation, some studies have pre-differentiated ES cells into appropriate cell lineages *in vitro* using gene transfection methods or growth factor induction prior to transplantation [102;103].

The use of transgenic hES cell lines for clinical transplantation also poses the theoretical risk that transgene insertion into a cell regulatory site may negatively alter cellular properties that affect cell proliferation, migration, differentiation or programmed cell death [104]. The use of viral vectors also poses a theoretical risk of transmitting viral particles that could then produce replication competent viruses [105]. Pre-clinical research is thus necessary to assess the risk of tumor formation using transgenic hES cells to ensure that any potential changes in cell biology do not pose further clinical risks to transplant recipients [104]. Tumor formation in the long term may be difficult to assess using animal models of disease due to the difference in life span between animals and humans [86]. Furthermore, any potential differences in the microenvironment between animal species and humans may also make tumor formation assessment difficult. Both of these risks may to some extent be reduced through studies using non-human primates, although the use of non-human primates for ES cell research requires greater costs and is ethically contentious.

Another risk associated with the clinical application of ES cells is the possibility of improper cellular differentiation following cellular induction *in vitro* or following transplantation. Specifically, ES cells may de-differentiate or differentiate into the wrong cell type [86]. The potential risks to transplant recipients are difficult to predict. Studies on the transplantation of stem cells into the brain have shown extensive migrational capacity; undifferentiated neural stem cells have been observed to migrate from the site of transplantation to non-target sites of the brain via white matter tracts [106], raising concerns about the generation of neurological disorders [104]. While offering significant promise for the treatment of otherwise intractable illnesses, research on the utility of hES cell transplantation must be complemented by research into measures to control their biological properties post-transplantation.

The Use of ES Cells in Biomedical Research

Along with cell replacement or regenerative strategies, ES cells could provide an unlimited source of cells for use in studies in cellular and developmental biology, genetics, cancer biology, and for toxicity testing during drug development.

Cell and Developmental Biology

Due to their ability to maintain a pluripotent state and differentiate into all cell types, ES cells provide useful tools to understand basic cell and developmental biology [107]. Specifically, extrinsic cytokine and growth factor assessment may provide a mechanism to study environmental cues for lineage restriction [8;108-110]. The potential for ES cells to undergo gene manipulation also allows for the assessment of genes critical to lineage restriction, such as the expression of Nurr-1 and the differentiation of ES cells into dopaminergic neurons [103].

The differentiation of ES cells into cell types such as cardiomyocytes, hepatocytes, and neurons suggests that they can be used to understand signaling pathways and gene expression profiles during cellular differentiation at different developmental stages. As such, a deeper understanding of the developmental profile of genes expressed in ES cells compared to other stem cells or tumor lines may be envisaged [111-115]. The expression of tissue-restricted genes can be assessed by growth factor addition and activation of receptors present on ES cells with established effects on *in vivo* development [110;116]. ES cells can also be engineered to restrict expression of green fluorescent protein, or other molecular markers, in germ cells allowing for a bioassay to study germ cell development of oocyte-like [117] and spermatozoon-like cells [118;119]. Such ES cell-based bioassays may prove useful for the study of germ cell development and epigenetic reprogramming [120] as well as the study of germ cell tumors [121].

Genetic Diseases

The analysis of hES cell lines with genetic or chromosomal abnormalities may also provide an *in vitro* tool to study primary phenotypic disturbances in cellular processes and progression. Currently, there is a vast array of pre-implantation genetic tests available to identify and isolate pre-implantation embryos with either genetic or chromosomal abnormalities [122;123]. This analysis may allow for the identification of molecular mechanisms that might be blocked or downregulated to prevent disease progression, thereby enabling the development of possible treatments [124]. Human ES cell lines have been created to reproduce genetic diseases such as cystic fibrosis (specifically the mutation ΔF508) [125], X-linked disorders [123], Huntington's disease, Marfan syndrome, fragile-X syndrome, adrenoleukodystrophy, Duchenne and Beckers muscular dystrophy [126;127].

Cancer

ES cells can be used to improve our understanding of embryonic cell carcinomas, as well as provide new insights into the molecular mechanisms of different cancers and potential therapeutic approaches to cancer treatment [128]. Embryonic stem cells have been shown to give rise to teratocarcinomas *in vivo* whose tumors comprise cells of all three germ layers [129;130]. Embryonic carcinoma cells isolated from teratocarcinomas may be used to model and thus better understand the self-renewal of stem cells and the key genetic and cellular events that cause oncogenecity [128].

Human cancers in various organ systems have been shown to possibly result from the transformation of stem cells or progenitors [128;131;132]. Genetic mutations or epigenetic changes may affect various oncogenic signaling pathways that alter the biology of stem cells resulting in transformation. Such activated cancer progenitor cells may give rise to different cancer cells which can grow uncontrollably and display decreased apoptosis. In fact, many of the properties of cancer cells are present in stem cells, such as a high propensity for self-renewal and the expression of key cellular markers. It is through developing a better understanding of stem cell properties, that it may be possible to gain further insight into cancer progression and the potential to develop novel cancer therapeutic strategies.

Embryo Toxicology

Mouse ES cells have been used in an *in vitro* system to test for the embryotoxicity of chemical compounds, known as the embryonic stem cell test (EST). The EST measures the ability of pharmaceutical compounds to prohibit the differentiation of ES cells into cardiomyocytes and is used to test cellular toxicity for the use of a drug during embryonic development. At present, embryotoxicity tests are performed *in vivo* using cell lines or cultures of dissociated cells from rat embryo limb buds, from midbrains known as micromass (MM) or the whole rat embryo culture (WEC) as well as other systems. The EST seems to have a predictive value similar to WEC, while both tests have a slightly higher predictive value when compared to MM. The EST employs the mouse D3 ES cell line and 3T3 fibroblasts [133]. Upon LIF withdrawal from the culture medium, mouse ES cells differentiate into embryoid bodies that form cells of the three germ layers. Cardiomyocytes are the main cell type formed during this process. The EST takes advantage of ES cell biology and uses it to assess the extent of inhibition of ES cell differentiation into cardiomyocytes [134]. Along with measuring the differentiation of ES cells into cardiomyocytes, the EST measures cytotoxicity by assessing growth inhibition of ES cells and fibroblasts. The advantage of the EST is that it uses an established ES cell line, so additional embryos are not needed nor are animals sacrificed. Despite the immediate and potential value of hES cells for basic and applied research and clinical applications, several ethical concerns in the use of hman embryos to derive hES cells have been raised. The major focus of ethics discourse on the use of human embryos to derive hES cells, or other embryo research, focuses on the moral status of human embryos and uses such arguments to influence debate either in favor or against hES cell research.

The Moral Status of Human Embryos

The moral status of human embryos has been a focal point for political and academic debate over their use as a means for research or therapy. It is worth noting that the same debate on the moral status of the human fetus, instead of the embryo also underscored the earlier issue of fetal abortion. Therefore, the politics of hES cell ethics is rooted in the politics of abortion, even though the fundamental question of the moral status of the embryo or fetus predates both issues. This link between abortion and hES cell research is noted, for example, in a comparative study of the politics of and policies around biotechnology in the United States, Germany and Britain by Sheila Jasanoff. She described the politics of abortion as forming "an essential node" in the more far-reaching politics and debate about reproductive technologies [135]. Discourse on the permissibility and moral acceptability of abortion served as an underlying framework that significantly constrained the course of the debate on the implementation of new human biotechnologies. At the core of both debates were the same non-resolvable questions, (i.e., when does life begin? or what is the moral status of the embryo?). Thus, the abortion debates in effect "created some of the conceptual and political resources that actors later drew on as they sought to expand or contract the range of application of the new human biotechnologies" [135].

The question of the moral status of the fetus and the resulting need to articulate criteria for personhood and having the right to life became a focal point for discussion in large part because it was perceived, particularly by opponents of abortion, to be the key to winning the debate. However, no argument has yet succeed in getting opponents and proponents of abortion to agree on the moral status of the fetus in part because the question of when life begins cannot be addressed strictly by science. Another reason why the abortion issue has not been won on these grounds, as noted by the bioethicist Dan Marquis, is that the incredible symmetry of the standard moral arguments for and against the fetus' right to life rendered the debate intractable [136]. Indeed, many of those who weighed in on the issue, individuals and institutions alike, appealed to other values or principles in order to make their case. For example, in the landmark 1973 US Supreme court case of *Roe v. Wade*, the Court did not attempt to resolve the question of the legality of abortion by determining the moral status or personhood of embryos or fetuses; instead the Court made a woman's right to privacy and control of her body the locus for debate, ultimately deciding in favor of strong rights to privacy and autonomy [137]. In the case of hES cell research, however, the question of the embryo's moral status cannot be addressed along the lines of privacy and autonomy. Decisions about the use of embryos in hES research have very little to do with a woman's control over her body or access to abortion (although the issue of control remains in a different sense, and will be discussed below) since the embryos are created and grown *in vitro*.

Advocates on both sides of the debate about the moral status of the embryo/fetus have often considered their arguments to be "morally self-evident" – the embryo is a person or it is not [138]. However, it does not necessarily follow that simply by establishing that an embryo is a person, that destroying that embryo to obtain stem cells is therefore morally impermissible. It must be shown, some commentators suggest, that destroying the embryo violates its right to life, i.e., that it is *unjust* killing. Conversely, even if one decides that the embryo is not a person, this does not imply that we may do with it whatever we wish as our society's concern for the humane treatment of animals generally suggests [139]. Nonetheless, much of the ethics literature on the use of hES cells and human embryos has focused on attempts to define (or limit) the moral status of human embryos and their connection to personhood. In the following section, we examine several normative views on the criteria for personhood and show their application in the context of hES cell research.

Defining Personhood

Generally, individuals who are persons deserve and are ascribed certain fundamental human rights, such as the right to life, freedom from persecution, freedom of speech, to name a few [140]. Defining or establishing the boundaries of personhood is often necessary for making decisions about how to treat persons and non-persons. The distinction between persons and non-persons is thus a potential solution to debates about the moral permissibility of stem cell research.

Often, the first relationship to be drawn by opponents of stem cell research is that being human is a criterion for personhood. However, upon reflection simple taxonomical membership in the species *Homo sapiens* does not necessarily imply personhood and along with it, the attribution of moral and legal rights [141]. This error in reasoning is likely committed because people often conflate two or more meanings of the word human. Mary Anne Warren distinguishes between being biologically human on one hand and being a member of the moral community on the other; only members of the moral community are persons with full moral rights [138]. Dan Marquis points out that this is essentially a problem of scope: the identity claim that what is genetically human is a person includes far too much. If we claim that whatever is genetically human has a right to life then we are led to falsely conclude that human cancer cells in culture should also have a right to life [136]. Also, many non-humans are granted some moral consideration, e.g., those that engender prohibitions on animal cruelty even if animals are not also considered persons. Conversely, proponents of stem cell research tend to define personhood in narrower terms. They too face the problem of scope in that their criteria for personhood tend to exclude too much [136]. For example, many claim that rational thought and self-awareness are necessary capacities for personhood. However, such psychological capacities may then exclude those humans with severe cognitive disabilities or young infants from being considered full persons [142]. Thus, the connection between the psychological traits and personhood is no more conspicuous than that between what is genetically human and a person.

Many argue that we cannot adequately define personhood and thus it cannot be invoked to provide a rationale for granting strong moral status to the embryo [139]. While there is a general understanding of what it means to be a person, there is no single (universally accepted) core of *necessary* and *sufficient* features which we can use as specific criteria to test or evaluate personhood [139]. Attempts to define personhood typically comprise of a number of factors including a wide range of biological, psychological, rational, social, and legal characteristics; however, the embryo (or fetus) falls into a "penumbra region" where there is no conclusive answer to the question of its humanity – it is not a person in the same sense that babies and adults are persons, but neither is it completely free of personal characteristics [139]. Warren suggests that developing a universally valid set of criteria for personhood is essentially problematic (because it raises the specter of racism, sexism, disability discrimination, etc.), even though the general concept of a person appears to be nearly universally understood [138].

Moreover, though detailed facts of embryonic and fetal development are well known and deeply embedded in biology, there is no distinct biological time point at which an embryo clearly becomes a person worthy of moral status and possessing human rights nor can embryology ever elucidate such a time point. According to Ronald Green, it is our own moral values regarding the nature of personhood (whether these are religious or secular) that are ascribed to specific events during embryonic development. Yet embryonic development is clearly a continuous process – any discrete or identifiable events are scientific impositions to help understand and explain the developmental process, and as our understanding of developmental biology increases, the number of distinct events increases [143]. These events are nonetheless ascribed (differing) moral value or importance.

The official Catholic doctrine, for example, is that life, and thus moral status, begins at conception [144]. Conception can be described as the event when a sperm penetrates the zona pellucida (outer membrane) of an oocyte, triggering the acrosome reaction where the sperm head carrying its haploid payload of genes enters the ooplasm and results in the formation of a zygote. *Prima facie*, this description coheres with the belief that conception is the moment where a new individual is created who will develop into a human being. Yet at this point, the pronucleus from the male sperm is still separate from the pronucleus of the female oocyte and the nuclear genetic material has yet to combine. In this sense, it may be difficult to argue biologically that an individual is created because almost all human cells from individuals are known to possess a diploid set of chromosomes, one from each parent. Perhaps, then, it is shortly after fertilization when the two pronuclei combine and the genetic material from both parents are mixed (a process known as syngamy) that life begins and personhood is achieved. However, natural or artificial embryo splitting can still occur at this stage which can then lead to the birth of identical twins, each of whom would be regarded as different individuals /persons. Experiments with mouse, pig and cow embryos have shown that a totipotent embryo is capable of developing into two embryos through bisection to produce monozygotic twins [145-147]. In some jurisdictions, artificial embryo splitting may be offered as an infertility procedure for individuals with reduced reproductive capacity [148] whereas in other jurisdictions, this procedure would be prohibited [149]. Thus the apparently simple idea that personhood begins at conception is complicated by the biological reality of two individuals/persons being formed from a single entity.

Arguments for the position that life begins at conception, and thus embryos must be granted moral status and deserve protection, are often premised on the view that there is no event after this point to warrant the destruction of the embryo [138;150]. For proponents of this view, conception is the only event with any substantive moral significance in the continuous development of a human being and, furthermore, to draw a line at any point between conception and birth is to make an arbitrary choice. Thomson, however, provides a famous counter example to this view. She argues by analogy that the development of an acorn into an oak tree is really no different from that of an embryo into a new born baby. "It does not follow that acorns are oak trees, or that we had better say they are," thus an embryo is "no more a person than an acorn is an oak tree." Thomson rejects the slippery slope argument that conception is the beginning of an inevitable and uninterruptible path to birth and personhood [150].

Many religious faiths believe that human life begins fourteen days after conception. The biological reasoning behind this phenomenon is that this point marks the beginning of gastrulation and the formation of the three germ layers and the primitive streak (the latter signifies the formation of the primitive nervous system) where the embryo loses its potential to split into more than one entity. This is one of the main justifications behind many national policies and legislation prohibiting the culturing of an embryo *in vitro* beyond fourteen days of development. However, as Green argues, the variety and continuity of developmental phenomena make it difficult to determine when a biological or genetic individual comes into being during the developmental process [143]. The fourteen day limit is no less arbitrary than choosing other events during early embryonic development, such as conception or birth, to ascribe personhood to human embryos [143].

To summarize, while the attribution of personhood has been a major argument in the abortion debate, it has had less traction in discussions about the ethics of stem cell research, if only because the embryo is destroyed in the earliest stages of development, well before it displays any overt human characteristics; as such, the adage that "abortion stops a beating heart" does not extend to hES cells. Nevertheless, if the concept of personhood is not sufficiently coherent to resolve the abortion debate, then neither will it be sufficient to address the moral impasse encountered in debates about stem cell research and the use of embryos. To determine the moral status of the embryo in terms of the concept of personhood is *obscurum per obscurius* – like trying to explain something obscure by means of the more obscure. Put slightly differently, the concept of personhood is really more difficult to comprehend than which it purports to illuminate. Proponents of stem cell research may have to respond to opponents by other means than a determination of the moral status of the human embryo.

Potentiality Argument

An important question to be answered is why the killing of an individual who is clearly a person is seemingly not in the same moral category as the destruction of an embryo or a fetus?

According to Marquis, killing persons is unjust because it deprives them of a future conscious life, aspects of which the person would come to value. Potential persons[1], like actual living persons, also have a future of value, which Marquis has termed a future like ours (FLO) [136]. Thus, it is equally wrong to kill potential persons as it is kill actual persons. Marquis' FLO theory is one of the strongest examples of potentiality arguments, which generally hold that if an organism has a future where it will have rights, such as the right to life, then there is no one point in its development that it acquires those rights but rather it has them from the beginning. An embryo is alive just like every other cell in the mother's body, but it is not just like every other cell because, if left to develop properly, it may become a full fledged member of humanity [150]. The potentiality argument has a significant intuitive appeal and may be associated with the sense of loss or tragedy that some people experience when an embryo is destroyed or spontaneously miscarried. Potentiality arguments also have the advantage of accounting for common intuitions in many life and death cases. For example, it can explain why euthanasia may be considered permissible in situations where the patient has no hope of regaining consciousness or is in severe intractable pain; patients either do not have a future that they could come to value or they have a future without any positive value [136].

However, as noted previously, the continuous development of the fetus makes the rational identification one key event for the attribution of moral status difficult to justify. Thus some have advocated a gradualist position (as opposed to a potentialist view) such that the rights of a fetus develop in the same way as the organism develops biologically, in a continuous and uninterrupted fashion. The more the embryo, and then the fetus, comes to resemble an adult person, the more rights it acquires until birth when it becomes a consummate member of the moral community. Copland and Gillett try to give a metaphysical basis for the gradualist argument, which they ground in recent developments in modern biology [151]. According to Copland and Gillett, an outdated understanding of the role of genetics in embryonic development has led people to conflate personal identity with biological identity. The cases of twins and clones show, first of all, that the very early embryo is not necessarily an individual and secondly, that individual identity is underdetermined by genetic identity [151]. Moreover, a newly formed embryo in the uterus may yet become a tumor, showing the importance of processes occurring after conception. Their essential point, however, is that research in developmental biology suggests that the genome may not be the primary driver of the developmental process. Differentiation of a cell appears to be determined more by its micro-environment and less by its ancestry as the removal of one cell in any animal embryo results in compensation in the fate of neighboring cells. Furthermore, cell function has been shown to be very sensitive to the presence and concentration of various stimuli. Thus, this view holds that an early embryo lacks adequate form to be considered truly

---

[1] Note that Marquis does not consider embryos to be potential persons prior to the 14th day of development as they are not definite individuals at this point, see section on the formation of the primitive streak above.

human let alone a person in the full moral sense [151], but it nonetheless may have the potential.

The Cognitive Capacities Argument

As alluded to earlier, Warren contends that merely being a member of the human species is not sufficient to warrant full human rights; one must also be a member of the "moral community" to hold such rights. Warren outlines five criteria for moral community membership: the being must be conscious and have the capacity to feel pain; it must have a developed reasoning ability to solve complex problems; it must display self-motivated activity that is independent of genetic and external controls; it must have the capacity to communicate messages on an indefinite variety of topics; and it must show the presence of self-concepts and self-awareness. Warren claims that none of the conditions are independently necessary or sufficient; however, a being that lacks *all* of them cannot possibly be considered a person. In general, a mental profile resembling that of a morally engaged being and a brain capable of some form of sentience [151] are features that often figure into the conditions for personhood in cognitive capacity arguments.

Lisa Bortolotti and John Harris offer an argument to this effect, claiming that only beings capable of taking an interest in their own well-being are appropriate candidates for personhood [141]. Having such an interest in oneself requires at minimum the possession of sentience. Sentient creatures have an interest in avoiding pain and we have a corresponding duty not to make them suffer. Sentient creatures that are also rational and self-aware are capable of an even more sophisticated interest, viz. that of their own continued existence, thus we should not take steps to terminate their existence, except in order to protect other moral beings (e.g., right to self-defense). Early human embryos do not possess sentience, let alone the other relevant mental capacities to qualify as persons, thus proponents of this approach can support as permissible research on early human embryos.

The Respect Argument

According to Bonnie Steinbock, respect for human embryos is not contingent on said embryos having rights, interests or moral status [152]. Steinbock argues that preimplantation embryos deserve respect and moral consideration even if they lack moral status since an embryo, as a developing human life, possesses intrinsic moral value [153]. As such, an embryo's potential to become a person with full rights is precluded from consideration. This would not mean that all embryo research is impermissible, but rather that their use in research should be justified for purposes with inherent value. Trivial research pursuits such as the testing of new cosmetics might not be considered a sufficiently valuable pursuit to warrant the use of human embryos. Valuable research will benefit society and includes such projects as understanding and treating disease, understanding developmental biology, and improving or validating existing clinical procedures. This argument raises several questions: could embryos be created specifically for research purposes if those research objectives were to be for socially valuable pursuits? How will we determine in an ethical and democratic manner what those pursuits should be? And does the intent to create embryos for research modify our level of respect for them?

The Symbolic Value Argument

John A. Robertson notes that many people who do not view the early embryo as a person with full moral rights feel, nevertheless, that it deserves some form of special respect, possibly even to the point of restricting embryonic research. Yet this view seems paradoxical; how can an entity that lacks rights or interests deserve any form of respect on our part? This view only makes sense, Robertson argues, if one sees it as a demonstration of respect for a very salient symbol of human life. How we treat a human being in the earliest stages of development "reflects and even defines the value that we place on human life generally" [154].

It has been argued that the many restrictions and/or prohibitions on embryo experimentation constitute evidence of a desire in society to demonstrate some form of respect for the embryo as more than just human tissue [154]. Restrictions, such as the prohibition of research on embryos after the fourteenth day of development, show how their symbolic status is at the same time non-trivial yet not equivalent to the full moral status accorded to persons. For many people who hold something akin to the symbolic view, the creation of embryos merely for research purposes is unacceptable treatment of an entity that symbolizes human life [155]. An embryo should not be used in such an instrumental manner, viz. as a mere means to an end. Embryo experimentation involving spare embryos from *in vitro* fertilization (IVF) for example is more acceptable from this perspective. The basis for this judgment is embodied in an Australian report from 1984 by the Victorian Government's Committee to Consider the Social, Ethical, and Legal Issues Arising from In Vitro Fertilization that said: "Where the formation occurs in the course of an IVF procedure for the treatment of infertility, the reasons which lead to the embryo's existence are not 'means to an end' ones" [discussed in 156].

Instrumental Use of Human Embryos

The symbolic argument highlights the issue of the instrumental use of human embryos by drawing a distinction between the permissibility of experimentation on surplus embryos[2] on the one hand, and possibly the intolerance towards experimentation on embryos created exclusively for research purposes on the other. This distinction is made despite the fact that in either case, embryo experimentation results in the instrumental use of embryos. Therefore, it would seem that the intention behind the creation of the source embryos matters a great deal with respect to the endorsement of embryonic experimentation. Creating embryos with the intention to use them for instrumental purposes such as research means that the reason for its existence is directly related to its instrumental value. By contrast, the primary reason for the existence of surplus embryos, i.e., from fertility clinics, is the desire of an individual(s) to

[2] Surplus embryos, also known as excess or spare embryos, are those that were originally created for reproductive purposes, but after time and due to inefficiencies of IVF technologies (see text below for details) are not required for reproductive use and can be donated for third party reproductive use, donated to research or destroyed.

begin a family. The source of embryos used for research is contentious for other important reasons as well. As a key component in potentially marketable research applications, embryos could become a valuable resource for private for-profit fertility clinics, many of which have already been actively involved in the commercialization of reproductive technologies such as IVF [154;157]. Some social scientists predict that if the derivation of embryos and obtaining of ova is not appropriately regulated, then it is likely that "the demand for eggs will greatly exceed the supply...[and] the price of eggs will be determined by the market" [157]. Furthermore, they argue that there needs to be some review of the affects of reproductive procedures on women as well as on offspring resulting from successful infertility treatments. For example, feminist critics have been concerned with the possible exploitation of women as suppliers of ova, doubting the possibility of truly voluntary participation under such circumstances given the grossly exaggerated (commercial) importance of the status of the embryo [158]. Indeed, there are many ethical considerations aside from the moral status of the human embryo that need to be addressed with regards to embryo research and which should not be masked by overemphasizing the potential human health benefits [157].

Harms to Women

A study examining women's experiences with oocyte donation revealed that none of the research participants had a regrettable experience. Nonetheless, the participants were concerned with reducing the risk of hyperstimulation syndrome, the compensation received, and the respectful treatment of donors [159]. For our purposes, it is important to consider the potential risks to women who are the donors of the source biological material necessary for hES cell research. Women may experience several risks during ovarian stimulation and oocyte retrieval. Clinical risks associated with ovarian stimulation include ovarian hyperstimulation syndrome (OHSS) as well as the possible development of cancers from long term use of stimulatory drugs. Oocyte retrieval itself carries surgical risks in association with anesthesia, hemorrhage, bleeding and pelvic injury. Large payments to women for oocytes or embryos for hES cell research may further fuel the possible solicitation and exploitation of impoverished young women.

Ovarian Stimulation

Hormone drugs are given to women to stimulate ovarian follicular growth and development, thereby facilitating the procurement of several mature oocytes that can then be fertilized either by IVF technologies or *in vivo* by gamete intrafallopian transfer. In the case of IVF, the objective of ovarian stimulation (depending on the individual and clinical situation) is to maximize the number of oocytes retrieved. Lower doses and durations of ovulatory stimulation cycles are also used to facilitate artificial insemination procedures such as intrauterine insemination or for timed intercourse. As such, ovulatory drugs are used as a treatment for infertility due to abnormal menstrual cycles or obstructed Fallopian tubes.

The use of more aggressive drug regimens for IVF may be associated with health risks to women. OHSS is one of the most immediate risks of ovarian stimulation and occurs after follicular rupture and administration of gonadotrophins or by using clomiphene citrate [160]. OHSS occurs through loss of control over the timed ovarian stimulation process, resulting in hyperstimulation [161]. OHSS is characterized by the presence of luteinized cysts within ovaries, hematological changes and, in rare cases, respiratory difficulty or thromboembolic episodes. Mild forms of OHSS include enlargement of the ovaries with minor abdominal distension, and possible diarrhea [162], whereas more severe forms cause increased abdominal pain, lower urine production, blood clots, and respiratory distress. Severe OHSS can even lead to hospitalization and has resulted in death. Mild OHSS occurs in 20-33% of IVF cycles [163]. The incidence of moderate OHSS is between 3-6% and for the severe form between 0.5-5% [160;164]. Women who are less than 35 years of age, with low body weight, polycystic ovary syndrome, higher than normal doses of exogenous gonadotrophins, high or rapidly rising estradiol levels, or previous episodes of OHSS are at greater risk of having OHSS [165]. OHSS can be managed through the identification of high risk donors such that drug regimens can be tailored appropriately and close monitoring implemented throughout their cycle [164]. The risk of OHSS can be reduced dramatically through unstimulated cycles and *in vitro* maturation of oocytes.

Another potential harm to women undergoing ovarian stimulation is the risk of developing ovarian cancer [166]. There are some reports that link ovarian cancer and fertility drugs, although others have found no such association. One study showed a 2.67 fold increase in the risk of ovarian cancer of nulligravid women who had tried for more than five years to become pregnant, as compared with women who had only tried for one year [167]. One study found an increased risk of ovarian cancer with the use of clomiphene citrate for more than a year [168]. In contrast, a subsequent study did not show an increased risk following a 12 month examination, but interestingly did report a significant increase in a low malignant form of ovarian cancer in women injected with ovulation-inducing human menopausal gonadotropin [169]. Other studies show no difference in the risk of ovarian cancer in women who underwent treatment with fertility drugs [170]. More recently, Althuis *et al.* showed that clomiphene citrate can increase the risk of uterine cancers in women [171]. Beeson and Lippman suggest that there may be a historical pattern of hormonal overuse by women and associated health concerns [172]. Discussing examples of diethylstilbestrol (DES) therapy and more recently, hormone replacement therapy, they cite the long term study from the Women's Health Initiative showing that women who have used estrogen with progestin have a higher rate of breast cancer [173], a slight increase in risk for heart attack and stroke [174;175] as well as a slightly higher risk for dementias [176].

Given the current scientific uncertainty, a strong link still cannot be made between the use of fertility drugs and cancer. Nevertheless, since fertility drugs have been used for several decades in assisted reproduction, long term and more comprehensive prospective and retrospective studies are required to investigate the health implications of fertility drugs to ensure that risks are clearly identified, mitigated where possible, and acknowledged to the patient or research subject [172].

Surgical Risks of Oocyte Retrieval

Oocyte retrieval is a surgical procedure used to obtain mature oocytes from ovarian follicles and is performed after ovarian stimulation. Oocytes are generally retrieved through transvaginal follicular aspiration using ultrasound guidance under sedation. In instances where the ovaries are not accessible from the vagina, oocytes can be retrieved laparoscopically under light anesthesia. If no oocytes are found after aspiration of a few follicles, the follicles may be flushed to facilitate the retrieval of oocytes. As a surgical procedure, the general risks of bleeding, vaginal hemorrhage and low dose anesthetics are present during oocyte retrieval. There is a minor risk for pelvic infections after the operation that could be due to a contaminated collecting needle. Pelvic injuries may also occur in 0.001% of cases [177]. Oocyte retrieval can be a very painful process for women and one that carries with it a risk of infection and injury.

Solicitation and Exploitation of Women

Oocytes and embryos can be donated for reproductive use, or may be destroyed, kept for future reproductive purposes, or provided to researchers. However, the oocyte donation process is physically demanding on women and as such, some have argued that remuneration is owed to women as a just compensation for their participation, if not directly for their oocytes. In 1999, individual egg donors in the US typically received $2,000 to $3500 [178] with costs ranging over $7,500 more recently [179]. However, some have reported financial incentives of $25,000 and even as high as $80,000 [180].

A major concern is that the introduction of substantial financial incentives for oocyte or embryo donors may influence women, particularly those in financial need, to assume risks, such as those associated with superovulation and oocyte retrieval, which might otherwise preclude their participation [180]. For example, young women at college or university might find the idea of donating oocytes (for a sizeable fee) worth the risk in order to pay for tuition, and not surprisingly, there have been a number of documented instances of advertisements for oocyte donation on college campuses [181]. Similarly, infertile women who require assisted reproduction services, but who cannot afford the cost for treatment have also been encouraged to share their excess oocytes in exchange for reduced costs for IVF treatment [181]. The worry about these situations is that significant financial inducements to women in already challenging situations may compromise their ability to make genuinely informed and autonomous decisions about whether they ought to take on the risks of oocyte donation.

The issue of remuneration also raises concerns about what constitutes reasonable compensation for services rendered, and the possibility that payment will become a commercial exchange. Is payment inherently problematic? What is wrong or unethical about the explicit commodification of oocytes? And what moral values are preserved by preventing such commodification? Clearly, commercial transactions are not by their very nature unethical; one can quite legitimately sell a variety of goods, such as a car or a house (with certain restrictions). But commercial exchanges of certain products, such as blood, organs, gametes, or embryos have been widely considered unethical as the exchange is between a special or sacred entity (the oocyte/embryo) and a profane entity (money) [182]. Altruistic donation of oocytes or embryos, however, is considered morally justifiable since it attempts to provide someone with something that they cannot create by themselves. This offers them something special, which is a chance to create a child. As such, like (sacred-sacred) exchanges are morally justifiable because they do not treat a sacred resource as a commodity [182]. The commercialization of oocytes and embryos and their associated ethical concerns will be discussed more fully below, but for this section, the important point is that the introduction of financial compensation for services rendered (i.e., inconvenience of donation) could look very much like the sale of eggs (and thus ultimately the sale of embryos or children) if compensation is overtly generous.

By extension from the case of the for profit infertility industry, the need for oocytes or embryos for hES cell research may result in the further exploitation of young women [172]. If commodification of oocytes and embryos is to be prevented and the negative affects mitigated, then some commentators suggest that financial reimbursements should be modest and only reflect the cost of the inconvenience of donation, thereby maintaining the fundamental altruistic motivation of donors. However, is it fair to say that financial incentives will prevent any woman from making autonomous decisions? In that sense, what is so morally repulsive that larger financial reimbursements ought not to be provided? If it seems ethically permissible that models can sell their looks, academics sell their minds and athletes sell their physical abilities, then why is it unethical for a fecund woman to sell her oocytes? In other words, what is so wrong with the commodification of oocytes or embryos? Some commentators suggest that special resources such as blood or blood products, organs and reproductive material (oocytes, sperm and embryos) should be exchanged for morally important reasons, such as altruism; the idea is that donors of special resources such as gametes should be cognizant about the implications of their donation [183]. For example, the altruistic donation of gametes to provide others the opportunity to experience child bearing and rearing seems more ethically satisfying than donation for financial gain. Nevertheless, this issue of altruistic donation remains contentious and as such, further discourse and ethical reflection on issues associated with the procurement of oocytes and embryos will be critical for the future public acceptability and ethical practice of hES cell research.

Issues in Informed Consent

The derivation of hES cells and their possible use for research poses some important questions with regards to informed consent. Informed consent is a process designed to respect and promote research participant autonomy and protect their interests. Thus all the relevant aspects of a medical procedure or clinical research project are described both verbally and through a written document, such that the participant is fully informed and understands the risks and benefits of a procedure(s), prior to the intervention. Because consent is an active and ongoing process rather than a static one, research subjects may also modify or rescind their consent during a trial; for example, they retain the right to withdraw from a trial or project at any point. All of this information and more is provided to the participant prior to obtaining their informed consent. Most developed and developing countries have research ethics boards – e.g., institutional review boards (IRB) in the US, research ethics boards (REB) in Canada, and research ethics committees (REC) in the UK – to review clinical research project proposals (to ensure a positive risk-benefit ratio) and informed consent amongst other criteria for ethics approval.

Informed consent in research and clinical practice has several limitations. There is increasing awareness that informed consent is often treated as a document to be signed, and not as a process of providing information and discussing the research with participants to fully obtain 'informed consent' [184]. Moreover, patients or research subjects often may not fully understand what they are being told or for what they are being asked to give consent [185]. In relation to embryo research, two ethical issues of particular importance in informed consent are the avoidance of therapeutic misconception of the anticipated benefits of hES cell research and which person is most suitable to provide the information and explain the research study to potential embryo donors.

An important issue in the description of the benefits of research is therapeutic misconception. A therapeutic misconception arises in the case where a research subject does not realize they may be part of a randomized clinical trial and therefore may receive a placebo that would not provide any net therapeutic benefit [186]. By virtue of their participation in research, research subjects believe that they may receive therapeutic benefit when in fact clinical research, like other types of experimentation, is about generating generalizable knowledge. In the case of donating eggs or embryos for the derivation of hES cell lines, there exists a slightly different therapeutic misconception associated with the promissory nature of the research [172;187]. First, researchers should inform subjects of the type of research their embryos would be used for, such as the derivation of hES cells [188]. The description of the research to donors about the potential uses of hES cells should not be exaggerated. Donors may have (intentionally or not) over-inflated expectations about the potential of their individual donation to lead to a therapeutically beneficial intervention in the near future. To avoid such a misconception, the information provided to donors about possible therapeutic benefit should not contain misleading language that, for example, implies that the derivation of hES cells will predictably result in future therapies [172]. Grandiose statements about identifying cures for degenerative diseases make it seem that stem cell research will lead directly to clinical interventions [187], thus misleading oocyte or embryo donors. The problem with this therapeutic misconception is that donors may genuinely believe that the ES cells derived from their donation will be used clinically to assist patients with debilitating disease, as would be the case with an organ donation. Yet given the present state of stem cell research, it is highly unlikely that hES cells will be used clinically in the near future. As such, hES cells will be of use only for basic research to yield generalizable scientific knowledge that in the future may be used for clinical therapies. A description of the benefits in any informed consent procedures dealing with hES research should thus include discussion about the early stage of hES cell research, the generalizable knowledge that will be obtained with the derivation of novel hES cell lines, and the potential for the donation to contribute to the advancement of scientific research that may produce clinical benefits in years or decades [187]. A direct and clear description of the potential and immediate and long-term benefits of hES cell research to potential embryo donors should help to reduce risk of therapeutic misconception.

In addition to avoiding therapeutic misconception, informed consent must be voluntarily provided and the consent obtained from the participant should be free of deception or coercion [189]. Clinical studies have traditionally involved the treating physician as the person responsible for informing the patient of the clinical study, addressing their concerns, and obtaining their consent to enroll, or not, in the study. In the case of donating embryos for research, who would be the most suitable individual to provide the information to patients and to obtain consent? For most clinical research studies, physicians inform their patients about the risks and the probability of benefits of enrolling in a research study. Physicians may infrequently justify the use of paternalism in cases concerning the patient's well-being, but should never be used for the benefit of a research project. However, physicians do have a fiduciary relationship with their patients. Heng argues that infertile couples who have favorable outcomes from their IVF experience may be so overwhelmed with gratitude that they are liable to consent to anything asked for by their infertility treatment physician, and that they may not be making a truly informed choice [190]. In such instances, health professionals may (perhaps inadvertently) be able to exercise influence that can sway the decision of the patients to consent for embryo research [190].

Yet it may be argued that a physician is the ideal person to provide information to a patient for hES cell research since they have a relationship with their patient and are familiar with their medical history [191]. Obstetricians-Gynaecologists and other infertility specialists do provide counseling and are accustomed to respecting a woman's choices and values [192]. A physician may be mindful of the patient's interests since their knowledge of the patient's infertility issues may be used to better inform patients of their future reproductive choices. For example, it has been argued that the donation of fresh embryos limits the reproductive choices for a woman [193] which is especially important in cases where a woman has limited reproductive capabilities; in such cases, the infertility treatment physician would be the most suitable person to inform the woman of her future reproductive options and possibly recommend cryopreservation of oocytes or embryos as the case may be. However, exceptions can be reasonable if the infertility physician is also involved in research [192]. Financial and other conflicts of interest should be made explicit. As such, it remains unclear whether physicians, or other parties such as nurses or researchers who derive the hES cell lines, should obtain consent. It could be argued that researchers are better suited to explain the field of stem cell research more than an infertility specialist who may not be as well informed. To avoid therapeutic misconception, perhaps a researcher may be a more suitable person to deliver information on the use of potential hES cell lines created from a donor's embryos. As such, it remains unclear as to which individual may be the best person to deliver information to patients and obtain their consent.

Several important pieces of information pertinent to embryo donors when deciding whether to donate their embryos for research should be disclosed. First, patients should be informed that their embryos will be destroyed in the research [192]. Second, informed consent for embryo research should ensure that individuals know that they may change their minds about their participation in the research at any point [194]. This may be of great importance since many couples may be unwilling to donate their embryos or have changed their minds after experiencing IVF [195;196]. However, time limits may be placed on the withdrawal of consent especially after the procedure to create hES cell lines has begun since at this point the researchers have invested their efforts to the derivation of a cell line [191]. Thirdly, patients should also be informed that their decision to participate in research will not be affected by their treatment [192]. Lastly, many people that attribute special moral and emotional significance on their reproductive material and embryos may only want to donate them for specific research categories such as infertility, human development and disease, and regenerative medicine [188;192;197]. Disclosure of such information will be helpful to potential embryo donors when deciding on whether to donate their embryos for research and will allow patients to make reasonable and well informed choices.

Issues in informed consent related to the donation of embryos for research requires the disclosure of specific information. Moreover, who would be the most suitable individual to deliver the information to patients and obtain their consent is also an issue. This issue is also important because the delivery of the potential benefits of the research to patients should not be inflated and perhaps someone other than a physician may be better suited to provide such information. Although informed consent is one of the most widely discussed topics in research ethics, the moral status of the embryo and the ethics surrounding the destruction of the human embryo has been the major focus of ethics discourse, and recent scientific inquiry as well.

EMBRYO ETHICS

Embryos can be created through insemination of an oocyte with sperm using IVF technologies, and then at various stages of development be used to isolate hES cells. Although traditionally hES cells were derived from the ICM of the blastocyst, pluripotent stem cells can also now be created from morulas [34] and from cleavage stage blastomeres [199]. Pluripotent stem cells can also be derived from late stage epiblasts of post-implantation mouse and rat embryos [200]. Embryos can also be created by artificial means such as parthenogenesis, either with or without nuclear transfer. The ethics of using embryos created for different purposes, and in different ways, all play a key role in determining their ethical acceptability for use in hES cell research.

Embryos Created by Insemination: Surplus Embryos and Fresh Embryos in Research

In vitro human embryos can be created through different methods and with different motives. It is said that embryos created specifically for research purposes violate the moral principle in research ethics of having a favorable risk-benefit calculus [201]. In many cases, the risks of clinical research must be weight against the larger social benefit of obtaining generalizable knowledge and the possible benefits of regenerative medicine to patients. George argues that the donation of oocytes to create embryos specifically for research places too many short term risks related to ovarian stimulation and oocyte retrieval, and potential long term risks of neoplasias, to women with no foreseeable direct benefits [201]; as such, the creation of embryos for research does not consider the well-being of the subject and places greater interests for science and society.

More common is the donation of surplus embryos by donors in IVF clinics. Surplus embryos were originally created for reproductive purposes by assisted reproductive technologies, but are no longer required for the creation of children and can be donated for research. A surplus number of embryos are created in order to maximize the chances of a successful pregnancy, to limit the number of ovulation cycles performed, and because IVF technologies like oocyte cryopreservation remain ineffective. Ovarian stimulation results in the maturation and release of multiple (5-15) oocytes depending on the woman and the drug regimen. Excess embryos can be cryopreserved, destroyed, donated to others for their reproductive needs, or donated for research. Surplus human embryos can be donated for research either fresh or cryopreserved.

However, the use of embryos for research, whether they are fresh or frozen, or whether they were originally created for reproductive or research purposes, does not avoid the ethical problem of destroying human embryos for the derivation of hES cells. Those that attribute significant weight to the moral status of early human embryos would oppose research on the derivation of hES cells regardless of any intention for its creation as it leads to using embryos only as a means for research ultimately resulting in their destruction.

Of major interest is the use of fresh embryos for the derivation of hES cells. The reasons for using fresh sources of embryos are due to concerns about the diminished utility and survival capacity of cryopreserved-thawed or genetically compromised embryos. However, it remains unclear whether fresh embryos are actually more useful for creating hES cell lines. The rates for the establishment of hES cell lines from fresh human blastocysts vary between 7.5% to 16.6% [21;24] whereas cryopreserved embryos have an establishment rate of 12.5% [24]. However, Nisker and White argue that the obligations of physicians to consider the well-being of their patients, and to prevent harm are violated if physicians allow their patients to donate fresh embryos for research [193]. A woman's chance of having a successful pregnancy may decrease if cryopreservation is not an option and may then put her at greater risks if another IVF treatment cycle is required [193].

The donation of fresh and frozen embryos may be especially sensitive for women and couples, given the often lengthy and close relationships formed during treatment for infertility with their physicians. Some women may feel pressure to donate their fresh embryos for research, both as a measure of recompense for continued professional support, but also to ensure that they will remain in 'good graces' with the IVF clinic throughout the course of their fertility treatment [193]. The use of fresh embryos for research, when compared to surplus embryos created for reproductive purposes also ties in concerns discussed previously about autonomous decision making, having appropriate informed consent, and the exploitation of women. But in some cases, fresh embryos will not even be cryopreserved for future reproductive purposes as they will be unlikely to survive cryopreservation and thaw and would also not be transferred due to their poor morphological quality after assessment. These embryos can only be discarded or donated to research. Moreover, fresh embryos from patients that tested positive for a disease gene using preimplantation genetic diagnosis (PGD) which would otherwise be discarded can also be used for the derivation of hES cells and would serve as important reagents to study the mechanisms of disease [24;124]. Lastly, fresh embryos may be donated for research in cases where women choose to only undergo one infertility treatment cycle irrespective of the outcomes or who cannot afford to cryopreserve excess embryos. Although in many cases offering women the choice of embryo cryopreservation is important to ensure that use of their embryos for reproductive purposes is fulfilled prior to donation, an overarching limitation of fresh embryos for hES cell research to prevent undue influence to women may however not capture all of the reasons for donating fresh embryos for research.

Rescuing Embryos from Destruction for hES Cell Research

Concerns about the destruction of embryos have lead to the introduction of experimental methods to create human embryos that would seemingly allow for the derivation of hES cells without embryo destruction. Generally, the idea is to take an embryo created *in vitro* for reproductive purposes and then subject it to an additional procedure that involves taking part(s) of the embryo for the creation of human pluripotent stem cells while the remainder of the embryo is cultured and transferred into a woman to create a child.

In the first method, pluripotent stem cells were derived from blastomeres that were inseminated *in vitro*. Blastomere or cleavage stage biopsy involves the removal of one or two blastomeres of an approximate eight cell embryo. The blastomeres are subjected to culture conditions in order to derive a pluripotent stem cell line, a method successfully demonstrated with both mouse [198] and human [199] embryos. Blastomere biopsy has already been successfully used for PGD: single blastomeres are removed and subjected to genetic testing for chromosomal abnormalities or single gene defects, and only those embryos with the selected genotype are then implanted. Many healthy children have been born from IVF with PGD. However, it must be noted that the remaining embryos after blastomere removal in these experiments were destroyed [199;202;203]; yet in theory, blastomere biopsy may be one method to yield pluripotent stem cells without destroying the embryo. However, the possibility of using blastomere biopsy to avoid the destruction of the embryo comes with two important caveats: 1) it is certain that the isolated blastomere cannot develop on its own into a new individual. It is known that blastomeres from 4 and 8 cell stage mouse embryos are totipotent and can result in the creation of live animals [204]. A blastomere may be totipotent, but it is functionally not similar to a blastocyst in that it is unlikely to implant on its own. However, whether a single blastomere from a human embryo may be coaxed *in vitro* to develop into a blastocyst and then implanted into a woman remains unknown. If however, a blastomere can develop into a blastocyst and be implanted into a woman, then one is not truly avoiding the destruction of the embryo, but rather preventing the creation of an identical twin. 2) It remains unknown whether, as a micromanipulation technique, blastomere biopsy reduces the viability, developmental potential or implantation potential of the remaining embryo to be transferred [203]. Micromanipulation of the embryo may cause genetic perturbations or epigenetic changes that may manifest as harms to children [203]. As such, some believe that a precautionary approach is warranted until it is confirmed that the use of micromanipulative technologies on embryos are safe.

A second theoretical method of obtaining hES cells is the blastocyst transfer method (BTM) [205]. The goal of the BTM is to isolate cells from the ICM of a blastocyst and use them to derive pluripotent stem cells without destroying the embryo. Using a needle similar to the one used in intracytoplasmic sperm injection (ICSI), a day five human blastocyst can be injected and cells of the ICM isolated. The objective is to isolate enough ICM cells to derive pluripotent stem cell lines along with ensuring that the blastocyst continues to develop and can be transferred into a woman [205]. It has been argued that this technique, although theoretically sound, poses fundamental uncertainties with regards to its safety for human embryos due to the extensive micromanipulation involved [206]. Liao compares the BTM to PGD and ICSI, but this is not an accurate comparison as embryo biopsy involves extraction of a large blastomere from a cleavage stage embryo that is easily accessible and not tiny, compacted cells of the ICM after piercing through the trophectoderm layer as theorized by Liao [205]. The removal of cells from the ICM may result in changes in intracellular signaling or induce *de novo* gene mutations that could affect embryo viability or developmental potential. In the worst case situation, certain alterations may manifest as morphological abnormalities in the fetus or congenital malformations in children born from an embryo where the BTM was performed.

Both the BTM and blastomere biopsy use sophisticated micromanipulation techniques to isolate cells for stem cell derivation while attempting to maintain embryo viability and developmental potential for the eventual creation of healthy children. Both these methods target individuals seeking IVF treatment and offer potential benefits to both the child and to society. The child born after the BTM or blastomere biopsy may benefit only if: 1) a hES cell line can be created from the isolated blastomere or from a collection of cells from the ICM, 2) the original embryo is transferred into a woman and a child is born, and 3) the child (or adult) develops a disease where hES cell transplantation therapy is established for that disease. The benefits to the child require a sequence of events to occur which are unlikely especially because the efficiencies of creating pluripotent stem cells using these methods is either low or only theoretically possible. The major benefit to society would be the creation of pluripotent stem cells that could be used for other research to create generalizable knowledge or for potential therapeutic purposes. On the other hand, the primary concern for individuals seeking infertility treatment is to have a healthy child and they may not want to risk jeopardizing the possible health of their child or lower their chances for a successful pregnancy in order to help basic scientific research with the possibility of procuring a vial of stem cells for their resulting child [206]. A recent study examined factors that affected a patient's choice in single embryo versus two embryo implantation and showed that *cautious* patients prefer fewer embryos to be transferred given the likelihood of, and possible health risks associated with, multiple births [207]. In the same study, other patients who may be less cautious could have positive views about the possibility of having twins [207] since many male and female infertility patients desire multiple pregnancies [208]. This study can be extrapolated to show that cautious IVF patients may similarly not wish to undertake the risks associated with the use of various methods to derive pluripotent stem cells in order to have a child. The continued use of human embryos for purposes other than to create a child may contribute to a social climate in which embryos are viewed as instruments to better human lives. This in turn could lead to the commodification of oocytes and embryos unless constrained by public policy [149].

Artificial Embryos Created by Alternate Strategies

A variety of experimental methods have been used to create embryos that might be classified as artificial, defective, or non-human [209]. As previously discussed, embryos can be created through IVF or parthenogenesis; in the later case, embryonic-like development of an oocyte is induced, with or without SCNT. Parthenotes without SCNT cannot implant because they lack imprinted paternal genes that are necessary for placental growth [210]. Parthenotes from non-human primates have been created without SCNT and are used to derive ES cells [49;50]. More recently, human parthenotes have also been used to derive hES cells [211]. The creation and use of parthenotes could be a way to avoid the ethical objections to the derivation of hES cells from IVF embryos because parthenotes lack the potential to develop to term [212-214]. One research group has generated genetically matched ES cells from parthenogenically activated mouse oocytes having the full complement of major histocompatability complex (MHC) antigens [211]. Engraftment of these MHC matched ES cells into their respective recipient demonstrated proof of concept that parthenogenic ES cells can serve as a source of histocompatible tissue for transplantation [211].

Although ES cells derived from parthenotes may serve as a useful source to derive histocompatible pluripotent stem cells, the creation of parthenotes highlights some particular ethical challenges associated with the creation of embryos, or embryo-like entities, more generally. Does creating an embryo-like entity that cannot fully develop to term decrease the moral status of that embryo? And, would the intentional creation of artificial or defective embryos for research to derive hES cells, despite their social and scientific worth, make this creation ethically permissible? William Hurlbut has argued that embryos created through SCNT alone have the same moral status as embryos produced by natural fertilization or IVF despite the embryo having difficulties during gestation or the cloned offspring after birth [215]. Hurlbut proposes the creation of embryos that are gestationally incompetent, through altered nuclear transfer (ANT) – these embryos do not have the same moral status as embryos created by the combination of sperm and egg or by SCNT, and thus can be used for the derivation of hES cells [215].

Proof of concept of ANT was tested by Meissner and Jaenisch in the generation of mouse ES cells derived from cloned *Cdx2*-deficient blastocysts [216]. *Cdx2* encodes for the trophectoderm specific transcription factor that is first expressed in eight cell embryos and is required for the establishment and function of the trophectoderm lineage [217;218]. Mice engineered to lack *Cdx2* fail to maintain a blastocoel and cannot form cells of the trophectoderm lineage, but can form an ICM. Short hairpin RNAs against *Cdx2* were designed in lentiviral vectors that were used to infect fibroblasts and then used in nuclear transfer experiments to generate a *Cdx2*-deficient blastocyst from which ES cells were successfully derived [216]. The cloned blastocysts were morphologically abnormal and failed to form a trophoblast or to implant into the uterus of pseudo-pregnant mice [216].

Embryos created by parthenogenesis without nuclear transfer, by SCNT or by ANT, can be said to be created by artificial means [219]. Such artificial embryos cannot occur naturally and may require mechanical or chemical aid to initiate or continue embryonic development. Examples of artificial processes may include mimicking fertilization by parthenogenesis or by the use of ICSI that injects a male sperm into an ovum. The use of technology to inhibit the expression of certain genes in embryos can also be considered an artificial means of creating embryos. It can be argued that the use of parthenogenesis without nuclear transfer or by ANT can be interpreted as creating 'defective' embryos since they lack implantation potential; it would only be a slight stretch to also include embryos created by SCNT, since most clones die during gestation or after birth due to various physical defects. Whether artificial or defective embryos deserve the same moral status as those created through IVF is questionable.

Cheshire and Jones explain that a physicalist's view of non-viable or gestationally incompetent embryos would bar them from inclusion as fully human and would imply that they have reduced moral status. A physicalist defines human life by inclusion of a particular set of physical attributes to an embryo such as the ability to develop a functional trophectoderm and undergo implantation and formation of the placenta [220]. But how far can one stretch the meaning of 'defective'? Embryos created by SCNT can inefficiently implant and develop to full term. If human embryos created by SCNT were to develop to term and produce offspring which, like cloned non-human animals, died early in life, would such human entities also have reduced moral status? If defectiveness holds as an exclusion criterion for personhood, then children born through natural means with severe congenital anomalies, genetic diseases and therefore lacking certain physical attributes, mental capabilities and/or who have a diminished lifespan might then also be considered to have less moral worth than children born naturally without such characteristics [220]. Should embryos purposely created to be defective, i.e., incapable of continuing embryonic development, still be considered human but with brief human lives? Others may consider such entities as human life which possesses the potential to actualize the structures and functions consistent with humans [220]. In such circumstances, human embryos with short lives created artificially would have the same moral status as embryos created naturally.

Cheshire and Jones argue that the artificial creation of human embryos deemed to be defective is not sufficient grounds to limit the moral worth of human embryos [220]. They caution that the classification of embryos created via these various molecular technologies as non-human may have far reaching consequences for how society will view vulnerable human beings even at other stages of life [220]. Will classification of such embryos as non-human lead to the increased instrumentalization and or commodification of all human embryos? For Jones and Cheshire, the creation of new forms of human life should be approached with caution and concerted ethical reflection [219].

The Creation of Pluripotent Stem Cells from Non-Human Embryonic Sources

The creation of artificial embryos or the avoidance of destroying embryos poses several moral challenges as discussed previously. Similar to how scientific research attempts to bypass the destruction of embryos or devoid them of moral status, biomedical research has also developed strategies to avoid the problem of the moral status of human embryos by creating pluripotent stem cells from non-human embryonic sources. Whether the creation of such cells will be used for regenerative transplantation therapies in the future is questionable, but this demonstrates how science is influenced by academic discourse on morality by creating new types of hES cell-like cells from non-embryonic sources. Two new scientific developments that create pluripotent cells can occur through cell fusion of somatic cells with embryonic stem cells and the reprogramming of somatic cells through the induction of key factors.

Advances in SCNT technology has demonstrated the ability of a somatic nucleus to be reprogrammed. However, the use of SCNT into oocytes resulting in the creation of embryos raises several ethical issues. More recently, it has been reported that nuclear reprogramming can also occur through the cytoplasmic fusion of human fibroblasts with ES cells [221]. This hybrid cell maintained a stable tetraploid genome and contained expression patterns similar to hES cells that are capable of differentiation into several cell types from the embryonic germ layer [221]. Other studies demonstrated that hES cells can reprogram myeloid precursor cells [222] or neurospheres cells [223] following cell-cell fusion. These studies show proof-of-principle that nuclear genomes of partially or fully differentiated cells can be reprogrammed to an undifferentiated state offering greater potentiality to differentiate into other cell types.

It remains unclear however, the extent the somatic genomes have been fully reprogrammed in the above cell fusion experiments [224]. Further genetic and epigenetic analysis should reveal the extent of genomic reprogramming occurred by fusion of hES cells [224]. It remains to be determined the safety of these tetraploid cells if they are to one day be used for clinical purposes. It is also of concern as to whether these cells will bypass immune rejection since the hybrid cells contain chromosomes from hES cells. The hybrid cells from the fusion of an hES cell line and somatic cells from a donor may offer a novel way to create cells that may bypass immune rejection and have the potentiality to undergo selected differentiation to a specific cell type to be used for cell restorative therapies. Importantly, these hybrid cells do not use embryos directly and thus bypasses the ethical issue of destroying human embryos for research purposes.

Reprogramming somatic cells by fusion with hES cells indicates that ES cells may contain the factors that induce potentiality [224]. A second way to avoid the use of human embryonic material and the destruction of human embryos is reprogramming somatic cells using defined factors. A study by Takahashi and Yamanaka demonstrated that induction of Oct3/4, Sox2, c-myc and Klf4 into mouse fibroblasts from fetal and adult tissues can induce potentiality [225]. These factors were discovered through selection for targets that affect the expression of a gene necessary for pluripotency and mouse development. These cells were designated as induced pluripotent stem (iPS) cells and exhibited similar morphology, growth and gene marker expression to ES cells. Transplantation of iPS cells induced teratoma formation containing cells of all three germ layers [225]. Similarly, another group reprogrammed human somatic cells to induce potentiality and showed these iPS cells resemble ES cells through expression of Oct4, Sox2, Nanog and Lin28 [226]. Using a mouse model for human sickle cell anemia, mice can be rescued following the transplantation of hematopoietic progenitors from iPS cells that were genetically modified to correct for the human sickle hemoglobin gene [227]. Using a more stringent selection marker, other groups have generated iPS cells using Nanog as a target of Oct3/4 and Sox2 [228-230]. These studies demonstrated that key factors can induce reprogramming of somatic cells to confer greater potentiality in order to be used for transplantation therapies. These cells do not contain another cell's genome and thus less likely to be recognized by a donor's body as foreign and would not be immune rejected.

Together, all of these scientific studies provide proof-of-principle that the manipulation of somatic cells of the body can be coaxed to have greater potentiality and can be induced to differentiate and may be transplanted. However, these studies have not all been performed using human cells and much basic research is required to understand the genetic and epigenetic reprogramming of these various cells and their safety and efficacy to be used for regenerative medicine.

The Influence of Diverse Ethical Values on the Commercialization of Stem Cell Research

Stem cell research is a complex, international field that involves a diversity of stakeholders in a wide range of basic and applied research. Scientists, clinicians, and industry partners are increasingly collaborating with governments and civil society in the development of, and debate about, the potential medical applications (e.g., treatment of disease vs. enhancement) and the ethics of stem cell research. This type of complexity is increasingly the norm in the biosciences, but just because it is 'normal' does not mean that it is stable or free from ethical concern [231]. The very interconnectedness of local, national and international relations raises a host of challenging social, ethical, economic and political issues. How should the materials such as oocytes and embryos necessary for ES cell research be 'ethically sourced' so as to avoid exploitation of poor or disempowered women and couples? Should oocytes and embryos be treated as altruistic gifts to be used for public research that will benefit society, or can they be treated as property (but whose) and commercialized (by whom)? Given the diversity of values attributed to the moral status of the human embryo from different religious and political perspectives, how will governments take into account all of these views as they seek to regulate the use of embryos for research and compete in a growing market for hES cell research and development? If we accept that ES cell science will progress only with significant public and private financial investment, how are the inevitable conflicting interests of university researchers, industry and government to be resolved, in particular around the issues of intellectual property rights, academic freedom, and benefit sharing? These important issues are common to other fields of biotechnology research such as genetically modified agriculture, drug development, and genetic testing, but are particularly challenging in the case of ES cell research due to this field's early stage of development and the charged nature of discussions about the moral status of the human embryo. In this section, we sketch out some of these issues and point to the tensions and opportunities posed for the increasingly global field of ES cell research. We discuss the ethical sourcing and supply of embryos, property rights and patents and their role in ES cell research.

'Ethical Sourcing' and Supply of Embryos and Embryonic Tissue

A major issue for both ES cell research and commercialization is the supply chain and the ethical sourcing of reproductive cells and embryos. Unlike the valued use of excised or waste tissue in biomedical research (e.g., tumor biopsies), human embryos or reproductive cells used to create embryos for hES cell derivation are not considered waste and are thus invariably considered intrinsically valuable to the individuals from whom they are removed. Individual donors may (in some instances) claim to be owners of human gametes or embryos and assert a right to decide whether this material is maintained in cryopreservation (although often at a cost to the donor), destroyed, donated for research, or donated to help others with their reproductive needs. Gametes and embryos, unlike excised tumor tissue for the most part, are often imbued with a spiritual or genetic connection to the donor which gives the material a non-instrumental value. If the tissue comes to have an instrumental and potential commercial value, to whom does the tissue and any benefits belong? [232;233]. The question of appropriate research use and ownership of products of embryos depend, in part, on the sourcing of embryos for research.

Embryo sourcing for research is in part influenced by social policies that govern the use of embryos through allocation of research funds, statutory prohibitions on research practice, practice guidelines published by societies or accreditation by oversight bodies. Human ES cell research may yield direct and indirect social benefits, but different nations vary in their policies on embryo sourcing. As discussed previously, the moral status of the embryo is highly contested which has led to significant international variation in policies and regulations that facilitate, control, or limit hES cell research through, amongst others, prohibitions on the creation of human embryos [234]. In North America and Europe, embryos have tended, in public discourse and policy, to be treated as morally value laden and in need of special handling, e.g., limits on the types of embryos available for research such as surplus, fresh or frozen, or the creation of embryos specifically for research purposes [235]. By comparison, in the global South embryos tend not to have the same moral status and are thus often treated as waste, to be disposed of or translated into commodities [236]. As such, there is an opportunity for researchers in the North to participate in a global 'moral economy' in which they trade on the less contentious nature of embryos and hES cell research in the South in order to source material they could not otherwise obtain [236]. This moral economy has been most evident with the movement of embryo and stem cell researchers from the US (with its prohibition on the use of federal dollars for hES cell research) to more permissive environments, such as the UK or Asia [237], or between less well funded US states to California [238]. One might view this as a simple academic/economic reality and thus decide to let the market forces dictate. But this moral economy also raises concerns about the sourcing of material from developing countries that have less stringent ethical oversight (e.g., underfinanced or even corrupt ethics review boards), and the potential for exploitation of vulnerable populations, in particular the exploitation of ovum donors from these nations [239]. What then are the responsibilities for scientists and policy makers in countries with more stringent and/or restrictive criteria for the use of embryos in ES cell research? And how should economic potential or competitiveness fit into policies about the appropriate sourcing of embryos and ES cell material?

Social policies in some jurisdictions have prohibited the creation of embryos for research purposes; however, many nations have permitted the use of surplus embryos for hES cell research [235;240]. As mentioned previously, some commentators have argued that because surplus embryos would normally be destroyed, that it is appropriate (and even respectful) to use them for beneficial purposes such as ES cell research [241;242]. It has been proposed that we will see an emerging market and international trade in human oocytes and embryos that, without formal regulation [243], will exploit the economic dependency of women in both wealthy and poorer countries [244]. The details of the health risks posed to women have been discussed in previous sections, but here the issue is the possibility that poor and vulnerable women will bear the disproportionate burden of risk, and will not, as promised by advocates for a commercial trade in human tissue, benefit in any real sense [239].

This translation of surplus embryos into source material for research is also connected to complex relations of gift, donation and trade that differ somewhat from those relations associated with tissue donation such as blood or organs. Tissue donation has tended to be one-to-one (e.g., whole organ) or one-to-a-few (e.g., blood, partial lung/liver) transfers where donors could conceive of and might wish to build relations of gift or reciprocity, although such relations might also incur feelings of debt or guilt on the part of recipients. These feelings about gift and responsibility have been very important to the development of public blood banks [245;246], and the success (or lack thereof) of national organ transplant programs [247]. But surplus embryos and the cells taken from them can lead to the derivation of a wide range of tissues that exist over long time periods that can be taken up by many users for a variety of purposes [236]. In such circumstances, what feelings do donors have about the embryos and resulting cell types or cell lines? Do they have a 'connection' to the tissue and possible recipients, and does it matter if they do not? These questions bring to the fore the very personal nature, for some people, of their bodily tissues and the potential or limits on its transfer. These questions also highlight the complexity of the value(s) attributed to embryos and stem cells, whether by donors, scientists, or policy makers.

Property Rights

Governments in the UK, Canada, the US and Europe have tended (with some exceptions) to treat the sourcing of biological material such as blood, organs or other tissues as gifts. People can altruistically donate their biological material for scientific research, or for potential therapeutic benefit to themselves or others through the banking of blood, bone marrow, organs or stem cells. At the same time, however, the primacy of autonomy as a significant driving social value, particularly in North America, has meant that individuals are often portrayed as fully autonomous, private persons with strong controlling interests in their bodies. This strong emphasis on autonomy can be the basis for gift giving, but is also one of the main arguments in favour of establishing a commercial trade in organs and tissues.

Discussions of a commercial trade in tissue invariably turn on the notion of individual autonomy and the right to have strong controlling interests, and even property rights, in one's body. If women do have strong property rights in their bodies, and thus their ova, then arguably they should be able to dispose of them as they choose, either treating them as a gift, as waste to be destroyed and/or as valued material to be sold for reproductive or research purposes [239]. But the notion of granting individuals property rights in their bodies is not straightforward as the concept of property itself is complex. According to Radin, one means of gauging the significance of a person's relationship with an object is the type and level of pain suffered by the loss of the object. If the object is loosely held (e.g., one's car), then it can be freely exchanged, sold or replaced. The relationship to the object is close and personal if the pain of its loss cannot be alleviated by its replacement, i.e., the loss of a family heirloom [248;249]. This leads to a hierarchy of entitlements, so that the closer the connection with personhood, the stronger the entitlement. Some items (e.g., bodily organs), according to Radin and others, cannot be classified as property at all. To make organs and tissue fully alienable would, as Bourianoff Bray observes, "encourage a perception of body parts as interchangeable commodities and undermine the recognition of the human body as the physical embodiment of the personality" [250]. Further, by conceiving of the body as property, one does not protect people but instead risks legitimating the exploitation of people who are economically vulnerable.

Drawing on similar arguments, most governments around the world have limited the scope of their citizen's property rights for various forms of tissue. One cannot legally sell oneself into indentured servitude or slavery (although one can sell one's labour), and there is an international prohibition on organ sales. But for renewable tissues such as blood, hair, sperm and oocytes, the situation is much less certain. In Canada for example, the sale of such tissues is prohibited by law, yet in the US, commercial blood and sperm banks have been in operation for decades, and egg sales are increasingly common. In Waldby's terms (drawing on the work of Michel Foucault), biological material, including embryos, are increasingly imbued with 'biovalue' such that patients, donors, and scientists are participating in a developing global 'tissue economy' in which gifts are translated into commodities for research and ultimately commercialization [251].

To further complicate matters, court decisions in the US, Canada and Europe over the last few decades have ruled that while individuals cannot own or have strong enduring property rights in their bodies or tissues (although they can control and sell some types of tissue), other people, namely scientists and companies, can have such strong property rights once the tissue is excised and transformed [252]. For example, in the 1990 case of *John Moore v. Regents of*

University of California, the US Supreme Court rejected John Moore's claim that he had property rights in his spleen (or his body more generally) which Moore's doctor had extracted as part of treating Moore's leukemia, and used to develop and commercialize a cell line [233]. Moore was not entitled to royalties from the sale of the cell line because while he had contributed the source tissue, he had not contributed to its development and transformation into a socially useful product [233;253]. The legal reasoning was in part based on the influential theory of the political philosopher John Locke, which adopts a natural rights theory of property rights such that, in the context of contemporary bioscience research, it is the scientist's mixture of labour with an object (e.g., Moore's cells) that adds value, or 'biovalue', to the transformed product and thus the scientist as inventor then has legitimate ownership or property rights [254]. However, a transformed entity, such as a new hES cell line created from an *in vitro* embryo, might be thought to gain value both from the transformation process and from the donated source material, particularly if one ascribes labour-type values to a woman's production of her reproductive material [255]. The natural rights view is thus incapable of determining the exact nature of the property rights in hES cells [254].

Bjorkman and Hansson argue that property rights should be arranged such that they promote a proper combination of social goals, such as justice and economic productivity, and so adopt a social constructivist account of property and ownership that stipulates that ownership is the result of a series of social choices and events [254]. Instead of relying on a Lockean natural rights approach that views property rights as based on a strict relation between an owner and a product, Bjorkman and Hansson suggest that it may be helpful to view rights to biological material as part of a bundle of rights that may not necessarily include a strong property right (i.e., using the source material as property to be bartered/sold) [254]. Thus an individual donor would have the right to be treated with respect, and the removal of material from their body would necessitate valid and informed consent. The use of the material could be for therapeutic benefit to the individual or to others, but could not be obtained in an exploitive manner, and the distribution of the biological material for therapeutic purposes would have to be based on medical need (and not commercial transactions). For our purposes, the donation and use of embryos would invoke a different bundle of rights for either gamete donors and/or third party embryo donor(s) that would depend on the availability of biological material and its importance to the donor (e.g., respect, decision-making authority, etc.). But the transformation of the biological material for research and innovation would invoke property rights only for the scientific/technical creators (as discussed above), such that the main financial beneficiaries from the use of embryos for the derivation of hES cells would be the parties (scientists, universities, companies) involved in the subsequent research. The source donors would not have any rights to share in profits earned from the patenting or licensing of products derived from their donated tissue but would possess other moral rights as mentioned above.

Patents and Intellectual Property

The landmark 1980 US Supreme Court case of *Diamond v. Chakrabarty* allowed for the patenting of a genetically modified bacterium and opened the door for patents on a broad range of biological materials, including genes, proteins, bacteria and even multicellular organisms [256]. A biologically derived invention is considered patentable if it can be shown to be new, useful, inventive and non-obvious. Driven in part by permissive US patent policy and international trade and patent harmonization agreements such as the *Agreement on Trade-Related Aspects of Intellectual Property Rights* (TRIPS) and the *North American Free Trade Agreement* (NAFTA), the last two decades have seen an explosion of biological patents granted around the world [257]. In the late 1980s, US patents were extended to genetically engineered plants and animals, and the infamous Harvard 'Oncomouse' patent granted in 1988. While cellular and genomic patents have been granted internationally, many countries, including Canada and members of the European Union, have either refrained from granting or severely limited patents on higher life forms for ethical reasons [258], and have had similar concerns about the patenting of stem cells.

As with other areas of competitive bioscience research, intellectual property rights (usually in the form of patents) loom large in ES cell research. Patents are widely accepted as a necessary but not sufficient requirement for leveraging venture capital for biotechnology or pharmaceutical company research. But patents in stem cells and cell lines are complicated by questions about how one defines the cells, their moral or symbolic connection to the body and human dignity, and concerns about a slippery slope to the commodification of human beings [259]. Nevertheless, broad stem cell patents were granted in the US in 1999 to James Thomson and the Wisconsin Alumni Research Foundation (WARF), and to Geron Co. in California [260]. A recent paper by Taymor *et al.* discusses key patents on ES cells, and argues that pluripotent stem cells derived through blastomere biopsy would likely not infringe the Thomson/WARF patents. However, the authors note that the existing and new patent claims will depend to a large extent on how the embryo and ES cells were defined in the patent and are subsequently interpreted by the courts [261]. By limiting the definition of ES cells to their source material, i.e. the ICM, the derivation of pluripotent stem cells from stages earlier than the blastocyst may then be considered novel and thus permit the patenting of stem cells derived from parthenotes or altered nuclear transfer [261].

To date, no stem cell patents have been granted in Canada, although stem cells can be patented if they meet the criteria under the Canadian Patent Act [262]. Yet the patenting of stem cells remains controversial due to the issues in patenting living organisms. Furthermore, the 'ordre public' morality clause in European patent law will likely stymie such patents, not to mention the social controversy of such patents or European Directives excluding the commercial use of embryos [263]. The early US stem cell patents (e.g., to Thomson/WARF) may well be over turned because of their overly broad scope, opening the way for a diversity of more focused US patents on various aspects of stem cells, cell lines and derivative products [264]. From a public utility perspective, it is fair to ask what is the right balance to be struck between the protection of intellectual property as a means of encouraging innovation and economic development, and the production of public domain science and knowledge [265;266].

Research Environment

The stem cell research context – as is also the case with other biotechnologies, such as pharmacogenomics [267] – is a complex environment with diverse public and private sector stakeholders, and one marked by high hopes for health, social and economic benefits for both consumers and producers of stem cell research and its clinical applications.

Asian governments – particularly those of China, Japan, Taiwan, and Singapore – are investing substantial public funds in stem cell research. There is also significant commercial interest, with many small and mid size biotechnology companies being created, often at the behest and with the approval of national governments. These private laboratories and start-up companies are staffed by local technicians and scientists, and are also attracting ex-patriots trained abroad as well as international scientists [268]. Stem cell research in Asia is benefiting from a much less restrictive scientific and regulatory environment than is present in North America and Europe as well as the existence of high quality laboratories and low labour costs. But of concern for some scientists and investors is that there is often a lack of senior, international level scientists to lead Asian research teams; moreover, a widespread culture of secrecy due in part to different academic and political histories may limit innovation and research independence, something that is also exacerbated by strong commercial interests (and thus involvement) by local governments.

In the US, many state governments are actively supporting and encourage public and private stem cell research in order to grow local companies that compete with leaders in the field such as Geron and WARF. There are, for example, various plans to float state bonds to raise research dollars, and provide tax incentives for companies as a means of counteracting the National Institutes of Health (NIH) freeze on ES cell research funding [269]. The aim for these states is to build environments that are conducive to research and technological development that will hopefully result in measurable employment and economic development. Other US states, however, are actively moving away from stem cell research and implementing legislation to ban research in this field.

One concern about the NIH freeze on funding, and the subsequent privatization of stem cell research in the US and internationally, is the lack of oversight of down stream research at the stage of clinical trials. The worry is that with stem cell research moving from public laboratories to private laboratories (whether US-based or off-shore), clinical research trials will not meet the same standards of human subjects protection and oversight in university research programs. This is particularly an issue in the US where pharmaceutical companies often employ private IRBs to perform research ethics review; but concern extends to research in Asia, highlighted most recently by the South Korean scandal and science fraud, which was in part the result of enormous public and government pressure [270]. Private sector involvement in stem cell research also poses questions about the social responsibility of companies. Companies clearly have different interests, and these will also differ depending on the type of companies involved in research and development e.g., small and large biotechnology companies, and private laboratories [271].

Stem cell research is a field that likely still requires significant basic scientific research and research funding if it is to transition to the proof of concept stage and eventually technology development and clinical implementation. As such, it is important to put stem cell research in the context of biotechnology research more generally, and recognize the fact that for companies to receive venture capital funding, they must have products that are actually in development, preferably at least in phase 1 or 2 clinical trials [272]. One of the challenges, besides the issues of regulation, is the funding of basic stem cell research. While the promises of hES cell research may be significant, given the early stage of research, it may be very difficult to interest venture capitalists to invest because of the contentious ethical and religious issues associated with ES cell research as well as the significant time frame prior to clinical applications [273].

Conclusions

Stem cell research may be of tremendous social and scientific benefit. The use of hES cells may prove scientifically valuable to research in developmental biology and to understand the molecular mechanisms of disease, such as cancer, that may lead to the development of novel therapies. ES cells can also be used in drug toxicity testing and may one day be used clinically to treat degenerative diseases or destroyed tissue. Despite the potential benefits of hES cell research, opponents continue to employ arguments similar to those used in the abortion debate (particularly the moral status of the embryo) to justify the claim that personhood begins at or near conception and thus to limit what types of embryo research should be considered appropriate. Proponents of hES cell research restrict criteria for personhood to later developmental stages in order to sway the debate on the permissibility of using human embryos for research. As the debate on the ethics of using embryos for hES cell research honed in on the moral status of the human embryo, so too did the practice of science shift to create alternative types of embryos for hES cell research or means of deriving hES cells without destroying the embryo. As such, the potential harms to women participating in research, i.e., from the use of ovulatory drugs and from oocyte retrieval is starting to receive more attention. While these alternate means of creating embryos might mitigate or alter ethical arguments about the moral status of embryos or their destruction, they fail to account for the potential harms to women. Moreover, as the need for oocytes for research increases, the possible solicitation and exploitation of women for their eggs may also occur. The physical and psychological risks should be adequately and accurately conveyed to oocyte donors and the possible benefits should not be exaggerated so as to avoid therapeutic misconception.

The various diverse ethical views on the moral status of the human embryo, the harms to women and the value of ES cell research affects the commercialization of stem cell research in different jurisdictions. These differences in values influence the sourcing and supply of embryos and embryonic tissue and their status as property and the corresponding property rights of individuals. This review has attempted to provide a broad overview of the range of arguments and debate on the ethics of hES cell research and to demonstrate how ethical reflection and discourse has influenced scientific practice on embryo and hES cell research. The changes in scientific research have in turn influenced ethical discussion on embryo and hES cell research. Further reflection and deliberation by all interested parties on the various topics presented in this chapter are needed to determine how societies can maximize the benefits of hES cell research while respecting the diverse value of their citizens and minimizing the potential harms to the embryo, to women and to society as a whole.

Acknowledgments

This article has been slightly modified and was originally published in the *Journal of Stem Cells* Volume 3, Issue 2, pages 127-161. Dr. Bryn Williams-Jones received funds from the Canadian Institutes of Health Research and the Stem Cell Network, a network within the Networks of Centres of Excellence. We would like to thank Dr. M. William Lensch of the Department of Biological Chemistry and Molecular Pharmacology, Harvard Medical School for sharing his knowledge and thoughts on embryo and stem cell research. The views expressed here are strictly those of the authors and not those of Health Canada or the Government of Canada.

REFERENCES

[1] Evans,M.J. and Kaufman,M.H. (1981) Establishment in culture of pluripotential cells from mouse embryos. *Nature*, 292, 154-156.

[2] Martin,G.R. (1981) Isolation of a pluripotent cell line from early mouse embryos cultured in medium conditioned by teratocarcinoma stem cells. *Proc. Natl. Acad. Sci. USA*, 78, 7634-7638.

[3] Deacon,T., Dinsmore,J., Costantini,L.C., Ratliff,J., and Isacson,O. (1998) Blastula-stage stem cells can differentiate into dopaminergic and serotonergic neurons after transplantation. *Exp. Neurol.*, 149, 28-41.

[4] Thomson,J.A., Itskovitz-Eldor,J., Shapiro,S.S., Waknitz,M.A., Swiergiel,J.J., Marshall,V.S., and Jones,J.M. (1998) Embryonic stem cell lines derived from human blastocysts. *Science*, 282, 1145-1147.

[5] Pedersen,R.A. (2002) Feeding hungry stem cells. *Nat. Biotechnol.*, 20, 882-883.

[6] Richards,M., Fong,C.Y., Chan,W.K., Wong,P.C., and Bongso,A. (2002) Human feeders support prolonged undifferentiated growth of human inner cell masses and embryonic stem cells. *Nat. Biotechnol.*, 20, 933-936.

[7] Hovatta,O., Mikkola,M., Gertow,K., Stromberg,A.M., Inzunza,J., Hreinsson,J., Rozell,B., Blennow,E., Andang,M., and Ahrlund-Richter,L. (2003) A culture system using human foreskin fibroblasts as feeder cells allows production of human embryonic stem cells. *Hum. Reprod.*, 18, 1404-1409.

[8] Keller,G.M. (1995) In vitro differentiation of embryonic stem cells. *Curr. Opin. Cell Biol.*, 7, 862-869.

[9] Smith,A.G. (2001) Embryo-derived stem cells: of mice and men. *Annu. Rev. Cell Dev. Biol.*, 17, 435-462.

[10] Smith,D.A., Glover,J.L., Townsend,L.E., and Maupin,D.E. (1991) A method for the harvest, culture, and characterization of human adult atrial myocardial cells: correlation with age of donor. *In Vitro Cell Dev. Biol.*, 27A, 914-920.

[11] Wiles,M.V. and Johansson,B.M. (1999) Embryonic stem cell development in a chemically defined medium. *Exp. Cell Res.*, 247, 241-248.

[12] Bradley,A., Evans,M., Kaufman,M.H., and Robertson,E. (1984) Formation of germ-line chimaeras from embryo-derived teratocarcinoma cell lines. *Nature*, 309, 255-256.

[13] Smith,A.G., Heath,J.K., Donaldson,D.D., Wong,G.G., Moreau,J., Stahl,M., and Rogers,D. (1988) Inhibition of pluripotential embryonic stem cell differentiation by purified polypeptides. *Nature*, 336, 688-690.

[14] Rossant,J. (2001) Stem cells from the Mammalian blastocyst. *Stem Cells*, 19, 477-482.

[15] Pain,B., Clark,M.E., Shen,M., Nakazawa,H., Sakurai,M., Samarut,J., and Etches,R.J. (1996) Long-term in vitro culture and characterisation of avian embryonic stem cells with multiple morphogenetic potentialities. *Development*, 122, 2339-2348.

[16] Doetschman,T., Williams,P., and Maeda,N. (1988) Establishment of hamster blastocyst-derived embryonic stem (ES) cells. *Dev. Biol.*, 127, 224-227.
[17] Wheeler,M.B. (1994) Development and validation of swine embryonic stem cells: a review. *Reprod. Fertil. Dev.*, 6, 563-568.
[18] Thomson,J.A., Kalishman,J., Golos,T.G., Durning,M., Harris,C.P., Becker,R.A., and Hearn,J.P. (1995) Isolation of a primate embryonic stem cell line. *Proc. Natl. Acad. Sci. USA*, 92, 7844-7848.
[19] Thomson,J.A., Kalishman,J., Golos,T.G., Durning,M., Harris,C.P., and Hearn,J.P. (1996) Pluripotent cell lines derived from common marmoset (Callithrix jacchus) blastocysts. *Biol. Reprod.*, 55, 254-259.
[20] Reubinoff,B.E., Pera,M.F., Fong,C.Y., Trounson,A., and Bongso,A. (2000) Embryonic stem cell lines from human blastocysts: somatic differentiation in vitro. *Nat. Biotechnol.*, 18, 399-404.
[21] Lanzendorf,S.E., Boyd,C.A., Wright,D.L., Muasher,S., Oehninger,S., and Hodgen,G.D. (2001) Use of human gametes obtained from anonymous donors for the production of human embryonic stem cell lines. *Fertil. Steril.*, 76, 132-137.
[22] Mitalipova,M., Calhoun,J., Shin,S., Wininger,D., Schulz,T., Noggle,S., Venable,A., Lyons,I., Robins,A., and Stice,S. (2003) Human embryonic stem cell lines derived from discarded embryos. *Stem Cells*, 21, 521-526.
[23] Park,J.H., Kim,S.J., Oh,E.J., Moon,S.Y., Roh,S.I., Kim,C.G., and Yoon,H.S. (2003) Establishment and maintenance of human embryonic stem cells on STO, a permanently growing cell line. *Biol. Reprod.*, 69, 2007-2014.
[24] Pickering,S.J., Braude,P.R., Patel,M., Burns,C.J., Trussler,J., Bolton,V., and Minger,S. (2003) Preimplantation genetic diagnosis as a novel source of embryos for stem cell research. *Reprod. Biomed. Online.*, 7, 353-364.
[25] Cowan,C.A., Klimanskaya,I., McMahon,J., Atienza,J., Witmyer,J., Zucker,J.P., Wang,S., Morton,C.C., McMahon,A.P., Powers,D., and Melton,D.A. (2004) Derivation of embryonic stem-cell lines from human blastocysts. *N. Engl. J. Med.*, 350, 1353-1356.
[26] Stojkovic,M., Lako,M., Stojkovic,P., Stewart,R., Przyborski,S., Armstrong,L., Evans,J., Herbert,M., Hyslop,L., Ahmad,S., Murdoch,A., and Strachan,T. (2004) Derivation of human embryonic stem cells from day-8 blastocysts recovered after three-step in vitro culture. *Stem Cells*, 22, 790-797.
[27] Kim,N.W., Piatyszek,M.A., Prowse,K.R., Harley,C.B., West,M.D., Ho,P.L., Coviello,G.M., Wright,W.E., Weinrich,S.L., and Shay,J.W. (1994) Specific association of human telomerase activity with immortal cells and cancer. *Science*, 266, 2011-2015.
[28] Betts,D.H. and King,W.A. (1999) Telomerase activity and telomere detection during early bovine development. *Dev. Genet.*, 25, 397-403.
[29] Brenner,C.A., Wolny,Y.M., Adler,R.R., and Cohen,J. (1999) Alternative splicing of the telomerase catalytic subunit in human oocytes and embryos. *Mol. Hum. Reprod.*, 5, 845-850.
[30] Thomson,J.A. and Marshall,V.S. (1998) Primate embryonic stem cells. *Curr. Top. Dev. Biol.*, 38, 133-165.
[31] Hayflick,L. and Moorhead,P.S. (1961) The serial cultivation of human diploid cell strains. *Exp. Cell Res.*, 25, 585-621.

[32] Allsopp,R.C., Vaziri,H., Patterson,C., Goldstein,S., Younglai,E.V., Futcher,A.B., Greider,C.W., and Harley,C.B. (1992) Telomere length predicts replicative capacity of human fibroblasts. *Proc. Natl. Acad. Sci. U. S. A*, 89, 10114-10118.

[33] Counter,C.M., Avilion,A.A., LeFeuvre,C.E., Stewart,N.G., Greider,C.W., Harley,C.B., and Bacchetti,S. (1992) Telomere shortening associated with chromosome instability is arrested in immortal cells which express telomerase activity. *EMBO J.*, 11, 1921-1929.

[34] Strelchenko,N., Verlinsky,O., Kukharenko,V., and Verlinsky,Y. (2004) Morula-derived human embryonic stem cells. *Reprod. Biomed. Online.*, 9, 623-629.

[35] Mitsui,K., Tokuzawa,Y., Itoh,H., Segawa,K., Murakami,M., Takahashi,K., Maruyama, M., Maeda,M., and Yamanaka,S. (2003) The homeoprotein Nanog is required for maintenance of pluripotency in mouse epiblast and ES cells. *Cell*, 113, 631-642.

[36] Chambers,I., Colby,D., Robertson,M., Nichols,J., Lee,S., Tweedie,S., and Smith,A. (2003) Functional expression cloning of Nanog, a pluripotency sustaining factor in embryonic stem cells. *Cell*, 113, 643-655.

[37] Wiles,M.V. and Keller,G. (1991) Multiple hematopoietic lineages develop from embryonic stem (ES) cells in culture. *Development*, 111, 259-267.

[38] Li,M., Pevny,L., Lovell-Badge,R., and Smith,A. (1998) Generation of purified neural precursors from embryonic stem cells by lineage selection. *Curr. Biol.*, 8, 971-974.

[39] Dani,C., Smith,A.G., Dessolin,S., Leroy,P., Staccini,L., Villageois,P., Darimont,C., and Ailhaud,G. (1997) Differentiation of embryonic stem cells into adipocytes in vitro. *J. Cell Sci.*, 110 (Pt 11), 1279-1285.

[40] Rohwedel,J., Maltsev,V., Bober,E., Arnold,H.H., Hescheler,J., and Wobus,A.M. (1994) Muscle cell differentiation of embryonic stem cells reflects myogenesis in vivo: developmentally regulated expression of myogenic determination genes and functional expression of ionic currents. *Dev. Biol.*, 164, 87-101.

[41] Klug,M.G., Soonpaa,M.H., Koh,G.Y., and Field,L.J. (1996) Genetically selected cardiomyocytes from differentiating embronic stem cells form stable intracardiac grafts. *J. Clin. Invest*, 98, 216-224.

[42] Kramer,J., Hegert,C., Guan,K., Wobus,A.M., Muller,P.K., and Rohwedel,J. (2000) Embryonic stem cell-derived chondrogenic differentiation in vitro: activation by BMP-2 and BMP-4. *Mech. Dev.*, 92, 193-205.

[43] Lumelsky,N., Blondel,O., Laeng,P., Velasco,I., Ravin,R., and McKay,R. (2001) Differentiation of embryonic stem cells to insulin-secreting structures similar to pancreatic islets. *Science*, 292, 1389-1394.

[44] Surani,M.A. and Barton,S.C. (1983) Development of gynogenetic eggs in the mouse: implications for parthenogenetic embryos. *Science*, 222, 1034-1036.

[45] Hagemann,L.J., Peterson,A.J., Weilert,L.L., Lee,R.S., and Tervit,H.R. (1998) In vitro and early in vivo development of sheep gynogenones and putative androgenones. *Mol. Reprod. Dev.*, 50, 154-162.

[46] Ozil,J.P. and Huneau,D. (2001) Activation of rabbit oocytes: the impact of the Ca2+ signal regime on development. *Development*, 128, 917-928.

[47] Carroll,J. (2001) The initiation and regulation of Ca2+ signalling at fertilization in mammals. *Semin. Cell Dev. Biol.*, 12, 37-43.

[48] Mitalipov,S.M., Nusser,K.D., and Wolf,D.P. (2001) Parthenogenetic activation of rhesus monkey oocytes and reconstructed embryos. *Biol. Reprod.*, 65, 253-259.

[49] Vrana,K.E., Hipp,J.D., Goss,A.M., McCool,B.A., Riddle,D.R., Walker,S.J., Wettstein,P.J., Studer,L.P., Tabar,V., Cunniff,K., Chapman,K., Vilner,L., West,M.D., Grant,K.A., and Cibelli,J.B. (2003) Nonhuman primate parthenogenetic stem cells. *Proc. Natl. Acad. Sci. U. S. A*, 100 Suppl 1, 11911-11916.

[50] Cibelli,J.B., Grant,K.A., Chapman,K.B., Cunniff,K., Worst,T., Green,H.L., Walker,S.J., Gutin,P.H., Vilner,L., Tabar,V., Dominko,T., Kane,J., Wettstein,P.J., Lanza,R.P., Studer,L., Vrana,K.E., and West,M.D. (2002) Parthenogenetic stem cells in nonhuman primates. *Science*, 295, 819.

[51] Paffoni,A., Brevini,T.A., Somigliana,E., Restelli,L., Gandolfi,F., and Ragni,G. (2006) In vitro development of human oocytes after parthenogenetic activation or intracytoplasmic sperm injection. *Fertil. Steril.*

[52] Lanza,R.P., Cibelli,J.B., and West,M.D. (1999) Prospects for the use of nuclear transfer in human transplantation. *Nat. Biotechnol.*, 17, 1171-1174.

[53] Wakayama,T., Tabar,V., Rodriguez,I., Perry,A.C., Studer,L., and Mombaerts,P. (2001) Differentiation of embryonic stem cell lines generated from adult somatic cells by nuclear transfer. *Science*, 292, 740-743.

[54] Solter,D. (2000) Mammalian cloning: advances and limitations. *Nat. Rev. Genet.*, 1, 199-207.

[55] Rideout,W.M., III, Eggan,K., and Jaenisch,R. (2001) Nuclear cloning and epigenetic reprogramming of the genome. *Science*, 293, 1093-1098.

[56] Rideout,W.M., III, Hochedlinger,K., Kyba,M., Daley,G.Q., and Jaenisch,R. (2002) Correction of a genetic defect by nuclear transplantation and combined cell and gene therapy. *Cell*, 109, 17-27.

[57] Lanza,R.P., Cibelli,J.B., Blackwell,C., Cristofalo,V.J., Francis,M.K., Baerlocher,G.M., Mak,J., Schertzer,M., Chavez,E.A., Sawyer,N., Lansdorp,P.M., and West,M.D. (2000) Extension of cell life-span and telomere length in animals cloned from senescent somatic cells. *Science*, 288, 665-669.

[58] Tian,X.C., Xu,J., and Yang,X. (2000) Normal telomere lengths found in cloned cattle. *Nat. Genet.*, 26, 272-273.

[59] Wakayama,T., Shinkai,Y., Tamashiro,K.L., Niida,H., Blanchard,D.C., Blanchard,R.J., Ogura,A., Tanemura,K., Tachibana,M., Perry,A.C., Colgan,D.F., Mombaerts,P., and Yanagimachi,R. (2000) Cloning of mice to six generations. *Nature*, 407, 318-319.

[60] Betts,D., Bordignon,V., Hill,J., Winger,Q., Westhusin,M., Smith,L., and King,W. (2001) Reprogramming of telomerase activity and rebuilding of telomere length in cloned cattle. *Proc. Natl. Acad. Sci. U. S. A*, 98, 1077-1082.

[61] Miyashita,N., Shiga,K., Yonai,M., Kaneyama,K., Kobayashi,S., Kojima,T., Goto,Y., Kishi,M., Aso,H., Suzuki,T., Sakaguchi,M., and Nagai,T. (2002) Remarkable differences in telomere lengths among cloned cattle derived from different cell types. *Biol. Reprod.*, 66, 1649-1655.

[62] Simerly,C., Dominko,T., Navara,C., Payne,C., Capuano,S., Gosman,G., Chong,K.Y., Takahashi,D., Chace,C., Compton,D., Hewitson,L., and Schatten,G. (2003) Molecular correlates of primate nuclear transfer failures. *Science*, 300, 297.

[63] Booth,P.J., Viuff,D., Tan,S., Holm,P., Greve,T., and Callesen,H. (2003) Numerical chromosome errors in day 7 somatic nuclear transfer bovine blastocysts. *Biol. Reprod.*, 68, 922-928.

[64] Dean,W., Santos,F., Stojkovic,M., Zakhartchenko,V., Walter,J., Wolf,E., and Reik,W. (2001) Conservation of methylation reprogramming in mammalian development: aberrant reprogramming in cloned embryos. *Proc. Natl. Acad. Sci. USA*, 98, 13734-13738.

[65] Humpherys,D., Eggan,K., Akutsu,H., Hochedlinger,K., Rideout,W.M., III, Biniszkiewicz,D., Yanagimachi,R., and Jaenisch,R. (2001) Epigenetic instability in ES cells and cloned mice. *Science*, 293, 95-97.

[66] Kang,Y.K., Koo,D.B., Park,J.S., Choi,Y.H., Chung,A.S., Lee,K.K., and Han,Y.M. (2001) Aberrant methylation of donor genome in cloned bovine embryos. *Nat. Genet.*, 28, 173-177.

[67] Humpherys,D., Eggan,K., Akutsu,H., Friedman,A., Hochedlinger,K., Yanagimachi,R., Lander,E.S., Golub,T.R., and Jaenisch,R. (2002) Abnormal gene expression in cloned mice derived from embryonic stem cell and cumulus cell nuclei. *Proc. Natl. Acad. Sci. USA*, 99, 12889-12894.

[68] Kang,Y.K., Park,J.S., Koo,D.B., Choi,Y.H., Kim,S.U., Lee,K.K., and Han,Y.M. (2002) Limited demethylation leaves mosaic-type methylation states in cloned bovine pre-implantation embryos. *EMBO J.*, 21, 1092-1100.

[69] McGrath,J. and Solter,D. (1983) Nuclear transplantation in the mouse embryo by microsurgery and cell fusion. *Science*, 220, 1300-1302.

[70] Willadsen,S.M. (1986) Nuclear transplantation in sheep embryos. *Nature*, 320, 63-65.

[71] Prather,R.S., Barnes,F.L., Sims,M.M., Robl,J.M., Eyestone,W.H., and First,N.L. (1987) Nuclear transplantation in the bovine embryo: assessment of donor nuclei and recipient oocyte. *Biol. Reprod.*, 37, 859-866.

[72] Stice,S.L. and Robl,J.M. (1988) Nuclear reprogramming in nuclear transplant rabbit embryos. *Biol. Reprod.*, 39, 657-664.

[73] Prather,R.S., Sims,M.M., and First,N.L. (1989) Nuclear transplantation in early pig embryos. *Biol. Reprod.*, 41, 414-418.

[74] Campbell,K.H., McWhir,J., Ritchie,W.A., and Wilmut,I. (1996) Sheep cloned by nuclear transfer from a cultured cell line. *Nature*, 380, 64-66.

[75] Hochedlinger,K. and Jaenisch,R. (2006) Nuclear reprogramming and pluripotency. *Nature*, 441, 1061-1067.

[76] Rhind,S.M., Taylor,J.E., De Sousa,P.A., King,T.J., McGarry,M., and Wilmut,I. (2003) Human cloning: can it be made safe? *Nat. Rev. Genet.*, 4, 855-864.

[77] Rhind,S.M., King,T.J., Harkness,L.M., Bellamy,C., Wallace,W., DeSousa,P., and Wilmut,I. (2003) Cloned lambs--lessons from pathology. *Nat. Biotechnol.*, 21, 744-745.

[78] Hill,J.R., Roussel,A.J., Cibelli,J.B., Edwards,J.F., Hooper,N.L., Miller,M.W., Thompson,J.A., Looney,C.R., Westhusin,M.E., Robl,J.M., and Stice,S.L. (1999) Clinical and pathologic features of cloned transgenic calves and fetuses (13 case studies). *Theriogenology*, 51, 1451-1465.

[79] Chavatte-Palmer,P., Heyman,Y., Richard,C., Monget,P., LeBourhis,D., Kann,G., Chilliard,Y., Vignon,X., and Renard,J.P. (2002) Clinical, hormonal, and hematologic characteristics of bovine calves derived from nuclei from somatic cells. *Biol. Reprod.*, 66, 1596-1603.

[80] Cibelli,J.B., Stice,S.L., Golueke,P.J., Kane,J.J., Jerry,J., Blackwell,C., Ponce de Leon,F.A., and Robl,J.M. (1998) Cloned transgenic calves produced from nonquiescent fetal fibroblasts. *Science*, 280, 1256-1258.

[81] Ogonuki,N., Inoue,K., Yamamoto,Y., Noguchi,Y., Tanemura,K., Suzuki,O., Nakayama,H., Doi,K., Ohtomo,Y., Satoh,M., Nishida,A., and Ogura,A. (2002) Early death of mice cloned from somatic cells. *Nat. Genet.*, 30, 253-254.

[82] Hynes,M. and Rosenthal,A. (2000) Embryonic stem cells go dopaminergic. *Neuron*, 28, 11-14.

[83] Svendsen,C.N. and Smith,A.G. (1999) New prospects for human stem-cell therapy in the nervous system. *Trends Neurosci.*, 22, 357-364.

[84] Bjorklund,L.M., Sanchez-Pernaute,R., Chung,S., Andersson,T., Chen,I.Y., McNaught,K.S., Brownell,A.L., Jenkins,B.G., Wahlestedt,C., Kim,K.S., and Isacson,O. (2002) Embryonic stem cells develop into functional dopaminergic neurons after transplantation in a Parkinson rat model. *Proc. Natl. Acad. Sci. USA*, 99, 2344-2349.

[85] Rezzani,R. (2004) Cyclosporine A and adverse effects on organs: histochemical studies. *Prog. Histochem. Cytochem.*, 39, 85-128.

[86] Dawson,L., Bateman-House,A.S., Mueller,A.D., Bok,H., Brock,D.W., Chakravarti,A., Greene,M., King,P.A., O'Brien,S.J., Sachs,D.H., Schill,K.E., Siegel,A., Solter,D., Suter,S.M., Verfaillie,C.M., Walters,L.B., Gearhart,J.D., and Faden,R.R. (2003) Safety issues in cell-based intervention trials. *Fertil. Steril.*, 80, 1077-1085.

[87] Gruen,L. and Grabel,L. (2006) Concise review: scientific and ethical roadblocks to human embryonic stem cell therapy. *Stem Cells*, 24, 2162-2169.

[88] Martin,M.J., Muotri,A., Gage,F., and Varki,A. (2005) Human embryonic stem cells express an immunogenic nonhuman sialic acid. *Nat. Med.*, 11, 228-232.

[89] Genbacev,O., Krtolica,A., Zdravkovic,T., Brunette,E., Powell,S., Nath,A., Caceres,E., McMaster,M., McDonagh,S., Li,Y., Mandalam,R., Lebkowski,J., and Fisher,S.J. (2005) Serum-free derivation of human embryonic stem cell lines on human placental fibroblast feeders. *Fertil. Steril.*, 83, 1517-1529.

[90] Inzunza,J., Gertow,K., Stromberg,M.A., Matilainen,E., Blennow,E., Skottman,H., Wolbank,S., Ahrlund-Richter,L., and Hovatta,O. (2005) Derivation of human embryonic stem cell lines in serum replacement medium using postnatal human fibroblasts as feeder cells. *Stem Cells*, 23, 544-549.

[91] Simon,C., Escobedo,C., Valbuena,D., Genbacev,O., Galan,A., Krtolica,A., Asensi,A., Sanchez,E., Esplugues,J., Fisher,S., and Pellicer,A. (2005) First derivation in Spain of human embryonic stem cell lines: use of long-term cryopreserved embryos and animal-free conditions. *Fertil. Steril.*, 83, 246-249.

[92] Lee,J.B., Lee,J.E., Park,J.H., Kim,S.J., Kim,M.K., Roh,S.I., and Yoon,H.S. (2005) Establishment and maintenance of human embryonic stem cell lines on human feeder cells derived from uterine endometrium under serum-free condition. *Biol. Reprod.*, 72, 42-49.

[93] Cheng,L., Hammond,H., Ye,Z., Zhan,X., and Dravid,G. (2003) Human adult marrow cells support prolonged expansion of human embryonic stem cells in culture. *Stem Cells*, 21, 131-142.

[94] Beattie,G.M., Lopez,A.D., Bucay,N., Hinton,A., Firpo,M.T., King,C.C., and Hayek,A. (2005) Activin A maintains pluripotency of human embryonic stem cells in the absence of feeder layers. *Stem Cells*, 23, 489-495.

[95] Amit,M., Shariki,C., Margulets,V., and Itskovitz-Eldor,J. (2004) Feeder layer- and serum-free culture of human embryonic stem cells. *Biol. Reprod.*, 70, 837-845.

[96] Kallos,M.S., Behie,L.A., and Vescovi,A.L. (1999) Extended serial passaging of mammalian neural stem cells in suspension bioreactors. *Biotechnol. Bioeng.*, 65, 589-599.

[97] Sen,A., Kallos,M.S., and Behie,L.A. (2002) Passaging protocols for mammalian neural stem cells in suspension bioreactors. *Biotechnol. Prog.*, 18, 337-345.

[98] Sen,A., Kallos,M.S., and Behie,L.A. (2004) New tissue dissociation protocol for scaled-up production of neural stem cells in suspension bioreactors. *Tissue Eng*, 10, 904-913.

[99] Draper,J.S., Smith,K., Gokhale,P., Moore,H.D., Maltby,E., Johnson,J., Meisner,L., Zwaka,T.P., Thomson,J.A., and Andrews,P.W. (2004) Recurrent gain of chromosomes 17q and 12 in cultured human embryonic stem cells. *Nat. Biotechnol.*, 22, 53-54.

[100] Inzunza,J., Sahlen,S., Holmberg,K., Stromberg,A.M., Teerijoki,H., Blennow,E., Hovatta,O., and Malmgren,H. (2004) Comparative genomic hybridization and karyotyping of human embryonic stem cells reveals the occurrence of an isodicentric X chromosome after long-term cultivation. *Mol. Hum. Reprod.*, 10, 461-466.

[101] Roy,N.S., Cleren,C., Singh,S.K., Yang,L., Beal,M.F., and Goldman,S.A. (2006) Functional engraftment of human ES cell-derived dopaminergic neurons enriched by coculture with telomerase-immortalized midbrain astrocytes. *Nat. Med.*, 12, 1259-1268.

[102] Lee,S.H., Lumelsky,N., Studer,L., Auerbach,J.M., and McKay,R.D. (2000) Efficient generation of midbrain and hindbrain neurons from mouse embryonic stem cells. *Nat. Biotechnol.*, 18, 675-679.

[103] Kim,J.H., Auerbach,J.M., Rodriguez-Gomez,J.A., Velasco,I., Gavin,D., Lumelsky,N., Lee,S.H., Nguyen,J., Sanchez-Pernaute,R., Bankiewicz,K., and McKay,R. (2002) Dopamine neurons derived from embryonic stem cells function in an animal model of Parkinson's disease. *Nature*, 418, 50-56.

[104] Master,Z., McLeod,M., and Mendez,I. (2007) Benefits, risks and ethical considerations in translation of stem cell research to clinical applications in Parkinson's disease. *Journal of Medical Ethics*, In Press.

[105] Glass,K.C., Weijer,C., Cournoyer,D., Lemmens,T., Palmour,R.M., Shapiro,S.H., and Freedman,B. (1999) Structuring the review of human genetics protocols, part III: gene therapy studies. *IRB.*, 21, 1-9.

[106] Modo,M., Mellodew,K., Cash,D., Fraser,S.E., Meade,T.J., Price,J., and Williams,S.C. (2004) Mapping transplanted stem cell migration after a stroke: a serial, in vivo magnetic resonance imaging study. *Neuroimage.*, 21, 311-317.

[107] Rathjen,P.D., Lake,J., Whyatt,L.M., Bettess,M.D., and Rathjen,J. (1998) Properties and uses of embryonic stem cells: prospects for application to human biology and gene therapy. *Reprod. Fertil. Dev.*, 10, 31-47.

[108] Dinsmore,J., Ratliff,J., Jacoby,D., Wunderlich,M., and Lindberg,C. (1998) Embryonic stem cells as a model for studying regulation of cellular differentiation. *Theriogenology*, 49, 145-151.

[109] Dani,C. (1999) Embryonic stem cell-derived adipogenesis. *Cells Tissues. Organs*, 165, 173-180.

[110] Schuldiner,M., Yanuka,O., Itskovitz-Eldor,J., Melton,D.A., and Benvenisty,N. (2000) Effects of eight growth factors on the differentiation of cells derived from human embryonic stem cells. *Proc. Natl. Acad. Sci. USA*, 97, 11307-11312.

[111] Sperger,J.M., Chen,X., Draper,J.S., Antosiewicz,J.E., Chon,C.H., Jones,S.B., Brooks,J.D., Andrews,P.W., Brown,P.O., and Thomson,J.A. (2003) Gene expression patterns in human embryonic stem cells and human pluripotent germ cell tumors. *Proc. Natl. Acad. Sci. USA*, 100, 13350-13355.

[112] D'Amour,K.A. and Gage,F.H. (2003) Genetic and functional differences between multipotent neural and pluripotent embryonic stem cells. *Proc. Natl. Acad. Sci. USA*, 100 Suppl 1, 11866-11872.

[113] Araki,R., Fukumura,R., Sasaki,N., Kasama,Y., Suzuki,N., Takahashi,H., Tabata,Y., Saito,T., and Abe,M. (2006) More than 40,000 transcripts, including novel and noncoding transcripts, in mouse embryonic stem cells. *Stem Cells*, 24, 2522-2528.

[114] Zeng,X., Miura,T., Luo,Y., Bhattacharya,B., Condie,B., Chen,J., Ginis,I., Lyons,I., Mejido,J., Puri,R.K., Rao,M.S., and Freed,W.J. (2004) Properties of pluripotent human embryonic stem cells BG01 and BG02. *Stem Cells*, 22, 292-312.

[115] Richards,M., Tan,S.P., Tan,J.H., Chan,W.K., and Bongso,A. (2004) The transcriptome profile of human embryonic stem cells as defined by SAGE. *Stem Cells*, 22, 51-64.

[116] D'Amour,K.A., Agulnick,A.D., Eliazer,S., Kelly,O.G., Kroon,E., and Baetge,E.E. (2005) Efficient differentiation of human embryonic stem cells to definitive endoderm. *Nat. Biotechnol.*, 23, 1534-1541.

[117] Hubner,K., Fuhrmann,G., Christenson,L.K., Kehler,J., Reinbold,R., De La,F.R., Wood,J., Strauss,J.F., III, Boiani,M., and Scholer,H.R. (2003) Derivation of oocytes from mouse embryonic stem cells. *Science*, 300, 1251-1256.

[118] Toyooka,Y., Tsunekawa,N., Akasu,R., and Noce,T. (2003) Embryonic stem cells can form germ cells in vitro. *Proc. Natl. Acad. Sci. USA*, 100, 11457-11462.

[119] Geijsen,N., Horoschak,M., Kim,K., Gribnau,J., Eggan,K., and Daley,G.Q. (2004) Derivation of embryonic germ cells and male gametes from embryonic stem cells. *Nature*, 427, 148-154.

[120] West,J.A. and Daley,G.Q. (2004) In vitro gametogenesis from embryonic stem cells. *Curr. Opin. Cell Biol.*, 16, 688-692.

[121] Master,Z. (2006) Embryonic stem-cell gametes: the new frontier in human reproduction. *Hum. Reprod.*, 21, 857-863.

[122] Jones,K.W., Singh,L., and Edwards,R.G. (1987) The use of probes for the Y chromosome in preimplantation embryo cells. *Hum. Reprod.*, 2, 439-445.

[123] Handyside,A.H., Kontogianni,E.H., Hardy,K., and Winston,R.M. (1990) Pregnancies from biopsied human preimplantation embryos sexed by Y-specific DNA amplification. *Nature*, 344, 768-770.

[124] Verlinsky,Y., Strelchenko,N., Kukharenko,V., Rechitsky,S., Verlinsky,O., Galat,V., and Kuliev,A. (2005) Human embryonic stem cell lines with genetic disorders. *Reprod. Biomed. Online.*, 10, 105-110.

[125] Pickering,S.J., Minger,S.L., Patel,M., Taylor,H., Black,C., Burns,C.J., Ekonomou,A., and Braude,P.R. (2005) Generation of a human embryonic stem cell line encoding the cystic fibrosis mutation deltaF508, using preimplantation genetic diagnosis. *Reprod. Biomed. Online.*, 10, 390-397.

[126] Verlinsky,Y. and Kuliev,A. (2003) Current status of preimplantation diagnosis for single gene disorders. *Reprod. Biomed. Online.*, 7, 145-150.

[127] Verlinsky,Y. (2005) Designing babies: what the future holds. *Reprod. Biomed. Online.*, 10 Suppl 1, 24-26.

[128] Mimeault,M. and Batra,S.K. (2006) Concise review: recent advances on the significance of stem cells in tissue regeneration and cancer therapies. *Stem Cells*, 24, 2319-2345.
[129] Chambers,I. and Smith,A. (2004) Self-renewal of teratocarcinoma and embryonic stem cells. *Oncogene*, 23, 7150-7160.
[130] Andrews,P.W., Matin,M.M., Bahrami,A.R., Damjanov,I., Gokhale,P., and Draper,J.S. (2005) Embryonic stem (ES) cells and embryonal carcinoma (EC) cells: opposite sides of the same coin. *Biochem. Soc. Trans.*, 33, 1526-1530.
[131] Kim,C.F., Jackson,E.L., Woolfenden,A.E., Lawrence,S., Babar,I., Vogel,S., Crowley,D., Bronson,R.T., and Jacks,T. (2005) Identification of bronchioalveolar stem cells in normal lung and lung cancer. *Cell*, 121, 823-835.
[132] Fang,D., Nguyen,T.K., Leishear,K., Finko,R., Kulp,A.N., Hotz,S., Van Belle,P.A., Xu,X., Elder,D.E., and Herlyn,M. (2005) A tumorigenic subpopulation with stem cell properties in melanomas. *Cancer Res.*, 65, 9328-9337.
[133] Piersma,A.H. (2004) Validation of alternative methods for developmental toxicity testing. *Toxicol. Lett.*, 149, 147-153.
[134] zur Nieden,N.I., Kempka,G., and Ahr,H.J. (2004) Molecular multiple endpoint embryonic stem cell test--a possible approach to test for the teratogenic potential of compounds. *Toxicol. Appl. Pharmacol.*, 194, 257-269.
[135] Jasanoff,S. (2005) *Designs on nature*. Princeton University Press, New Jersey.
[136] Marquis,D. (2002) An argument that abortion is wrong. In *Morality and Moral Controversies. Readings in Moral, Social and Political Philosophy* (Arthur,J., ed), pp. 218-227. Prentice Hall, New Jersey.
[137] Roe v.Wade (2002) The constitutional right to abortion. In *Morality and Moral Controversies. Readings in Moral, Social, and Political Philosophy* (Arthur,J., ed), pp. 190-195. Prentice Hall, New Jersey.
[138] Warren,M. (2002) On the moral and legal status of abortion. In *Morality and Moral Controversies. Readings in Moral, Social and Political Philosophy* (Arthur,J., ed), pp. 204-210. Prentice Hall, New Jersey.
[139] English,J. (1975) Abortion and the concept of a person. *Can. J. Philos.*, 5, 233-243.
[140] United Nations. Universal Declaration of Human Rights. General Assembly resolution 217A (III). 1948. Unenacted Bill/Resolution
[141] Bortolotti,L. and Harris,J. (2005) Stem cell research, personhood and sentience. *Reprod. Biomed. Online.*, 10 (Suppl 1), 68-75.
[142] Kittay,E.F. (2005) At the margins of moral personhood. *Ethics*, 116, 100-131.
[143] Green,R.M. (2002) Stem cell research: a target article collection: Part III--determining moral status. *Am. J. Bioeth.*, 2, 20-30.
[144] Pope John Paul II. (2003) The unspeakable crime of abortion. In *Ethical Issues in Modern Medicine* (Steinbock,B., Arras,J.D., and London, A. eds), pp. 461-463. McGraw-Hill, NewYork.
[145] Nagashima,H., Matsui,K., Sawasaki,T., and Kano,Y. (1984) Production of monozygotic mouse twins from microsurgically bisected morulae. *J. Reprod. Fertil.*, 70, 357-362.
[146] Williams,T.J., Elsden,R.P., and Seidel,G.E., Jr. (1984) Pregnancy rates with bisected bovine embryos. *Theriogenology*, 22, 521-531.
[147] Nagashima,H., Kato,Y., and Ogawa,S. (1989) Microsurgical bisection of porcine morulae and blastocysts to produce monozygotic twin pregnancy. *Gamete Res.*, 23, 1-9.

[148] American Medical Association. Pre-Embryo Splitting. 2007. E-2.145. Unenacted Bill/Resolution

[149] Bill C-6 (Royal Assent). (2004) An Act Respecting Assisted Human Reproduction and Related Research (Assisted Human Reproduction Act). Third Session, Thirty-seventh Parliament. http://www.parl.gc.ca/PDF/37/3/parlbus/chambus/house/bills/government/C-6_4.pdf.

[150] Thomson,J.J. (1971) A defense of abortion. *Philosophy and Public Affairs*, 1, 47-66.

[151] Copland,P. and Gillett,G. (2003) The bioethical structure of a human being. *J. Appl. Philos.*, 20, 123-131.

[152] Steinbock,B. (2001) Respect for human embryos. In *Cloning and the Future of Human Embryo Research* (Lauritzen,P., ed), pp. 21-33. Oxford University Press, New York.

[153] Steinbock,B. (1992) *Life before birth the moral and legal status of embryos and fetuses*. Oxford University Press, New York.

[154] Robertson,J.A. (1995) Symbolic issues in embryo research. *Hastings Cent. Rep.*, 25, 37-38.

[155] Ryan,M.A. (2001) Creating embryos for research: on weighing symbolic costs. In *Cloning and the Future of Human Embryo Research* (Lauritzen,P., ed), pp. 50-66. Oxford University Press, New York.

[156] Waller,L. (1987) Reproductive technology: in Australia, the debate moves to embryo experimentation. *Hastings Cent. Rep.*, 17, S21-S22.

[157] Krimsky,S. and Hubbard,R. (1995) The business of research. *Hastings Cent. Rep.*, 25, 41-43.

[158] Sullivan,L. (1993) In the path of Daedalus: middle-class Australians' attitudes to embryo research. *Br. J. Sociol.*, 44, 271-302.

[159] Kalfoglou,A.L. and Gittelsohn,J. (2000) A qualitative follow-up study of women's experiences with oocyte donation. *Hum. Reprod.,* 15, 798-805.

[160] Budev,M.M., Arroliga,A.C., and Falcone,T. (2005) Ovarian hyperstimulation syndrome. *Crit Care Med.*, 33, S301-S306.

[161] Delvigne,A. and Rozenberg,S. (2003) Review of clinical course and treatment of ovarian hyperstimulation syndrome (OHSS). *Hum. Reprod. Update.*, 9, 77-96.

[162] Golan,A., Ron-el,R., Herman,A., Soffer,Y., Weinraub,Z., and Caspi,E. (1989) Ovarian hyperstimulation syndrome: an update review. *Obstet. Gynecol. Surv.*, 44, 430-440.

[163] Mathur,R.S., Akande,A.V., Keay,S.D., Hunt,L.P., and Jenkins,J.M. (2000) Distinction between early and late ovarian hyperstimulation syndrome. *Fertil. Steril.*, 73, 901-907.

[164] Rizk,B. and Aboulghar,M. (2005) Classification, pathophysiology and management of ovarian hyperstimulation syndrome. In *Textbook of In Vitro Fertilization and Assisted Reproduction. The Bourn Hall Guide to Clinical and Laboratory Practice* (Brisden,P.R., ed), pp. 217-258. Taylor and Francis Group, New York.

[165] Practice Committee of the American Society of Reproductive Medicine. (2004) Ovarian hyperstimulation syndrome. *Fertil. Steril.*, 82 Suppl 1, S81-S86.

[166] Wakeley,K.E. and Grendys,E.C. (2000) Reproductive technologies and risk of ovarian cancer. *Curr. Opin. Obstet. Gynecol.*, 12, 43-47.

[167] Ness,R.B., Cramer,D.W., Goodman,M.T., Kjaer,S.K., Mallin,K., Mosgaard,B.J., Purdie,D.M., Risch,H.A., Vergona,R., and Wu,A.H. (2002) Infertility, fertility drugs, and ovarian cancer: a pooled analysis of case-control studies. *Am. J. Epidemiol.*, 155, 217-224.

[168] Rossing,M.A., Daling,J.R., Weiss,N.S., Moore,D.E., and Self,S.G. (1994) Ovarian tumors in a cohort of infertile women. *N. Engl. J. Med.*, 331, 771-776.

[169] Shushan,A., Paltiel,O., Iscovich,J., Elchalal,U., Peretz,T., and Schenker,J.G. (1996) Human menopausal gonadotropin and the risk of epithelial ovarian cancer. *Fertil. Steril.*, 65, 13-18.

[170] Venn,A., Watson,L., Lumley,J., Giles,G., King,C., and Healy,D. (1995) Breast and ovarian cancer incidence after infertility and in vitro fertilisation. *Lancet*, 346, 995-1000.

[171] Althuis,M.D., Moghissi,K.S., Westhoff,C.L., Scoccia,B., Lamb,E.J., Lubin,J.H., and Brinton,L.A. (2005) Uterine cancer after use of clomiphene citrate to induce ovulation. *Am. J. Epidemiol.*, 161, 607-615.

[172] Beeson,D. and Lippman,A. (2006) Egg harvesting for stem cell research: medical risks and ethical problems. *Reprod. Biomed. Online.,* 13, 573-579.

[173] Rossouw,J.E., Anderson,G.L., Prentice,R.L., LaCroix,A.Z., Kooperberg,C., Stefanick, M.L., Jackson,R.D., Beresford,S.A., Howard,B.V., Johnson,K.C., Kotchen, J.M., and Ockene,J. (2002) Risks and benefits of estrogen plus progestin in healthy postmenopausal women: principal results From the Women's Health Initiative randomized controlled trial. *JAMA*, 288, 321-333.

[174] Wassertheil-Smoller,S., Hendrix,S.L., Limacher,M., Heiss,G., Kooperberg,C., Baird,A., Kotchen,T., Curb,J.D., Black,H., Rossouw,J.E., Aragaki,A., Safford,M., Stein,E., Laowattana,S., and Mysiw,W.J. (2003) Effect of estrogen plus progestin on stroke in postmenopausal women: the Women's Health Initiative: a randomized trial. *JAMA*, 289, 2673-2684.

[175] Manson,J.E., Hsia,J., Johnson,K.C., Rossouw,J.E., Assaf,A.R., Lasser,N.L., Trevisan,M., Black,H.R., Heckbert,S.R., Detrano,R., Strickland,O.L., Wong,N.D., Crouse,J.R., Stein,E., and Cushman,M. (2003) Estrogen plus progestin and the risk of coronary heart disease. *N. Engl. J. Med.*, 349, 523-534.

[176] Shumaker,S.A., Legault,C., Rapp,S.R., Thal,L., Wallace,R.B., Ockene,J.K., Hendrix,S.L., Jones,B.N., III, Assaf,A.R., Jackson,R.D., Kotchen,J.M., Wassertheil-Smoller, S., and Wactawski-Wende,J. (2003) Estrogen plus progestin and the incidence of dementia and mild cognitive impairment in postmenopausal women: the Women's Health Initiative Memory Study: a randomized controlled trial. *JAMA*, 289, 2651-2662.

[177] Ludwig,A.K., Glawatz,M., Griesinger,G., Diedrich,K., and Ludwig,M. (2006) Perioperative and post-operative complications of transvaginal ultrasound-guided oocyte retrieval: prospective study of >1000 oocyte retrievals. *Hum. Reprod.*, 21, 3235-3240.

[178] Gabriel,T. High-Tech Pregnancies Test Hope's Limit. The New York Times Late Edition - Final, Section 1, Page 1, Column 1. 1999. New York, NY, The New York Times Company.

[179] Padawer,R. (2002) Soaring egg donation prices causing ethical concerns. http://www.gettingpregnantbook.com/EggDonationCostsSoar.htm.

[180] Steinbock,B. (2004) Payment for egg donation and surrogacy. *Mt. Sinai J. Med.*, 71, 255-265.

[181] The Ethics Committee of the American Society for Reproductive Medicine. (2000) Financial incentives in recruitment of oocyte donors. *Fertil. Steril.*, 74, 216-220.

[182] Hirschman,E.C. (1991) Babies for sale: market ethics and the new reproductive technologies. *J. Consum. Aff.*, 25, 358-390.

[183] Macklin,R. (2003) What is wrong with Commodification. In *Ethical Issues in Modern Medicine* (Steinbock,B., Arras,J.D., and London,A., eds), pp. 615-624. McGraw-Hill, New York.

[184] Corrigan,O. (2003) Empty ethics: the problem with informed consent. *Sociol. Health Illn.*, 25, 768-792.

[185] Ingelfinger,F.J. (1972) Informed (but uneducated) consent. *N. Engl. J. Med.,* 287, 465-466.

[186] Appelbaum,P.S., Roth,L.H., Lidz,C.W., Benson,P., and Winslade,W. (1987) False hopes and best data: consent to research and the therapeutic misconception. *Hastings Cent. Rep.*, 17, 20-24.

[187] Magnus,D. and Cho,M.K. (2005) Ethics. Issues in oocyte donation for stem cell research. *Science*, 308, 1747-1748.

[188] Ethics Committee of the American Society for Reproductive Medicine. (2002) Donating spare embryos for embryonic stem-cell research. *Fertil. Steril.*, 78, 957-960.

[189] Levine,R.J. (2003) Consent issues in human research. In *Ethical and regulatory aspects of clinical research* (Emanuel,E.J., Crouch,R.A., Arras,J.D., Moreno,J.D., & Grady,C., eds), pp. 197-201. The Johns Hopkins University Press, Baltimore.

[190] Heng,B.C. (2006) Donation of surplus frozen embryos for stem cell research or fertility treatment-should medical professionals and healthcare institutions be allowed to exercise undue influence on the informed decision of their former patients? *J. Assist. Reprod. Genet.*, 23, 381-382.

[191] Caulfield,T., Ogbogu,U., & Isasi,R.M. (2007) Informed consent in embryonic stem cell research: are we following basic principles? *CMAJ.*, 176, 1722-1725.

[192] Lo,B., Chou,V., Cedars,M.I., Gates,E., Taylor,R.N., Wagner,R.M., Wolf,L., & Yamamoto,K.R. (2004) Informed consent in human oocyte, embryo, and embryonic stem cell research. *Fertil. Steril.*, 82, 559-563.

[193] Nisker,J. & White,A. (2005) The CMA Code of Ethics and the donation of fresh embryos for stem cell research. *CMAJ.*, 173, 621-622.

[194] Ethics Committee of the American Society for Reproductive Medicine (2004) Informed consent and the use of gametes and embryos for research. *Fertil. Steril.*, 82 Suppl 1, S251-S252.

[195] Newton,C.R., McDermid,A., Tekpetey,F., & Tummon,I.S. (2003) Embryo donation: attitudes toward donation procedures and factors predicting willingness to donate. *Hum. Reprod.*, 18, 878-884.

[196] Nachtigall,R.D., Becker,G., Friese,C., Butler,A., & MacDougall,K. (2005) Parents' conceptualization of their frozen embryos complicates the disposition decision. *Fertil. Steril.*, 84, 431-434.

[197] Human Fertilisation and Embryology Act (c.37). c.37. 1990.

[198] Chung,Y., Klimanskaya,I., Becker,S., Marh,J., Lu,S.J., Johnson,J., Meisner,L., & Lanza,R. (2006) Embryonic and extraembryonic stem cell lines derived from single mouse blastomeres. *Nature*, 439, 216-219.

[199] Klimanskaya,I., Chung,Y., Becker,S., Lu,S.J., & Lanza,R. (2006) Human embryonic stem cell lines derived from single blastomeres. *Nature*, 444, 481-485.

[200] Brons,I.G., Smithers,L.E., Trotter,M.W., Rugg-Gunn,P., Sun,B., Chuva de Sousa Lopes SM, Howlett,S.K., Clarkson,A., Ahrlund-Richter,L., Pedersen,R.A., & Vallier,L. (2007) Derivation of pluripotent epiblast stem cells from mammalian embryos. *Nature*, 448, 191-195.
[201] George,K. (2007) What about the women? Ethical and policy aspects of egg supply for cloning research. *Reprod. Biomed. Online.*, 15, 127-133.
[202] Lewis,R. (2006) Blastomere blasphemy. *Am. J. Bioeth.*, 6, 1-3.
[203] Pearson,H. (2006) Early embryos can yield stem cells... and survive. *Nature*, 442, 858.
[204] Kelly,S.J. (1977) Studies on the developmental potential of 4- and 8-cell stage mouse blastomeres. *J. Exp. Zool.,* 200, 365-376.
[205] Liao,S.M. (2005) Rescuing human embryonic stem cell research: the Blastocyst Transfer Method. *Am. J. Bioeth.*, 5, 8-16.
[206] Master,Z. (2005) Can we really bypass the moral debate for embryo research? *Am. J. Bioeth.*, 5, 27-28.
[207] Newton,C.R., McBride,J., Feyles,V., Tekpetey,F., & Power,S. (2006) Factors affecting patients' attitudes toward single- and multiple-embryo transfer. *Fertil. Steril.*
[208] Child,T.J., Henderson,A.M., & Tan,S.L. (2004) The desire for multiple pregnancy in male and female infertility patients. *Hum. Reprod.*, 19, 558-561.
[209] President's Council on Bioethics. Alternative sources of human pluripotent stem cells. A white paper. 1-99. 2005.
[210] Lyle,R. (1997) Gametic imprinting in development and disease. *J. Endocrinol.*, 155, 1-12.
[211] Kim,K., Lerou,P., Yabuuchi,A., Lengerke,C., Ng,K., West,J., Kirby,A., Daly,M.J., & Daley,G.Q. (2007) Histocompatible embryonic stem cells by parthenogenesis. *Science*, 315, 482-486.
[212] Marchant,J. (2006) Human eggs supply 'ethical' stem cells. *Nature*, 441, 1038.
[213] Kiessling,A.A. (2005) Eggs alone. *Nature*, 434, 145.
[214] Fangerau,H. (2005) Can artificial parthenogenesis sidestep ethical pitfalls in human therapeutic cloning? An historical perspective. *J. Med. Ethics*, 31, 733-735.
[215] Hurlbut,W.B. (2005) Altered nuclear transfer as a morally acceptable means for the procurement of human embryonic stem cells. *Perspect. Biol. Med.*, 48, 211-228.
[216] Meissner,A. & Jaenisch,R. (2006) Generation of nuclear transfer-derived pluripotent ES cells from cloned Cdx2-deficient blastocysts. *Nature*, 439, 212-215.
[217] Chawengsaksophak,K., de Graaff,W., Rossant,J., Deschamps,J., & Beck,F. (2004) Cdx2 is essential for axial elongation in mouse development. *Proc. Natl. Acad. Sci. U. S. A*, 101, 7641-7645.
[218] Strumpf,D., Mao,C.A., Yamanaka,Y., Ralston,A., Chawengsaksophak,K., Beck,F., & Rossant,J. (2005) Cdx2 is required for correct cell fate specification and differentiation of trophectoderm in the mouse blastocyst. *Development*, 132, 2093-2102.
[219] Jones,N.L. & Cheshire,W.P. (2005) Can artificial techniques supply morally neutral human embryos for research? Part I. Creating novel categories of human embryos. *Ethics Med.*, 21, 29-40.
[220] Cheshire,W.P. & Jones,N.L. (2005) Can artificial techniques supply morally neutral human embryos for research? *Ethics Med.*, 21, 73-88.
[221] Cowan,C.A., Atienza,J., Melton,D.A., & Eggan,K. (2005) Nuclear reprogramming of somatic cells after fusion with human embryonic stem cells. *Science*, 309, 1369-1373.

[222] Yu,J., Vodyanik,M.A., He,P., Slukvin,I.I., & Thomson,J.A. (2006) Human embryonic stem cells reprogram myeloid precursors following cell-cell fusion. *Stem Cells*, 24, 168-176.

[223] Do,J.T. & Scholer,H.R. (2004) Nuclei of embryonic stem cells reprogram somatic cells. *Stem Cells*, 22, 941-949.

[224] Yamanaka,S. (2007) Strategies and new developments in the generation of patient-specific pluripotent stem cells. *Cell Stem Cell*, 1, 39-49.

[225] Takahashi,K. & Yamanaka,S. (2006) Induction of pluripotent stem cells from mouse embryonic and adult fibroblast cultures by defined factors. *Cell*, 126, 663-676.e

[226] Yu,J., Vodyanik,M.A., Smuga-Otto,K., Antosiewicz-Bourget,J., Frane,J.L., Tian,S., Nie,J., Jonsdottir,G.A., Ruotti,V., Stewart,R., Slukvin,I.I., & Thomson,J.A. (2007) Induced pluripotent stem cell lines derived from human somatic cells. *Science*, 318, 1917-1920.

[227] Hanna,J., Wernig,M., Markoulaki,S., Sun,C.W., Meissner,A., Cassady,J.P., Beard,C., Brambrink,T., Wu,L.C., Townes,T.M., & Jaenisch,R. (2007) Treatment of sickle cell anemia mouse model with iPS cells generated from autologous skin. *Science*, 318, 1920-1923.

[228] Maherali,N., Sridharan,R., Xie,W., Utikal,J., Eminli,S., Arnold,K., Stadtfeld,M., Yachechko,R., Tchieu,J., & Jaenisch,R.e.al. (2007) Directly reprogrammed fibroblasts show global epigenetic remodeling and widespread tissue contribution. *Cell Stem Cell*, 1, 55-70.

[229] Nakagawa,M., Koyanagi,M., Tanabe,K., Takahashi,K., Ichisaka,T., Aoi,T., Okita,K., Mochiduki,Y., Takizawa,N., & Yamanaka,S. (2008) Generation of induced pluripotent stem cells without Myc from mouse and human fibroblasts. *Nat. Biotechnol.*, 26, 101-106.

[230] Wernig,M., Meissner,A., Foreman,R., Brambrink,T., Ku,M., Hochedlinger,K., Bernstein,B.E., & Jaenisch,R. (2007) In vitro reprogramming of fibroblasts into a pluripotent ES-cell-like state. *Nature*, 448, 318-324.

[231] Atkinson-Grosjean,J. (2006) *Public science private interests: culture and commerce in Canada's Networks of Centres of Excellence*. University of Toronto Press, Toronto.

[232] Nelkin,D. & Andrews,L.B. (1998) Homo economicus: commercialization of body tissue in the age of biotechnology. *Hastings Center Report*, 28, 30-39.

[233] Annas,G.J. (1988) Whose waste is it anyway? The case of John Moore. *Hastings Cent. Rep.*, 18, 37-39.

[234] Isasi,R.M. & Knoppers,B.M. (2006) Mind the gap: policy approaches to embryonic stem cell and cloning research in 50 countries. *Eur. J. Health Law*, 13, 9-25.

[235] Knowles,L.P. (2004) A regulatory patchwork--human ES cell research oversight. *Nat. Biotechnol.*, 22, 157-163.

[236] Glasner,P. (2005) Banking on Immortality? Exploring the Stem Cell Supply Chain from Embryo to Therapeutic Application. *Current Sociology*, 53, 355-366.

[237] Fischbach,G.D. & Fischbach,R.L. (2004) Stem cells: science, policy, and ethics. *J. Clin. Invest*, 114, 1364-1370.

[238] Russo,E. (2005) Follow the money--the politics of embryonic stem cell research. *PLoS. Biol.*, 3, e234.

[239] Dickenson,D. (2002) Commodification of human tissue: implications for feminist and development ethics. *Developing. World Bioeth.*, 2, 55-63.

[240] Jain,K.K. (2005) Ethical and regulatory aspects of embryonic stem cell research. *Expert. Opin. Biol. Ther.*, 5, 153-162.
[241] de Wert,G. & Mummery,C. (2003) Human embryonic stem cells: research, ethics and policy. *Hum. Reprod.*, 18, 672-682.
[242] Harris,J. (2003) Stem cells, sex, and procreation. *Camb. Q. Healthc. Ethics*, 12, 353-371.
[243] Resnik,D.B. (1998) The commodification of human reproductive materials. *J. Med. Ethics*, 24, 388-393.
[244] Mahoney,J.D. (2000) The market for human tissue. *Va. Law Rev.*, 86, 163-223.
[245] Titmuss,R.M. (1971) *The gift relationship: from human blood to social policy*. Pantheon Books, New York.
[246] Sullivan,P. (2005) Developing an administrative plan for transfusion medicine--a global perspective. *Transfusion*, 45, 224S-240S.
[247] Lock,M. (2002) Human body parts as therapeutic tools: contradictory discourses and transformed subjectivities. *Qual. Health Res.*, 12, 1406-1418.
[248] Radin,M.J. (1982) Property and personhood. *Stanford Law Review*, 34, 957-1015.
[249] Radin,M.J. (1987) Market-inalienability. *Harvard Law Review*, 100, 1849-1937.
[250] Bray,M.B. (1990) Personalizing personality: toward a property right in human bodies. *Tex. Law Rev.*, 69, 209-244.
[251] Waldby,C. (2002) Stem Cells, Tissue Cultures and the Production of Biovalue. *Health*, 6, 305-323.
[252] Magnus,D., Caplun,A., & McGee,G. (2002) *Who owns life?* Prometheus Books, Amherst.
[253] Gilmour,J.M. (1993) Our bodies: property rights in human tissue. *Canadian Journal of Law and Society*, 8, 113-138.
[254] Bjorkman,B. & Hansson,S.O. (2006) Bodily rights and property rights. *J. Med. Ethics*, 32, 209-214.
[255] ickenson,D. (2006) The lady vanishes: what's missing from the stem cell debate. *Journal of Bioethical Inquiry*, 3, 43-54.
[256] Kevles,D. (1998) Diamond v. Chakrabarty and beyond: the political economy of patenting life. In *Private Science: Biotechnology and the Rise of the Molecular Sciences* (Thackray,A., ed), pp. 65-79. University of Pennsylvania Press, Pittsburgh.
[257] aulfield,T.A. & Gold,E.R. (2000) Whistling in the wind: patents on genetic research ara a reality. It's time to reframe the debate. *Form for Applied Research and Public Policy*, Spring, 75-79.
[258] Knowles,L.P. (2003) Of mice and men: patenting the oncomouse. *Hastings Cent. Rep.*, 33, 6-7.
[259] Resnik,D.B. (2002) The commercialization of human stem cells: ethical and policy issues. *Health Care Anal.*, 10, 127-154.
[260] Loring,J.F. & Campbell,C. (2006) Science and law. Intellectual property and human embryonic stem cell research. *Science*, 311, 1716-1717.
[261] Taymor,K.S., Scott,C.T., & Greely,H.T. (2006) The paths around stem cell intellectual property. *Nat. Biotechnol.*, 24, 411-413.
[262] Patent Act. P-4. 1985.
[263] Siegel,A.W. (2004) Temporal restrictions and the impasse on human embryonic stem-cell research. *Lancet*, 364, 215-218.

[264] Rabin,S. (2005) The gatekeepers of hES cell products. *Nat. Biotechnol.*, **23,** 817-819.

[265] Caulfield,T. (2006) Stem Cell Patents and Social Controversy: A Speculative View from Canada. *Medical Law International*, **7,** 219-232.

[266] Herder,M. (2006) Proliferating patent problems with human embryonic stem cell research. *Journal of Bioethical Inquiry*, **3,** 69-79.

[267] Williams-Jones,B. & Corrigan,O.P. (2003) Rhetoric and hype: where's the 'ethics' in pharmacogenomics? *Am. J. Pharmacogenomics.*, **3,** 375-383.

[268] Normile,D. & Mann,C.C. (2005) Cell biology. Asia jockeys for stem cell lead. *Science*, **307,** 660-664.

[269] De Trizio,E. & Brennan,C.S. (2004) The business of human embryonic stem cell research and an international analysis of relevant laws. *J. Biolaw. Bus.*, **7,** 14-22.

[270] Hyun,I. (2006) Magic eggs and the frontier of stem cell science. *Hastings Cent. Rep.*, **36,** 16-19.

[271] MacDonald,C. (2002) Stem cell ethics and the forgotten corporate context. *Am. J. Bioeth.*, **2,** 54-56.

[272] Giebel,L.B. (2005) Stem cells--a hard sell to investors. *Nat. Biotechnol.*, **23,** 798-800.

[273] Little,M., Hall,W., & Orlandi,A. (2006) Delivering on the promise of human stem-cell research. What are the real barriers? *EMBO Rep.*, **7,** 1188-1192.

In: Perspectives in Stem Cell Research ISBN: 978-1-61122-985-1
Editors: Brenda M. Davis and Christopher B. Halton © 2011 Nova Science Publishers, Inc.

Chapter XII

BACKGROUND AND LEGAL ISSUES RELATED TO STEM CELL RESEARCH*

Diane T. Duffy

SUMMARY

With certain restrictions, the President has announced that federal funds may be used to conduct research on human embryonic stem cells. Federal research is limited to 64 [1] existing stem cell lines that were derived (1) with the informed consent of the donors; (2) from excess embryos created solely for reproductive purposes; and (3) without any financial inducements to the donors. No federal funds will be used for the derivation or use of stem cell lines derived from newly destroyed embryos; the creation of any human embryos for research purposes; or cloning of human embryos for any purposes. Several lawsuits have been filed relating to stem cell research, and questions have been raised concerning access to existing stem cell lines by federal researchers.

Human Embryonic Stem Cells. Human embryonic stem cells are "master cells" and are able to develop into almost any cell in the human body. Building on earlier stem cell research, in 1998, researchers at the University of Wisconsin isolated cells from the inner cell mass of the early human embryo, called the blastocyst, and developed the first human embryonic stem cell lines. [2] Research has focused on the potential that these cells can offer to treat or mitigate diseases and conditions and to generate replacement tissues for disfunctioning cells or organs. [3] Research efforts have focused on spinal cord injury, multiple sclerosis, Parkinson's disease, Alzheimer's disease, diabetes, and other diseases or conditions. Scientists hope to use specialized cells to replace dysfunctional cells in the brain, spinal cord, pancreas, and other organs. [4] The sources for stem cells include: one week old embryos (blastocysts) created via in vitro fertilization (IVF) to treat infertility; five to nine week old embryos or fetuses obtained through elective abortion; embryos created through IVF for research

* Excerpted from CRS Report, updated June 12, 2002.

purposes; embryos created through cloning or somatic cell nuclear transfer (SCNT); and adult tissues (umbilical cord blood, bone marrow). Controversy surrounds the derivation of stem cells from human embryos and fetuses. In order to derive or extract the stem cells found within the embryo, the embryo is destroyed in the removal process. The earliest embryonic stem cells are called totipotent cells, which means they can develop into an entire organism, producing both the embryo and tissues required to support it in the uterus. At a later stage of development, pluripotent embryonic stem cells exist and can develop into almost any type of cell in the body. These stem cells cannot form the supporting tissues, as seen with totipotent cells. [5] Human embryonic stem cells found in the early stage embryo are believed to have a greater ability to become different types of body cells and have more uses than adult stem cells.

Background and Recent Presidential and Congressional Action

Executive Action. When President Bush took office in January, 2001, he announced he would conduct a review of the stem cell research issue and ordered the Department of Health and Human Services (HHS) to review the National Institutes of Health's (NIH) guidelines issued by the former administration. During the review period, NIH suspended its review of applications from researchers seeking federal funds to perform human embryonic stem cell research. On August 9, 2001, President Bush announced that federal funds would be available to support limited human embryonic stem cell research. The new policy provides that federal funds may be used for research on 64 existing stem cell lines that have already been derived or were already in existence as of the date of the announcement. In identifying the 64 stem cell lines as being eligible for federal funding, the President said these embryos, from which the existing stem cell lines were created, had been destroyed previously and could not develop as human beings.

Under the new policy, federal agencies, primarily NIH, will consider applications for funding if certain standards or eligibility criteria are met. The White House fact sheet setting forth the President's policy states: federal funds will only be used for research on existing stem cell lines that were derived (1) with the informed consent of the donors; (2) from excess embryos created solely for reproductive purposes; and (3) without any financial inducements to the donors. [6] The President directed NIH to examine the derivation of all existing stem cell lines and create a registry of those lines. Pursuant to this new policy, no federal funds will be used for: (1) the derivation or use of stem cell lines derived from newly destroyed embryos; (2) the creation of any human embryos for research purposes; or (3) cloning of human embryos for any purposes. The new policy replaces previously issued stem cell guidelines and policies. The policy also requires the creation of the President's Council on Bioethics to study stem cells and embryo research as well as other issues. NIH has listed entities that have developed stem cells lines that meet the President's criteria and are eligible for federal funding (the Human Embryonic Stem Cell Registry). The President also stated that in FY2001, the government will spend $250 million on research involving stem cells from other sources, *e. g.*, umbilical cord, placenta, adult and animal tissues.

Background and Congressional Activity. Prior to President Bush's stem cell announcement, and over the past years, federal law has prohibited HHS from funding human embryo research. No federal funds have been used to support research on stem cells derived from human embryos. Research in this area has been done through private funding. Subsequent to several phases of action, in December 1994, President Clinton, through an executive directive, prohibited federal funding on research to support the creation of human embryos for research purposes and directed NIH not to allocate resources for such research. [7] The order banning funding for such research was followed by a legislative ban in 1996 enacted in NIH's funding measure. [8] Congress has passed a similar ban annually since that time. The original congressional ban stated that federally appropriated funds could not be used for the creation of a human embryo or embryos for research purposes or for research in which a human embryo or embryos are destroyed, discarded, or knowingly subjected to risk of injury or death greater than that allowed for research on fetuses in utero under 45 C. F. R. 46.208(a)(2) and 42 U. S. C. § 289g(b). The ban defined "human embryo or embryos" to include any organism, not protected as a human subject under 45 C. F. R. 46 (Human Subject Protection regulations) that is derived by fertilization, parthenogenesis, cloning, or any other means from one or more human gametes (sperm or egg.) The rider language has not changed significantly over the years. In the subsequent fiscal years after FY1996, the rider was enacted in Title V (General Provisions) of the Labor, HHS and Education appropriations acts. [9] The prohibition does not ban fetal tissue research, although other restrictions apply. [10]

Advances in medical science proceeded and in 1998 critical developments were recognized by scientists at the University of Wisconsin. These researchers were able to isolate human embryonic stem cells and coax them to grow into specialized cells. In light of the presidential and legislative bans, NIH requested a legal opinion from the General Counsel of HHS on whether federal funds could be used to support research on human stem cells derived from embryos or fetal tissue. HHS' General Counsel, Harriet Rabb, concluded that then-current law prohibiting the use of HHS appropriated funds for human embryo research would not apply to research using stem cells "because such cells are not a human embryo within the statutory definition." [11] General Counsel Rabb determined that the statutory ban on human embryo research defines embryo as an "organism" that when implanted in the uterus is capable of becoming a human being. The opinion stated that pluripotent stem cells are not and cannot develop into an organism, as defined in the statute. HHS concluded that NIH could fund research that uses stem cells derived from the embryo by private funds. But, because of the language in the rider, NIH could not fund research that, with federal funds, derived the stem cells from embryos.

Some members of Congress strongly opposed HHS' view and believed that the legislative ban, that would continue through FY2001, covered and prohibited such research. Others supported both the administration's position and the funding of such research. In response to those opposed to the HHS opinion, and the subsequently published NIH guidelines, Secretary Shalala stated in a letter that the definition of embryo used in the HHS legal opinion relied on the definition of embryo in the statute and that the ban applied only to research in which human embryos are discarded or destroyed but not to research preceding or following "on such projects." [12] The letter stated: "Moreover... there is nothing in the legislative history to suggest that the provision was intended to prohibit funding for research in which embryos - organisms -are not involved."

After the HHS legal opinion, and despite expressions of congressional opposition, NIH indicated that it would fund research on pluripotent stem cells derived from human embryos and fetal tissue once guidelines were issued and an oversight committee was established. Draft guidelines were published in the *Federal Register* in December 1999 and final guidelines were issued in August 2000. [13] The guidelines provided that studies utilizing pluripotent stem cells derived from human embryos may be conducted using NIH funds only if the cells were derived, without federal funds, from human embryos that were created for the purposes of fertility treatment and were in excess of the clinical need of the individuals seeking such treatment. Based upon HHS's interpretation, funds could not be used to extract or derive the stem cells from the embryo, thereby destroying the embryo. NIH initiated the applications process but ultimately funding was not granted to the applications. The prior administration's process was then overtaken by events and the new policy was set.

In addition to President Bush's actions, congressional interest has continued into the 107th Congress. In July 2001, Senator Frist outlined a ten-point plan that favored stem cell research and included, in part, these points: (1) prohibit the creation of human embryos solely for research purposes; (2) strengthen and codify the ban on federal funding for the derivation of embryonic stem cells; (3) prohibit cloning to prevent the creation and exploitation of life for research purposes; (4) increase federal funding for adult stem cell research; (5) allow federal funding for research using only those embryonic stem cells derived from blastocysts that are left over after IVF and would otherwise be discarded; and other points.

Various bills or initiatives have been introduced in the 107th Congress on stem cell research or cloning, which in some cases would have an effect on stem cell research. The following highlights major legislation or other initiatives that are likely to receive additional legislative attention this session. On April 5, 2001, Senator Specter introduced S. 723, the Stem Cell Research Act of 2001, which would amend current law and authorize NIH to fund the derivation of stem cells from surplus IVF embryos. This type of research activity is prohibited under the current Labor/ HHS appropriation bill rider. The bill was referred to the Senate Committee on Health, Education, Labor, and Pensions. A companion bill to S. 723, H. R. 2059, was introduced by Rep. McDermott. On May 1, 2002, Senators Specter, Feinstein, Hatch and Kennedy, as well as other Senators, introduced S. 2439, the Human Cloning Prohibition Act of 2002. This bill would prohibit human reproductive cloning but would allow cloning for medical research purposes, including stem cell research. The bill was referred the Senate Committee on the Judiciary and is expected to receive heightened legislative attention. H. Res. 17 was introduced by Rep. Maloney on January 30, 2001, expressing the sense of the Congress supporting federal funding of pluripotent stem cell research. Other bills have been introduced on stem cell research, but have not received extensive legislative attention: the Responsible Stem Cell Research Act of 2001 (H. R. 2096; companion bill, S. 1349); the Stem Cell Research for Patient Benefit Act (H. R. 2747); the New Century Health Advantage Act (H. R. 2838); and the Science of Stem Cell Research Act (H. R. 4011), which was introduced in April 2002.

In addition to S. 2439, other cloning bills have been introduced that implicate stem cell research. For instance, H. R. 2505, the Human Cloning Prohibition Act of 2001 (Weldon) was introduced in July 2001 and would amend Title 18, U. S. Code, to prohibit human cloning. The bill was approved by voice vote by the House Judiciary Subcommittee on Crime on July 19, 2001 and approved by the full committee on July 24, 2001. [14] The House passed H. R. 2505 on July 31, 2001. The bill was received in the Senate, and the last action was August 8,

2001. [15] H. R. 2505 has received support from the Administration. While this bill is referred to as a cloning bill and would ban the process of human cloning called somatic cell nuclear transfer when used for reproductive purposes as well as for research and therapeutic uses, it would restrict stem cell research. In addition, Sen. Brownback's bill, S. 1899, the Human Cloning Prohibition Act of 2001, the companion bill to H. R. 2505, was introduced January 28, 2002 and is expected to receive legislative attention this session. As with H. R. 2505, the Administration has expressed support for S. 1899. The Senate also considered, but did not pass, Senator Lott's amendment to H. R. 10, the Railroad Retirement and Survivors' Improvement Act of 2001, which would have imposed a 6-month moratorium on all human cloning research and would have affected stem cell research.

Legal Activity. Several lawsuits have been filed relating to stem cell research issues. In March 2001, a lawsuit was filed in federal court to stop federal funding of human embryonic stem cell research and to overturn the NIH guidelines. In *Nightlight Christian Adoptions, et al. v. Thompson,* [16] the plaintiffs sought declaratory and injunctive relief and challenged the NIH guidelines for the public funding for research involving stem cells derived from human embryos. The plaintiffs, a non-profit adoption agency and others, claim that the NIH guidelines authorizing such research violate the legislative ban found in the appropriations rider which prohibits federal funding of research in which a human embryo is destroyed, discarded, or knowingly subjected to risk of injury or death greater than allowed for research on fetuses in utero under 45 C. F. R 46.208(a)(2) and 42 U. S. C. § 289g(b). [17] The plaintiffs challenge NIH's interpretation that the ban on funding of research using human embryos does not cover embryonic stem cell research, as long as the embryos are not destroyed using federal funds. The complaint states the NIH guidelines are arbitrary and capricious within the meaning of the Administrative Procedure Act, 5 U. S. C. § 706(2), not the product of reasoned decisionmaking, and inconsistent with scientific evidence. A stipulated motion to stay the case was issued in May, 2001, which essentially suspended the lawsuit while the President conducted his review of the NIH guidelines. Although events may have overtaken this lawsuit and rendered the claims moot, the case is still pending before the court. In May 2001, a federal lawsuit was filed claiming the Bush administration illegally withheld federal funding for stem cell research. In *Thomson v. Thompson* [18], actor Christopher Reeve and seven scientists filed suit in the U. S. District Court for the District of Columbia claiming the administration was doing irreparable harm by delaying the development of therapies that could, the plaintiffs argued, save lives. The case challenges new administration's decision to halt funding and the directive to Secretary Thompson to review the NIH guidelines. The plaintiffs claim that administrative procedures were not followed in halting the research that, they argue, is permissible under federal statute.

Another legal action involves licensing, patent, and intellectual property right issues relative to stem cell research. In 1999, Geron Corp. obtained an exclusive license from the Wisconsin Alumni Research Foundation (WARF) for human embryonic stem cell technology developed by Dr. Thomson of the University of Wisconsin. The license grants Geron exclusive commercial rights to develop six types of human cells, *e. g.,* nerve cells, heart and liver cells, derived from stem cells. Later, Geron attempted to exercise its option on commercial rights to additional (12) cell types but WARF countered that the option had expired. On August 13, 2001, the foundation filed a lawsuit [19] in U. S. District Court in Madison, Wisconsin asking the court to declare Geron's exercise of the option invalid. WARF later amended its complaint to ask the court to declare that Geron's license does not cover rights to research products that might be developed from the stem cells. Geron has asked the court to decide the dispute by discerning the meaning of the agreement without a trial. [20]

In September 2001, NIH began discussions with WARF concerning access by federally-funded researchers to human embryonic stem cells. WARF is said to hold patents affecting 64 stem cell lines, including absolute rights to five lines. [21] Secretary Thompson announced that an agreement has been reached with WARF that allows federal researchers access. Notwithstanding these developments, the *Geron* case raises legal questions concerning intellectual property rights, patents, licensing, and contract rights. The case also raises questions concerning the degree to which licensees or patent holders will make cells available or impose conditions on their use. Current guidelines on research do not reach the specifics of licensing agreements between grant applicants and patent holders. Those parties may negotiate agreements to license, share, and use the subject matter of the agreement.

REFERENCES

[1] The number was originally noted as 60 stem cell lines.
[2] "Stem cells: Scientific Progress and Future Research Directions," NIH, HHS, available at [*http:// www. nih. gov/ news/ stemcell/ scireport. htm*], Summary, p. 4.
[3] For more information on stem cell research, see CRS Report RL31015, Stem Cell Research.
[4] Id. at pp. 4-6.
[5] Generally, for human development, the term embryo is used for the first 8 weeks after fertilization and the term fetus for the 9 th week through birth. HHS regulations define fetus as "the product of conception from the time of implantation." 45 C. F. R. 46.203.
[6] President's embryonic stem cell research policy, Fact Sheet, White House, Office of the Press Secretary, August 9, 2001, [*http:// www. whitehouse. gov/ news/ releases/ 2001*].
[7] Statement, 30 Weekly Comp. Pres. Doc. 2459, Dec. 2, 1994.
[8] Balanced Budget Downpayment Act, 1996, Pub. L. No. 104-99, Sec. 128, 110 Stat. 26, 34 (1996).
[9] For the most recent rider, see, Pub. L. No. 106-554, § 510 (FY2001). For a list of all the annual riders, see CRS Report 31015, infra, footnote 12, p. 5. The current text adds at the end of the original language, "... or human diploid cells [cells that have two sets of chromosomes, such as somatic cells.] Federal funds have been provided for adult stem cell research.
[10] With respect to stem cells derived from fetal tissue, these cells and associated research would be subject to certain other restrictions that safeguard against the inappropriate use of fetuses
[11] Letter from HHS Gen. Counsel Harriet Rabb to Harold Varmus, Director, NIH, January 15, 1999.
[12] Letter from Secretary Shalala to the Honorable Jay Dickey, Feb. 23, 1999.
[13] 64 Fed. Reg. 67576 (1999); 65 Fed. Reg. 51976 (2000), respectively.
[14] The full committee defeated a substitute measure that was identical to H. R. 2608 (Greenwood).

[15] For additional and specific legislative details, including amendment and vote information, see CRS Report RL31015, *Stem Cell Research,* by Judith A. Johnson.

[16] Civ. No. 1: 01CV00502 (D. D. C. March 8, 2001).

[17] Omnibus Consolidated Appropriations Act of 2001, Pub. L. No. 106-554, § 510, 114 Stat. 2763.

[18] Civ. No. 1: 01CV00973 (D. D. C., May 8, 2001).

[19] *WARF v. Geron,* Civ. No. 01-C-459-C (D. Wis. Aug. 2001).

[20] Geron has received two patents for human embryonic germ cells. See, www. geron. com.

[21] *Marketletter,* Sept. 3, 2001. Other patent holders are Geron Corp., BresaGen of Australia and ES Cell International of Singapore as well as WARF's nonprofit subsidiary WiCell.

INDEX

A

C

F

G

H

I

J

K

L

M

N

O

P

S

U

V

W

X

Y

Z